Endothelin:
Role in Health and Disease

Endothelin: Role in Health and Disease

edited by

Anil Gulati

*University of Illinois
Chicago, USA*

harwood academic publishers

Australia • Austria • Belgium • China • France • Germany • India • Japan
Luxembourg • Malaysia • Netherlands • Russia • Singapore • Switzerland
Thailand • United Kingdom • United States

Copyright © 1995 by Harwood Academic Publishers GmbH.

All rights reserved.

No part of this book may be reproduced or utilized in any form or by any means, electronic or mechanical, including photocopying and recording, or by any information storage or retrieval system, without permission in writing from the publisher. Printed in Singapore.

British Library Cataloguing in Publication Data

Endothelin: Role in Health and Disease
  I. Gulati, Anil
  612.11

  ISBN 3-7186-5631-0

CONTENTS

Preface vii

Contributors ix

1. The Discovery of Endothelin: Impact on Biomedicine
   Tomoh Masaki 1
2. Endothelin Receptors and their Sub-Types
   Anthony P. Davenport, Janet J. Maguire and Fiona E. Karet 13
3. Endothelins: Transmembrane Signaling Mechanisms
   Mordechai Sokolovsky 25
4. Structure–Activity Relationship of Endothelin
   Om Prakash and Anil Gulati 35
5. Endothelin-Converting Enzyme and its Inhibitors: Pathophysiological Significances
   Yasuo Matsumura, Masanori Takaoka, Kazuhiro Hisaki and Shiro Morimoto 53
6. Pharmacological Interactions of Endothelin with Various Regulatory Agents
   Sam Rebello and Anil Gulati 69
7. Biological Activities of Endothelin and their Clinical Significance
   Govind Singh, Avadhesh C. Sharma, Sam Rebello and Anil Gulati 99
8. Endothelin Mechanisms in the Central Nervous System: Role in Pathophysiology
   Anil Gulati 117
9. Central Nervous System Actions of Endothelin in Cardiovascular Control
   Alastair V. Ferguson 143
10. Endothelin: Cerebrovascular Effects and Potential Role in Cerebral Vasospasm
    Robert N. Willette and Eliot H. Ohlstein 155
11. The Role of Endothelium and Endothelin in Subarachnoid Hemorrhage
    Ryuta Suzuki, Kimiyoshi Hirakawa and Yukio Hirata 167
12. Neurological and Psychiatric Aspects of Endothelin Research
    Toshihiro Yoshizawa and Ichiro Kanazawa 183
13. Endothelin Mechanisms in the Heart: Role in Pathophysiology
    Anil Gulati 193

14.	Role of Endothelin in Regional Vascular System	
	Avadhesh C. Sharma and Anil Gulati	215
15.	Role of Endothelin in Renal Disorders	
	Ananda P. Sen and Anil Gulati	233
16.	Role of Endothelin in Pulmonary Diseases	
	Douglas W. P. Hay and Roy G. Goldie	251
17.	Endothelin: Role in Endocrine Disorders	
	Elena I. Barengolts	279
18.	Endothelin: Role in Obstetrics and Gynecological Disorders	
	Annie L. Wrobel Eis, Murray D. Mitchell and Leslie Myatt	307
19.	Role of Endothelins in Neonatology	
	Ravi S. Iyer and Rama Bhat	327
20.	Role of Endothelin in Inflammatory Reactions	
	Maria das Graças M. O. Henriques and Giles A. Rae	339
21.	Pathophysiological Roles of Endothelin in the Liver	
	Namiki Izumi, Fumiaki Marumo and Chifumi Sato	353
22.	The Role of Endothelin in Skeletal Homeostasis	
	Mone Zaidi, Michael Pazianas, Vijai S. Shankar, Olugbenga A. Adebanjo,	
	Ali Zaidi and Christopher L.-H. Huang	361
Index		369

PREFACE

Endothelin exerts biological actions by acting on specific receptors on the cell membranes and increasing the intracellular calcium. Endothelin is widely distributed in various tissues and its binding sites have been identified in the heart, lung, kidneys, adrenal glands and central nervous system. Endothelin has several important cardiovascular, respiratory, renal, endocrine, hepatobiliary, neurological and behavioral functions. It has been implicated in skeletal homeostasis, inflammatory reactions and has an important role in neonatology, obstetrics and gynecological disorders.

The physiological effects of endothelin are complicated. Endothelin can act directly or in concert with other regulatory agents. Studies conducted in animal models and in patients clearly indicate that endothelin is increased in heart failure and after heart transplantation. Although the clinical significance of elevated levels of endothelin in these diseases is not clear, studies do indicate that endothelin has biological actions at pathophysiological concentration, suggesting a possible role of endothelin mechanisms in the pathogenesis of cardiovascular disorders. The role of endothelin in the pathophysiology of pulmonary hypertension and in acute myocardial infarction is becoming more evident. Endothelin has been shown to regulate the local cerebral blood flow and may be involved in conditions such as cerebral ischemia, subarachnoid hemorrhage and migraine where alteration in local cerebral blood flow may be the responsible factor. The functional importance of endothelin increases because of its mitogenic potential, which could contribute to structural changes. Endothelin-1 has been shown to be a smooth muscle mitogen and its synthesis can be increased by damage to the endothelium. Thus, it may play a role in genesis of atherosclerosis and in forms of hypertension in which smooth muscle proliferation has been implicated. Endothelin has also been reported to stimulate the proliferation of fibroblasts, glomerular mesangial and human carcinoma cells with the expression of proto-oncogenes (c-myc, c-fos) in these cells. Various strategies, including the development of endothelin-converting enzyme inhibitors, decreasing the stimuli to endothelin secretion and the development of specific endothelin receptor antagonists, are likely to be introduced as a new armamentarium for the treatment of at least some of the disease conditions. It is also possible that endothelin itself may find a place in the treatment of some clinical disorders.

An attempt has been made to describe in detail the role of endothelin in numerous clinical disorders involving various body systems. As endothelin acts in concert with other regulatory agents, a separate chapter has been included describing the interactions of endothelin with various regulatory agents. It must be pointed out that progress in endothelin research is so fast that newer concepts are likely to emerge in the near future. This book reviews the current situation and will provide a base for studying the emerging role of endothelin in various disease conditions.

Anil Gulati

CONTRIBUTORS

Adebanjo, Olugbenga A.
The Bone Research Unit
Department of Biochemical Medicine
St. George's Hospital Medical School
London SW17 0RE
UK

Barengolts, Elena I.
Department of Medicine
Section of Endocrinology
The University of Illinois College of
    Medicine at Chicago
820 South Wood Street
Chicago, IL 60612
USA

Bhat, Rama
Department of Pediatrics
The University of Illinois at Chicago
840 South Wood Street
Chicago, IL 60612
USA

Davenport, Anthony P.
Clinical Pharmacology Unit
University of Cambridge
Level 2, F & G Block
Addenbrooke's Hospital
Cambridge, CB2 2QQ
UK

Eis, Annie L. Wrobel
Department of Obstetrics & Gynecology
University of Cincinnati College of
    Medicine
231 Bethesda
Cincinnati, OH 45267
USA

Ferguson, Alastair V.
Department of Physiology
Queen's University
Kingston, Ontario
Canada K7L 3N6

Goldie, Roy G.
Department of Pharmacology
University of Western Australia, Perth
Nedlands 6009, Western Australia
Australia

Gulati, Anil
Department of Pharmaceutics &
    Pharmacodynamics
The University of Illinois at Chicago
833 South Wood Street
Chicago, IL 60612
USA

Hay, Douglas W. P.
Department of Inflammation & Respiratory
    Pharmacology
SmithKline Beecham Pharmaceuticals
709 Swedeland Road
King of Prussia, PA 19406
USA

Henriques, Maria das Graças M. O.
Department of Physiology &
  Pharmacodynamics
Oswaldo Cruz Foundation–IOC
Av. Brasil, 4365
P. O. Box 926, Rio de Janeiro
21045-900, RJ
Brazil

Hirakawa, Kimiyoshi
Department of Neurosurgery
Tokyo Medical & Dental University
1-5-45 Yushima Bunkyo-ku
Tokyo 113
Japan

Hirata, Yukio
2nd Department of Internal Medicine
Tokyo Medical & Dental University
1-5-45 Yushima Bunkyo-ku
Tokyo 113
Japan

Hisaki, Kazuhiro
Department of Pharmacology
Osaka University of Pharmaceutical
  Sciences
2-10-65 Kawai
Matsubara, Osaka 580
Japan

Huang, Christopher L. H.
The Bone Research Unit
Department of Biochemical Medicine
St. George's Hospital Medical School
London SW17 0RE
UK

Iyer, Ravi S.
Department of Pediatrics
The University of Illinois at Chicago
840 South Wood Street
Chicago, IL 60612
USA

Izumi, Namiki
Division of Gastroenterology
Department of Internal Medicine
Musashino Red Cross Hospital
Musashino-shi, Tokyo 180
Japan

Kanazawa, Ichiro
Department of Neurology
Institute of Brain Research
Faculty of Medicine
University of Tokyo
Tokyo 113
Japan

Karet, Fiona E.
Clinical Pharmacology Unit
University of Cambridge
Level 2, F & G Block
Addenbrooke's Hospital
Cambridge, CB2 2QQ
UK

Maguire, Janet J.
Clinical Pharmacology Unit
University of Cambridge
Level 2, F & G Block
Addenbrooke's Hospital
Cambridge, CB2 2QQ
UK

Marumo, Fumiaki
2nd Department of Internal Medicine
Tokyo Medical & Dental University
5-45 Yushima 1-chome
Bunkyo-ku, Tokyo 113
Japan

Masaki, Tomoh
Department of Pharmacology
Faculty of Medicine, Kyoto University
Kyoto 606
Japan

Matsumura, Yasuo
Department of Pharmacology
Osaka University of Pharmaceutical
 Sciences
2-10-65 Kawai
Matsubara, Osaka 580
Japan

Mitchell, Murray D.
Department of Obstetrics & Gynecology
University of Utah Medical Center
50 North Medical Drive
Salt Lake City, UT 84132
USA

Morimoto, Shiro
Department of Pharmacology
Osaka University of Pharmaceutical
 Sciences
2-10-65 Kawai
Matsubara, Osaka 580
Japan

Myatt, Leslie
Department of Obstetrics & Gynecology
University of Cincinnati College of
 Medicine
231 Bethesda
Cincinnati, OH 45267
USA

Ohlstein, Eliot H.
Department of Cardiovascular
 Pharmacology
SmithKline Beecham Pharmaceuticals
709 Swedeland Road
King of Prussia, PA 19406
USA

Pazianas, Michael
The Bone Research Unit
Department of Biochemical Medicine
St. George's Hospital Medical School
London SW17 0RE
UK

Prakash, Om
Department of Biochemistry
Kansas State University
Manhattan, Kansas 66506
USA

Rae, Giles A.
Department of Pharmacology CCB
Federal University of Santa Catarina
Rua Ferreira Lima 82
Florianopolis, 88015-420 SC
Brazil

Rebello, Sam
Department of Pharmaceutics &
 Pharmacodynamics
The University of Illinois at Chicago
833 South Wood Street
Chicago, IL 60612
USA

Sato, Chifumi
Division of Health Science
Tokyo Medical & Dental University
5-45 Yushima 1-chome
Bunkyo-ku, Tokyo 113
Japan

Sen, Ananda P.
Department of Pharmaceutics &
 Pharmacodynamics
The University of Illinois at Chicago
833 South Wood Street
Chicago, IL 60612
USA

Shankar, Vijay S.
The Bone Research Unit
Department of Biochemical Medicine
St. George's Hospital Medical School
London SW17 0RE
UK

Sharma, Avadhesh C.
Department of Pharmaceutics & Pharmacodynamics
The University of Illinois at Chicago
833 South Wood Street
Chicago, IL 60612
USA

Singh, Govind
Department of Pharmaceutics & Pharmacodynamics
The University of Illinois at Chicago
833 South Wood Street
Chicago, IL 60612
USA

Sokolovsky, Mordechai
Laboratory of Neurobiochemistry
Department of Biochemistry
The George S. Wise Faculty of Life Sciences
Tel Aviv University
Tel Aviv 69978
Israel

Suzuki, Ryuta
Department of Neurosurgery
Tokyo Medical & Dental University
1-5-45 Yushima Bunkyo-ku
Tokyo 113
Japan

Takaoka, Masanori
Department of Pharmacology
Osaka University of Pharmaceutical Sciences
2-10-65 Kawai
Matsubara, Osaka 580
Japan

Willette, Robert N.
Department of Cardiovascular Pharmacology
SmithKline Beecham Pharmaceuticals
709 Swedeland Road
King of Prussia, PA 19406
USA

Yoshizawa, Toshihiro
Department of Neurology
Institute of Clinical Medicine
University of Tsukuba
Tsukuba City 305

Zaidi, Ali
The Bone Research Unit
Department of Biochemical Medicine
St. George's Hospital Medical School
London SW17 0RE
UK

Zaidi, Mone
The Bone Research Unit
Department of Biochemical Medicine
St. George's Hospital Medical School
London SW17 0RE
UK

1 The Discovery of Endothelin: Impact on Biomedicine

Tomoh Masaki

Department of Pharmacology, Faculty of Medicine, Kyoto University, Kyoto 606, Japan

INTRODUCTION

In the past decade, there is an increasing body of evidence that vascular endothelium is an important factor in regulation of vascular tonus. This concept has emerged after discovery of endothelium-derived relaxing factor (EDRF) in 1980.

For many years, adrenergic nerve had been known as the most important factor in regulation of vascular tonus. In addition to this neuronic control, several circulating and locally produced vasoactive substances have been recognized as important factors in controlling the caliber of blood vessels.

From a more physiological standpoint, rate of blood flow has been known to be more natural and important factor in controlling the vascular tonus. For this function vascular endothelial cell has at least two mechanoreceptors, i.e. stretch receptor and shear stress receptor. Distension of the vessel wall, elicits contraction of vascular smooth muscle.[1] This constriction was later proved to be endothelium dependent,[2] and mediated by stretch receptor on the endothelial cells. On the other hand, the increase in blood flow caused enlargement of the caliber of the blood vessel, whereas the decrease caused its reduction. This mechanism is also endothelium dependent and mediated by activation of shear stress receptor on the endothelial cells.[3]

From the late 1970s to the early 1980s, it was discovered that prostacyclin and endothelium-derived relaxing factor (EDRF, characterized as nitric oxide later) were produced and released from endothelial cells in response to a variety of vasoactive substances.[4,5] The discovery led to an extensive investigation of the role of those factors in the mechanism of control of vascular caliber by blood flow. We know now that stretch receptor mediates release of vasoconstrictive prostanoid and shear stress receptor mediates release of vasodilators and vasoconstrictors including nitric oxide and some prostanoids that act on the underlying smooth muscle. Obviously regulatory mechanism of vascular tonus by physiological blood stream involves several chemical substances. In addition to the physical stimulus, chemical stimulus also modifies production and release of vasoconstrictors or vasodilators from endothelium. Endothelium is now an important source of generation of those vasoactive substances.

DISCOVERY OF ENDOTHELIN

Thus, vascular endothelium has appeared as a pivotal factor in regulation of vascular tonus. Numerous papers regarding the endothelium derived relaxing factors appeared in the beginning of the 1980s. However, less attention has been paid to the endothelium-derived constricting factor until mid-1980s. In 1985, Highsmith and his colleagues reported the existence of vasoconstrictive factor in a conditioned medium of cultured bovine endothelial cells.[6] They suggested that the factor was peptide since it was sensitive to trypsin. This paper evoked a quiet competition in this research field in the world.

In 1986, we attended a symposium on vascular endothelium held in the annual meeting of the Japanese Pharmacological Society at Nigata and were stimulated first by the rapid development of endothelial research. Our main interest at that time was the biochemistry and molecular biology of muscle proteins and we were looking for the more pharmacological project where our expertise in molecular and cellular biology could be utilized. We were interested in determination of the structure of EDRF. Purification and characterization of EDRF was thought to be one of the most interesting project at that time. However, survey of the published literatures revealed that EDRF had extremely short half life and might not be a peptide. Just at that time, Tomobe, a research student at the Tsukuba University introduced the Highsmith's paper in a seminar of our laboratory. In contrast to EDRF, the peptidergic vasoconstrictor was an excellent target of our interest. In May 1987, Yanagisawa who was my student and Dr. Kurihara who came from University of Tokyo were also interested in this problem and started to identify the vasoconstrictor in our lab.. Kimura, the excellent biochemist who discovered neurokinin, is the most important member at the initial step. Goto, a vascular pharmacologist was also an excellent expert in this project. The conditioned medium of cultured porcine aortic endothelial cells was concentrated by reverse-phase column. The concentrated material was purified sequentially by anion-exchange chromatography and two steps of reverse-phase column chromatographies. Porcine coronary artery strips was used for the assay system.

The purification of this peptide was accomplished by the end of July. Both Dr. Yazaki's and Dr. Mitsui's group helped in supplying the conditioned medium of the cultured endothelial cells. The Applied Biosystem Co., Ltd. was asked to analyse the sequence of the peptide, because our university had no peptide sequencer at that time. The whole sequence, except five residues, was determined by the middle of August. Kimura thought that those undetermined residues were cysteines. After modification of cysteine residues, the sequence was again analysed by a new apparatus in the National Institute of Basic Biology at Okazaki. The whole sequence of the peptide was determined by the next day. Yanagisawa started the molecular cloning of the peptide, and finished the determination of the whole sequence of the preproform of the peptide within 3 weeks. At the end of August, we asked Dr. Fujino of Takeda

Chemical Industries Ltd. to make a 20 amino acid residue peptide. They synthesized it within one week. The biological activity was tested, but the results were negative. Kimura determined amino acid composition of the peptide again and looked for tryptophan. Also tryptophan residue at the 21st residue of the peptide was confirmed according to the result of the sequence of the preproform of the peptide. The 21 residue peptide, including tryptophan at the 21st position, was synthesized and exactly matched the native peptide both by chemical and pharmacological analyses. The results of purification and pharmacological properties of the peptide was first reported in a local meeting of Japanese Pharmacological Society at Jichi Medical School in Tochigi, Japan on October 10, 1987. It was named "endotheline (ET)" and a paper describing whole results was sent to and published in March 1988 in Nature.[8]

EXPLOSION OF ENDOTHELIN RESEARCH

This paper stimulated worldwide interest particularly for cardiologists, since the peptide had a unique sequence and interesting pharmacological properties. As the worldwide interest in the peptide was expected at the point of the discovery, I intended to expedite the progress of ET research extensively with distributing the synthetic ET to investigators who were interested in the peptide before publication of the first paper, resulting in explosion of the research of ET. Of course, this was reinforced by the rapid commercial availability of the peptide later.

The peptide had the most potent vasoconstrictive activity so far known and induced a sustained pressor response when administered intravenously into animal. The sustained increase in blood pressure by the peptide suggested an involvement of the peptide in mechanisms of hypertension, or maintenance of blood pressure. In fact, detailed cardiovascular studies on the peptide have confirmed its vasoconstrictor actions in most vascular beds. However, a great number of subsequent papers revealed that the mechanisms are not so simple. In maintenance of blood pressure, many factors may be involved. ET is not only the factor involved in this system. The role of ET in the mechanism is still remained to be solved. However, several recent reports on clinical significance of ET and effectiveness of ET-receptor antagonists in some pathological state suggest an importance of ET in maintenance of blood pressure as described below. Many investigators again think that the peptide plays some role in cardiovascular system under some conditons.

ENDOTHELIN FAMILY

Endothelin comprises 21 amino acid residues including four cysteine residues (Figure 1.1).[8] The four cysteine residues form two intramolecular disulfide bonds. Theoretically there are three ways of intramolecular disulfide bridges. Natural product showed the most potent vasoconstrictive activity. After submission of our initial manuscript to the journal, the disulfide bonds described in the manuscript were proved to be wrong. Then the manuscript was revised before the publication. This

```
ET-1     C S C S S L M D K E C V Y F C H L D I I W
ET-2     C S C S S W L D K E C V Y F C H L D I I W
ET-3     C T C F T Y K D K E C V Y Y C H L D I I W
STXa     C S C K D M T D K E C L N F C H Q D V I W
STXb     C S C K D M T D K E C L Y F C H Q D V I W
STXc     C T C N D M T D E E C L N F C H Q D V I W
STXd     C T C K D M T D K E C L Y F C H Q D I I W
```

Figure 1.1. Structures of endothelins and sarafotoxins. Amino acids written by white boldface are different from those of ET-1. All of endothelins and sarafotoxins have two disulfide bonds (1–15, 3–11).

error was pointed out by Peptide Institute in Osaka and was confirmed by Kimura at the Tsukuba University.

One of the most remarkable steps in the progress of ET research, following the initial publication, was the discovery of isotypes of ET. Analysis of human genome revealed the existence of three distinct genes of ET, which encode three distinct ET peptides, designated ET-1, ET-2 and ET-3.[9] Endothelin that was discovered initially in the conditioned medium of the cultured endothelial cells was ET-1. The existence of the isopeptides had been already known before the summer in 1988. However, the result was veiled until the end of 1988 when the First International Conference on Endothelin (The First William Harvey Workshop on Endothelin) was held at London.

Soon after the discovery of ET, structure of the rare snake venom (venom toxins of *Atractaspis engaddensis*) sarafotoxin (STX) was published. Surprisingly, it was very similar to ETs in its structure. It consists of 21 amino acid residues including four cysteine residues. Seven amino acid residues of sarafotoxin 6b were replaced by those of the ET-1. So far, four sarafotoxins (STXa, STXb, STXc and STXd) were reported.[10] Structures of those four peptides were shown in Figure 1.1.

ENDOTHELIN RECEPTOR AND ANTAGONIST

Detailed pharmacological studies on vasoconstriction and vasodilation of ET *in vitro* and *in vivo* have confirmed diverse responses to the ET depending on the isopeptides and the vascular beds used. In addition, pharmacological responses of various tissues of non-vascular system to the isopeptides were also diverse. Those pharmacological responses were divided into two classes (Type I and II).[11] In type I response, ET-1 and ET-2 are more potent than ET-3, while in type II response, all of the three isotypes are equally potent. Experiments on replacement of iodine-labeled ET-1 bound to the ET receptor by non-labeled isopeptides demonstrated the existence of several distinct binding sites of ET.[11] These results strongly suggest multiplicity of ET receptor. Indeed, similar but distinct two cDNAs for ET receptor were isolated, designated ET_A

Table 1.1 Character of endothelin receptor subtypes

Receptor subtype	ET_A	ET_B
Ligand affinity	ET-1 = ET-2 ≫ ET-3	ET-1 = ET-2 = ET-3
Cellular Distribution	Vascular smooth muscle Neuroblast chromaffine cells	Vascular endothelial cell Glia cells
Antagonist Selective for Subtype	BQ-123 FR-139317 50-235 TTA-386	IRL-1038
Non-selective	PD145065 RO46-2005	

and ET_B, and published at the end of 1990 when the Second International Conference on Endothelin was held at Tsukuba.[12,13] Both subtypes belong to the seven membrane-spanning-receptor coupled with G-proteins. ET_A has a high affinity to ET-1 and ET-2, but has a low affinity to ET-3. ET_B has an equipotent affinity to all of the three isopeptides (Table 1.1). ET_A has been thought to exist on the smooth muscle cells and to mediate vasoconstriction.[12,13] In contrast, ET_B was thought to exist on the endothelial cells and mediate release of prostacyclin and/or EDRF. However, recently, ET_B was reported to exist also in some blood vessels and to mediate vasoconstriction. As described later, both types of the receptor distribute in a variety of tissue in different proportion.[14]

Existence of the third type of ET receptor, ETc, that has high affinity to ET-3 but low to ET-1 and ET-2, was demonstrated pharmacologically on mammalian cells, i.e. bovine endothelial cells[15] and lactotrophs[16] within the anterior pituitary. So far, no report has demonstrated the cloning of cDNA for the ETc receptor. Analysis of gene for ET receptor revealed also existence of only two subtypes of the receptor. This fact suggests that the third type of ET receptor must be a quite different type. However, very recently, cDNA cloning of ETc receptor from a frog, *Xenopus lavies* was demonstrated.[17] The receptor also belongs to the seven transmembrane domain G-protein-coupled receptor. In this case, displacing of ^{125}I-ET-3 bound to the receptor by ET-3 or ET-1 revealed only four times stronger affinity of the receptor to ET-3 than ET-1. I have to point out a fact that nobody demonstrated the existence of ET_A or ET_B on the frog cells.

First antagonist for ET receptor, BQ-123, was reported in 1991.[18] Subsequently several antagonists have come out. Chemistry and pharmacology of most of those antagonists were presented in the Third International Conference on Endothelin held at Houston in 1993. Interestingly, most of the antagonists are ET_A antagonists, for instance, BQ-123, FR139317,[19] 50-235[20] and TTA-386.[21] Up to now, only one ET_B-antagonist, IRL1038, was reported.[22] This peptidergic ET_B-antagonist has the same amino acid sequence of the carboxyl terminal side of the ET-1 from Cys 11 to Trp 21, but it has a disulfide bond between two cysteine residues in the sequence. Non-selective antagonists that react to both ET_A and ET_B receptors are also reported, for instance, [Thr^{18}, gMeLeu^{19}] ET-1,[23] PD145065[24] and Ro46-2005.[25] Among others, Ro-46-2005 is a non-peptidergic and orally administrable non-selective antagonist.

Additionally, pharmacological experiments using several types of antagonist suggested that there may be several subtypes of ET_A or ET_B, or another type of ET receptor other than ET_A and ET_B.[26,27,28,29]

ENDOTHELIN CONVERTING ENZYME

In the first paper on discovery of ET, it was described that ET-1 is produced by an unusual pathway.[8] In case of human ET-1, it is produced from a precursor, 212 amino acid preproform of ET-1, via a 38-amino acid intermediate form named big ET-1. Big ET-1 is processed from preproET-1 by a conventional processing enzyme, i.e. an endopeptidase specific for a pair of dibasic amino acid residues. Subsequent experiments demonstrated the existence of equimolar big ET-1 and ET-1 in both cytosolic and extracellular medium of cultured endothelial cells, and also in human plasma.[30,31] It is clear that the enzyme converting big ET-1 to ET-1 exists. However, several enzymes that showed ET converting activity were demonstrated. Among others, a metalloprotease that is inhibited by phosphoramidon is currently the most probably candidate for the converting enzyme.[32] Very recently, several reports have demonstrated the cDNA cloning of this enzyme.

CARDIOVASCULAR SIGNIFICANCE OF ENDOTHELIN

To elucidate physiological and pathophysiological significance of ET, measurement of the concentration of ET-1 in blood stream was thought to be important. This method had already been established in 1988.[33] Using this method, it was demonstrated that circulating ET-1 in the blood stream of normal subject was very low, approximately 1 pg/ml.[33] The low circulating levels of ET may be attributable to its very short half-life in blood probably because of the rapid clearance of ET through lung and kidney. Since the plasma concentration of ET-1 is not sufficient to elicit constriction of smooth muscle layer of the vascular beds, ET may not be a circulating hormone, but a local hormone. Since ET-1 is released from endothelium mainly abluminally and acts on the underlying smooth muscle,[34,35] and small artery and vein have a high sensitivity to ET,[36] ET may control peripheral blood flow in paracrine manner.

ET-1 seems to be produced in peripheral vascular beds. Probably the released ET-1 acts on the underlying smooth muscle, resulting in a significant increase in peripheral vascular resistance.[38] This concept is supported by the fact that in normal subjects venous plasma concentration of ET is slightly higher than in arterial blood.[37] In patients undergoing upon chest surgery, plasma ET-1 level increased remarkably in vein than in artery during the operation,[38] suggesting also that the ET-1 produced in peripheral vascular beds. It was also demonstrated that level of plasma ET-1 increases in response to the postural change in biphasic manner, probably in response to the systemic blood pressure.[39] The first phase occurs quickly within a few minutes, suggesting an existence of ET-pool. Probably ET-1 plays some compensatory role for haemodynamic stress.

Plasma ET-1 level increases in various pathological conditions of cardiovascular system.[40] Among others, vasospasm after subarachnoid haemorrhage[41] and pulmonary hypertension[42] are the cases where ET-1 may play a primary role in the pathogenesis. Several cases of endothelin-dependent hypertension were also reported, such as hemangioendotheliomas, disseminated intravascular coagulation and cyclosporin-induced hypertension.[43]

Opinion is divided on a problem of plasma level of ET-1 in essential hypertension.[43] ET may not be the primary cause of essential hypertension. However, elevation of plasma level of ET-1 and the blunted ET-induced responses of the vascular beds in severe hypertensive patients[44] suggest an increased local vascular production of ET-1. In some cases, there is a good correlation between plasma levels of ET-1 and elevated blood pressure values. ET may play some role in generation of hypertension.

In congestive heart failure and atherosclerosis, plasma ET-1 level also increases as a consequence of imbalance between EDRF and ET production, resulting in progress of the diseases. In those cases, vascular endothelial dysfunction may be the major factor in increase in plasma ET-1 level.

ENDOTHELIN RESEARCH IN NON-CARDIOVASCULAR SYSTEM

At the very early stage of ET research, autoradiographic experiment using radioligand ET-1 demonstrated that ET-1 binding sites are distributed not only on vascular system but also on other organs including brain, adrenal gland, lung, kidney, intestine, etc.[45,46] This suggested the existence of ET-receptor in unexpected regions and predicted the multiple function of ET. Later this supposition was proved by numerous reports showing a variety of actions of ET in various tissues and organs. Subsequently, northern blot analysis of mRNAs from those tissues probed with cDNAs for three isopeptides of ETs revealed a wide distribution of the endogenous agonists in a variety of tissues and organs in different proportions[46] (Table 1.2). Those results indicated that endogenous agonists, ETs, are produced by cells located near to their effector cells, showing that ET is a local hormone. Now we know that the peptide has a variety of pharmacological actions not only in cardiovascular but also non-cardiovascular system.[11,46]

Some of the non-vascular actions of ET are extremely important. ET may be an important regulator of functions in central nervous system, maintenance of volume and composition of body fluids, hormone secretion, etc. However, at present, reports on those problems are few and far between.

There are several evidences that ET is a neuropeptide, probably a transmitter or modulator of the nervous transmission.[46] In central nervous system, both ET and ET-receptor are distributed in neuron and glia cell as well as vascular bed. Regarding ET-receptor, ET_A and ET_B are distributed separately. In contrast, endogenous ET in brain is mostly ET-1.[47] Probably ET shows different function depending on the neuron or glia cell. There are several reports on a regulatory action of ET in

Table 1.2 Distribution of endogenous ETs and subtypes of ET receptors in various tissues

Tissues	ET-1	ET-2	ET-3	ET$_A$	ET$_B$
Vascular tissue					
Endothelium	++++				+
Smooth muscle	+			++	
Brain	+++		+	+	+++
Lung	++		+	+++	+++
Heart	+			+++	++
Kidney	++	++	+	+	++
Intestines	+	+	+++	+	+++
Liver	+			++	+
Thyroid	++			?	+
Parathyroid	+	?	?	+	?
Adrenal gland	+		+++	+	++
Spleen	+		++	+	
Uterus	++		+	++	+
Placenta	++			++	+++
Amnion	+++	?	?	?	?
Ovary	++	?	?	++	?

++++, Highest; +++ high; ++ moderate; and +, low levels of expression of ETs or ET receptor mRNA and/or immunoreactive ETs.

vasomotor neuron,[48] and in water balance through central nervous system,[49] suggesting important roles of ET in central nervous system.

Kidney will also be an interesting target of the endothelin research. In fact, many nephrologists are interested in ET. *In situ* hybridization of kidney tissues revealed an interesting distribution of ET$_A$ and ET$_B$ receptors.[14] Kohan *et al.* demonstrated that renal inner medullary collecting duct produced ET-1 and ET$_A$ receptor,[50,51] suggesting again paracrine or autocrine action of ET. ET exerts a number of biological activities in the kidney, including regulation of sodium reabsorption and water absorption, vasoconstriction, mesangial cell contraction, inhibition of vasopressin action in collecting tubules, and inhibition of Na$^+$, K$^+$-ATPase activity through increased prostaglandin E$_2$ formation in papillary collecting duct cells.[52,53]

It is also known that ET is a potent constrictor of airway smooth muscle.[54] Mechanism of the ET-induced bronchoconstriction seems to be different from that of vasoconstriction. Endothelin may regulate the bronchial tonus. Probably it plays some role in bronchoconstriction at the inflammatory lesion and might therefore play a role in the pathogenesis of asthma.

Another important property of ET is the mitotic action on various types of cell.[55,56] Endothelin also stimulates RNA and protein synthesis.[57,58] In addition, ET transforms cells from a differentiated state into an undifferentiated state.[59] On the other hand, it is well known that blood flow affects production of ET-1 in endothelial cells. Decrease in rate of blood flow induces production and release of ET-1 from endothelial cells. The released ET-1 probably changes phenotype and elicits proliferation of underlying smooth muscle cells by the aid of other growth factor concomitantly expressed in endothelial cells by the decrease in rate of blood flow.[55] Moreover, it was reported that oxidized LDL stimulates production of ET-1 in endothelial cells.[60] These results strongly suggest an involvement of ET in generation of atherosclerosis. Indeed, concentration of ET-1 in plasma of patients with atherosclerosis is higher than that of the normal subject.[61]

Endothelin and its receptor exist in various endocrine organs including adrenal gland, thyroid, ovary, etc. In accordance with this fact, ET shows many actions on those endocrine organs such as aldosterone release, inhibition of renin release and stimulation of gonadotropines at pituitary. Endothelin may play some role in those endocrine organs as a local hormone.

Findings of those multiple functions of the ETs now open a new field where ET shows important physiological and pathophysiological significance.

References

1. Bayliss, W. M. (1902) On the local reactions of the arterial wall to changes of internal pressure. *Journal of Physiology*, **28**, 220–231.
2. Katusic, Z. S., Shepherd, J. T. and Vanhoutte, P. M. (1986) Endothelium-dependent contraction to stretch in canine basilar arteries. *American Journal of Physiology*, **252**, H1–H3.
3. Bassenge, E., Busse, R. and Pohl, U. (1988) *Relaxing and Contracting Factors*, edited by P.M. Vanhoutte, pp. 189–217. Clifton New Jersey: The Human Press Inc.
4. Moncada, S., Gryglewski, R., Bunting, S. and Vane, J. R. (1976) An enzyme isolated from arteries transforms prostaglandin endoperoxidase to an unstable substance that inhibits platelet aggregation. *Nature*, **263**, 663–665.
5. Furchgott, R. F. and Zawadzki, J. V. (1980) The obligatory role of endothelial cells in the relaxation of arterial smooth muscle by acetylcholine. *Nature*, **288**, 373–376.
6. Hickey, K. A., Rubany, G. M., Paul, R. and Highsmith, R. F. (1985) Characterization of a coronary vasoconstrictor produced by cultured endothelial cells. *American Journal of Physiology*, **248**, C550–556.
7. O'Brien, R., Robbins, R. J. and McMurtry, I. F. (1987) Endothelial cells in culture produce a vasoconstrictor substance. *Journal of Cell Physiology*, **135**, 263–270.
8. Yanagisawa, M., Kurihara, H., Kimura, S., Tomobe, Y., Kobayashi, M., Mitsui, Y. et al. (1988) A novel potent vasoconstrictor peptide produced by vascular endothelial cells. *Nature*, **332**, 411–415.
9. Inoue, A., Yanagisawa, M., Kimura, S., Kasuya, Y., Miyauchi, T., Goto, K. et al. (1989) The human endothelin family: three structurally and pharmacologically distinct isopeptides predicted by three separate genes. *Proceedings of National Academy of Science USA*, **86**, 2863–2867.
10. Landan, G., Bdolah, A., Wollberg, Z., Kochva, E. and Graur, D. (1991) Evolution of the sarafotoxin/endothelin superfamily of proteins. *Toxicon*, **29**, 237–244.
11. Sakurai, T., Yanagisawa, M. and Masaki, T. (1992) Molecular characterization of endothelin receptor. *Trends in Pharmacological Science*, **13**, 103–108.
12. Arai, H., Hori, S., Aramori, I., Ohkubo, H. and Nakanishi, S. (1990) Cloning and expression of a cDNA encoding an endothelin receptor. *Nature*, **348**, 730–732.
13. Sakurai, T., Yanagisawa, M., Takuwa, Y., Miyazaki, H., Kimura, S., Goto, K. et al. (1990) Cloning of a cDNA encoding a non-isopeptide-selective subtype of the endothelin receptor. *Nature*, **348**, 732–735.
14. Hori, S., Komatsu, Y., Shigemoto, R., Mizuno, N. and Nakanishi, S. (1992) Distinct tissue distribution and cellular localization of two messenger ribonucleic acids encoding different subtypes of rat endothelin receptors. *Endocrinology*, **130**, 1885–1895.
15. Emori, T., Hirata, Y. and Marumo, F. (1990) Specific receptors for endothelin-3 in cultured bovine endothelial cells and its cellular mechanism of action. *FEBS Letters*, **263**, 261–264.
16. Samson, W. K., Skala, K. D., Alexander, B. and Huang, F. L. S. (1991) Possible neuroendocrine actions of endothelin-3. *Endocrinology*, **128**, 1465–1473.
17. Karne, S., Jayawickreme C. K. and Lerner, M. R. (1993) Cloning and characterization of an endothelin-3 specific receptor (ETc receptor) from xenopus laevis dermal melanophores. *The Journal of Biological Chemistry*, **268**, 19126–19133.
18. Ihara, M., Noguchi, K., Saeki, T., Fukuroda, T., Tsuchida, S., Kimura, S., et al., (1991) Biological profiles of highly potent novel endothelin antagonists selective for the ETA receptor. *Life Science*, **50**, 247–255.
19. Aramori, I., Nirei, H., Shoubo, M., Sogabe, K., Nakamura, K., Kojo, H., et al. (1993) Subtype selectivity of a novel endothelin antagonist, FR139317, for the two endothelin receptors in transfected chinese hamster ovary cells. *Molecular Pharmacology*, **43**, 127–131.

20. Fujimoto, M., Mihara, S., Nakajima, S., Ueda, M., Nakamura, M. and Sakurai, K. (1992) A novel non-peptide endothelin antagonist isolated from bayberry, *Myrica cerifera*. *FEBS Letters*, **305**, 41–44.
21. Kitada, C., Ohtaki, T., Masuda, Y., Masuo, Y., Nomura, H., Asami, T. *et al.* (1993) Design and synthesis of ETA-receptor antagonists and study of ETA-receptor distribution. *Abstract of 3rd International Conference on Endothelin*, pp. 59.
22. Urade, Y., Fujitani, Y., Oda, K., Watakabe, T., Umemura, I. M. Takai, T., *et al.* (1992) An endothelin B receptor-selective antagonist: IRL 1038, [Cys 11–Cys 15]-endothelin-1 (11–21). *FEBS Letters*, **311**, 12–16.
23. Wakimasu, M., Kikuchi, T., Kubo, K., Asami, T., Ohtaki, T. and Fujino, M. (1993) Studies on endothelin antagonists. Perspectives. In *Medicinal Chemistry*, edited by B. Testa, E. Kyburz, W. Fuhrer and R. Giger. pp. 165–177. Verlag. Helvetica Chemical Acta, Basel.
24. Doherty, A. M., Cody, W. L., He, J. X., Depue, P. L., Welch, K. M., Flynn, *et al.* (1993) *In vitro* and *in vivo* studies with a series of hexapeptide endothelin antegonists. *Abstract of 3rd International Conference of Endothelin*, pp. 25.
25. Clozel, M., Breu, V., Burri, K., Cassal, J., Fischli, W., Gray, G.A. *et al.*, (1993) Pathophysiological role of endothelin revealed by the first orally active endothelin receptor antagonist, *Nature*, **365**, 759.
26. Sumner, M. J., Cannon, T. R., Mundin, J. W., White, D. G. and Watts, I. S. (1992) Endothelin ETA and ETB receptors mediate vascular smooth muscle contraction. *British Journal of Pharmacology*, **107**, 858–860.
27. Moreland, S., McMullen, D. M., Delaney, C. L., Lee, V. G. and Hunt, J. T. (1992) Venous smooth muscle contains vasoconstrictor ETB-like receptors. *Biochemical and Biophysical Research Communications*, **184**, 100–106.
28. D'Orléans-Juste, P., Télémaque, S., Claing, A., Ihara, M. and Yano, M. (1992) Human big-endothelin-1 and endothelin-1 release prostacyclin via the activation of ETA receptors in the rat perfused lung. *British Journal of Pharmacology*, **105**, 773–775.
29. Sudjarwo, S. A., Hori, M., Takai, M., Urade, Y., Okada, T. and Karaki, H. (1993) A novel subtype of endothelin B receptor mediating contraction in swine pulmonary vein. *Life Science*, **53**, 431–437.
30. Sawamura, T., Kimura, S., Shinmi, O., Sugita, Y., Yanagisawa, M. and Masaki, T. (1989) Analysis of endothelin related peptides in culture supernatant of porcine aortic endothelial cells: evidence for biosynthetic pathway of endothelin-1. *Biochemical and Biophysical Research Communications*, **162**, 1287–1294.
31. Miyauchi, T., Yanagisawa, M., Tomizawa, T., Sugishita, Y., Suzuki, N., Fujino, M. *et al.* (1989) Increased plasma concentrations of endothelin-1 and big endothelin-1 in acute myocardial infarction. *Lancet*, **2**, 53–54.
32. Okada, K., Miyazaki, Y., Takada, J., Matsuyama, K., Yamaki, T. and Yano, M. (1990) Conversion of big endothelin-1 by membrane-bound metalloendopeptidase in cultured bovine endothelial cells. *Biochemical and Biophysical Research Communications*, **171**, 1192–1198.
33. Suzuki, N., Matsumoto, H., Kitada, C., Kimura, S., Miyauchi, T. and Fujino, M. (1989) A sensitive sandwich-enzyme immunoassay for human endothelin. *Journal of Immunological Method*, **118**, 245–250.
34. Masaki, T., Kimura, S., Yanagisawa, M. and Goto, K. (1991) Molecular and cellular mechanism of endothelin regulation. *Circulation*, **84**, 1457–1462.
35. Wagner, O. F., Christ, G., Wojta, J., Vierhapper, H., Parzer, S., Nowotny, P. J. *et al.* (1992) Polar secretion of endothelin-1 by cultured endothelial cells. *The Journal of Biological Chemistry*, **267**, 16066–16068.
36. Honma, S., Miyauchi, T., Goto, K., Sugishita, Y., Sato, M. and Oshima, N. (1991) Effects of endothelin-1 on coronary microcirculation in isolated beating hearts of rats. *Journal of Cardiovascular Pharmacology*, **17 (Supplement 7)**, S276–S278.
37. Wagner, O. F., Nowotny, P., Vierhappeer, H. and Waldhausl, W. (1990) Plasma concentrations of endothelin in man: arterio-venous differences and release during venous stasis. *European Journal of Clinical Investigation*, **20**, 502–505.
38. Onizuka, M., Miyauchi, T., Mitsui, K., Suzuki, N., Masaki, T., Goto, K., *et al.* (1992) Endothelin-1 mediates regioned blood flow during and after pulmonary operations. *Journal of Thoracic and Cardiovascular Surgery*, **104**, 1696–1701.
39. Stewart, D. J., Cernacek, P., Costells, K. B. and Rouleau, J. L. (1992) Elevated endothelin-1 in heart failure and loss of normal response to postural change. *Circulation*, **85**, 510–517.
40. Battistini, B., D'Orléans-Juste, P. and Sirois, P. (1993) Biology of Disease: Endothelins: Circulating plasma levels and presence in other biologic fluids. *Laboratory Investigation*, **68**, 600–628.
41. Mima, T., Takakura, K., Shigeno, T., Yanagisawa, M., Saito, A., Goto, K. *et al.* (1989) Endothelin induces sustained constriction of feline and canine basilar arteries *in vivo*, when administered cisternally but not intraarterially. *Stroke*, **20**, 1553–1556.

42. Giad, A., Yanagisawa, M., Langleben, D., Michel, R., Levy, R., Shennib, et al. (1993) Expression of endothelin-1 in the lungs of patients with pulmonary hypertension. *The New England Journal of Medicine*, **328**, 1732–1739.
43. Lüscher, T. F., Seo, B. and Bühler, F. R. (1993) Potential role of endothelin in hypertension; Controversy on endothelin in hypertension. *Hypertension*, **21**, 752–757.
44. Masaki, T. (1993) Reduced sensitivity of vascular response to endothelin. *Circulation*, **87**, V-33–V35.
45. Koseki, C., Imai, M., Hirata, Y., Yanagisawa M. and Masaki, T. (1989) Autoradiographic distribution in rat tissues of binding sites for endothelin: a neuropeptide? *American Journal of Physiology*, **256**, R858–R866.
46. Masaki, T. (1993) Endothelins: Homeostatic and compensatory actions in the circulatory and endocrine system. *Endocrine Reviews*, **14**, 256–268.
47. MacCumber, M. W., Ross, C. A., Glaser, B. M. and Snyder, S. H. (1990) Endothelin: Visualization of mRNAs by *in situ* hybridization provides evidence for local action. *Proceedings of National Academy of Science USA*, **86**, 7285–7289.
48. Kuwaki, T., Cao, W. H., Yamamoto, M., Terui, N. and Kumada, M. (1991) Cardiorespiratory effects of topical application of endothelin-1 to the ventral surface of the rat medulla. *Journal of Cardiovascular Pharmacology*, **17 (Supplement 7)**, S343–S345.
49. Yoshizawa, T., Shinmi, O., Giad, A., Yanagisawa, M., Gibson, S., Kimura, J. S. et al. (1990) Endothelin: a novel peptide in the posterior pituitary system. *Science*, **247**, 462–464.
50. Kohan, D. E., (1991) Endothelin synthesis by rabbit renal tubule cells. *American Journal of Physiology*, **261**, F221–F226.
51. Kohan, D. E., Huges, A. K. and Perkins, S. L. (1992) Characterization of endothelin receptors in the inner medullary collecting duct of the rat. *The Journal of Biological Chemistry*, **267**, 12336–12340.
52. Harris, P. J., Zhuo, J., Mendelsohn, P. A. O. and Skinner, S. L. (1991) Haemodynamic and renal tubular effects of low doses of endothelin in anaesthetized rats. *Journal of Physiology*, **433**, 25–39.
53. Kohn, V. and Badr, K. (1991) Biological actions and pathophysiologic significance of endothelin in the kidney. *Kidney International*, **40**, 1–12.
54. Grunstein, M. M., Rosenberg, S. M., Schramm, C. M. and Pawlowski, N. A. (1991) Mechanisms of action of endothelin 1 in maturing rabbit airway smooth muscle. *American Journal of Physiology*, **260**, L434–L443.
55. Masaki, T. Endothelin in vascular biology. *Annals of The New York Academy of Sciences*, in press.
56. Takuwa, N., Takuwa, Y., Yanagisawa, M., Yamashita, K. and Masaki, T. (1989) A novel vasoactive peptide endothelin stimulates mitogenesis through inositol lipid turnover in Swiss 3T3 fibroblasts. *The Journal of Biological Chemistry*, **264**, 7856–7861.
57. Chua, B. H. L., Krebs, C. J., Chua, C. C. and Diglio, C. A. (1992) Endothelin stimulates protein synthesis in smooth muscle cells. *American Journal of Physiology*, **262**, E412–416.
58. Shubeita, H. E., McDonough, P. M., Harris, A. N., Knowlton, K. U., Glembotski, C. C., Brown, J. H. et al. (1990) Endothelin induction of inositol phospholipid hydrolysis, sarcomere assembly, and cardiac gene expression in ventricular myocytes. *The Journal of Biological Chemistry*, **265**, 20555–20562.
59. Hama, H., Sakurai, T., Kasuya, Y., Fujiki, M., Masaki, T. and Goto, K. (1992) Action of endothelin-1 on rat astrocytes through the ETB receptor. *Biochemistry and Biophysiology of Research Communications*, **186**, 355–362.
60. Boulanger, C. M., Tanner, F. C., Béa, M. L., Hahn, A. W. A., Werner, A. and Lüscher, T. F. (1992) Oxidized low density lipoproteins induce mRNA expression and release of endothelin from human and porcine endothelium. *Circulation Research*, **70**, 1191–1197.
61. Lerman, A., Edwards, B. S., Hallett, J. W., Heublein, D. M., Sandberg, S. M. and Burnett Jr., J. C. (1991) Circulating and tissue endothelin immunoreactivity in advanced atherosclerosis. *The New England Journal of Medicine*, **325**, 997–1001.

2 Endothelin Receptors and their Sub-Types

Anthony P. Davenport, Janet J. Maguire and Fiona E. Karet

Clinical Pharmacology Unit, University of Cambridge, Box 110 Level 2, F & G Block, Addenbrooke's Hospital, Cambridge, CB2 2QQ, UK

INTRODUCTION

Endothelin (ET) receptors belong to the superfamily of seven transmembrane domain-spanning receptors linked to G-proteins. Their actions are mediated via several intracellular messengers but mainly inositol phosphates. Two ET receptor sub-types, ET_A and ET_B, have been isolated and cloned from human tissue and have been classified according to the rank order of their affinity for the three ET isoforms. ET-1 and ET-2 show similar affinity for the ET_A sub-type whilst ET-3 has little or no affinity. All three isoforms have similar affinity for ET_B. ET receptors are unusual in that sub-types were cloned *before* the development of sub-type selective ligands. Although ET-1 was first described in 1988[1], triggering an explosion of research, the precise physiological function in man of this family of peptides, or pathological conditions associated with a change in the ET system, are still unclear. In part, this has been due to the lack of specific pharmacological tools to delineate the actions of ET *in vitro* or *in vivo*.

This review focuses on the characterization of human ET receptors, particularly within cardiovascular tissue, since this system is a major target for ET-1. When systemically infused into volunteers to produce an increase in basal plasma concentrations from 1 to about 60 pmol/l, ET-1 produces a significant 10% increase in blood pressure[2]. *In vitro*, ET-1 potently constricts isolated human vessels by interacting with vascular smooth muscle cell receptors[3-5]. In addition, human heart muscle is exquisitely sensitive: ET-1 is a potent positive inotropic agent by direct action on cardiac muscle, with a threshold of about 10 pM and an EC_{50} value of 2 nM[3].

ET RECEPTORS

ET receptors have been studied in a range of human tissues (Table 2.1)[3,5-28] using [^{125}I]ET-1 in saturation binding experiments. In these assays, partially purified

Table 2.1 Receptor binding affinities (K_D) and densities (B_{max}) for [^{125}I]E-1 in normal and pathological human tissues

	K_D (pM)	B_{max} (fmol/mg protein)	Rank order isoform affinity	Ref.
Cardiovascular:				
atrium	595	153		6
	350	1166	ET-1 > ET-3	7
ventricle	354	64		6
	30	7	ET-1 > ET-3	8
Arteries (media):				
aorta	507	9	ET-1 > ET-3	5
pulmonary	845	15		5
coronary	141	71		5
Brain:				
brain stem	45	5052	ET-1 = ET-3	9
hypothalamus	34	963	ET-1 = ET-3	9
hippocampus	34	278	ET-1 = ET-3	10
pituitary[a]	59	418	ET-1 = ET-3	9
	652	1717	ET-1 = ET-3	9
cortex(normal)	1500	15	ET-1 = ET-3	11
astroglioma	2100	30	ET-1 = ET-3	11
glioblastoma	2500	60	ET-1 = ET-3	11
Spinal cord (thoracic):				
laminae I-III	194	12	ET-1 = ET-3	12
lamina X	256	14	ET-1 = ET-3	12
intermedio-lateral nucleus	265	12	ET-1 = ET-3	12
Kidney:				
medulla				
adult	139	360		13
adult	3460	4[b]		14
adult	170	58		15
cortex				
adult	91	165		13
adult	5590	3[b]		14
glomeruli	42			16
Liver:	100	361	ET-1 = ET-3	7
Lung:				
	1330	9610		17
	153	6	ET-1 > ET-3	8
Parathyroid:	62	77	ET-1 > ET-3	18
Adrenal:				
cortex(normal)	65	60	ET-1 = ET-3	19
adenoma	70	226	ET-1 = ET-3	19
Placenta:	80	113	ET-1 = ET-3	8
	36	185	ET-1 > ET-3	20
	24	240		21
	34	93		22
stem villi				
vessels	26	681	ET-1 > ET-3	23
ateries	45	602	ET-1 > ET-3	24
veins	45	619	ET-1 > ET-3	24

Table 2.1 (*Continued*)

	K_D (pM)	B_{max} (fmol/mg protein)	Rank order isoform affinity	Ref.
microvillus membranes	26	50	ET-1 = ET-3	23
basal plasma membrane	12	150	ET-1 > ET-3	23
Uterus:				
myometrium	1190	37		25
endometrium	1390	181		25
Colon:				
myenteric plexus	350			26
Bladder:				
base	4	3		27
dome	7	47		27

[a]Two sites.
[b]fmol/mg tissue equivalents.

plasma membrane fractions from tissue homogenates or cryostat sections of fresh-frozen tissue are incubated with increasing concentrations of [^{125}I] ET-1. An appropriate incubation period to allow the assay to reach equilibrium should be determined (although this information is not always given) but about 2 hours at 25°C is usually sufficient. The equilibrium is rapidly broken by washing to separate free [^{125}I] ET-1 and the amount of radioactivity bound to the tissue is measured. Non-specific binding is determined using a 1000 fold excess of unlabelled ET-1 over the K_D (usually 1 µM). Hill slopes, initial estimates for the equilibrium dissociation constant (receptor affinity) K_D, and density, B_{max} are calculated using Scatchard plots. Further analysis of the binding data are carried out using iterative curve fitting programmes to obtain final values[5,28].

Binding parameters may be altered by numerous factors. Most studies use rapidly processed surgical samples of human tissue to avoid delays inevitable with post-mortem material. Variation may occur with the increased tissue processing necessary when using homogenates compared with cryostat sections. No standard buffer has emerged for ET binding assays but buffers such as HEPES are preferred, containing magnesium ions to promote agonist binding to G-protein-coupled receptors[5,28]. Peptidase inhibitors are sometimes included. In human cardiovascular tissue, under non-physiological binding conditions, no degradation of labelled ET-1 can be detected by high performance liquid chromatography indicating the peptide is stable. However, the stability of receptor protein has not been investigated. Finally, not all binding sites detected in ligand binding experiments are necessarily functional receptors.

Comparison of results must therefore be undertaken with caution, although some general patterns do emerge. Since ET-1 is a potent constrictor of all human vessels examined and a ubiquitous endothelium-derived constricting factor, it is not surprising that ET receptors have been detected in all tissues studied. In human tissues for which information is available, [^{125}I] ET-1 binds with Hill slopes close to unity indicating the presence of either a single population of receptors or a heterogeneous population with the same affinity for the peptide, i.e. [^{125}I] ET-1 binds to both ET$_A$ and ET$_B$ sub-types with equal affinity. An exception would appear to be the pituitary where [^{125}I] ET-1 binds with high affinity to about 20% of the receptors but has an order of magnitude lower affinity for the remaining receptors[9]. This might be an artefact of post mortem delay (10–24 h) but this is unlikely as labelled ET bound with a single affinity elsewhere in the brain in this study. The significance of these findings is unclear and intriguingly, human pituitary contains mainly ET-3[9].

The kinetics of ET binding in human tissues have not been extensively studied, but the association rate is typically slow. In sections of cardiac tissue, labelled peptide has an observed association rate constant value of 0.077 per minute at 22 °C. Dissociation rates are very slow, with only about 5% dissociation after 15 minutes[6].

In human tissue, labelled ET-1 binds with affinities ranging from about 10 pM to 10 nM and densities of 10 to 10,000 fmol/mg protein. Lungs[8,17] (as in animals) appear to have the highest density of receptors although labelled ET-1 binds with lower affinity (in the nM range). In contrast, low density, but high affinity, sites have been detected in the bladder[27]. Brain stem and hypothalamus[9] also have a high density of receptors, and as in the rat brain[29], densities decrease caudally. In the brain, reported K_D values vary 100-fold but it is unclear whether these differences can be explained by interassay variation or whether they reflect true biological differences. Low receptor densities are also present in the spinal cord[12].

Labelled ET-1 binds with similar affinity to cardiac atrium and ventricle[6,28]. High affinity sites are present in the media of vessels (aortic, pulmonary, coronary) containing predominantly vascular smooth muscle cells[5]. A similar density of receptors was detected in the media of these vessels and myometrial smooth muscle cells. Placenta is the most studied tissue and consistent results have been obtained by different groups for both affinity and density of ET receptors[8,21–22]. Receptors have been localized to placental veins and arteries as well as membranes. In the kidney, two studies using different tissue preparations gave similar results, with higher densities in medulla than cortex[3,15]. A third study[14], claiming lower affinities, is difficult to interpret.

ET RECEPTOR SUB-TYPES

Sub-type sequences

Human, bovine and rat receptor sub-types have been isolated and cloned (Tables 2.2, 2.3). The aligned primary amino acid sequences for the human ET$_A$[30] and ET$_B$[31] receptors (including putative N-terminal signal sequences of 20 and 26 amino acids respectively), are shown in Table 2.2 together with the proposed seven hydrophobic regions (I–VII) that are thought to form transmembrane helices. The human ET$_A$ deduced sequence is 95% identical to bovine and 93% to rat, with the N-terminus showing the least homology between species[32]. Human ET$_B$ has 88% sequence homology with rat[31]. It is possible that these variations between species may explain observed inter-species differences in the selectivity of ligands.

Table 2.2 Alignment of the primary amino acid sequences for human ET_A and ET_B receptor sub-types.

```
A  M----------------------------------------------ETLCLRASF  10
B  MQPPPSLCGRALVALVLACGLSRIWGEERGFPPDRA----TP--LLQTAEIMTPPTKTL  53

A  WLALVGCVISDNPERYSTNLSNHVDDFTTFRGTELSFLVTTHQPTNLVLPSNGSMHNYC  69
B  W-----------PKGSNASLARSLAPAEVPKGDR----TAGSPPRTISPPP-------C  90
                                                  I
A  PQQTKITSAFKYINTVISCTIFIVGMVGNATLLRIIYQNKCMRNGPNALIASLALGDLI  128
B  QGPIEIKETFKYINTVVSCLVFVLGIIGNSTLLRIIYKNKCMRNGPNILIASLALGDLL  149
           II                               III
A  YVVIDLPINVFKLLAGRWPFDHNDFGVFLCKLFPFLQKSSVGITVLNLCALSVDRYRAV  187
B  HIVIDIPINVYKLLAEDWPFGAE-----MCKLVPFIQKASVGITVLSLCALSIDRYRAV  203
                                        IV
A  ASWSRVQGIGIPLVTAIEIVSIWILSFILAIPEAIGFVMVPFEYRGEQHKTCMLNATSK  246
B  ASWSRIKGIGVPKWTAVEIVLIWVVSVVLAVPEAIGFDIITMDYKGSYLRICLLHPVQK  262
                 V
A  --FMEFYQDVKDWWLFGFYFCMPLVCTAIFYTLMTCEMLNRRNGSLRIALSEHLKQRRE  303
B  TAFMQFYKTAKDWWLFSFYFCLPLAITAFFYTLMTCEML-RKKSGMQIALNDHLKQRRE  320
              VI                                    VII
A  VAKTVFCLVVIFALCWFPLHLSRILKKTVYNEMDKNRCELLSFLLLMDYIGINLATMNS  362
B  VAKTVFCLVLVFALCWLPLHLSRILKLTLYNQNDPNRCELLSFLLVLDYIGINMASLNS  379

A  CINPIALYFVSKKFKNCFQSCLCCCCYQSKSLMTSVPMNGTSIQWKNHDQNNHNTDRSS  421
B  CINPIALYLVSKRFKNCFKSCLCCWCQSFEEKQSLEEKQSCLKFKANDHGYDNFRSSNK  438

A  HKDSMN                                                      427
B  YSSS                                                        442
```

The extracellular N-terminal sequence is shorter in the ET_A receptor compared to ET_B with only 4% homology[33] in contrast with the much greater similarity within the seven transmembrane domains. Truncation of the entire N-terminal extracellular or the intracellular C-terminal domain of ET_A abolishes binding of ET-1. However, binding activity is retained following deletion of a 25 amino acid N-terminal segment (residues 25–49). Part of the N-terminus may therefore be important for ligand binding[34].

Sequences were aligned using the programme CLUSTAL. The predicted transmembrane domains (I–VII) are shown by underlining.

Chimeric receptor studies

ET receptors have been expressed in cultured cells and the primary sequences modified to identify possible amino acids important for ligand binding[34,35]. An important caveat is that expressed receptors may not behave in the same way as native receptors. Chimeric receptors have been constructed in which each of the four extracellular regions of ET_A was replaced with the corresponding ET_B sequence. The reverse process was carried out by replacing each ET_B extracellular domain with an ET_A sequence. The results suggest that transmembrane domains I, II, III and VII are of importance for ET_A binding whereas IV, V and VI are necessary for ET_B binding.

Table 2.3 Classification of ET receptors and selective ligands[a]

	ET_A	ET_B
Primary[b] amino acid sequence	427(human) 427(bovine) 426(rat)	442(human) 441(bovine) 441(rat)
Potency order	ET-1 = ET-2 ≫ ET-3	ET-1 = ET-2 = ET-3
Peptides: selective agonists	—	[Ala^{1,3,11,15}]ET-1 [Ala^{11,15}]Ac-ET-1$_{(6-21)}$ (BQ3020) Sarafotoxin S6c
selective antagonists	BQ123 FR139317	[Cys^{11}–Cys^{15}]ET$_{(11-21)}$ (IRL1038)
non-selective antagonist	PD142893	
Non-peptides: selective antagonist	50235	—
non-selective antagonists	RO462005	
Radioligands:	[^{125}I]ET-1 [^{125}I]ET-2 —	[^{125}I]ET-1 [^{125}I]ET-2 [^{125}I]ET-3
selective	[^{125}I]PD 151242	[^{125}I]-[Ala^{1,3,11,15}]ET-1 [^{125}I]-[Ala^{11,15}] Ac-ET-1$_{(6-21)}$ ([^{125}I] BQ3020)

[a] Nomenclature agreed by receptor subcommittee of IUPHAR, 2nd International Endothelin Meeting, Tskuba, Japan, 1990.
[b] Includes putative signal sequence.

Receptor sub-type studies

Using the present classification scheme (Table 2.3) the two known sub-types can be distinguished by the affinity of ET-3 compared to ET-1 in competion binding assays. This method compares the ability of increasing concentrations of unlabelled ET-1 or ET-3 to compete for the binding of a fixed concentration of [^{125}I] ET-1. Because tissues contain a heterogeneous population of cells, sub-type ratios may vary. ET$_A$ receptors would be expected to be present in most if not all tissues as they are predicted to predominate in vascular smooth muscle cells. Using this classification scheme (Table 2.1) some general patterns emerge. The cardiovascular system contains predominantly ET$_A$, whereas in placenta, kidney, lung, adrenal cortex and brain, ET$_B$ is more abundant. However, a limitation of this method is that it is difficult to calculate the ratio of the two sub-types. This has required the development of selective ligands.

Endothelin receptors

ET$_A$ selective compounds

BQ123 is a cyclic pentapeptide[36] (Table 2.3, Figure 2.1) containing three D-isomers rather than the naturally occurring L-form, a common strategy used to increase antagonist activity in peptides. BQ123 is highly selective for human ET$_A$ receptors

ET$_A$ antagonists

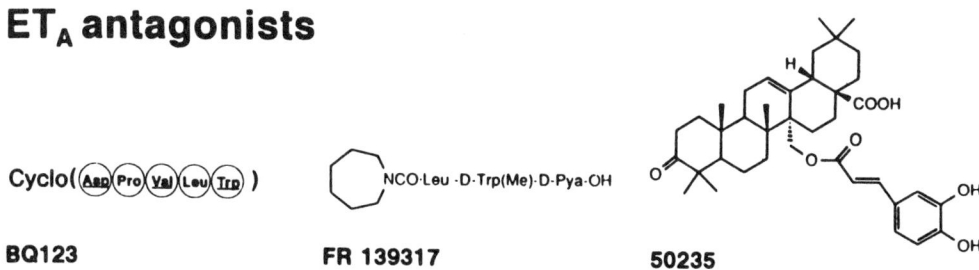

BQ123   FR 139317   50235

ET$_B$ antagonist

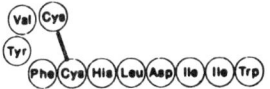

IRL-1038

ET$_B$ agonists

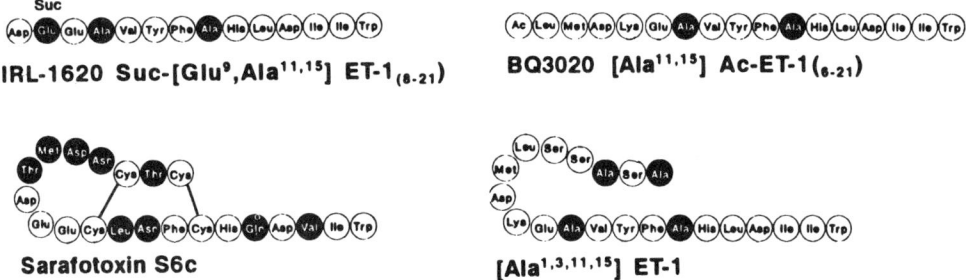

IRL-1620 Suc-[Glu^9,Ala^{11,15}] ET-1$_{(8-21)}$ BQ3020 [Ala^{11,15}] Ac-ET-1$_{(6-21)}$

Sarafotoxin S6c   [Ala^{1,3,11,15}] ET-1

Non-selective antagonists

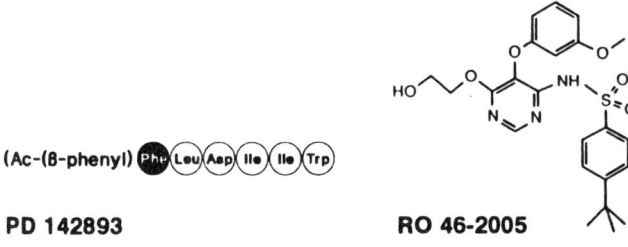

(Ac-(β-phenyl)) Phe Leu Asp Ile Ile Trp

PD 142893   RO 46-2005

Figure 2.1. Schematic diagram showing the structure of some selective ET compounds. Filled circles indicate differences in amino-acids from ET-1. The position of D-amino acids in BQ123 has been indicated by underlining the residues.

Table 2.4 Receptor binding affinities (K_D) for sub-type-selective ligands and percentage of ET_A and ET_B receptors in human tissue

	$K_D ET_A$	$K_D ET_B$	$ET_A:ET_B$	
ET_A selective	(nM)	(µM)	(%)	Ref.
BQ123				
ventricle	0.7	24.3	57:43	6
myocytes	2.2	179.0	92:8	6
coronary	0.9	7.6	87:13	5
kidney				
medulla	11.8	32.8	24:76	15
cortex	26.0	6.5	26:74	15
FR139317				
ventricle	1.2	287.0	62:38	a
50235				
ventricle	150.0	165.0	54:46	a
coronary	9.0	11.0	80:20	b
ET_B selective	(µM)	(nM)	(%)	
BQ3020				
ventricle	2.0	1.4	67:33	6
coronary:	0.2	0.8	62:38	5
kidney				
medulla	5.0	3.0	37:63	15
cortex	2.1	4.9	37:63	15
IRL1038				
ventricle	32.6	4860	63:37	a

[a] Peter, M. and Davenport, A. P. (Unpublished)
[b] Bacon, C. M. and Davenport, A. P. (Unpublished)

expressed in cardiovascular and renal tissue (Table 2.4) with affinities in the sub-nanomolar range and has up to 30,000-fold affinity for ET_A versus ET_B[5,6]. FR139317 (Figure 2.1) is a modified tripeptide with Leu and D-Trp residues in common with BQ123. The compound was originally shown to be selective for animal ET_A receptors[37] and shows ten-fold higher affinity for human cardiac ET_A receptors (Table 2.4).

Although BQ123 and FR139317 are highly selective for human ET_A receptors, they are peptides and whilst useful as tools to delineate sub-types, they are not orally active and are thus unlikely to have therapeutic use. 50235 (myricerone caffeoyl ester)[38] extracted from bayberry bark was the first potent non-peptide compound to be described with selectivity for the human ET_A receptor (Table 2.4). This compound demonstrates that the carbon-nitrogen peptide bond is not crucial for antagonist activity, and this structure may help to determine the functional groups important for ET_A binding. To date, no selective ET_A agonist has been described.

ET_B selective compounds

These include sarafotoxin S6c (Table 2.3, Figure 2.1), isolated from a snake venom, and modified linear analogues of ET-1 in which disulphide bridges are removed by substituting alanine residues (IRL1620, [Ala[1,3,11,15]]ET-1 and BQ3020). BQ3020 has up to 1,500-fold selectivity for cardiovascular and renal ET_B receptors[5,6,15]. Radio-labelled BQ3020 and [Ala^{1,3,11,15}]ET-1 have also been used to characterize ET_B receptors. Both bind with high affinity in left ventricle, with K_D of 0.1 and 0.2 nM, respectively[28].

IRL1038 contains the C-terminal sequence of ET-1$_{(11-21)}$ and is a highly selective ET_B antagonist in rat tissue[39]. However in receptor binding assays using human heart, IRL1038 competed with only μM affinity for human ET_B and had only about 10-fold selectivity over ET_A (Table 2.4). These results suggest that the compound is less effective for human receptors and this could reflect inter-species differences. PD142893 also has the C-terminal Leu^{17}-Trp^{21} of ET-1 and is suggested to be a non-selective antagonist[40]. RO462005, a sulphonamide derivative, is the first orally active non-peptide to be disclosed. In rat, it inhibits ET-1 action *in vivo* and *in vitro*, where it is a competitive but non-selective antagonist with comparatively low pA_2 values (6.6 and 6.1 at ET_A and ET_B respectively)[41]. The compound will provide the stimulus for the development of more potent oral agents.

FUNCTION OF ET RECEPTOR SUB-TYPES IN VASCULAR TISSUE

ET-1 infused into human vessels causes an initial vasodilatation before higher concentrations produce vasoconstriction[2]. This dilatation is probably ET_B-mediated via the release of endothelium derived relaxing factors. Reverse-transcriptase PCR assays have detected mRNA encoding ET_B but not ET_A in human endothelial cells[6] together with ET_B receptor protein. Human vascular smooth muscle cells express mRNA encoding both receptor sub-types. Competition binding assays show that ET_A predominates in the media of coronary arteries with only about 13% ET_B[5]. However [Ala^{1,3,11,15}] ET-1, which potently constricts some vascular beds when infused into rats[42], had no constrictor activity at concentrations up to 10 μM in a range of isolated human vessels[5,43-45]. These results suggest that an important species difference exists. In rats, constriction occurs via both sub-types whereas in man, ET-1 mediates vasoconstriction mainly if not exclusively via ET_A. An ET_A selective antagonist would therefore have potential therapeutic value since the beneficial vasodilator response would be preserved, despite animal studies suggesting that a non-selective compound would be preferable.

CONCLUSION

ET receptors are widely distributed in human tissues, supporting the hypothesis that ET-1 functions as a ubiquitous endothelium derived vasoconstrictor. Significant species differences exist between the function of ET_B receptors expressed by vessels which has important implications for the development of novel therapeutic agents. With the development of sub-type selective agonists and antagonists, ET research is entering a new phase in which it may be possible to elucidate the role of ET and its receptors in man.

Acknowledgements

We thank the British Heart Foundation, National Kidney Research Fund, Royal Society and Newton Trust for research grants.

References

1. Yanagisawa, M., Kurihara, H., Kimura, S., Tomobe, Y., Kobayashi, M., Mitsui, Y. et al. (1988) A novel potent vasoconstrictor peptide produced by vascular endothelial cells. Nature, 332, 411–415.
2. Vierhapper, H., Wagner, O., Nowotny, P. and Waldhäusl, W. (1990) Effect of endothelin in man. Circulation, 81, 1415–1418.
3. Davenport, A. P., Nunez, D. J., Hall, J. A., Kaumann, A. J. and Brown, M. J. (1989) Autoradiographical localisation of binding sites for [^{125}I] endothelin-1 in humans, pigs and rats: functional relevance in man. Journal of Cardiovascular Pharmacology, 13 (5), S166–170.
4. Howard, P. G., Plumpton, C. and Davenport, A. P. (1992) Anatomical localisation and pharmacological activity of mature endothelins and their precursors in human vascular tissue. Journal of Hypertension, 10, 1379–1386.
5. Davenport, A. P., O'Reilly, G., Molenaar, P., Maguire, J. J., Kuc, R. E., Sharkey, A., et al. (1993) Human endothelin receptors characterised using reverse-transcriptase polymerase chain reaction, in situ hybridization and sub-type selective ligands BQ123 and BQ3020: evidence for expression of ET$_B$ receptors in human vascular smooth muscle. Journal of Cardiovascular Pharmacology, 22(S8), 22–25.
6. Molenaar, P., O'Reilly, G., Sharkey, A., Kuc, R. E., Harding, D. P., Plumpton, C. et al. (1993) Characterization and localization of endothelin receptor subtypes in the human atrioventricular conducting system and myocardium. Circulation Research, 72, 526–538.
7. Takayanagi, R., Ohnaka, K., Takasaki, C., Ohashi, M. and Nawata, H. (1991) Multiple subtypes of endothelin receptors in human and porcine tissues: characterization by ligand binding, affinity labelling, and regional distribution. Journal of Cardiovascular Pharmacology, 17, (7), S127–130.
8. Hemsen, A. (1991) Biochemical and functional characterization of endothelin peptides with special reference to vascular effects. Acta Physiologica Scandinava Suppl., 602, 1–61.
9. Takahashi, K., Ghatei, M. A., Jones, P. M., Murphy, J. K., Lam, H. C., O'Halloran, D. J. et al. (1991) Endothelin in human brain and pituitary gland: presence of immunoreactive endothlin, endothelin messenger ribonucleic acid, and endothelin receptors. Journal of Clinical Endocrinology & Metabolism, 72, 693–699.
10. Williams, D. L., Jones, K. L., Colton, C. D. and Nutt, R. F. (1991) Identification of high affinity ET-1 receptor subtypes in human tissues. Biochemical Biophysical Research Communications, 180, 475–480.
11. Kurihara, M., Ochi, A., Kawaguchi, T., Niwa, M., Kataoka, Y. and Mori, K. (1990) Localization and characterization of endothelin receptors in human gliomas: a growth factor? Neurosurgery, 27, 275–281.
12. Niwa, M., Kawaguchi, T., Himeno, A., Fujimoto, M., Kurihara, M., Yamashita, K. et al. (1992) Specific binding sites for ^{125}I-endothelin-1 in the porcine and human spinal cord. European Journal of Pharmacology, 225, 281–289.
13. Nambi, P., Pullen, M., Wu, H. L., Aiyar, N., Ohlstein, E. H. and Edwards, R. M. (1992) Identification of endothelin receptor subtypes in human renal cortex and medulla using subtype-selective ligands. Endocrinology, 131, 1081–1086.
14. Grone, H. J., Laue, A. and Fuchs, E. (1990) Localization and quantification of [^{125}I]-endothelin binding sites in human fetal and adult kidneys-relevance to renal ontogeny and pathophysiology. Klinische Wochenschrift, 68, 758–767.
15. Karet, F. E., Kuc, R. E. and Davenport, A. P. (1993) Novel Ligands BQ123 and BQ3020 characterise endothelin receptor subtypes ET$_A$ and ET$_B$ in human kidney. Kidney International, 44, 36–42.
16. Rebibou, J. M., He, C. J., Delarue, F., Peraldi, M. N., Adida, C., Rondeau, E et al. (1992) Functional endothelin 1 receptors on human glomerular podocytes and mesangial cells. Nephrology, Dialysis & Transplantation, 7, 288–292.
17. Brink, C., Gillard, V., Roubert, P., Mencia-Huerta, J. M., Chabrier, P. E. et al. (1991) Effects and specific binding sites of endothelin in human lung preparations. Pulmonary Pharmacology, 4, 54–59.
18. Eguchi, S., Hirata, Y., Imai, T., Kanno, K., Akiba, T., Sakamoto, A., et al. (1992) Endothelin receptors in human parathyroid gland. Biochemical Biophysical Research Communications, 184, 1448–1455.
19. Imai, T., Hirata, Y., Eguchi, S., Kanno, K., Ohta, K., Emori, T. et al. (1992) Concomitant expression of receptor subtype and isopeptides of endothelin by human adrenal gland. Biochemical Biophysical Research Communications, 182, 1115–1121.
20. Wilkes, B. M., Mento, P. F., Hollander, A. M., Maita, M. E., Sung, S. and Girardi, E. P. (1990) Endothelin receptors in human placenta: relationship to vascular resistance and thromboxane release. American Journal of Physiology, 258, E864–870.
21. Fischli, W., Clozel, M. and Guilly, C. (1989) Specific receptors for endothelin on membranes from human placenta. Characterization and use in a binding assay. Life Science, 44, 1429–1436.
22. Kalina, B. and Loffler, B. M. (1992) Crosslinking analysis of an endothelin receptor protein from human placenta. Biochemistry International, 27, 735–744.

23. Mondon, F., Malassine, A., Robaut, C., Vial, M., Bandet, J., Tanguy, G. et al. (1993) Biochemical characterization and autoradiographic localization of [^{125}I] endothelin-1 binding sites on trophoblast and blood vessels of human placenta. *Journal of Clinical Endocrinolgy and Metabolism*, **76**, 237–244.
24. Robaut, C., Mondon, F., Bandet, J., Ferre, F. and Cavero, I. (1991) Regional distribution and pharmacological characterization of [^{125}I]endothelin, 1 binding sites in human fetal placental vessels. *Placenta*, **12**, 55–67.
25. Bacon, C. R., O'Reilly, G., Cameron, I. T. and Davenport, A. P. (1993) Endothelin receptor sub-types in human myometrium characerized by BQ123 and BQ3020. *British Journal of Pharmacology*, 110S, P45.
26. Inagaki, H., Bishop, A. E., Yura, J. and Polak, J. M. (1991) Localization of endothelin-1 and its binding sites to the nervous system of the human colon. *Journal of Cardiovascular Pharmacology*, **17**(7), S455–457.
27. Kondo, S., Fushimi, E., Morita, T. and Tashima, Y. (1992) Direct measurement of endothelin receptor in human bladder base and dome using ^{125}I-endothelin. *Tohoku Journal of Experimental Medicine*, **167**, 159–161.
28. Molenaar, P., Kuc, R. E. and Davenport, A. P. (1992) Characterization of two new ETB selective radioligands, [^{125}I]-BQ3020 and [^{125}I]-[Ala1,3,11,15]ET-1 in human heart. *British Journal of Pharmacology*, **107**, 637–639.
29. Davenport, A. P. and Morton, A. J. (1991) Binding sites for ^{125}I ET-1, ET-2, ET-3 and vasoactive intestinal contractor are present in adult rat brain and neurone-enriched primary cultures of embryonic brain cells. *Brain Research*, **554**, 278–285.
30. Adachi, M., Yang, Y., Furuichi, Y. and Miyamoto, C. (1991) Cloning and characterization of cDNA encoding human A-type endothelin receptor. *Biochemical Biophysical Research Communications*, **180**, 1265–1272.
31. Ogawa, Y., Nakao, K., Arai, H., Nakagawa, O., Hosoda, K., Suga, S. et al. (1991) Molecular cloning of a non-isopeptide-selective human endothelin receptor. *Biochemical Biophysical Research Communications*, **178**, 248–255.
32. Cyr, C., Huebener, K., Druck, T. and Kris, R. (1991) Cloning and chromosomal localization of the human endothelin ET$_A$ receptor. *Biochemical Biophysical Research Communications*, **181**, 184–190.
33. Hashido, K., Gamou, T., Adachi, M., Tabuchi, H., Watanabe, T., Furuichi, Y. and Miyamoto, C. (1992) Truncation of N-terminal extracellular or C-terminal domains of human ET$_A$ receptor abrogate the binding activity to ET-1. *Biochemical Biophysical Research Communications*, **187**, 1241–1248.
34. Adachi, M., Yang, Y., Trzeciak, A., Furuichi, Y. and Miyamoto, C. (1992) Identification of a domain of ET$_A$ receptor required for ligand binding. *FEBS*, **311**, 179–183.
35. Sakamoto, A., Yanagisawa, M., Sawamura, T., Enoki, T., Sakurai, T. et al. (1993) Distinct sub-domains of human endothelin receptors determine their selectivity to endothelin(A)-selective antagonists and endothelin(B)-selective agonists. *Journal of Biological Chemistry*, **268**, 8547–8553.
36. Nakamichi, K., Ihara, M., Kobayashi, M., Saeki, T., Ishikawa, K. and Yano, M. et al. (1992) Different distribution of endothelin receptor sub-type in pulmonary tissue revealed by the novel selective ligands BQ123 and BQ3020. *Biochemical Biophysical Research Communications*, **182**, 144–150.
37. Doherty, A. M. (1992) Endothelin: a new challenge. *Journal of Medicinal Chemistry*, **35**, 1493–1508.
38. Fujimoto, M., Mihara, S., Nakajima, N., Ueda, M., Nakamura, M. and Sakurai, K. (1992) A novel non-peptide endothelin antagonist isolated from bayberry Myrica cerifera. *FEBS*, **305**, 41–44.
39. Urade, Y., Fuitani, Y., Oda, K., Watakable, T., Umemura, I., Takai, M. et al. (1992) An endothelin B receptor-selective antagonist:IRL1038 [Cys^{11}–Cys^{15}]-endothelin(11–21). *FEBS*, **311**, 12–16.
40. Hingorani, G., Major, T., Panek, R., Flynn, M., Reynolds, E., He, X. et al. (1992) *In vitro* pharmacology of a non-selective (ET$_A$/ET$_B$) endothelin receptor antagonist, PD142893. *FASEB Journal*, **6**(4), A1003.
41. Haynes, W. G., Davenport, A. P. and Webb, D. J. (1993) Endothelins: progress in pharmacology and physiology. *Trends in Pharmacological Sciences*, **14**, 225–228.
42. Gardiner, S. M., Kemp, P. A., Bennett, T. and Davenport, A. P. (1992) Regional haemodynamic responses to [Ala^{1,3,11,15}] Endothelin-1 in conscious rats. *British Journal of Pharmacology*, 107S, P145.
43. Davenport, A. P. and Maguire, J. J. Is endothelin-induced vasoconstriction mediated only by ET$_A$ receptors in man? *Trends in Pharmacological Sciences*, **15**, 9–11.
44. Maguire, J. J. and Davenport, A. P. (1993) Endothelin-induced vasoconstriction in human isolated vasculature is mediated predominantly via activation of ET$_A$ receptors. *British Journal of Pharmacology*, 110S, P47.
45. Maguire, J. J., Kuc, R. E., O'Reilly, G. and Davenport, A. P. (1994) Vasoconstrictor endothelin receptors characterised in human renal artery and vein *in vitro*. *British Journal of Pharmacology*, **113**, 49–54.

3 Endothelins: Transmembrane Signaling Mechanisms

Mordechai Sokolovsky

*Laboratory of Neurobiochemistry, Department of Biochemistry,
The George S. Wise Faculty of Life Sciences,
Tel Aviv University, Tel Aviv 69978, Israel*

INTRODUCTION

The endothelins (ETs) and the sarafotoxins (SRTXs) are two structurally related families of potent vasoactive peptides[1,2]. Although it is still too early to define the precise physiological role for endothelins, these peptides regulate a surprisingly diverse array of biological actions, such as contraction of vascular and nonvascular smooth muscle, neuromodulation and neurotransmission, and secretion of effectors. In addition, they exhibit growth factor properties.

The diversity of action of the ETs and SRTXs may be explained in terms of (i) the existence of several receptor subtypes and/or (ii) the activation of different signal transduction pathways[1,5]. Most of the reports point to similar patterns of signal transduction induced by the two families of peptides. For simplicity, in the following we shall refer to the peptides as one family, namely, the endothelins.

Transmembrane signaling systems relay information from the exterior to the interior of a cell through a series of complex protein-protein interactions and second-messenger cascades. One such system involves the coupling of receptors to a family of heterotrimeric G-proteins; activation through G-proteins is initiated upon agonist binding to the receptor. The coupling activates an effector molecule, thereby leading to a second-messenger cascade[6]. Two types of signaling have been described: short-term action, which is characterized by responses such as contraction and/or secretion, and long-term responses that are adaptive in nature, such as cell growth. Numerous studies have focused on the second-messenger cascades responsible for the short-term effects, whereas the pathways of cytosolic and nuclear signaling involved in the long-term changes have only recently attracted attention[3,7,8]. For example, Wang et al.[7] have shown that mitogen-activated protein kinases in rat mesangial cells are rapidly activated by ET-1, a regulatory process that induces activation of protein kinase C and also of a tyrosine kinase. The focus of this review is on the effectors associated with ET receptors (ET-R) in various tissues and species. A schematic representation of some of the pathways described is given in Figure 3.1.

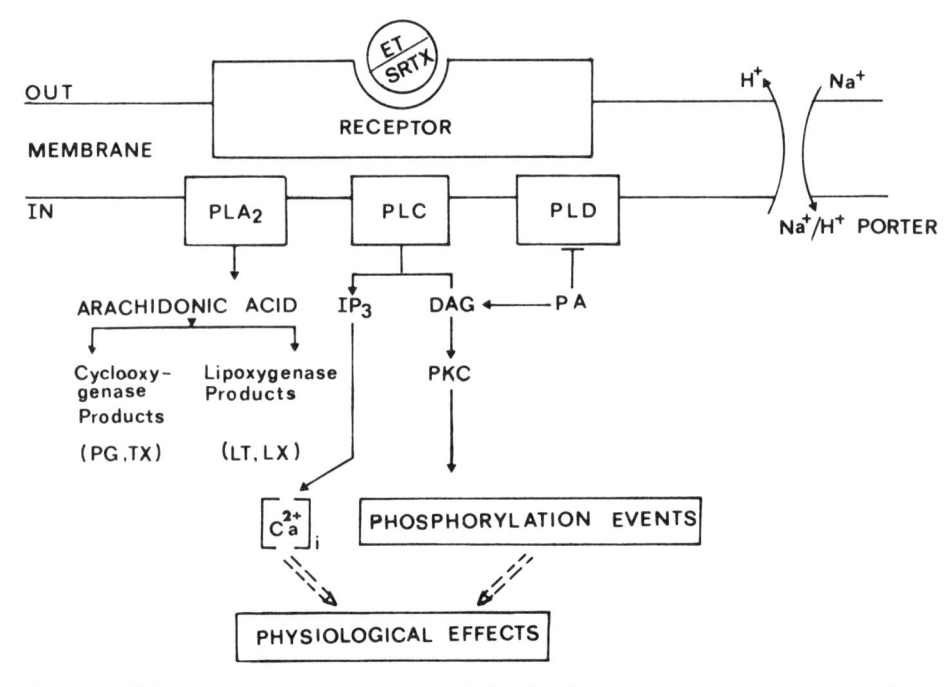

Figure 3.1. Schematic representation of some of the signal transduction pathways associated with activation of the ET/SRTX receptor. IP$_3$, inositol-1,4,5-trisphosphate; LT, Leukotriene; LX, lipoxin; PA, phosphatidic acid; PG, prostaglandin; PKC, protein kinase C; PLA$_2$, Phospholipase A$_2$; PLC, phosphoinositide-specific phospholipase C; PLD, phospholipase D; TX, thromboxane.

COUPLING OF RECEPTORS TO G-PROTEINS

As with most G-protein-coupled receptors (see review[9,10]), activated ET receptors couple to a number of effector systems to produce a complicated network of second messengers. It is now generally accepted that receptors which consist of single polypeptides, and which are likely to traverse the plasma membrane seven times, all achieve regulation of an effector system through activation of a family of heterotrimeric G-proteins. Recent ET-R cloning experiments support the existence of such an interaction[11–13]. It is interesting to note that the third intracellular loop of the ET-R, which is a portion of the receptor considered to be part of the receptor – G-protein interaction site, is relatively small (as a comparison the third intracellular loop of the muscarinic receptor, M1, is about five times longer), thus offering an attractive site for future structure-activity relationship studies. A major signal transduction pathway for the ET-R was found to be the system involving activation of phospholipase C (PLC) via G-protein(s). Interaction of this system with the receptor could be directly assessed by measurement of receptor-stimulated GTPase activity. Recently, stimulation of GTPase activity by ET-1, ET-3, SRTX-b and SRTX-c in rat cerebellum preparation[14] and in rat heart myocytes[15], demonstrated directly the functional coupling between ET_B-R (cerebellum) or ET_A-R (myocytes) and G-protein(s). In both preparations the G-protein involved in the PLC activation was insensitive to pertussis toxin (PT) and was probably Gq/11. These experiments also showed that the phosphoinositide hydrolysis resulting from agonist-induced stimulation of pertussis toxin treated preparations is enhanced by the toxin, suggesting that PT-sensitive inhibitory G-proteins (Gil/2-like and/or Go-like) may normally act to repress PLC activity.

PHOSPHOLIPASE C

As already indicated, the major signal transduction pathway for ET-R was established as the system involving activation of phosphatidylinositol 4,5-bisphosphate (PIP_2)-specific PLC. Activation of PLC by ETs leads to the cleavage of membrane-bound phosphoinositides into inositol 1,4,5-trisphosphate (IP_3) and diacylglycerol (DAG), each of which subsequently activates separate signal transduction pathways. DAG activates protein kinase C (PKC) while IP_3, which binds to a high-affinity receptor on endoplasmic reticulum, triggers the rapid mobilization of intracellular Ca^{2+}[16]. An increase in intracellular Ca^{2+} can directly activate Ca^{2+}-dependent protein kinases as well as Ca^{2+}-sensitive PLC and phospholipase A_2 (PLA_2), leading to the release of arachidonic acid. The Ca^{2+}, often in association with calmodulin, triggers or modulates processes such as secretion (including transmitter release) and activates enzymes such as myosin light chain kinase, which regulates cellular contractile mechanisms. An increase in $[Ca^{2+}]_i$, as well as enhanced contraction and secretion, are therefore expected responses to ET-R activation.

Stimulation of ET-R is followed by a rapid increase in the activity of PLC, and several tissues show a dose-dependent increase in the hydrolysis of phosphoinositides[17,18] (and refs. therein).

In a number of studies[17,18] (and refs. therein), stimulation of PLC activity by ETs occurred at higher concentrations than their K_d values for binding. This apparent inconsistency might be explained by (i) the different conditions employed in the binding experiments and the PI experiments, (iii) coupling of only a fraction of the receptors to PLC, and/or (iii) different ligand receptor complexes.

Recently, a new subtype of endothelin receptor was described[3,14,15,18] with K_d values in the pM range, as distinct from the previously identified ET_A-R and ET_B-R with K_d values in the nM range. Both ET_A-R and ET_B-R have been shown to mediate the stimulation of phosphoinositide hydrolysis in various tissues and cell types (see reviews[1,3,18]). Phosphoinositide hydrolysis induced by ET-1 and ET-3, for example, was observed only with ET concentrations higher than 500 pM, indicating that the sites coupled to this pathway are not those with EC_{50} values in the pM range.

It is interesting to note the interaction of endothelins with pituitary cells[19,20]. Since pituitary cells are heterogeneous, it was decided to investigate the effects of endothelins on pituitary cell lines representing gonadotrophs (αT3-1 cell line) and mammotrophs (GH_3 cell line); in both cell lines PLC activation was confirmed[20]. Interestingly, thyrotropin releasing hormone (TRH), which also binds to pituitary mammotrophs and activates PLC, stimulates prolactin release, whereas activation of the same pathway by endothelins results in inhibition of basal and TRH-induced prolactin release[20]. It was therefore proposed that biochemical events subsequent to phosphoinositide turnover in the signal transduction cascade are critical in determining whether stimulation or inhibition of prolactin release will occur. Also, the nanomolar concentration range needed to stimulate PLC and to inhibit prolactin secretion, together with the finding that ETs are present in the hypothalamo-pituitary axis[21], suggest that ETs might participate in the neuroendocrine modulation of pituitary function.

Recent investigations of the signaling cascade in rat mesangial and vascular smooth muscle cells showed that IP_3 formation, which results in mobilization of $[Ca^{2+}]_i$, is followed by activation of chloride channels[22]. The ensuing Cl^- efflux causes membrane depolarization and, in turn, activation of voltage-dependent Ca^{2+} channels, resulting in sustained elevation of $[Ca^{2+}]_i$.

CALCIUM FLUX

ET induces a substantial and sustained increase in intracellular Ca^{2+}. Studies with the fluorescent probes quin 2, indo 1, and fura 2 demonstrate that the concentration of intracellular Ca^{2+} increases rapidly in a concentration-dependent manner, when the cells are exposed to ET[23,24]. ET can produce an increase in intracellular Ca^{2+} even in the absence of extracellular Ca^{2+}, though the increase is less pronounced[24]. ET appears to increase PI turnover and liberate intracellular Ca^{2+}, in addition to increasing plasmalemmal Ca^{2+} permeability[3]. ET affects both voltage-operated channels and receptor-operated channels, which can be opened directly through the involvement of cellular second messengers[3]. Nishimura et al.[25] studied the effect of ET on neurons, using an intracellular, single-electrode voltage-clamp technique with sodium and potassium channels blocked. The inward current induced by ET had two components, a predominant component mediated by calcium ions and a calcium-insensitive component mediated by chloride ions.

PHOSPHOLIPASE A2

ET was also found to activate phospholipase A_2 (PLA_2) in several tissues, leading to the release of arachidonic acid. This is then metabolized to prostaglandins, thromboxanes and leukotrienes[24,26,27], suggesting that eicosanoid metabolites of arachidonic acid may play an important role as second messengers in mediating some of the biological activities of ETs. Two mechanisms might be responsible for the induced generation of arachidonic acid by ETs in various cells: (i) activation of PLA_2 and direct formation of arachidonic acid; and (ii) an indirect pathway via PLC. The former mechanism leads to an increase in $[Ca^{2+}]_i$, thereby activating Ca^{2+}-sensitive PLA_2, while the latter stimulates production of e.g. DAG, which might act as a substrate for lipases producing arachidonic acid (see review[28]).

PHOSPHOLIPASE D

Phospholipase D (PLD) hydrolyzes phospholipids such as phosphatidylcholine and phosphatidylethanolamine, producing phosphatidic acid and releasing the free polar head-groups, e.g. choline and ethanolamine. Some of the biochemical signals, such as the biphasic elevation of intracellular Ca^{2+} induced by ET-1[23,24,31,32] and the biphasic elevation of diacylglycerol in ET-1 stimulated cells[33,34], might result from the formation of more than one second messenger. Recent evidence suggests that the activation of PLD by neurotransmitters, hormones and growth factors may represent a novel and ubiquitous signal transduction pathway in mammalian cells, mediated by accumulation of phosphatidic acid and/or diacylglycerol[29]. Stimulation by ET-1 of choline generation from phosphatidylcholine was recently discovered in Rat-1 fibroblasts[30], leading to the suggestion that ET activates PLD by both PKC-dependent and PKC-independent mechanisms.

The activation of PLD and PLC by ETs was recently described in three cell lines[18], namely, C6-glioma cells and Rat-1 and Swiss 3T3 fibroblasts. The activation of PLC or PLD by ETs in all three cell lines was mediated by the sites in the nanomolar but not in the picomolar range. The EC_{50} values were similar in all cases and were not significantly affected be either extracellular or intracellular Ca^{2+}. The ET-R- induced activation of both PLD and PLC has led some authors to suggest that PLC activation (thought to be the first event induced by ET-R[30,35]) can stimulate PLD through its two second messengers, DAG and Ca^{2+}[36]. The data reported by Ambar and Sokolovsky[18] appear to indicate that ET-R induces PLD activation directly and not through activation of PLC. This conclusion is supported by the finding that ET-1 stimulation of PLD in rabbit iris sphincter smooth muscle[37] occurs independently of PKC, PLC and PLA_2 activation and intracellular Ca^{2+} mobilization.

PLD-related second messengers, such as choline and phosphatidic acid (which can be metabolized to DAG by phosphatidic acid hydrolase), may participate in the regulation of several cell functions[38,39] and play an important role in ET-mediated signal transduction. For example, ET-R-induced activation of PLD may explain the sustained generation of DAG and hence the prolonged maintenance of PKC activation. Phosphatidic acid, as a second messenger derived from PLD activation, may be involved in some of the observed ET-1-induced cellular responses, such as the sustained increase in intracellular Ca^{2+} which is not mediated via IP_3[41], long-lasting contraction of smooth muscles, and rapid DNA synthesis and cell proliferation (see review[3]). It was recently suggested that stimulation of ET_A-R causes inhibition of adenylate cyclase activated by cholera toxin[42]. This could be explained by the presence of phosphatidic acid, which in turn may stimulate receptors that mediate adenylate cyclase inhibition in 3T3 fibroblasts[43].

The role of PLD-related second messengers has intriguing implications especially in the brain, which is a rich source of PLD[44]. For example, choline—a product of PLD activity—can serve as a source of free choline for the synthesis of acetylcholine in the brain[45]. Moreover, ethanol-intoxicated rats produce large quantities of phosphatidylethanol (PEt) (an exclusive product of PLD) in various organs, including the brain[46]. Another relevant finding is that PEt can substitute for phosphatidylserine in activating a brain-specific PKC[47]. These observations indicate that PLD-catalyzed transphosphatidylation may play a role in the development of alcohol dependency and alcohol-related pathology. Because of the wide distribution of ET receptors in the brain, it will be interesting to investigate the effect of ET-R activation in relation to this pathology.

Na$^+$/H$^+$ EXCHANGE

Receptor-mediated regulation of Na$^+$/H$^+$ exchange activity has been described for a number of polypeptide growth factors, vasoactive agents and hormones (see review[48]). Multiple intracellular pathways are thought to be involved in the coupling of receptors to Na$^+$/H$^+$ exchange mechanisms, including possible mediation by G-proteins.

Simonson et al.[49] have shown that ET activates Na$^+$/H$^+$ exchange and induces cytoplasmic alkalinization. The alkalinization is preceded by a short, transient acidification, probably the result of an increase in intracellular Ca^{2+}[49,50]. Vigne et al.[51] have described two types of receptors in brain capillary endothelial cells: those with high affinity for ET-1 and low affinity for ET-3, and those with high affinity for both ET-1 and ET-3. The latter receptor is thought to control Na$^+$/H$^+$ exchange via PKC-independent mechanism.

Kramer et al.[52] investigated the role of intracellular alkalysis by activation of PKC-dependent of Na$^+$/H$^+$ exchange in adult rat ventricular myocytes. They concluded that the positive inotropic action of ET is due in part to stimulation of the sacrolemmal Na$^+$/H$^+$ exchanges by a PKC-mediated pathway, resulting in a rise in pHi and sensitization of cardiac myofilaments to intracellular Ca^{2+}. It should be noted that ET concentrations in the experiments performed by Simonson et al.[49] were above 10 nM, whereas in those of Kramer et al.[52] they were below 1 nM. This suggests that in the latter work the receptors involved have affinities in the pM range[4] (i.e., not those involved in PLC activation). At high ET concentrations, activation of the PLC pathway leads to activation of PKC, which in turn presumably leads to phosphorylation of Na$^+$/H$^+$ antiporter resulting in the observed intracellular alkalinization[52]. As indicated, the use of lower concentrations of ETs leads to an increase in contractile function and an intracellular alkalinization that could facilitate the development of myocyte hypertrophy.

ADENYLATE AND GUANYLATE CYLASES

As discussed above, a large body of literature describes the involvement of ETs in lipases stimulation. In contrast the mediation of e.g. adenylate cyclase activity by ETs has only recently been described. In several tissues ETs have shown to inhibit cyclic AMP (cAMP) formation, while in a few systems they stimulate it. For example, in brain capillary endothelial cells[42] ETs, via ET$_A$-R, inhibit cAMP formation. In adult rat cardiac myocytes ET-1 reduces cAMP formation in response to isoproteranol and forskolin[53]. The cAMP-lowering effect of ET-1 is sensitive to pertussis toxin and appears to be mediated by Gi. These data indicate that the effects of ET on adult cardiac myocytes involve multiple signaling pathways, including enhanced activity of the inositol phosphate pathway and a decrease in cAMP-mediated responses, neither of which seems likely to account for the positive contractile effects of endothelin[53].

On the other hand, ETs stimulate cAMP generation in several other systems such as cultured rat epididymal cells[54], rat glomerular mesangial cells[40] and cultured embryonic bovine tracheal cells[55]. In all cases, simultaneous action of ETs on PI hydrolysis and cellular cAMP was observed.

It should be noted that the effects of ETs on cAMP metabolism may be difficult to detect in the absence of concurrent stimulation of adenylate cyclase, (e.g. by β-adrenergic agonists). In addition, it should be noted that the accumulation of cAMP might result from the stimulation of adenylate cyclase not directly, but rather indirectly via the activation of PLC[56], or as in rat glomerular mesangial cells in which ET-1 amplified β-adrenergic mediated cAMP accumulation by a PGE_2-dependent mechanism[40].

The question then arises: why, in some preparations does the same signal activate opposing pathways (inhibition and stimulation of cAMP formation)? An elegant solution was recently advanced by Aramori and Nakanishi[57], who examined the intracellular signal transduction of ET_A-R and ET_B-R by transfection and stable expression of individual receptor cDNAs in Chinese hamster ovary cells. While both receptors exhibited a rapid and pronounced stimulation of phosphatidylinositol hydrolysis and arachidonic acid release in response to agonist interaction, they showed different responses in the cAMP transduction cascades. ET_A-R mediated cAMP formation (noted also by Oda et al.[55]), whereas ET_B-R inhibited it. It should however be pointed out that these conclusions are not in agreement with data obtained by Hilal-Danan et al. in rat cardiomyocytes[53], where the majority of the receptors are of the ET_A-R subtype[17], and where ET was found to inhibit cAMP formation. These apparently contradictory findings probably reflect the complexity of the signaling pathway. Other critical factors could be the nature of the G-proteins involved and the ratio of the various ET-R subtypes. Thus the presence of ET_A-R and ET_B-R in the same preparation might lead to cancellation of the effect; however, potentiation cannot be ruled out.

Aramori and Nakanishi[57] found that in each of the two receptor subtypes, the responses of phosphatidylinositol hydrolysis, arachidonic acid release, and cAMP formation were induced in complete agreement with its ET-binding selectivity. ET, added together with GTP, activated adenylate cyclase activity in membrane preparations of cells that express ET_A-R, indicating a direct linkage of ET_A-R to the adenylate cyclase system. Pertussis toxin treatment of cells that express ET_A-R resulted in partial inhibition ET-induced cAMP accumulation, whereas the same treatment of cells that express ET_B-R completely abolished the ET-induced inhibition of cAMP formation.

ET increases cGMP levels in glomeruli by stimulating the formation of a nitricoxide-like factor that activates soluble guanylate cyclase. This effect of ET appears to be mediated by ET_B-R and may serve to modulate the contractile effects of ET[58].

CONCLUSION

From the information reviewed above, it appears that the complexity of ET activity can be explained by the existence of four or five receptor subtypes that are coupled to multiple but distinct signal transduction cascades through different G-proteins, producing a complicated network of second messengers. Further characterization of the mode of interaction of each ET-R subtype is a prerequisite for elucidation of the possible interaction and integration of the various pathways. Pathophysiological consequences might result from the simultaneous actions of ETs leading to activation of two or more signal transduction pathways.

References

1. Sokolovsky, M. (1992) Endothelins and sarafotoxins: physiological regulation, receptor subtypes and transmembrane signaling. *Pharmac. Ther.*, **54**, 129–149.
2. Yanagisawa, M. and Masaki, T. (1989) Molecular biology and biochemistry of the endothelins. *Trends Pharmac. Sci.*, **10**, 374–378.
3. Simonson, M. S., Wang, Y. and Dunn, M. J. (1992) Cellular signaling by endothelin peptides: pathways to the nucleus. *J. Amer. Soc. Nephrol.*, **2**, S116–S125.
4. Sokolovsky, M., Ambar, I. and Galron, R. (1992) A novel subtype of endothelin receptors. *J. Biol. Chem.*, **267**, 20551–20554.
5. Kloog, Y., Bousso-Mittler, D., Bdolah, A. and Sokolovsky, M. (1989) Three apparent receptor subtypes for the endothelin/sarafotoxin family. *FEBS Lett.*, **253**, 199–202.
6. Gilman, A. (1987) G-proteins: transducers of receptor-generated signals. *Annu. Rev. Biochem.*, **56**, 615–649.
7. Wang, Y., Simonson, M. S., Pouyssegur, J. and Dunn, M. J. (1992) Endothelin rapidly stimulates mitogen-activated protein kinase activity in rat mesangial cells. *Biochem. J.*, **287**, 589–594.
8. Pribnow, D., Muldoon, L. L., Fajardo, M., Theodorf, L., Chen, L-Y. S. and Magun, B. E. (1992) Endothelin induces transcription of fos/jun family genes: a prominent role for calcium ion. *Mol. Endocrinol.*, **6**, 1003–1012.
9. Downes, C. P. (1989) G protein-dependent regulation of phospholipase C. *Trends Pharmac. Sci.*, **10**, 39–42.
10. Ross, E. M. (1989) Signal sorting and amplification through G protein-coupled receptors. *Neuron*, **3**, 141–152.
11. Arai, H., Hori, S., Aramori, I., Ohkuno, H. and Nakanishi, S. (1990) Cloning and expression of a cDNA encoding an endothelin receptor. *Nature*, **348**, 730–732.
12. Sakurai, T., Yanagisawa, M., Takuwa, Y., Miyazaki, H., Kimura, S., Goto, K. and Masaki, T. (1990) Cloning of a cDNA encoding non-isopeptide-selective subtype of the endothelin receptor. *Nature*, **348**, 732–735.
13. Lin, H. Y., Kaji, E. H., Winkel, G. K., Ives, H. E. and Lodish, H. E. (1991) Cloning and functional expression of a vascular smooth muscle endothelin 1 receptor. *Proc. Natl. Acad. Sci. USA*, **88**, 3185–3189.
14. Sokolovsky, M. (1993) Endothelin receptors in rat cerebellum: activation of phosphoinositide hydrolysis is transduced by multiple G-protein. *Cell. Signal.*, **5**, 473–483.
15. Sokolovsky, M. (1993) Functional coupling between endothelin receptors and multiple G-proteins in rat heart myocytes. Receptors and Channels, **1**, 295–304.
16. Nishizuka, Y. (1988) The molecular heterogeneity of protein kinase C and its implications for cellular regulation. *Nature*, **334**, 661–665.
17. Galron, R., Kloog, Y., Bdolah, A. and Sokolovsky, M. (1989) Functional endothelin-sarafotoxin receptors in rat heart myocytes: structure-activity relationships and receptor subtypes. *Biochem. Biophys. Res. Commun.*, **163**, 936–943.
18. Ambar, I. and Sokolovsky, M. (1993) Endothelin receptors stimulate both phospholipase C and phospholipase D activities in different cell lines. *Eur J. Pharmacol.-Mol. Pharmacol. section*, **245**, 31–41.
19. Stojilkovic, S. S., Merelli, F., Iida, T., Krsmanovic, L. Z. and Catt, K. J. (1990) Endothelin stimulation of cytosolic calcium and gonadotropin secretion in anterior pituitary cells. *Science*, **248**, 1663–1666.

20. Lewy, H., Galron, R., Bdolah, A., Sokolovsky, M. and Naor, Z. (1992) Paradoxical signal transduction mechanism of endothelins and sarafotoxins in cultured pituitary cells: stimulation of phosphoinositide turnover and inhibition of prolactin release. *Mol. Cell. Endocrinol.*, **89**, 1–9.
21. Yoshizawa, T., Shimmi, O., Glaid, A., Yanagisawa, M., Gibson, S. J., Kimuna, S., Uchiyama, Y., Polak, J. M., Masaki, T. and Konazawa, I. (1990) Endothelin: a novel peptide in the posterior pituitary system. *Science*, **247**, 462–464.
22. Iijima, K., Lin, L., Nasjletti, A. and Goligorsky, M. S. (1991) Intracellular ramification of endothelin signal. *Amer. J. Physiol.*, **260**, C982–C992.
23. Miasiro, N., Yamamoto, H., Kanaide, H. and Nakamura, M. (1988) Does endothelin mobilize calcium from intercellular store sites in rat aortic vascular smooth muscle cells in primary culture? *Biochem. Biophys. Res. Commun.*, **156**, 312–317.
24. Marsden, P. A., Danthuluri, R., Brenner, B., Ballerman, N. J. and Brock, T. A. (1989) Endothelin action on vascular smooth muscle involves inosito ltrisphosphate and calcium mobilization. *Biochem. Biophys. Res. Commun.*, **158**, 86–93.
25. Nishimura, T., Akasu, T. and Kraier, J. (1991) Endothelin modulates calcium channel current in neurons of rabbit pelvic parasu, pathetic ganglia. *Br. J. Pharmacol.*, **103**, 1242–1250.
26. Resink, T. J., Scott-Burden, T. and Buhler, F. R. (1989) Activation of phospholipase A2 by endothelin in cultured vascular smooth muscle cells. *Biochem. Biophys. Res. Commun.*, **158**, 279–286.
27. Reynolds, E. E. and Mok, L. L. S. (1990) Role of thromboxane A_2/Prostaglandin H_2 receptor in the vasoconstrictor response of rat aorta to endothelin. *J. Pharmac. Exp. Ther.*, **252**, 915–921.
28. Burgoyne, R. D. and Morgan, A. (1990) The control of free arachidonic acid levels. *Trends Biochem. Sci.*, **15**, 365–366.
29. Dennis, E. A., Rhee, S. G., Billah, M. M. and Hannun, Y. A. (1991) Role of phospholipases in generating lipid second messengers in signal transduction. *FASEB J.*, **5**, 2068–2077.
30. MacNulty, E. E., Plevin, R. and Wakelam, M. J. D. (1990) Stimulation of hydrolysis of phosphatidylinositol 4,5-biphosphate and phosphatidylcholine by endothelin, a complete mitogen for Rat-1 fibroblasts. *Biochem. J.*, **272**, 761–766.
31. Marsault, R., Vigne, P., Breittmayer, J. P. and Frelin, C. (1990) Astrocytes are target cells for endothelins and sarafotoxin. *J. Neurochem.*, **54**, 2142–2144.
32. Marin, P., Delumeau, J. C., Durieu-Trautmann, O., Le Nguyen, D., Premont, J., Strosberg, A. D. and Couraud, P. O. (1991) Are several G-proteins involved in the different effects of endothelin-1 in mouse striatal astrocytes? *J. Neurochem.*, **56**, 1270–1275.
33. Griendling, K. K., Tsuda, T. and Alexander, R. W. (1989) Endothelin stimulates diacylglycerol accumulation and activates protein kinase C in cultured vascular smooth muscle cells. *J. Biol. Chem.*, **264**, 8237–8240.
34. Sunako, M., Kawahara, Y., Hirata, K., Tsudo, T., Yokoyama, M., Fukuzaki, H. and Takai, Y. (1990) Mass analysis of 1,2-diacyglycerol in cultured rabbit vascular smooth muscle cells. *Hypertension*, **15**, 84–88.
35. Muldoon, L., Pribnow, D., Rodland, K. D. and Magnum, B. E. (1990) Endothelin-1 stimulates DNA synthesis and anchorage-independent growth of Rat-1m fibroblasts through a protein kinase C-dependent mechanism. *Cell Regul.*, **1**, 379–390.
36. Shukla, S. D. and Halenda, S. P. (1991) Phospholipase D in cell signaling and its relationship to phospholipase C. *Life Sci.*, **48**, 851–866.
37. Zhang, Y. and Abdel-Latif, A. A. (1992) Activation of phospholipase D by endothelin-1 and other pharmacological agents in rabbit iris sphincter smooth muscle. *Cell. Signal.*, **4**, 777–786.
38. Loffelholz, J. (1989) Receptor regulation of choline phospholipid hydrolysis. A novel source of diacylglycerol and phosphatidic acid. *Biochem. Pharmacol.*, **38**, 1543–1549.
39. Exton, J. H. (1990) Signaling through phosphatidylcholine breakdown. *J. Biol. Chem.*, **165**, 1–2.
40. Simonson, M. S. and Dunn, M. J. (1990) Endothelin-1 stimulates contraction of rat glomerular cells and potentitates β-adrenergic-mediated cyclic adenosine monophosphate accumulation. *J. Clin. Invest.*, **85**, 790–797.
41. Lin, W. W., Kiang, J. G. and Chuang, D. (1992) Pharmacological characterization of endothelin-stimulated phosphoinositide breakdown and cytosolic Ca^{2+} rise in rat C6 glioma cells. *J. Neurosci.*, **12**, 1077–1085.
42. Ladoux, A. and Frelin, C. (1991) Endothelins inhibit adenylate cyclase in brain capillary endothelial cells. *Biochem. Biophys. Res. Commun.*, **180**, 169–173.
43. Murayama, T. and Ui, M. (1987) Phosphatidic acid may stimulate membrane receptors mediating adenylate cyclase inhibition and phospholipid breakdown in 3T3 fibroblasts. *J. Biol. Chem.*, **262**, 5522–5529.
44. Chalifour, B. J. and Kanfer, J. N. (1980) Microsomal phospholipase D of rat brain and lung tissues. *Biochem. Biophys. Res. Commun.*, **96**, 742–747.

45. Hattori, H. and Kanfer, J. N. (1985) Synaptosomal phospholipase D potential role in providing choline for acetylcholine synthesis. *J. Neurochem.*, **45**, 1578–1583.
46. Alling, C., Gustavsson, L. and Anggard, E. (1983) An abnormal phospholipid in rat organs after ethanol treatment. *FEBS Lett.*, **152**, 24–28.
47. Asaoka, Y., Kikkawa, U., Sekiguchi, K., Shearman, M. S., Kosaka, Y., Nakano, Y., Satoh, T. and Nishizuka, Y. (1988) *FEBS Lett.*, **231**, 221–224.
48. Moolenaar, W. H. (1986) Effects of growth factors on intracellular pH regulation. *Annu. Rev. Physiol.*, **48**, 363–376.
49. Simonson, M. S., Wann, S., Mene, P., Dubyak, G. R., Kester, M., Nakazato, Y., Sedor, J. R. and Dunn, M. J. (1989) *J. Clin. Invest.*, **83**, 708–712.
50. Meyer-Lehnert, H., Wanning, C., Predel, H-G., Backer, A., Stelkens, H. and Kramer, H. J. (1989) Effects of endothelin on sodium transport mechanisms: potential role in cellular Ca^{2+} mobilization. *Biochem. Biophys. Res. Commun.*, **163**, 458–465.
51. Vigne, P., Ladoux, A. and Frelin, C. (1991) Endothelins activate Na^+/H^+ exchange in brain capillary endothelial cells via a high affinity endothelin-3 receptor that is not coupled to phospholipase C. *J. Biol. Chem.*, **266**, 5925–5928.
52. Kramer, B. K., Smith, T. W. and Kelly, R. A. (1990) Endothelin and increased contractility in adult rat ventricular myocytes: role of intracellular alkalosis induced by activation of the protein kinase C-dependent Na^+-H^+ exchanger. *Circul. Res.*, **68**, 269–279.
53. Hilal-Dandan, R., Urasawa, K. and Brunton, L. L. (1992) Endothelin inhibits adenylate cyclase and stimulates phosphoinositide hydrolysis in adult cardiac myocytes. *J. Biol. Chem.*, **267**, 10620–10624.
54. Wong, P. Y. D. and Huang, S. J. (1990) Secretory agonists stimulate a rise in intracellular cyclic AMP but not Ca^{2+} and inositol phosphates in cultured rat epididymal epithelium. *Exp. Physiol.*, **75**, 321–337.
55. Oda, K., Fujitani, Y., Watakabe, T., Inui, T., Okada, T. Urade, Y., Okuda-Ashitaka, E. and Ito, S. (1992) Endothelin stimulates both cAMP formation and phosphatidylinositol hydrolysis in cultured embryonic bovine tracheal cells. *FEBS Lett.*, **299**, 187–191.
56. Felder, C. C., Kanterman, R. Y., Ma, A. L. and Axelrod, J. (1989) A transfected m1 muscarinic acetylcholine receptor stimulates adenylate cyclase via phosphatidylinositol hydrolysis. *J. Biol. Chem.*, **264**, 20356–20362.
57. Aramori, I. and Nakanishi, S. (1992) Coupling of two endothelin receptor subtype to differing signal transduction in transfected chinese hamster ovary cells. *J. Biol. Chem.*, **267**, 12468–12474.
58. Edwards, R. M., Pullen, M. and Nambi, P. (1992) Activation of endothelin ETB receptors increases a glomerular cGMP via on L-arginine-dependent pathway. *Am. J. Physiol.*, **263**, F1020–F1025.

4 Structure–Activity Relationship of Endothelin

Om Prakash[1] and Anil Gulati[2]

[1]*Department of Biochemistry, Kansas State University, Manhattan, Kansas 66506, USA*
[2]*Department of Pharmaceutics and Pharmacodynamics (m/c 865), The University of Illinois at Chicago, 833 South Wood Street, Chicago, IL 60612, USA*

INTRODUCTION

Endothelin (ET), a polypeptide composed of 21 amino acid, is one of the most potent constrictor of the vascular smooth muscle. The amino acid residues of ET are sequenced in a unique bicyclic motif formed by two disulfide bridges between Cys^1, Cys^{15} and Cys^3, Cys^{11}, respectively. It is known that ET has a potent vasoconstrictor effect. It is also recognized that such vasoconstriction is caused by binding of ET to its receptors on the vascular smooth muscles[1–3]. Patients with hypertension, coronary vasospasm or acute myocardial infarction have increased levels of ET in their blood stream[4,5] and in the washing fluids of respiratory tract of patients of bronchial asthma[6]. ET has been found to produce cerebral vasospasm in several species when administered directly in the central nervous system or on the cerebral blood vessels[7,8]. An improved renal function by the ET antibody in an animal model of acute renal failure has also been observed[9]. ET is assumed to be one of the mediators causing acute renal failure or cerebral vasospasm following subarachnoid hemorrhage. Tracheal epithelial cells or kidney cells have also been found to secrete ET[10,11]. ET also causes contraction of the gastrointestinal tract and the uterine smooth muscles[12–14]. ET has been found to control the release of physiologically active substances like renin, endothelium-derived relaxing factor (EDRF), thromboxane A2, prostacyclin, noradrenaline, angiotensin II and substance P[15–18].

ET receptors are present in a high concentration not only in the peripheral tissues but also in the central nervous system. Central administration of ET produces cardiovascular and behavioral changes in animals[19]. ET is likely to play an important role for controlling nervous functions[20]. ET has been characterized as one of the important mediators for endotoxin induced disease conditions[21,22]. In a recent study, ET has been found to be involved in the control of blood flow and vascular tone in human skin, and also in the abnormal vasoconstrictor response in primary Raynaud's phenomenon and systemic sclerosis. Specific ET-1 and ET-3 binding sites have been localized to microvessels of the sub-epidermal plexus and dermal papillae, larger blood vessels, sweat glands, epidermis, and hair follicles[23]. An increased ET secretion is observed when cyclosporine is added to the renal cell culture (LLC-PKI cells)[24]. ET appears to have a pivotal role in pathophysiology and cyclosporine-induced acute renal vasoconstrictor and glomerular dysfunction. The cyclosporine induced renal failure can be suppressed by the administration of ET antibody[25]. Thus ET, directly or indirectly induces sustained contraction of vascular or non vascular smooth muscles as an endogenous substance. Increased production or secretion of ET is believed to be one of the mechanisms contributing to hypertension, bronchial asthma, acute renal failure, myocardial infarction, angina pectoris, cerebral vasospasm and cerebral infarction. It also serves as an important mediator in conditions such as endotoxin shock, endotoxin-induced multiple organ failure and cyclosporine-induced renal failure or hypertension.

ET was originally discovered and isolated from the supernatant of cultured bovine aortic endothelial cells[1,26]. The primary sequence of human ET has been deduced from a human placental cDNA library and found to be identical to that of porcine ET, which is now known as ET-1[2], Two other 21-amino acids containing peptides have been reported and designated as ET-2 and ET-3. These related peptides are differing by 2 and 6 amino acid residues respectively from ET-1[27,28]. ET-1, 2, and 3 are distinct gene products[29]. Sarafotoxins, isolated from snake venom are a group of cardiotoxic homologous peptides showing strong resemblance to ETs, suggesting an ancient and common evolutionary origin[30-34]. A feature similar to ET is also shared by another peptide whose gene has been identified in the mouse genome and expressed in the intestine, subsequently referred to as "vasoactive intestinal contractor" (VIC)[35]. These peptides, containing 21 amino-acid residues, show high sequence homology. Furthermore, disulfide bonds are formed similar to ET-1 at Cys^1-Cys^{15} and Cys^3- Cys^{11}. These resemblances indicate that endogenous ETs should play an important role in many functions of the mammalian body.

ET is the expression product of prepro ET gene. The prepro ET gene produces prepro ET mRNA which in turn produces an approximately 200 residue precursor peptide prepro ET. The prepro ET is proteolytically cleaved to form pro ET also known as big ET[1,2,36]. A protease enzyme called "ET converting enzyme" (ECE) cleaves Trp^{21}-Val^{22} of big ET to form the mature ET peptide. Synthetic big ET-1(1-39) and big ET-1(1-25) induced a slow, long lasting and potent vasoconstriction like ET-1(1-21). However, the contractile molar potencies of big ET-1(1-39) and big ET-1(1-25) were found to be 140 and 50 fold lower than that of ET-1(1-21), respectively. The conversion of big ET-1 to mature ET-1 is essential for the expression of full biological activity[37]. Phosphoramidon (N-α-L-rhamnopyranosyloxyhyroxyphosphinyl)-L-leucyl-L-tryptophan) effectively antagonized the effects of big ET-1[38-41] suggesting that a phosphoramidon-sensitive metalloproteinase contributes to the conversion of big ET-1 to ET-1. This protease is different from enkephalinase since thiorphan which inhibits enkephalinase activity does not affect the conversion of big ET-1 to ET-1[42]. Analogues of phosphoramidon lacking the rhamnose group were found to be potent inhibitors of metallopeptidases similar to phosphoramidon, indicating that the carbohydrate group is not important for recognition and binding to the enzyme[43,44]. Similarly, like phosphoramidon an analog of phosphoramidon lacking the rhamnose group (phosphoryl-leu-trp-OH) significantly attenuated the pressor effect of big ET-1[45]. These studies clearly indicate that the rhamnose moiety of phosphoramidon is not responsible for distinguishing this compound as an inhibitor of ECE.

STRUCTURAL AND CONFORMATIONAL STUDIES

The nuclear magnetic resonance spectroscopy (NMR), molecular dynamics simulation, and circular dichroism (CD) studies have been carried out to determine the three dimensional structure of ET[46–51]. NMR studies of ET-1 have been carried out in dimethyl sulfoxide[52,53], aqueous acetic acid, acetonitrile as well as in aqueous ethylene glycol[54–57]. Recently, preliminary X-ray crystallography data of human ET has also been reported[58]. The NMR studies in DMSO-d6 have suggested a well defined conformation in the N-terminal core region (residues 1-15). The three dimensional structural studies of ET-1 in an aqueous solution by combination of two-dimensional NMR and distance geometry calculations have indicated an alpha helix comprising residue Lys^9 to Cys^{15}. A series of NOE connectivities have been observed between NH(i) and NH(i + 1), d_{NN}, for the residue Lys^9 to Cys^{15}. These observations suggest the existence of a helical conformation in this region. This fact has been further confirmed by the proximities between αH(i) and βH(i + 3), as well as between αH(i) and NH(i + 3), dαN(i, i + 3) based on nuclear Overhauser enhancement studies. Other characteristic NOEs i.e. dβN(i, i + 2) between Ser^5 and Met^7, and dβN(i, i + 3) between Ser^5 and Asp^8 along with the coupling constant $^3J_{HN\alpha}$ of Leu^6 and Met^7, the values of which are 5 and 8 Hz respectively, also suggest a type-I β-turn configuration in this segment of the polypeptide. In the remaining parts of the polypeptide, particularly C-terminal region beyond His^{16}, which showed a series of strong NOEs of dαN, peptide bonds exist in an extended or random structure. These secondary structural features, the alpha helical conformation in the sequence in Cys-X-X-X-Cys, and the extended structure in Cys-X-Cys are homologous to those found commonly in several neurotoxic peptides[59]. For biological evaluation such a homologous profile should be of great interest. Conformational analysis of this group of peptides is quite interesting to determine specific conformational features that may be important to receptor binding and vasoconstrictor activity. CD studies showed a negative band at 223 nm and a positive band around 192 nm. These CD results supports the helical structure as determined by NMR and indicate that ET-1 is about 30–35% helical, and although there are some variations, the helical region is generally considered to exist between residue Lys^9 and Cys^{15}. The fully linear peptide [Ala^{1,3,11,15}]ET-1 shows no helical character and thus disulfide arrangement seems to induced this helicity. There have been conflicting reports regarding the conformation of the biologically important C-terminal hexapeptides. In some reports this hexapeptide of ET-1 has been suggested to be folded back towards the main bicyclic region of the molecules. Other studies suggest a random conformation for C-terminus portion of ET-1. However most studies are unable to define this apparently flexible region[57,60].

Molecular dynamics calculations have been carried out to study the conformational preferences for ET. These studies suggest suitable places for the introduction of conformational constraints, such as cyclization or turns, in the search for receptor antagonists. The entire conformational space accessible to the ET has been searched by (I) Monte Carlo search in torsion angle space followed by energy minimization (II) annealing of snapshots from high temperature molecular dynamics by gradually cooling to 300 K followed by energy minimization and (III) systematic forcing of selected pairs of correlated interatomic distances followed by molecular dynamics and energy minimization annealing. Such studies reveal that there are four possible conformational families and one of these conformational families consisting of the lowest energy conformer indicates a helical conformation in the region consisting residue 9 through 13[61,62]. Furthermore, molecular dynamic studies also suggest aromatic ring of Trp^{21} residue is located close to His^{16}, Asp^{18} pair such that it may be stabilizing the donation transfer of a proton between these residues. Thus, these three residues may also play an important function in the biological response of ET. It has also been suggested that hydrogen bond formation may occur between the His^{16} and Asp^{18} residues[63,64].

STRUCTURE-ACTIVITY RELATIONSHIP

ETs and sarafotoxins consist of more than eight compounds forming a super family (Figure 4.1) with four isopeptides in each of the two family. Differences in biological responses of these two families have been ascribed to heterogeneity of amino acids residue at position 4–7 in the N-terminal region of the peptides[65,66]. However among ETs there is a very high degree of sequence similarity particularly the four cysteine residues Cys^1, Cys^3, Cys^{11}, Cys^{15}, the C-terminal residues His^{16}-Leu^{17}-Asp^{18}-Ile^{19}-Ile^{20}-Trp^{21}, aromatic residues at 13 and 14 and the charged loop region Asp^8-Lys^9-Glu^{10} are conserved. The structure activity relationship studies with the C-terminal hexapeptide of ETs have shown that this peptide is capable of discriminating between different ET receptors[67,68]. Structure-activity studies of the C-terminal hexapeptide of ET have also been carried out to elucidate the amino acids that are important for receptor binding and agonist or antagonist activity. A mono D-amino acid scan of the ET(16-21) has revealed that substitution at His^{16} gives rise to analogues with significant binding affinity[69]. In the intact molecule, the indole group of Trp^{21} has been found to be important for both binding and vasoconstrictor activities of ET[70]. L-stereochemistry of this residue also seems to be important[71]. Replacement of L-Trp^{21} by D-Trp^{21} markedly reduces binding and contractile activity[72]. Removal of Trp^{21} residue decreases the vasconstrictor potency in porcine coronary artery strips by 3 orders of magnitude. The replacement of this residue by other aromatic amino acids such as Phe or Tyr is poorly tolerated[73]. It has been found that sequential removal of C-terminal residues in ET decreases receptor binding and vasoconstrictor activity. The ET(1-15) has been found totally inactive[74]. In another study, C-terminal elongated peptides have been found to be weaker agonists during receptor binding in cultured rat smooth muscle cells[75]. Recently, a series of ET analogues has been synthesized in which each non-cysteinyl residue is substituted individually with Ala residue. These analogues have been studied to understand the importance of each side chain functionality for receptor binding without affecting the overall backbone

Structure activity relationship   39

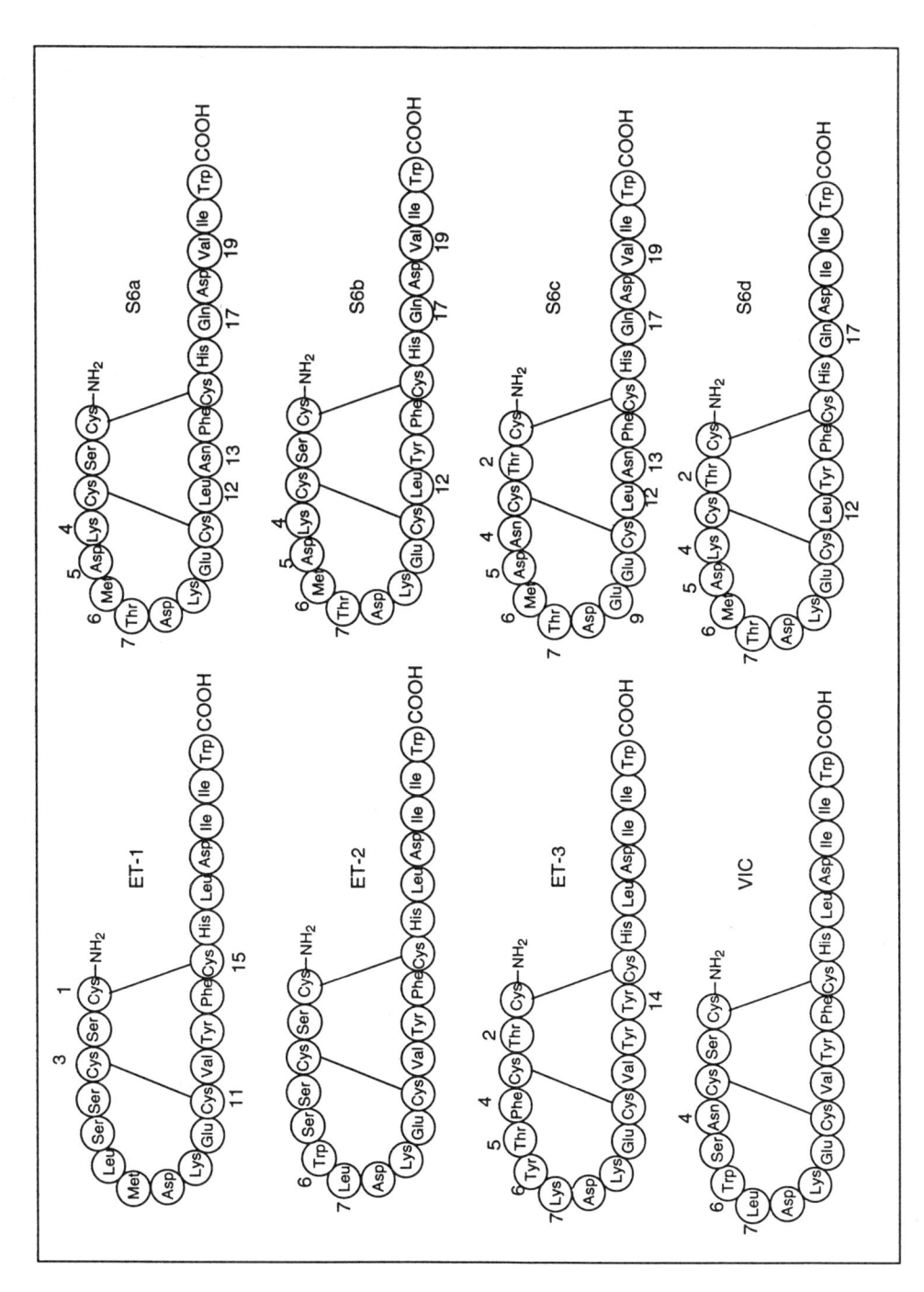

Figure 4.1. Structures of endothelins and sarafotoxins.

conformation. The isomers with disulfide pairing of natural ET are always more potent than the corresponding inverted one with the only exception of Asp[8] substitution, in which both the isomers display practically the same marginal activity on the smooth muscle contraction[76]. These studies suggest that the nature of protecting groups on the cysteins rather than the reduction of the disulfide bonds, is responsible for the marked decrease in biological activity and that the disulfide bonds themselves are not the absolute requirement for receptor recognition. Among the ET peptides, ET-3 is not only the weakest vasoconstrictor but it also acts as a vasodilator in some vascular beds. In ET-3 the Lys at position 9 is retained, indicating that other factors may account for the reduced vasoconstrictor activity of this compound. One of the important differences of this polypeptide from other ET is the replacement of Ser[2] with Thr[2] similar to two weak constrictor peptides in sarafotoxin family, S6c and S6d, suggesting its importance[77]. [Thr^2]ET-1 has been shown to be a potent agonist with only slightly reduced potency and binding affinity[76]. Another suggestion that the net charge within the interior loop (Cys[3]-Cys[11]) can play an important role for biological activity has been ruled out by extremely low biological activity of S6f[49].

STRUCTURE-ACTIVITY RELATIONSHIP OF MONOCYCLIC ANALOGUES

Removal of one or the other of the disulfide bridges of ET-1 reduces the potency of the peptide. The monocyclic ET-1 retaining 1-15 disulfide bridge has been found to maintain 10% of activity. The analogue retaining only 3-11 disulfide bridge has been found to be about 200-fold less active than the bicyclic ET-1[78]. The initial structure-activity relationship studies of ET have been reported on monocyclic analogues with the 1-15 disulfide bridge due to simplicity of their synthesis and maintaining of respectable activity. In order to determine the role of each residue of ET in receptor binding and receptor activation, a number of monocyclic analogues has been synthesized. A series of monocyclic analogues, ET-1(Ala^{3,11}, Nle^7) with each amino acid in turn substituted with alanine has been studied. Receptor binding (A10 vascular smooth muscle cell membranes, ET$_A$) and vasoconstrictor activity (rabbit, carotid rings) assay of these polypeptides have indicated that Glu^{10}, Phe^{14}, Leu^{17}, and Asp^{18} may be important for agonist activity, while Asp^8, Tyr^{13}, Ile^{20} and Trp^{21} are important for binding[79]. The residues Ser^2, Val^{12}, His^{16} and Ile^{19} were less important for binding and have been therefore identified as tolerant sites. An earlier study has suggested that the vasoconstrictor activity of ET-1 is unaffected by a Leu replacement at position 9 identifying Lys^9 as a tolerant site also. It is possible that these tolerant sites may influence subtype selectivity. Recent identification of sarafotoxin-b and sarafotoxin-c as selective ET$_B$ agonist suggests that site 9 is a determinant for this subtype[80]. Therefore, while ET$_A$ appears to tolerate replacement of Lys^9 with Ala or Leu, this position is not tolerant of a Glu substitution. The role of individual amino acids in ET binding and function at ET$_A$ receptor is being clarified while studies using the ET$_B$ receptor agonists or antagonists are in their initial stages. Therefore, much work remains before any selective peptidic ET receptor antagonist can be discovered for specific ET receptor subtype. In order to investigate the effect of ET-1 analogues on the pulmonary vasodilator, intralobar injection of ET(16-21) and (Ala[1,3,11,15]) ET-1 to the intact cat did not alter arterial blood pressure while ET-1 itself and ET(1-15) caused a decrease in lobar arterial blood pressure[81]. Thus, it is clear that intact amino terminus and intra chain disulfide bridges are necessary for pulmonary vasodilation.

ET RECEPTORS

Two types of ET receptors classified as ET_A and ET_B have been cloned. One of the receptors was found to be specific for ET-1. It causes vasoconstriction when bound to ET in vascular smooth muscle[3,82-85]. Both have characteristics of G-protein coupled receptors revealed by their amino acids sequence consisting of seven transmembrane domains. Their structure has been studied by cloning of cDNA and their expression in mammalian cell lines. Particularly cDNAs from bovine lung and from smooth muscle cell line have been found to be highly specific for ET-1 (ET-1 = ET-2 > ET-3). It has been defined as ET_A receptor. ET_B receptor is nonselective for ET-1 (ET-1 = ET-2 = ET-3) and binds with equal affinity to all the three ETs[86-90]. ET_B receptor has been reported to be commonly found in the lung parenchyma and in many other tissues including brain, kidney and liver[91]. It has also been found in human and porcine endothelial cells and evoked the production of EDRF[80,92,93]. The ET_B receptor is responsible for vasodilator effects due to the release of endothelium derived relaxing factor/nitric oxide. The ET_B receptor also mediates vasoconstriction of various vessels such as the rabbit and dog saphenous vein, rat and dog coronary resistance bed and renal vasculature of rat. The nonselectivity of ET_B receptor has been attributed to the fact that it mainly recognizes the identical C-terminal region of ETs[94]. Many studies in a variety of animal tissues are being carried out to determine the existence and distribution of ET receptor subtypes. There is now evidence for the involvement of more than two receptors in mediating ET responses obtained through the use of the available selective and nonselective receptor antagonists. It appears that the recognized ET_A and ET_B receptor classification will certainly change in future. Even though 80% of the ET binding in dog kidney is to ET_A receptor, ET_B receptor also mediates the vasoconstriction. Therefore, the ratio of ET_A/ET_B receptors varies between tissues and species-related differences are observed. There are reports for an ET-3 specific receptor subtype which is found in brain and in endothelial cells although this receptor subtype has not been cloned[95-97]. Furthermore these receptors are regulated by a number of vasoactive substances such as angiotensin II, Arg-vasopressin and TPA besides ET-1 itself[3,98]. Recently, two types of ET_A receptors (ET_{A1} which are BQ-123 sensitive and ET_{A2} which are BQ-123 insensitive) have been described based on the sensitivity of ET_A receptors to BQ-123[99-101] and two types of ET_B receptors (ET_{B1} sensitive to IRL 1038 and RES 701-1 and ET_{B2} insensitive to IRL 1038 and RES 701-1) have been described based on the sensitivity of ET_B receptors to conventional ET_B antagonists[100,102,103].

ET RECEPTOR AGONISTS AND ANTAGONISTS

A number of selective ET receptor antagonists have been developed and these compounds have been studied to understand the nature of ET_A and ET_B receptors that mediate various effects of ETs (Table 4.1). The reports of a variety of receptor antagonists have appeared over the last few years. ET-1[Dpr^1-Asp^{15}] has been reported as specific ET antagonist[104] (Figures 4.2 and 4.3). This compound may be a nonselective ET_A/ET_B receptor antagonist, but binding results have not been reported in a known ET_B tissue preparation. A detailed study on competitive inhibition of [^{125}I]ET-1 binding to membranes from rat aorta, rat atria, rat cerebellum and rat hippocampus respectively, has indicated that sarafotoxin S6c is a highly selective agonist for ET_B receptors.

Furthermore, S6c is also a potent pressor agent in the pithed rat, indicating that the ET_B receptor subtype is also important in cardiovascular functions[105]. Like sarafotoxin S6c, ($Ala^{1,3,11,15}$) ET-1 has also been found to have greater ET_B receptor selectivity. This compound is five times more potent in binding to rabbit pulmonary artery compared with rat aorta and left atria[90]. Saeki et al.[106] have observed that

Table 4.1 Peptide agonists and antagonists of selective/nonselective endothelin receptors

Name	Formula	Reference
ET-A Selective Antagonists:		
BQ-123	Cyclo(-D-Trp-D-Asp-L-Pro-D-val-L-Leu-)	Ihara et al., 1992; Hiley et al., 1992
FR-139317 (Tripeptides)	Perhydrazepin-1-ylcarbonyl-L-leucyl-(1-methyl)-D-tryptophyl-[3-(2-pyridyl)]-D-alanine	Hemmi et al., 1991; European Patent 91107554.7
BE-18257B	Cyclo(-D-Glu-L-Ala-allo-D-Ile-L-Leu-D-Trp-)	Ihara et al., 1991
BMS	($Pen^{3,15}$, Nle^7, N^α-Me-Ile^{20})-ET-1(1-21)	Hunt et al., 1993
ET-B-Selective Antagonist:		
IRL-1038	($Cys^{11,15}$)-ET-1(11-21)	Urade et al., 1992
ET-A/ET-B Nonselective Antagonists:		
PD-142893	Ac-(3,3-diphenyl-D-alanine)-leu-Asp-Ile-Ilu-Trp	Doherty et al., 1993
(Dpr^1, Asp^{15})ET-1	(Dpr^1, Asp^{15})-ET-1(1-21)	Spinella et al., 1991
PD-145065	AC-[2-(R)-(10,11)-dihydro-5H-dibenzo[a,d]cycloheptan-5yl]Gyl-L-Leu-L-Asp-L-Ile-L-Trp	McMurdo et al., 1993
Cyclic depsipeptide	N-(pyrrol-2-carboxy)-Phe-[D-allo-Thr-D-Phe-D-Als-D-dihydroxyphenyl glycine-D(L)-dihydroxyphenylglycine]	Lam et al., 1992; European Patent No 92200111.0
TM-ET	(Thr18, gamma-Me-Leu19)-ET-1(1-21)	Kikuchi et al., 1993
ET-B Agonists:		
IRL-1620	Suc-(Glu^9, $Ala^{11,15}$)-ET-1(8-21)	Takai et al., 1992
4 Ala-ET-1	($Ala^{1,3,11,15}$)-ET-1(1-21)	Panek et al., 1992
Sarafotoxin 6c	(Thr^2, Asn^4, Asp^5, Met^6, Thr^7, Leu^{12}, Asn^{13}, Gln^{17}, Val^{19})-ET-1(1-21)	Williams et al., 1991
BQ-3020	N-Acetyl-NH_2($Ala^{11,15}$)-Et-1(6-21)	Molenaar et al., 1992

Structure activity relationship 43

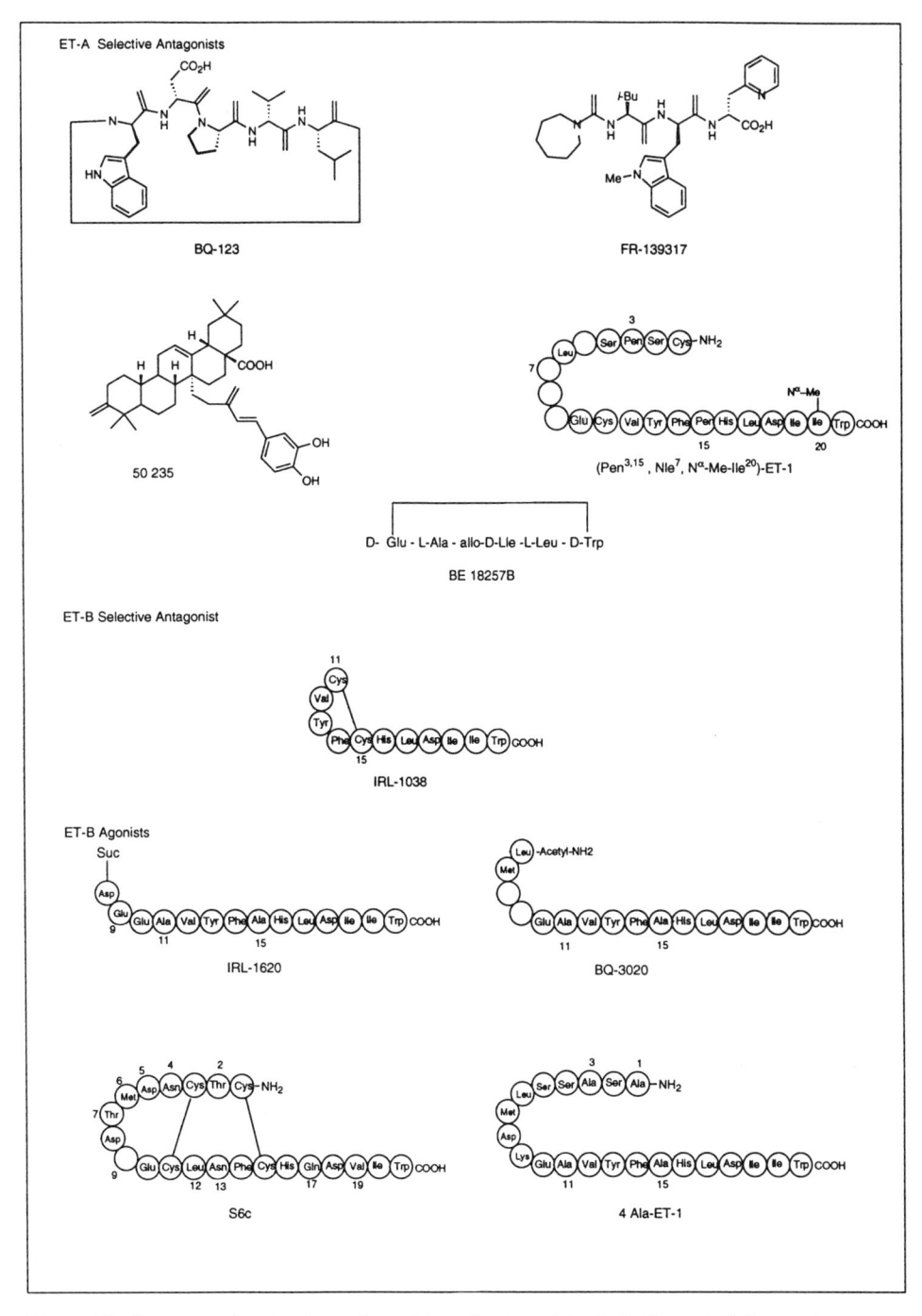

Figure 4.2. Representative structures of agonists and antagonists of selective endothein receptor.

(Ala[1,3,11,15]) ET-1 is a potent agonist in producing endothelium dependent relaxation of norepinephrine precontracted porcine pulmonary artery rings. The binding affinity studies of Suc-(Glu[9], Ala[11,15])ET-1 (IRL-1620) for ET_A and ET_B receptor in porcine lung membranes have suggested that it is a potent and specific ligand for ET_B receptor. IRL-1620 induces contractions of the guinea pig trachea with a comparable potency to those of ET-1 or ET-3 indicating that it is a potent ET_B receptor agonist[107].

A novel cyclic pentapeptide (BE-18257B), a competitive ET_A receptor antagonist, isolated from fermentation products from Streptomyces misakiensis was reported a few years ago[108,109]. Detailed structure-activity relationship studies on this peptide (BE-18257B) resulted into a highly ET_A selective antagonist known as BQ-123[110]. BQ-123 was found to possess high binding affinity to cardiac tissue (ET_A) (with a 1000 fold selectivity) over binding to rat cerebellum (ET_B)[111-113]. The detailed NMR and molecular modelling studies[114-117] on BQ-123 have suggested that the solution conformation of this molecule consists of a type-II β-turn and a γ-turn. Based on molecular modelling studies Satoh and Barlow[118] have suggested that its conformation is similar to that reported for residues Leu[6]-Met[7]-Asp[8] of ET-1. It has been proposed that ET_A receptor recognition requires two hydrogen bond donor sites, two non specific hydrophobic-binding sites and a third site bearing a positive charge. Interestingly, a recent study on BE18257B using NMR spectroscopy and simulated annealing calculations based on NOE constraints have shown similar backbone conformation of this cyclic peptide[119]. Comparisons of structure activity data suggest that these peptides may mimic structural features of the C-terminal tail of the ETs. A number of non-peptide ET_A/ET_B – nonselective antagonists have been reported in a recent patent[120]. These molecules have been discovered through random screening of natural product libraries. A potent compound of this series, isolated from a streptomyces strain and known as FR901367, possesses a binding affinity in porcine aorta of 670 nM and inhibits the contractions induced by ET-1 in rabbit thoracic aorta at high concentrations. Recently, a cyclic depsipeptide series of nonselective ET-receptor antagonists isolated from a Microbispora sp. culture have also been reported[121]. In another study, the replacement of Asp[18] with the Thr[18] and of Ile[19] with a hydrophobic amino acid whose side chain branches on the γ-carbon such as Leu, cyclohexylalanine, and γ-methylleucine (γ-MeLeu) resulted in loss of biological activity of ET-1, while high affinity for the ET_A ($IC_{50} = 0.42$–0.70 nM) ET_B ($IC_{50} = 0.17$–0.43 nM) receptor was retained. These compounds were shown to have high antagonist activities in ET-1 induced vasoconstriction of porcine coronary artery (pA_2 7.4–7.7) and in sarafotoxin 6c induced vasoconstriction of rabbit pulmonary artery ([Thr[18], γ- MeLeu[19]]ET-1: pA_2 8.4) indicating potent antagonistic activity at both subtypes (ET_A and ET_B) of receptors[122]. A series of linear smaller tripeptides have been reported to possess ET antagonist activity. The compounds are reported to be active in a tissue contraction assay and produced 100% inhibition of ET-1 pressor response at 10 mg/kg in rats[123]. A potent non-peptide ET receptor antagonist, myriceron caffeoyl ester (50-235), isolated from the methanol extract of the bark of the bayberry, Myrica cerifera, has been reported. This compound selectively antagonized specific binding of [^{125}I]ET-1, but not of [^{125}I]ET-3. This is the first reported non-peptide ET_A receptor antagonist[123,125].

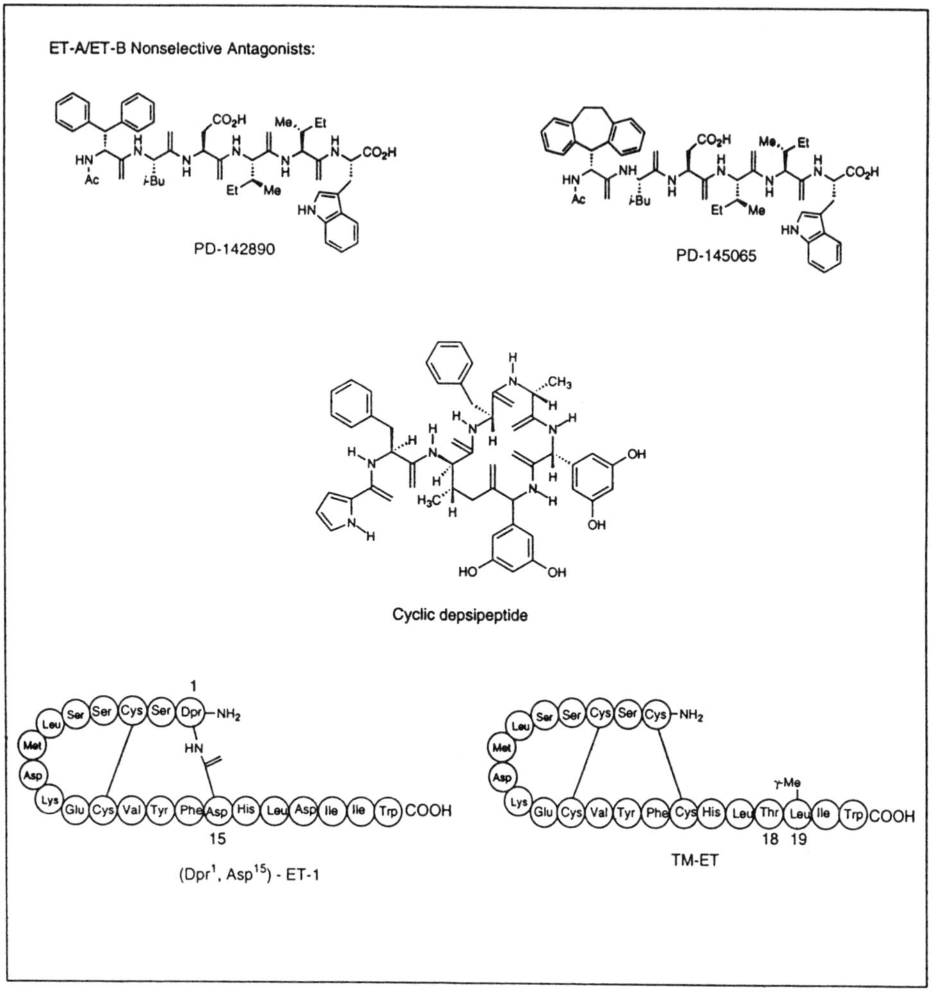

Figure 4.3. Representative structures of antagonists of nonselective endothelin receptor.

Recently, International Research Laboratories (IRL) in Japan have reported [Cys^{11}-Cys^{15}]ET-1(11-21) (IRL 1038) as a ET$_B$ receptor selective antagonist. This peptide is almost 100 times selective for ET$_B$ than ET$_A$ receptors[126]. Importance of ETs in physiology and pathology as well as its role in various diseases is now entering an exciting new phase with the development of new selective and nonselective ET receptor agonists and antagonists[69,107,122,127-130].

CONCLUSIONS

ET has attracted considerable research since its discovery and numerous compounds believed to be acting on or through ET mechanisms have been synthesized and their pharmacological activities determined. The interest in this field has increased mainly because of the involvement of ET in numerous body functions including cardiovascular, central nervous system, endocrinal, renal, skeletal, hepatobiliary, perinatal and many others. Understanding the role of ET in the pathophysiology of diseases can be greatly increased as a result of the discovery of new, potent and selective ET agonists and antagonists. These studies will ultimately lead to possible therapeutic use of ET agonists and antagonists in disease conditions.

Acknowledgement

The authors are grateful to Dr. Andrew S. Borovik and Ms. C. Ruth for help in preparation of this manuscript. This is contribution 94-596-B of the Kansas Agriculture Experiment Station.

References

1. Yanagisawa, M., Kurihara, H., Kimura, S., Tomobe, Y., Kobayashi, M., Mitsui, Y., Yazaki, Y., Goto, K. & Masaki, T. (1988) A novel potent vasoconstrictor peptide produced by vascular endothelial cells. *Nature*, **332**, 411–415.
2. Itoh, Y., Yanagisawa, M., Ohkubo, S., Kimura, C., Kosaka, T., Inoue, A., Ishida, N., Mitsui, Y., Onda, H., Fujino, M. & et al. (1988) Cloning and sequence analysis of cDNA encoding the precursor of a human endothelium-derived vasconstrictor peptide, endothelin: identity of human and porcine endothelin. *FEBS Lett*, **231**, 440–444.
3. Hirata, Y., Yoshimi, H., Takata, S., Watanabe, T. X., Kumagai, S., Nakajima, K. & Sakakibara, S. (1988) Cellular mechanism of action by a novel vasoconstrictor endothelin in cultured rat vascular smooth muscle cells. *Biochem Biophys Res Commun*, **154**, 868–875.
4. Matsuyama, K., Yasue, H., Okumura, K., Saito, Y., Nakao, K., Shirakami, G. & Imura, H. (1991) Increased plasma level of endothelin-1-like immunoreactivity during coronary spasm in patients with coronary spastic angina. *Am J Cardiol*, **68**, 991–995.
5. Salminen, K., Tikkanen, I., Saijonmaa, O., Nieminen, M., Fyhrquist, F. & Frick, M. H. (1989) Modulation of coronary tone in acute myocardial infarction by endothelin, *Lancet*, **2**, 747.
6. Mattoli, S., Soloperto, M., Marini, M. & Fasoli, A. (1991) Levels of endothelin in the bronchoalveolar lavage fluid off patients with symptomatic asthma and reversible airflow obstruction. *J Allergy Clin Immunol*, **88**, 376–384.
7. Macrae, I. M., Robinson, M. J., Graham, D. I., Reid, J. L. & McCulloch, J. (1993) Endothelin-1-induced reductions in cerebral blood flow: dose dependency, time course, and neuropathological consequences. *J Cereb Blood Flow Metab*, **13**, 276–284.
8. Fuxe, K., Kurosawa, N., Cintra, A., Hallström, A., Goiny, M., Rosén, L., Agnati, L. F. & Ungerstedt, U. (1992) Involvement of local ischemia in endothelin-1 induced lesions of the neostriatum of the anaesthetized rat. *Exp Brain Res*, **88**, 131–139.
9. Miller, W. L., Redfield, M. M. & Burnett, J. C. J. (1989) Integrated cardiac, renal, and endocrine actions of endothelin, *J Clin Invest*, **83**, 317–320.
10. Black, P. N., Ghatei, M. A., Takahashi, K., Bretherton Watt, D., Krausz, T. & Dollery, C. T. (1989) Formation of endothelin by cultured airway epithelial cells. *FEBS Lett*, **255**, 129–132.
11. Kosaka, T., Suzuki, N., Matsumoto, H., Itoh, Y., Yasuhara, T., Onda, H. & Fujino, M. (1989) Synthesis of the vasoconstrictor peptide endothelin in kidney cells. *FEBS Lett*, **249**, 42–46.
12. Ishida, N., Tsujioka, K., Tomoi, M., Saida, K. & Mitsui, Y. (1989) Differential activities of two distinct endothelin family peptides on ileum and coronary artery. *FEBS Lett*, **247**, 337–340.
13. Uchida, Y., Ninomiya, H., Saotome, M., Nomura, A., Ohtsuka, M., Yanagisawa, M., Goto, K., Masaki, T. & Hasegawa, S. (1988) Endothelin, a novel vasoconstrictor peptide, as potent bronchoconstrictor. *Eur J Pharmacol*, **154**, 227–228.
14. Kozuka, M., Ito, T., Hirose, S., Takahashi, K. & Hagiwara, H. (1989) Endothelin induces two types of contractions of rat uterus: phasic contractions by way of voltage-dependent calcium channels and developing contractions through a second type of calcium channels. *Biochem Biophys Res Commun*, **159**, 317–323.

15. Takagi, M., Matsuoka, H., Atarashi, K. & Yagi, S. (1988) Endothelin: a new inhibitor of renin release. *Biochem Biophys Res Commun*, **157**, 1164–1168.
16. Fukuda, Y., Hirata, Y., Yoshimi, H., Kojima, T., Kobayashi, Y., Yanagisawa, M. & Masaki, T. (1988) Endothelin is a potent secretagogue for atrial natriuretic peptide in cultured rat atrial myocytes. *Biochem Biophys Res Commun*, **155**, 167–172.
17. Yoshizawa, T., Kimura, S., Kanazawa, I., Uchiyama, Y., Yanagisawa, M. & Masaki, T. (1989) Endothelin localizes in the dorsal horn and acts on the spinal neurones: possible involvement of dihydropyridine-sensitive channels and substance P release. *Neurosci Lett*, **102**, 179–184.
18. Rubanyi, G. M. & Botelho, L. H. (1991) Endothelins, *FASEB J*, **5**, 2713–2720.
19. Gultai, A. & Srimal, R. C. (1992) Endothelin mechanisms in the central nervous system: A target for drug development. *Drug Develop Res*, **26**, 361–387.
20. Jones, C. R., Hiley, C. R., Pelton, J. T. & Mohr, M. (1989) Autoradiographic visualization of the binding sites for [^{125}I]endothelin in rat and human brain. *Neurosci Lett*, **97**, 276–279.
21. Sugiura, M., Inagami, T. & Kon, V. (1989) Endotoxin stimulates endothelin-release *in vivo* and *in vitro* as determined by radioimmunoassay. *Biochem Biophys Res Commun*, **161**, 1220–1227.
22. Pernow, J., Hemsen, A. & Lundberg, J. M. (1989) Increased plasma levels of endothelin-like immunoreactivity during endotoxin administration in the pig. *Acta Physiol Scand*, **137**, 317–318.
23. Knock, G. A., Terenghi, G., Bunker, C. B., Bull, H. A., Dowd, P. M. & Polak, J. M. (1993) Characterization of endothelin-binding sites in human skin and their regulation in primary Raynaud's phenomenon and systemic sclerosis. *J Invest Dermatol*, **101**, 73–78.
24. Nakahama, H. (1990) Stimulatory effect of cyclosporine A on endothelin secretion by a cultured renal epithelial cell line, LLC-PK1 cells. *Eur J Pharmacol*, **180**, 191–192.
25. Kon, V., Sugiura, M., Inagami, T., Harvie, B. R., Ichikawa, I. & Hoover, R. L. (1990) Role of endothelin in cyclosporine-induced glomerular dysfunction. *Kidney Int*, **37**, 1487–1491.
26. Hickey, K. A., Rubanyi, G., Paul, R. J. & Highsmith, R. F. (1985) Characterization of a coronary vasoconstrictor produced by cultured endothelial cells. *Am J Physiol*, **248**, C550–C556.
27. Shinmi, O., Kimura, S., Sawamura, T., Sugita, Y., Yoshizawa, T., Uchiyama, Y., Goto, K., Masaki, T. & Kanazawa, I. (1989) Endothelin-3 in a novel neuropeptide: isolation and sequence determination of endothelin-1 and endothelin-3 in porcine brain. *Biochem Biophys Res Commun*, **164**, 587–593.
28. Inoue, A., Yanagisawa, M., Kimura, S., Kasuya, Y., Miyauchi, T., Goto, K. & Masaki, T. (1989) The human endothelin family: three structurally and pharmacologically distinct isopeptides predicted by three separate genes. *Proc Natl Acad Sci USA*, **86**, 2863–2867.
29. Yanagisawa, M., Inoue, A., Ishikawa, T., Kasuya, Y., Kimura, S., Kumagaye, S., Nakajima, K., Watanabe, T. X., Sakakibara, S., Goto, K. *et al.* (1988) Primary structure, synthesis, and biological activity of rat endothelin, an endothelium-derived vasoconstrictor peptide. *Proc Natl Acad Sci USA*, **85**, 6964–6967.
30. Kloog, Y., Ambar, I., Sokolovsky, M., Kochva, E., Wollberg, Z. & Bdolah, A. (1988) Sarafotoxin, a novel vasoconstrictor peptide: phosphoinositide hydrolysis in rat heart and brain. *Science*, **242**, 268–270.
31. Lee, S.-Y. & Chiappinelli, V. A. (1989) Similarity of endothelin to snake venom toxin. *Nature*, **335**, 303.
32. Wolberg, Z., Shabo-Shina, R., Intrator, N., Bdolah, A., Kochva, E., Shavit, G., Oron, Y., Vidne, B. A. & Gitter, S. (1988) A novel cardiotoxic polypeptide from the venom of *Atractaspis engaddensis* (burrowing asp): Cardiac effects in mice and isolated rat and human heart preparations. *Toxicon*, **26**, 525–534.
33. Bdolah, A., Wollberg, Z., Fleminger, G. & Kochva, E. (1989) SRTX-d, a new native peptide of the endothelin/sarafotoxin family. *FEBS Lett*, **256**, 1–3.
34. Takasaki, C., Tamiya, N., Bdolah, A., Wollberg, Z. & Kochiva, E. (1988) Sarafotoxins S6: Several isotoxins from Atractaspis engaddensis (burrowing Asp) venom that affect the heat. *Toxicon*, **26**, 543–548.
35. Saida, K., Mitsui, Y. & Ishida, N. (1989) A novel peptide, vasoactive intestinal contractor, of a new (endothelin) peptide family. Molecular cloning, expression, and biological activity. *J Biol Chem*, **264**, 14613–14616.
36. Yanagisawa, M. & Masaki, T. (1989) Endothelin, a novel endothelium-derived peptide. Pharmacological activities, regulation and possible roles in cardiovascular control. *Biochem Pharmacol*, **38**, 1877–1883.
37. Kimura, S., Kasuya, Y., Sawamura, T., Shinimi, O., Sugita, Y., Yanagisawa, M. & Goto, K. (1989) Conversion of big endothelin-1 to 21-residue endothelin-1 is essential for expression of full vasoconstrictor activity: structure-activity relationships of big endothelin-1. *J Cardiovasc Pharmacol*, **13 (Suppl 5)**, S5–S7.
38. Shinyama, H., Uchida, T., Kido, H., Hayashi, K., Watanabe, M., Ikegawa, R., Takaoka, M. & Morimoto, S. (1991) Phosphoramidon inhibits the conversion of intracisternally administered big endothelin-1 to endothelin-1. *Biochem Biophys Res Commun*, **178**, 24–30.

39. Matsumura, Y., Hisaki, K., Takaoka, M. & Morimoto, S. (1990) Phosphoramidon, a metalloproteinase inhibitor, suppresses the hypertensive effect of big endothelin-1. *Eur J Pharmacol*, **185**, 103–106.
40. McMahon, E. G., Palomo, M. A. & Moore, W. M. (1991) Phosphoramidon blocks the pressor activity of big endothelin[1-39] and lowers blood pressure in spontaneously hypertensive rats. *J Cardiovasc Pharmacol*, **17 (Suppl 7)**, S29–S33.
41. Pollock, D. M. & Opgenorth, T. J. (1991) Comparison of the hemodynamic effects of endothelin-1 and big endothelin-1 in the rat. *Biochem Biophys Res Commun*, **179**, 1122–1126.
42. Sawamura, T., Kasuya, Y., Matsushita, Y., Suzuki, N., Shinmi, O., Kishi, N., Sigita, Y., Yanagisawa, M., Goto, K., Masaki, T. & Kimura, S. (1991) Phosphoramidon inhibits the intracellular conversion of big endothelin-1 to endothelin-1 in cultured endothelial cells. *Biochem Biophys Res Commun*, **174**, 779–784.
43. Kam, C. M., Nishino, N. & Powers, J. C. (1979) Inhibition of thermolysin and carboxypeptidase A by phosphoramidates. *Biochemistry*, **18**, 3032–3038.
44. Altstein, M., Bachar, E., Vogel, Z. & Blumberg, S. (1983) Protection of enkephalins from enzymatic degradation utilizing selective metal-chelating inhibitors. *Eur J Pharmacol*, **91**, 353–361.
45. Pollock, D. M., Shiosaki, K., Sullivan, G. M. & Opgenorth, T. J. (1992) Rhamnose moiety of phosphoramidon is not required for *in vivo* inhibition of endothelin converting enzyme. *Biochem Biophys Res Commun*, **186**, 1146–1150.
46. Brown, S. C., Donlan, M. E. & Jeffs, P. W. (1990) Structural studies of endothelin by CD and NMR. In: *Peptides: Chemistry, structure and biology*, pp. 595–597. Ed. Rivier, J. E. & Marshall, G. R. ESCOM, Leiden, The Netherlands.
47. Perkins, T. D., Hider, R. C. & Barlow, D. J. (1990) Proposed solution structure of endothelin. *Int J Pept Protein Res*, **36**, 128–133.
48. Saudek, V. Hoflack, J. & Pelton, J. T. (1989) 1H-NMR study of endothelin, sequence-specific assignment of the spectrum and a solution structure. *FEBS Lett*, **257**, 145–148.
49. Endo, S., Inooka, H., Ishibashi, Y., Kitada, C., Mizuta, E. & Fujino, M. (1989) Solution conformation of endothelin determined by nuclear magnetic resonance and distance geometry. *FEBS Lett*, **257**, 149–154.
50. Bennes, R., Calas, B., Chabrier, P. E., Demaille, J. & Heitz, F. (1990) Evidence for aggregation of endothelin 1 in water. *FEBS Lett*, **276**, 21–24.
51. Tamaoki, H., Kyogoku, Y., Nakajima, K., Sakakibara, S., Hayashi, M. & Kobayashi, Y. (1992) Conformational study of endothelins and sarafotoxins with the cystine-stabilized helical motif by means of CD spectra. *Biopolymers*, **32**, 353–357.
52. Munro, S., Craik, D., McConville, C., Hall, J., Searle, M., Bicknell, W., Scanlon, D. & Chandler, C. (1991) Solution conformation of endothelin, a potent vasocontricting bicyclic peptide: A combined use of H NMR spectroscopy and distance geometry calculations. *FEBS Lett*, **278**, 9–13.
53. Saudek, V., Hoflack, J. & Pelton, J. T. (1991) Solution conformation of endothelin-1 by 1H NMR, CD, and molecular modeling. *Int J Pept Protein Res*, **37**, 174–179.
54. Tamaoki, H., Kobayashi, Y., Nishimura, S., Ohkubo, T., Kyogoku, Y., Nakajima, K., Kumagaye, S., Kimura, T. & Sakakibara, S. (1991) Solution conformation of endothelin determined by means of 1H-NMR spectroscopy and distance geometry calculations. *Protein Eng*, **4**, 509–518.
55. Donlan, M. L., Brown, F. K. & Jeffs, P. W. (1992) Solution conformation of human big endothelin-1, *J Biomol NMR*, **2**, 407–420.
56. Krystek, S. R., Bassolino, D. A., Novotny, J., Chen, C., Marschner, T. M. & Andersen, N. H. (1991) Conformation of endothelin in aqueous ethylene glycol determined by H-NMR and molecular dynamics simulations. *FEBS Lett*, **281**, 212–218.
57. Reily, M. D. & Dunbar, J. B. J. (1991) The conformation of endothelin-1 in aqueous solution: NMR-derived constraints combined with distance geometry and molecular dynamics calculations. *Biochem Biophys Res Commun*, **178**, 570–577.
58. Wolff, M., Day, J., Greenwood, A., Larson, S. & McPherson, A. (1992) Crystallization and preliminary X-ray analysis of human endothelin. *Acta Crystallogr Sect B, Struct Sci*, **48**, 239–240.
59. Kobayashi, Y., Sato, A., Takashima, H., Tamaoki, H., Nishimura, S., Kyogoku, Y., Ikenaka, K., Kondo, T., Mikoshiba, K., Hojo, H., Aimoto, S. & Moroder, L. (1991) A new α-helical motif in membrane active peptides. *Neurochem Int*, **18**, 525–534.
60. Andersen, N. H., Chen, C. P., Marschner, T. M., Krystek, S. R., Jr. & Bassolino, D. A. (1992) Conformational isomerism of endothelin in acidic aqueous media: a quantitative NOESY analysis. *Biochemistry*, **31**, 1280–1295.
61. Hemple, J. C., Ghoul, W. A., Wurtz, J. M. & Hagler, A. T. (1990) Energy-based modelling studies of endothelin. In: *Peptides: Chemistry, structure and biology*, pp. 279, Ed. Rivier, J. E. & Marshall, J. R. ESCOM, Leiden, The Netherlands.

62. Hassan, M., Hempel, J. C., Li, Z. & Hagler, A. T. (1992) Distance-energy maps in peptide conformational search: application to cyclosporin and endothelin-1. In: *Peptides: Chemistry, structure and biology*, pp. 283–284. Ed. Smith, J. A. & Rivier, J. E. ESCOM, Leiden, The Netherlands.
63. Spinella, M. J., Krystek, S. R., Jr., Peapus, D. H., Wallace, B. A., Bruner, C. & Andersen, T. T. (1989) A proposed structural model of endothelin. *Pept Res*, **2**, 286–291.
64. Topiol, S. (1987) The deletion model for the origin of receptors. *Trends Biochem Sci*, **12**, 419–421.
65. Kloog, Y. & Sokolovsky, M. (1989) Similarities in mode and sites of action of sarafotoxins and endothelins. *Trends Pharmacol Sci*, **10**, 212–214.
66. Nakajima, K., Kumagaye, S., Nishio, H., Kuroda, H., Watanabe, T. X., Kobayashi, Y., Kimura, T. & Sakakibara, S. (1989) Synthesis of endothelin-1 analogues, endothelin-3, and sarafotoxin S6b: structure-activity relationships. *J Cardiovasc Pharmacol*, **13 (Suppl 5)**, S8–12.
67. Doherty, A. M., Cody, W. L., Leitz, N. L., DePue, P. L., Taylor, M. D., Rapundalo, S. T., Hingorani, G. P., Major, T. C., Panek, R. L. & Taylor, D. G. (1991) Structure-activity studies of the C-terminal region of the endothelins and the sarafotoxins. *J Cardiovasc Pharmacol*, **17 (Suppl 7)**, S59–S61.
68. Maggi, C. A., Giuliani, S., Patacchini, R., Santicioli, P., Rovero, P., Giachetti, A. & Meli, A. (1989) The C-terminal hexapeptide, endothelin-(16-21), discriminates between different endothelin receptors. *Eur J Pharmacol*, **166**, 121–122.
69. Doherty, A. M., Cody, W. L., DePue, P. L., He, J. X., Waite, L. A., Leonard, D. M., Leitz, N. L., Dudley, D. T., Rapundalo, S. T. & Hingorani, G. P. (1993) Structure-activity relationships of C-terminal endothelin hexapeptide antagonists. *J Med Chem*, **36**, 2585–2594.
70. Koshi, T., Suzuki, C., Arai, K., Mizoguchi, T., Torii, T., Hirata, M., Ohkuchi, M. & Okabe, T. (1991) Syntheses and biological activities of endothelin-1 analogs. *Chem Pharm Bull Tokyo*, **39**, 3061–3063.
71. Kimura, S., Kasuya, Y., Sawamura, T., Shinmi, O., Sugita, Y., Yanagisawa, M., Goto, K. & Masaki, T. (1988) Structure-activity relationships of endothelin: importance of the C-terminal moiety. *Biochem Biophys Res Commun*, **156**, 1182–1186.
72. Galatino, M., De Castiglione, R., Tam, J. P., Liu, W., Zhang, J. W., Cristiani, C. & Vaghi, F. (1992) D-amino acid scan of endothelin. In: *Peptides: Chemistry, structure and biology*, pp. 404–405. Ed. Smith, J. A. & Rivier, J. E. ESCOM, Leiden, The Netherlands.
73. Nakajima, K., Kubo, S., Kumagaye, S., Nishio, H., Tsunemi, M., Inui, T., Kuroda, H., Watanabe, T. X., Kimura, T. et al. (1989) Structure-activity relationship of endothelin: importance of charged groups. *Biochem Biophys Res Commun*, **163**, 424–429.
74. Kitazumi, K., Shiba, T., Nishiki, K., Furukawa, Y., Takasaki, C. & Tasaka, K. (1990) Structure-activity relationship in vasoconstrictor effects of sarafotoxins and endothelin-1. *FEBS Lett*, **260**, 269–272.
75. Yogo, K., Yano, S. & Watanabe, K. (1990) Vasoconstrictor effect of endothelin in isolated perfused stomach of the rat. *Jpn J Pharmacol*, **52**, 160–163.
76. De Castiglione, R., Tam, J. P., Liu, W., Zhang, J. W., Galatino, M., Bertolero, F. & Vaghi, F. (1992) Alanine scan of endothelin. In: *Peptides: Chemistry, structure and biology*, pp. 402–403. Ed. Smith, J. A. & Rivier, J. E. ESCOM, Leiden, The Netherlands.
77. Landan, G., Bdolah, A., Wollberg, Z., Kochva, E. & Graur, D. (1991) The evolutionary history of the sarafotoxin/endothelin/endothelin-like superfamily. *J Cardiovasc Pharmacol*, **17 (Suppl 7)**, S517–S519.
78. Topouzis, S., Pelton, J. T. & Miller, R. C. (1989) Effects of calcium entry blockers on contractions evoked by endothelin-1, [Ala^{3,11}]endothelin-1 and [Ala^{1,15}]endothelin-1 in rat isolated aorta. *Br J Pharmacol*, **98**, 669–677.
79. Hunt, J. T., Lee, V. G., Stein, P. D., Hedberg, A., Liu, E. C., McMullen, D. & Moreland, S. (1991) Structure-activity relationship of monocyclic endothelin analogs. *Bioorg & Med Chem Letts*, **1**, 33–38.
80. Takayanagi, R., Kitazumi, K., Takasaki, C., Ohnaka, K., Aimoto, S., Tasaka, K., Ohashi, M. & Nawata, H. (1991) Presence of non-selective type of endothelin receptor on vascular endothelium and its linkage to vasodilation. *FEBS Lett*, **282**, 103–106.
81. Cohen, G., Knight, M., Lippton, H. & Hyman, A. (1990) Structural requirements for pulmonary vasodilation by endothelin. *Circulation*, **82**, III-227.
82. Arai, H., Hori, S., Aramori, I., Ohkubo, H. & Nakanishi, S. (1990) Cloning and expression of a cDNA encoding an endothelin receptor. *Nature*, **348**, 730–732.
83. Sakurai, T., Yanagisawa, M., Takuwa, Y., Miyazaki, H., Kimura, S., Goto, K. & Masaki, T. (1990) Cloning of a cDNA encoding a non-isopeptide-selective subtype of the endothelin receptor. *Nature*, **348**, 732–735.
84. Schvartz, I., Ittoop, O. & Hazum, E. (1991) Direct evidence for multiple endothelin receptors. *Biochemistry*, **30**, 5325–5327.
85. Mizuno, T., Imai, T., Itakura, M., Hirose, S., Hirata, Y., Marumo, F. & Hagiwara, H. (1992) Structure of the bovine endothelin-B receptor gene and its tissue-specific expression revealed by northern analysis. *J Cardiovasc Pharmacol*, **20 (Suppl 12)**, S8–10.

86. Lin, H. Y., Kaji, E. H., Winkel, G. K., Ives, H. E. & Lodish, H. F. (1991) Cloning and functional expression of a vascular smooth muscle endothelin 1 receptor. *Proc Natl Acad Sci USA*, **88**, 3185–3189.
87. Kozuka, M., Ito, T., Hirose, S., Lodhi, K. M. & Hagiwara, H. (1991) Purification and characterization of bovine lung endothelin receptor. *J Biol Chem*, **266**, 16892–16896.
88. Nakamichi, K., Ihara, M., Kobayashi, M., Saeki, T., Ishikawa, K. & Yano, M. (1992) Different distribution of endothelin receptor subtypes in pulmonary tissues revealed by the novel selective ligands BQ-123 and [Ala^{1,3,11,15}]ET-1. *Biochem Biophys Res Commun*, **182**, 144–150.
89. Williams, D. L., Jr., Jones, K. L., Colton, C. D. & Nutt, R. F. (1991) Identification of high affinity endothelin-1 receptor subtypes in human tissues. *Biochem Biophys Res Commun*, **180**, 475–480.
90. Panek, R. L., Major, T. C., Hingorani, G. P., Doherty, A. M., Taylor, D. G. & Rapundalo, S. T. (1992) Endothelin and structurally related analogs distinguish between endothelin receptor subtypes. *Biochem Biophys Res Commun*, **183**, 566–571.
91. Gomez Sanchez, C. E., Cozza, E. N., Foecking, M. F., Chiou, S. & Ferris, M. W. (1990) Endothelin receptor subtypes and stimulation of aldosterone secretion. *Hypertension*, **15**, 744–747.
92. Masaki, T., Kimura, S., Yanagisawa, M. & Goto, K. (1991) Molecular and cellular mechanism of endothelin regulation. Implications for vascular function. *Circulation*, **84**, 1457–1468.
93. Sakamoto, A., Yanagisawa, M., Sakurai, T., Takuwa, Y., Yanagisawa, H. & Masaki, T. (1991) Cloning and functional expression of human cDNA for the ET$_B$ endothelin receptor. *Biochem Biophys Res Commun*, **178**, 656–663.
94. Sakurai, T., Yanagisawa, M. & Masaki, T. (1992) Molecular characterization of endothelin receptors. *Trends Pharmacol Sci*, **13**, 103–108.
95. Nambi, P., Pullen, M. & Feuerstein, G. (1990) Identification of endothelin receptors in various regions of rat brain. *Neuropeptides*, **16**, 195–199.
96. Emori, T., Hirata, Y. & Marumo, F. (1990) Specific receptors for endothelin-3 in cultured bovine endothelial cells and its cellular mechanism of action. *FEBS Lett*, **263**, 261–264.
97. Harrison, V. J., Randriantsoa, A. & Schoeffter, P. (1992) Heterogeneity of endothelin-sarafotoxin receptors mediating contraction of pig coronary artery. *Br J Pharmacol*, **105**, 511–513.
98. Roubert, P., Gillard, V., Plas, P., Guillon, J. M., Chabrier, P. E. & Braquet, P. (1989) Angiotensin II and phorbol-esters potently down-regulate endothelin (ET-1) binding sites in vascular smooth muscle cells. *Biochem Biophys Res Commun*, **164**, 809–815.
99. Bax, W. A., Bos, E. & Saxena, P. R. (1993) Heterogeneity of endothelin/sarafotoxin receptors mediating contraction of the human isolated saphenous vein. *Eur J Pharmacol*, **239**, 267–268.
100. Sudjarwo, S. A., Hori, M., Tanaka, T., Matsuda, Y., Okada, T. & Karaki, H. (1994) Subtypes of endothelin ET$_A$ and ET$_B$ receptors mediating venous smooth muscle contraction. *Biochem Biophys Res Commun*, **200**, 627–633.
101. Eglezos, A., Cucchi, P., Patacchini, R., Quartara, L., Maggi, C. A. & Mizrahi, J. (1993) Differential effects of BQ-123 against endothelin-1 and endothelin-3 on the rat vas deferens: evidence for an atypical endothelin receptor. *Br J Pharmacol*, **109**, 736–738.
102. Karaki, H., Sudjarwo, S. A., Hori, M., Takai, M., Urade, Y. & Okada, T. (1993) Induction of endothelium-dependent relaxation in the rat aorta by IRL 1620, a novel and selective agonist at the endothelin ET$_B$ receptor. *Br J Pharmacol*, **109**, 486–490.
103. Sudjarwo, S. A., Hori, M., Takai, M., Urade, Y., Okada, T. & Karaki, H. (1993) A novel subtype of endothelin B receptor mediating contraction in swine pulmonary vein. *Life Sci*, **53**, 431–437.
104. Spinella, M. J., Malik, A. B., Everitt, J. & Andersen, T. T. (1991) Design and synthesis of a specific endothelin-1 antagonist: effects on pulmonary vasoconstriction. *Proc Natl Acad Sci USA*, **88**, 7443–7446.
105. Williams, D. L., Jr., Jones, K. L., Pettibone, D. J., Lis, E. V. & Clineschmidt, B. V. (1991) Sarafotoxin S6c: an agonist which distinguishes between endothelin receptor subtypes. *Biochem Biophys Res Commun*, **175**, 556–561.
106. Saeki, T., Ihara, M., Fukuroda, T., Yamagiwa, M. & Yano, M. (1991) [Ala1,3,11,15]endothelin-1 analogs with ETB agonistic activity. *Biochem Biophys Res Commun*, **179**, 286–292.
107. Takai, M., Umemura, I., Yamasaki, K., Watakabe, T., Fujitani, Y., Oda, K., Urade, Y., Inui, T., Yamamura, T. & Okada, T. (1992) A potent and specific agonist, Suc-[Glu^9,Ala^{11,15}]-endothelin-1(8-21), IRL 1620, for the ETB receptor. *Biochem Biophys Res Commun*, **184**, 953–959.
108. Ihara, M., Fukuroda, T., Saeki, T., Nishikibe, M., Kojiri, K., Suda, H. & Yano, M. (1991) An endothelin receptor (ETA) antagonist isolated from Streptomyces misakiensis. *Biochem Biophys Res Commun*, **178**, 132–137.
109. Nakajima, S., Niiyama, K., Ihara, M., Kojiri, K. & Suda, H. (1991) Endothelin-binding inhibitors, BE-18257A and BE-18257B II. Structure determination. *J Antibiot Tokyo*, **44**, 1348–1356.
110. Ishikawa, K., Fukami, T., Hayama, T., Niiyama, K., Nagase, T., Mase, T., Fujita, K., Kumagai, U., Urakawa, Y., Kimura, S., Ihara, M. & Yano, M. (1992) Endothelin antagonistic cyclic pentapeptides

with high selectivity for ET_A receptor. In: *Peptides: Chemistry and Biology*, pp. 812–813. Ed. Smith, J. A. & Rivier, J. E. ESCOM, Leiden, The Netherlands.
111. Ihara, M., Noguchi, K., Saeki, T., Fukuroda, T., Tsuchida, S., Kimura, S., Fukami, T., Ishikawa, K., Nishikibe, M. & Yano, M. (1992) Biological profiles of highly potent novel endothelin antagonists selective for the ETA receptor. *Life Sci*, **50**, 247–255.
112. Ihara, M., Saeki, T., Fukuroda, T., Kimura, S., Ozaki, S., Patel, A. C. & Yano, M. (1992) A novel radioligand [125I]BQ-3020 selective for endothelin (ETB) receptors. *Life Sci*, **51**, PL47–PL52.
113. Hiley, C. R., Cowley, D. J., Pelton, J. T. & Hargreaves, A. C. (1992) BQ-123, cyclo(-D-Trp-D-Asp-Pro-D-Val-Leu), is a non-competitive antagonist of the actions of endothelin-1 in SK-N-MC human neuroblastoma cells. *Biochem Biophys Res Commun*, **184**, 504–510.
114. Atkinson, R. A. & Pelton, J. T. (1992) Conformational study of cyclo[D-Trp-D-Asp-Pro-D-Val-Leu], an endothelin-A receptor-selective antagonist. *FEBS Lett*, **296**, 1–6.
115. Reily, M. D., Thanabal, V., Omecinsky, D. O., Dunbar, J. B., Jr., Doherty, A. M. & DePue, P. L. (1992) The solution structure of a cyclic endothelin antagonist, BQ-123, based on 1H-1H and 13C-1H three bond coupling constants. *FEBS Lett*, **300**, 136–140.
116. Krystek, S. R., Jr., Bassolino, D. A., Bruccoleri, R. E., Hunt, J. T., Porubcan, M. A., Wandler, C. F. & Andersen, N. H. (1992) Solution conformation of a cyclic pentapeptide endothelin antagonist. Comparison of structure obtained from constrained dynamics and conformational search. *FEBS Lett*, **299**, 255–261.
117. Gonnella, N. C., Zhang, X., Jin, Y., Prakash, O., Paris, C. G., Kolossvary, I., Guida, W. C., Bohacek, R. S., Vlattas, I. & Sytwu, T. (1994) Solvent effects on the conformation of cyclo(-D-Trp-D-Asp-Pro-D-Val-Leu): An NMR spectroscopy and molecular modelling study. *Int J Pept Protein Res*, **43**, 454–462.
118. Satoh, T. & Barlow, D. (1992) Molecular modelling of the structures of endothelin antagonists. Identification of a possible structural determinant for ET-A receptor binding. *FEBS Lett*, **310**, 83–87.
119. Coles, M., Sowemino, V., Scanlon, D., Munro, S. L. A. & Craik, D. J. (1993) A conformation study by ^{1}H NMR of a cyclic pentapeptide antagonist of endothelin. *J Med Chem*, **36**, 2658–2665.
120. Oohata, N., Nishikawa, M., Kiyoto, S., Takase, S., Hemmi, K., Murai, H. & Okuhara, M. (1990) Anthraquinone derivatives and preparation thereof. *European Patent Application*, **90112076.6**, (Filed 26 June 1990)
121. Lam, Y. K. T., Hensens, O. D., Liesch, J. M., Zink, D. M., Huang, L., Williams, D. L. J. & Genilloud, O. R. (1992) Cyclic depsipeptide endothelin receptor antagonist isolated from Microbispora. *European Patent Application*, **EP 496,452**, (Filled 29 July 1992)
122. Kikuchi, T., Kubo, K., Ohtaki, T., Suzuki, N., Asami, T., Shimamoto, N., Wakimasu, M. & Fujino, M. (1993) Endothelin-1 analogues substituted at both position 18 and 19: highly potent endothelin antagonists with no selectivity for either receptor subtype ETA or ETB. *J Med Chem*, **36**, 4087–4093.
123. Keji, H., Masahiro, N., Naoki, F., Masashi, H., Tanaka, H. & Kayakiri, N. (1991) Peptides having endothelin antagonist activity, a process for the preparation thereof and pharmaceutical compositions comprising the same. *EPA*, **457 195 A2** (Filed 9 May 1991)
124. Fujimoto, M., Mihara, S., Nakajima, S., Ueda, M., Nakamura, M. & Sakurai, K. (1992) A novel non-peptide endothelin antagonist isolated from bayberry, Myrica cerifera. *FEBS Lett*, **305**, 41–44.
125. Mihara, S. & Fujimoto, M. (1993) The endothelin ETA receptor-specific effect of 50-235, a nonpeptide endothelin antagonist. *EUR J Pharmacol*, **246**, 33–38.
126. Urade, Y., Fujitani, Y., Oda, K., Watakabe, T., Umemura, I., Takai, M., Okada, T., Sakata, K. & Karaki, H. (1992) An endothelin B receptor-selective antagonist: IRL 1038, [Cys^{11}-Cys^{15}]-endothelin- 1(11-21). *FEBS Lett*, **311**, 12–16.
127. Watakabe, T., Urade, Y., Takai, M., Umemura, I. & Okada, T. (1992) A reversible radioligand specific for the ETB receptor: [^{125}I]Tyr13-Suc-[Glu^9,Ala^{11,15}]-endothelin-1(8-21), [^{125}I]IRL 1620. *Biochem Biophys Res Commun*, **185**, 867–873.
128. Hunt, J. T., Lee, V. G., Liu, E. C., Moreland, S., McMullen, D., Webb, M. L. & Bolgar, M. (1993) Control of peptide disulfide regioisomer formation by mixed cysteine-penicillamine bridges. Application to endothelin-1. *Int J Pept Protein Res*, **42**, 249–258.
129. Molenaar, P., Kuc, R. E. & Davenport, A. P. (1992) Characterization of two new ETB selective radioligands, [^{125}I]-BQ3020 and [^{125}I]-[Ala1,3,11,15]ET-1 in human heart. *Br J Pharmacol*, **107**, 637–639.
130. McMurdo, L., Lidbury, P. S., Thiemermann, C. & Vane, J. R. (1993) Mediation of endothelin-1-induced inhibition of platelet aggregation via the ETB receptor. *Br J Pharmacol*, **109**, 530–534.

5 Endothelin-Converting Enzyme and its Inhibitors: Pathophysiological Significances

Yasuo Matsumura, Masanori Takaoka, Kazuhiro Hisaki and Shiro Morimoto

Department of Pharmacology, Osaka University of Pharmaceutical Sciences, 2-10-65 Kawai, Matsubara, Osaka 580, Japan

INTRODUCTION

Endothelin-1 (ET-1), a highly potent vasoconstrictor peptide with 21-amino acid residue, has been identified in the culture supernatant of porcine aortic endothelial cells (ECs).[1] Sequence analysis of porcine cDNA encoding ET-1 revealed the existence of a 203-residue prepro-form.[1] From the deduced amino acid sequence, Yanagisawa *et al.*[1] proposed the possible biosynthetic pathway for the production of the 21-amino acid mature ET-1, i.e., the prepro-form is initially processed by dibasic pair specific proteolysis to produce a 39-amino acid intermediate form, termed big ET-1, and the big ET-1 is converted to the mature form by an unusual proteolytic processing between Trp-21 and Val-22. Since the vasoconstrictor activity of big ET-1 is much lower than that of ET-1,[2,3] this final step for the ET-1 biosynthesis has been considered to be essential for the pathophysiological significance of ET-1. Subsequently, two groups independently found that the carboxy-terminal fragment of big-ET-1 (22–39) as well as ET-1 and big ET-1, were detected in the culture supernatant of ECs,[4,5] thereby strongly suggesting that the mature ET-1 is generated from big ET-1 by a putative ET-1 converting enzyme (ECE) in ECs. Thereafter, a number of experimental groups including us have indicated the existence of ECE in vascular and nonvascular tissues. Although several kinds of endopeptidases have been reported to convert big ET-1 to the mature form, a phosphoramidon-sensitive and membrane-bound metalloproteinase is regarded as the most plausible candidate for a physiological ECE (Figure 5.1). In this review, we summarize recent efforts on the identification and characterization of ECE and focus on the pathophysiological significance of ECE in ET-1 biosynthesis.

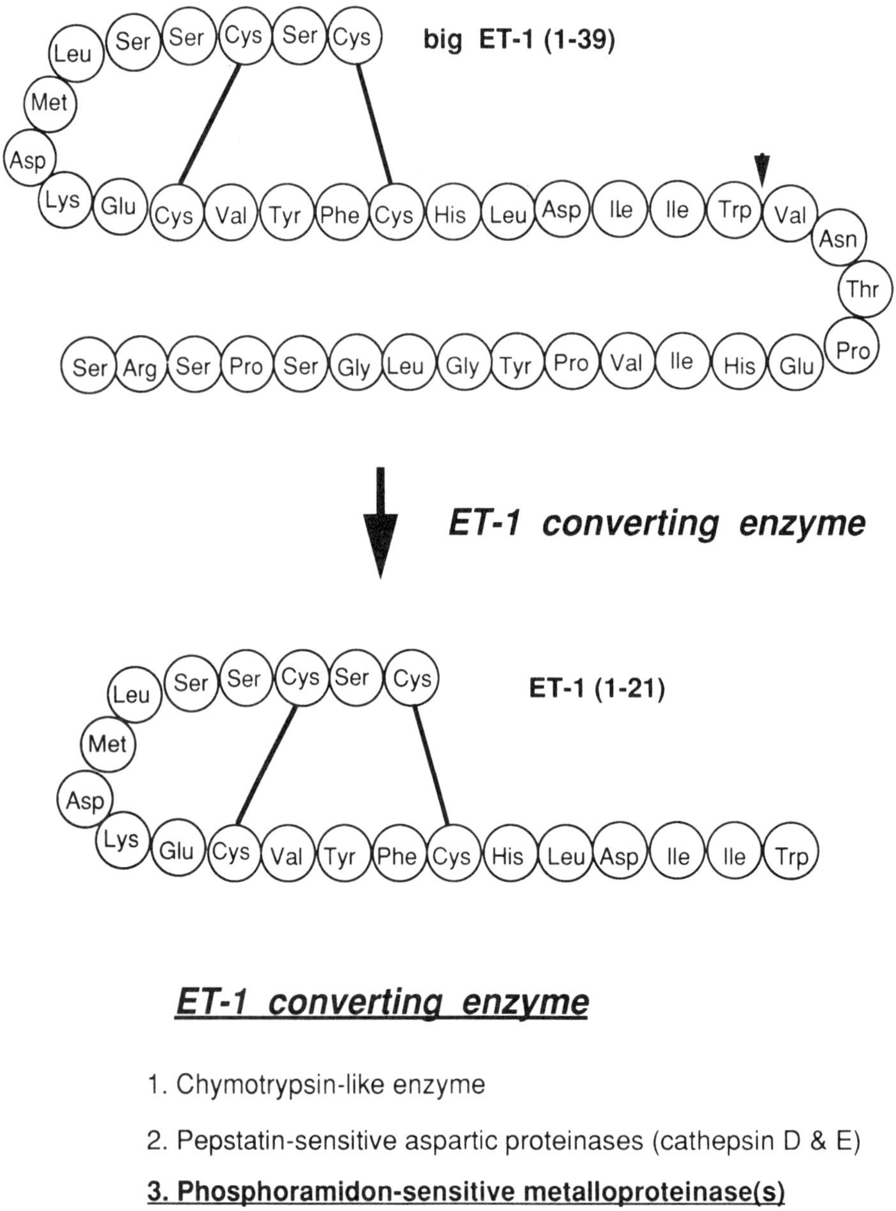
big ET-1 (1-39)
Leu Ser Ser Cys Ser Cys
Met
Asp
Lys Glu Cys Val Tyr Phe Cys His Leu Asp Ile Ile Trp Val
Asn
Thr
Ser Arg Ser Pro Ser Gly Leu Gly Tyr Pro Val Ile His Glu Pro
ET-1 converting enzyme
ET-1 (1-21)
Leu Ser Ser Cys Ser Cys
Met
Asp
Lys Glu Cys Val Tyr Phe Cys His Leu Asp Ile Ile Trp
ET-1 converting enzyme
1. Chymotrypsin-like enzyme
2. Pepstatin-sensitive aspartic proteinases (cathepsin D & E)
3. Phosphoramidon-sensitive metalloproteinase(s)

Figure 5.1. Processing of big endothelin-1 to the mature endothelin-1.

ENDOPEPTIDASES POSSESSING ET-CONVERTING ACTIVITIES

Chymotyrpsin-like enzyme(s)

In the original report by Yanagisawa *et al.*,[1] a putative ECE was postulated to be a chymotrypsin-like enzyme, based on the amino acid moiety of the cleavage site.

McMahon et al.[6] found that chymotrypsin-treated big ET-1 (1–40) produced an ET-1-like contraction of isolated rat aortic rings, and a characteristic ET-1-like effect on blood pressure *in vivo*. In their work, however, the mode of conversion of big ET-1 to ET-1 was not described. We[7] examined the chymotryptic-cleavage sites of big ET-1 and found that this enzyme cleaved initially the Tyr-31–Gly-32 bond of big ET-1, followed by cleavage between Trp-21 and Val-22. In addition, chymotrypsin hydrolysed the generated ET-1, producing Tyr-13-nicked form of ET-1. From these findings, we proposed that a chymotrypsin-like proteinase might be involved not only in the production but also in the degradation of ET-1.

Recently, Wypij et al.[8] reported that a chymostatin-sensitive enzyme chymase is involved in the extracellular processing of big ET-1 to ET-1 in the perfused rat lung. In their study, however, the pressor responses to big ET-1 was not documented. We have most recently evaluated whether the chymostatin-sensitive enzyme is responsible for the functional conversion of big ET-1 to ET-1 using the isolated perfused rat lung.[9] Results indicated that during perfusion of big ET-1, chymostatin descreased the accumulation of ET-1-like materials in perfusate but failed to suppress the big ET-1-induced pressor action, thereby suggesting that chymostatin-sensitive enzyme does not play a major role in functional conversion of big ET-1 in rat lung. Whether a chymostatin-sensitive enzyme, probably chymase, has a functional role in the production of ET-1 would need to be ruled out.

Pepstatin-sensitive aspartic proteinase(s)

We have provided the first evidence that a pepstatin-sensitive aspartic proteinase from porcine vascular ECs can convert big ET-1 to the mature form, via single cleavage between Trp-21 and Val-22.[10,11] Thereafter, several experimental groups observed the pepstatin-sensitive ECE activities in bovine vascular ECs,[12,13] in bovine adrenal medulla[14] and in rat lung.[15] In addition, pure enzymes such as pepsin[16] and cathepsin E[17] were reported to convert efficiently big ET-1 to ET-1. From these findings, it has been postulated that some pepstatin-sensitive aspartic proteinase may be a possible candidate for physiologically relevant ECE *in vivo*. However, Sawamura et al.[18] demonstrated that an aspartic proteinase cathepsin D, which was identified as an ECE in ECs and adrenal medulla, cleaved Asn-18–Ile19 bond in addition to Trp-21–Val-22 bond of big ET-1 and therefore suggested that cathepsin D was not a physiological ECE. Similar proteolytic responses of big ET-1 to cathepsin D of bovine spleen was also observed by us.[19] Thus, lysosomal cathepsin D may act as an ET-1-degrading enzyme rather than ECE. Shields et al.[20] suggested that pepstatin-sensitive aspartic proteinase is not an ECE, based on the findings that pepstatin did not alter the secretion ratio of ET-1 to big ET-1 in cultured vascular ECs. Furthermore, Bird et al.[21] found using conscious rats that potent inhibitors of cathepsin E did not specifically suppress the big ET-1-induced pressor responses, suggesting that this type of proteinase is not a physiologically relevant ECE. At present, it becomes infeasible that pepstatin-sensitive aspartic proteinase(s) is a physiologically relevant ECE. However, there are findings indicating that the activities of lysosomal enzymes, including cathepsin D, increase in aortic ECs isolated from hypertensive animals and that these increased lysosomal enzymes seem to be

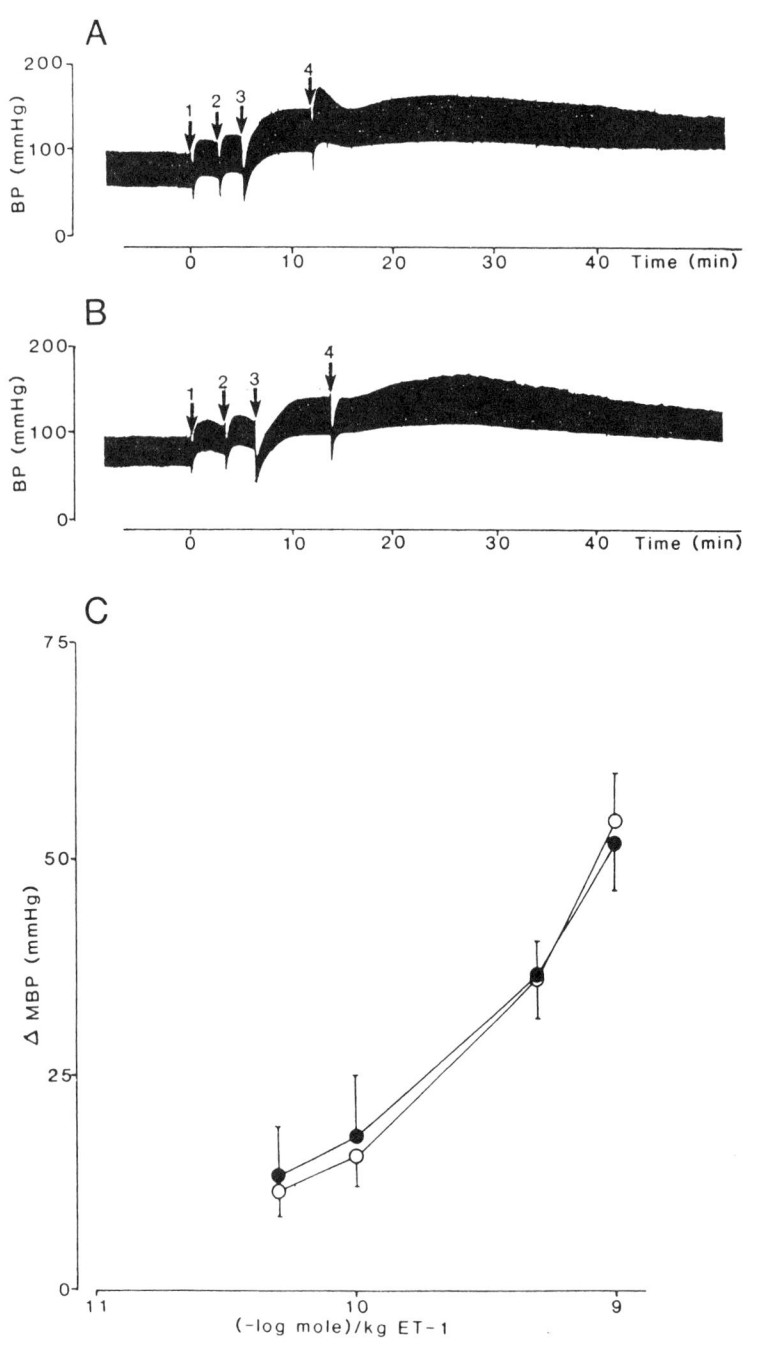

Figure 5.2. (A, B) A typical pattern of changes in blood pressure after administration of big ET-1 (left) or ET-1 (right), with (B) or without (A) an i.v. infusion of phosphoramidon (0.25 mg/kg per min). At the time indicated by the arrows, big ET-1 or ET-1 was cumulatively injected i.v.; (1) 0.05 nmol/kg; (2) 0.1 nmol/kg; (3) 0.5 nmol/kg; (4) 1.0 nmol/kg. (C) Dose-response curves for increases in mean arterial blood pressure after

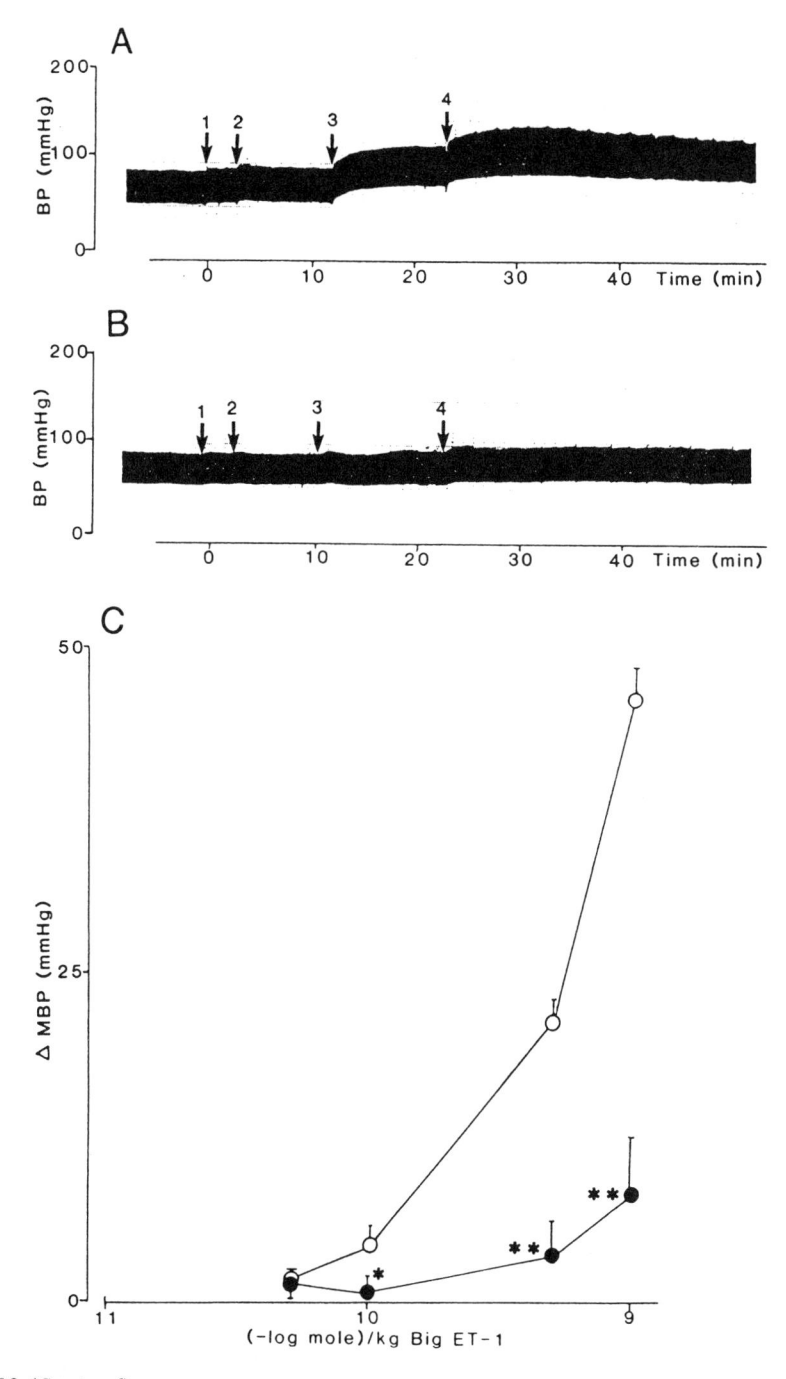

Figure 5.2 (*Continued*)
administration of big ET-1 (left) or ET-1 (right), with (·) or without (∘) infusion of phosphoramidon. Each point and bar represents the mean ± S.E. (n = 5). *P < 0.05; **P < 0.01, compared with values obtained in the absence of phosphoramidon infusion.

involved in the developmental mechanism of arterial ECs injury in hypertension and in further development of hypertensive vascular changes.[22] In such a case, ET-1 might be non-specifically produced from big ET-1 by cathepsin D which is increased in vascular ECs with development of hypertension, and subsequently is responsible for the maintenance of hypertension.

Phosphoramidon-sensitive metalloproteinase(s)

It has been acknowledged that an intravenous injection of big ET-1 causes almost the same dose-dependent pressor effect as ET-1 in anesthetized rats.[2,3] Since the vasoconstrictor activity of big ET-1 *in vitro* is much lower than that of ET-1,[2,3] the above pressor effect of big ET-1 has been regarded to be due to the proteolytic processing of this precursor to the mature ET-1. This notion was strongly supported by the evidence that plasma ET-1 levels remarkably increased following the bolus injection of big ET-1 to anesthetized rabbits.[23]

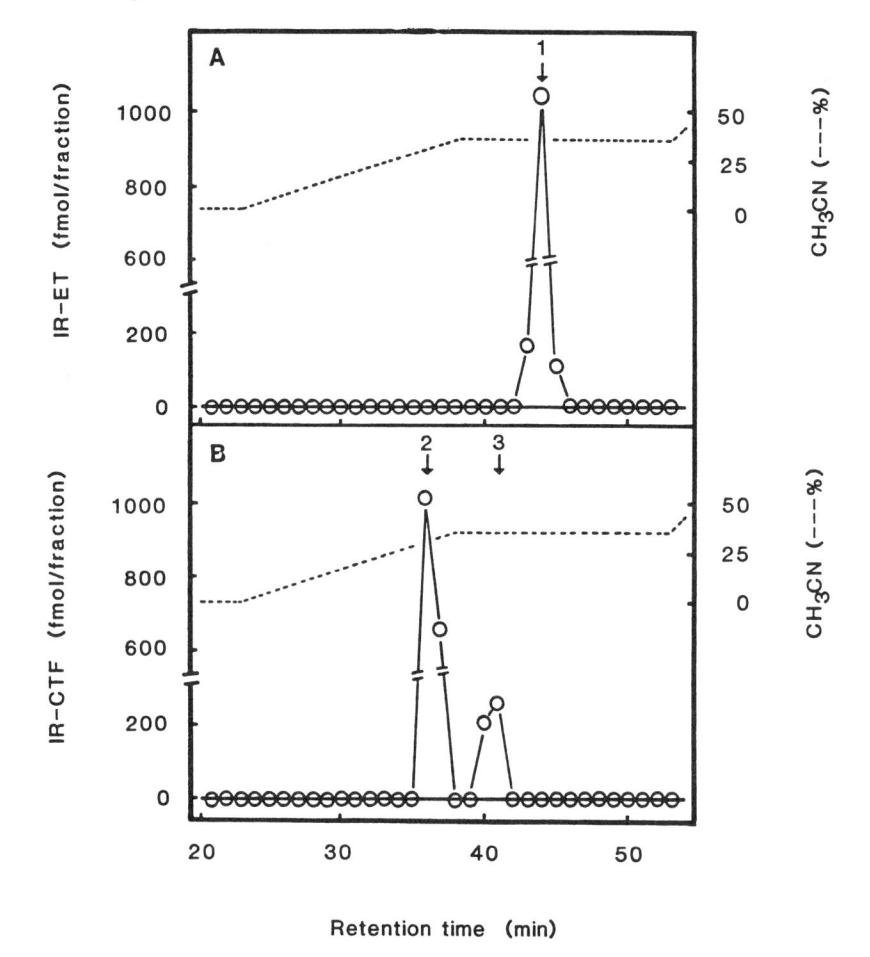

Fig. 5.3. (*Continued*)

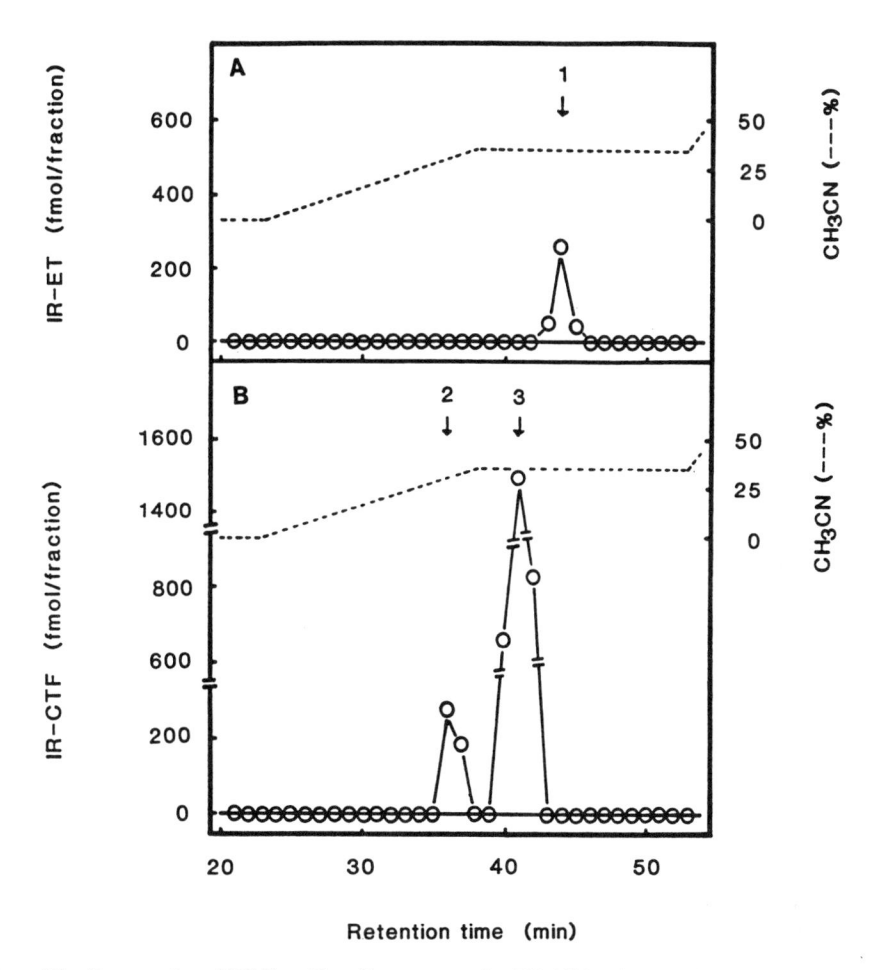

Figure 5.3. Reverse-phase HPLC profiles of immunoreactive-ET-1 (A) and -C-terminal fragment (CTF) of big ET-1 (B) in the EC-conditioned medium. ECs was incubated for 12 hr in the absence (left) or presence (right) of 10^{-4} M phosphoramidon. Arrows indicate the elution positions of synthetic ET-1 (1), CTF (2) and big ET-1 (3).

We first demonstrated that phosphoramidon, a metalloproteinase inhibitor, markedly suppressed the big ET-1-induced hypertensive action without affecting the action of the mature ET-1 in anesthetized rats (Figure 5.2).[24] From these findings, we proposed that big ET-1 was converted to ET-1 in the circulation by a phosphoramidon-sensitive metalloproteinase. Fukuroda et al.[25] also provided similar pharmacological actions of phosphoramidon, using conscious rats. Thereafter, a number of studies have indicated the inhibitory action of phosphoramidon on big ET-1-induced hypertension.[26-34] We and others[35,36] independently reported that the membrane fraction of cultured ECs possessed big ET-1-converting activities, which are specifically inhibited by phosphoramidon, suggesting that membrane-bound and phosphoramidon-sensitive ECE is involved in the production of ET-1 in ECs. Moreover, we noted that the addition of phosphoramidon to the monolayer of cultured ECs significantly reduced the secretion of ET-1 from ECs with a concomitant increase in the secretion of big ET-1 (Figure 5.3).[37] Taken together, it is reasonable to consider that a membrane-bound and phosphoramidon-sensitive metalloproteinase functions as a physiological ECE in ECs. In addition, this phosphoramidon-sensitive ECE is distinct from a neutral endopeptidase 24.11. Several experimental groups including us obtained evidences that specific inhibitors of neutral endopeptidase 24.11 such as thiorphan and kelatorphan did not influence the *in vivo* action of big ET-1, ET-1 secretion from cultured ECs and the ECE activities of the membrane fraction of ECs.[26,35,37,38] Angiotensin converting enzyme (a well-known metalloproteinase) inhibitor captopril was also without effect on ECE activities.[36,38] Thus, it seems likely that phosphoramidon-sensitive ECE is an unreported novel metalloproteinase.

IMPORTANCE OF PHOSPHORAMIDON-SENSITIVE METALLOPROTEINASE AS A PHYSIOLOGICAL ECE

Phosphoramidon-sensitive conversion of big ET-1 in vascular tissues

There are now accumulating evidences that *in vivo* effect of big ET-1 is inhibited by the treatment with phosphoramidon[24–34] and that the membrane fraction of cultured ECs contain a phosphoramidon-sensitive metalloproteinase(s) which convert big ET-1 to the mature ET-1.[35,36,38–43] However, informations whether or not the inhibitory action of phosphoramidon on big ET-1-induced pressor effect correlates to the decrease in ET-1 converted from big ET-1, have not been available. To clarify this problem, we examined the effects of phosphoramidon on ET-1 generation and the pressor responses during perfusion of big ET-1 in isolated rat mesenteric artery.[44] Results clearly indicated that both the big ET-1-induced pressor action and the accumulation of ET-1 in perfusate during perfusion of big ET-1 were markedly suppressed by phosphoramidon. These findings strongly suggest the importance of phosphoramidon-sensitive metalloproteinase for functional conversion of big ET-1 in vascular tissues.

Since the pressor activity of big ET-1 in the above preparation is not attenuated by the removal of endothelium,[45] the endothelium seems not to be essential for the functional conversion of big ET-1 in vascular tissues. Fukuroda *et al.*[25] also noted that the big ET-1-induced vasoconstriction of porcine coronary arteries, which is markedly inhibited by phosphoramidon, was not affected by the endothelium removal. We[46] and others[47] observed the phosphoramidon-sensitive ECE activities in the membrane fraction of cultured and non-cultured vascular smooth muscle cells (VSMCs), respectively, although the enzyme activities were considerably less potent than those seen with cultured ECs. Taken together, phosphoramidon-sensitive ECEs, which exist in both ECs and VSMCs, seem to be involved in the production of the mature ET-1 in vascular tissues. Furthermore, it is likely that these ECEs function as an ectoenzyme, based on the evidences that exogenously applied big ET-1 to the monolayer of cultured ECs[48] and VSMCs[46] is converted to ET-1 in phosphoramidon-sensitive fashion.

Using conscious rats, Gardiner et al.[29] investigated the hemodynamic responses of various organs to an intravenous bolus injection of big ET-1, and noted the different patterns of pressor responses to big ET-1 in the effector tissues studied (heart, renal, mesenteric and hindquarters vascular beds). In addition, the differential degrees of inhibition of pressor responses by phosphoramidon were observed. We also found that the pressor molar potency of big ET-1 is only about 5-fold less potent than that seen with ET-1, in isolated lung and hind leg preparations, in contrast to that in the isolated mesenteric artery big ET-1 has a 20–40-fold less potent pressor molar potency than ET-1.[9] Thus, it is likely that the pressor potencies of big ET-1 depend on its local conversion to the mature form by processes with differing degrees of susceptibility to phosphoramidon, as suggested by Gardiner et al.[29]

Phosphoramidon-sensitive conversion of big ET-1 in nonvascular tissues

Phosphoramidon-sensitive ECE activities have been observed in several nonvascular tissues. Sessa et al.[49] indicated that the incubation of big ET-1 with non-activated human polymorphonuclear leukocytes (PMNLs) generated ET-1-like vasoconstrictor activity, which was inhibited by phosphoramidon, and suggested that this ECE-like activity of PMNLs may contribute to the pressor effects of big ET-1 *in vivo* and to the pathogenesis of some vascular diseases. Noguchi et al.[50] found the phosphoramidon-sensitive ECE activity in isolated guinea pig bronchus. Since ET-1 has a potent bronchoconstrictor activity, they suggested that this activity may be involved in the regulation of bronchomotor tone and/or the pathogenesis of respiratory disorders such as asthma. Other nonvascular tissues (renal epithelial cells, rat vas deferens, rat lung, rat brain etc.) have been also indicated to contain the phosphoramidon-sensitive ECE activities.[51–56] Thus, this type of enzyme seems to be widely distributed in the nonvascular tissues.

Biochemical characteristics of phosphoramidon-sensitive ECE

A number of reports have indicated that phosphoramidon-sensitive ECE is present as a membrane-bound form, in various organs including vascular tissues.[35,36,38–56] On the other hand, there is some discrepancy with respect to the cytosolic ECE activities. Takada et al.[57] noted that the cytosol from bovine cultured ECs also contains a phosphoramidon-sensitive ECE with an apparent molecular weight of 540 kD, which is 5–6 times greater than that of the membranous enzyme isolated by the same experimental groups.[36] In contrast, using the cytosol of porcine cultured ECs, we observed a metal-dependent ECE activity insensitive to phosphoramidon.[35] This enzyme activity in the cytosol was completely inhibited by N-ethylmaleimide, a sulfhydryl blocking reagent.[38] Irrespective of the sensitivity to phosphoramidon, there seems to be an cytosolic ECE, which is distinct from the membranous enzyme.

Okada et al.[36] initially indicated using gel filtration HPLC that an apparent molecular weight of the membrane-bound and phosphoramidon-sensitive ECE is 100 kD. Using the same techniques, we[58] and others[59] partially purified a membranous ECE with an apparent molecular weight of 500 kD and 300 kD, respectively, using rat

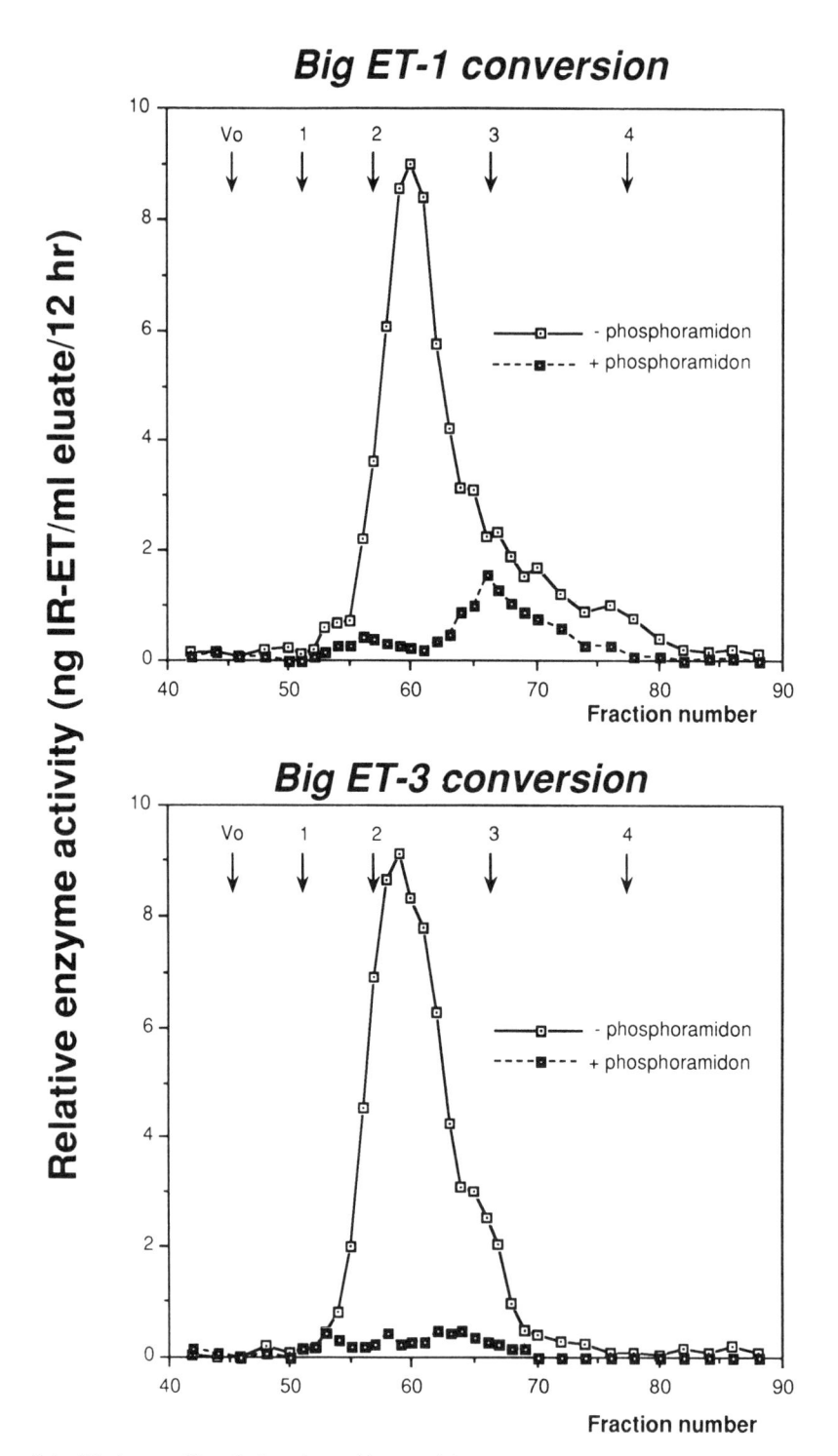

Figure 5.4. Elution profiles of phosphoramidon-sensitive ECE by gel filtration on a Superdex 200 pg column. Each eluate was incubated with big ET-1 or big ET-3 in the presence of 1 mM N-ethylmaleimide for 12 hr. Arrows indicate the elution positions of void volume (Vo) and molecular weight standards: 1, thyroglobulin (669 kD); 2, ferritin (440 kD); 3, catalase (232 kD); 4, bovine serum albumin (67 kD).

lung homogenate. Similar great size of membranous ECE was also found in porcine ECs by us.[60]

Several recent studies[59,61] characterized the membranous ECE as a glycoprotein, based on that ECE activities were able to bind to a concanavalin A-Sepharose column and were eluted by α-methyl-D-glucoside. Ohnaka *et al.*[62] separated a 2100-fold purified ECE from porcine ECs, using sequential chromatography; in their procedure, a lectin (*Ricinus communis* agglutinin) affinity column chromatography was an useful step for the partial purification of ECE. Hence, these affinity column procedures may be a powerful method for the further purification of ECE.

Does phosphoramidon-sensitive ECE convert big ET-2 and big ET-3?

Subsequent to the original discovery of ET-1,[1] an analysis of a human genomic library showed the possible existence of three structurally distinct isopeptides, termed ET-1, ET-2 and ET-3.[63] Several studies have indicated the presence of immunoreactive ET-1, ET-2 and ET-3 in mammalian tissues.[64-66] Based on findings that ET-2 and ET-3 are derived from big ET-2 (1–37) and big ET-3 (1–41), as deduced from sequence analyses of cDNA,[67-69] one can speculate on the possible biosynthetic pathway for ET-2 and ET-3 analogous to ET-1.

In contrast to the conversion of big ET-1, results with regard to the conversion of big ET-3 are conflicting. Okada *et al.*[36] reported that big ET-3 is much less susceptible than big ET-1 to the membrane-bound and phosphoramidon-sensitive ECE of cultured bovine ECs. Takada *et al.*[57] also found no substantial big ET-3-converting activity of cytosolic ECE obtained from cultured bovine ECs. In contrast, using intact cultured bovine ECs, Ohnaka *et al.*[70] noted that exogenously applied big ET-3 (also big ET-2) is converted to the mature ET-3 at a high affinity and that this conversion is abolished by phosphoramidon, in the same manner as seen with big ET-1. We[60] found that partially purified phosphoramidon-sensitive ECE from ECs, with an apparent molecular mass of 300–350 kD, can convert both big ET-1 and big ET-3 to their mature forms, thereby suggesting that enzymes involved in the conversion of big ET-1 and big ET-3 are identical (Figure 5.4). This notion is strongly supported by our recent study indicating that the ECE activity for big ET-1 was inseparable from the big ET-3-converting activity, in four types of chromatography on Cosmogel QA, phenyl-Sepharose, concanavalin A-Sepharose and Superdex 200 pg columns.[61] The apparent K_m and $V_{max.}$ values for big ET-1 (K_m, 1.85 μM; $V_{max.}$, 604 pmol ET-1/mg protein/hr) were about 4-fold higher than those for big ET-3 (K_m, 0.4 μM; $V_{max.}$, 144 pmol ET-3/mg protein/hr).[61]

In vivo studies, using conscious[71] and anesthetized rats,[72,73] demonstrated the pressor effects of big ET-3, which were inhibited efficiently by phosphoramidon. Thus, the phosphoramidon-sensitive ECE appears to be involved at least in the extracellular conversion of big ET-3 to the mature form.

With respect to the biosynthetic pathway for ET-2, a recent paper by Yorimitsu *et al.*[74] demonstrated that big ET-2 (1–38) was converted to ET-2 by phosphoramidonsensitive ECE in cultured human renal adenocarcinoma cells.

ARE ECE INHIBITORS USEFUL TO VASCULAR DISEASES?

It has been documented that ET-1 might participate in various vascular disorders, including coronary vasospasm, cerebral vasospasm following subarachnoid hemorrhage, ischemic acute renal failure, pulmonary hypertension and atherosclerosis.[75,76] Thus, ET-1 receptor antagonists and/or ECE inhibitors may be a novel class of therapeutic drugs for the treatment of such cardiovascular diseases. Discussion on receptor antagonists as therapeutic agents will be made in detail in another chapter. In this section, we describe recent experimental evidences which suggest the usefulness of ECE inhibitors on the cardiovascular diseases.

We first demonstrated that the intracisternal administration of phosphoramidon potently prevents delayed cerebral vasospasm following subarachnoid hemorrhage in a two-hemorrhage canine model,[77] suggesting that ECE inhibitors may be useful as a therapeutic tool for the treatment of the cerebral vasospasm. To determine whether ET-1 is a key factor related to vasospasm after subarachnoid hemorrhage and the effects of phosphoramidon, the local levels of ET-1 in cerebral spastic arteries would need to be determined. Recent study by Clozel and Watanabe[78] using BQ-123, a peptidic ET_A receptor antagonist, also indicated a possible role of ET-1 in the pathogenesis of the cerebral vasospasm.

The relationships between the pathogenesis of myocardial ischemia and ET-1 have been documented.[79] Grover et al.[80] noted that an intravenous administration of phosphoramidon significantly reduced infarct size in a rat model of myocardial ischemia and reperfusion.

Vemulapalli et al.[81] found that phosphoramidon attenuates efficiently the increases in ET-1 release and in pulmonary insufflation pressure induced by ischemia-hypoxia in isolated perfused guinea pig lungs.

Although the role of ET-1 as a causal factor in ischemic or hypoxic injury is still obscure, the above findings suggest a possible usefulness of ECE inhibitors as a therapeutic agent on such cardiopulmonary diseases.

CONCLUSION

It seems likely that ETs play a role as an importnat regulatory factor in various cardiovascular dysfunctions. Since the conversion of big ETs to mature ETs is a rate-limiting factor for the expression of biological actions, specific inhibitors of ECE must be a useful tool for the treatment of cardiovascular diseases. Phosphoramidon-sensitive metalloproteinase, which is not a neutral endopeptidase 24.11, is considered to be the most plausible candidate for physiologically relevant ECE. This type of ECE seems to be a membrane-bound ectoenzyme and widely distributed in vascular and nonvascular tissues, in which it may be responsible for the extracellular conversion of big ETs. Phosphoramidon is an only available inhibitor of this type of ECE. Since phosphoramidon inhibits potently also neutral endopeptidase 24.11, a development of pure ECE inhibitors is necessary to clarify the pathophysiological significance of ETs. Furthermore, the elucidation of biosynthetic mechanisms of ETs must await the purification of ECE and/or cloning of the ECE gene.

References

1. Yanagisawa, M., Kurihara, H., Kimura, S., Tomobe, Y., Kobayashi, M., Mitsui, Y., Yazaki, Y., Goto, K. and Masaki, T. (1988) A novel vasoconstrictor peptide produced by vascular endothelial cells. *Nature*, **332**, 411–415.
2. Kimura, S., Kasuya, Y., Sawamura, T., Shinmi, O., Sugita, Y., Yanagisawa, M., Goto, K. and Masaki, T. (1989) Conversion of big endothelin-1 to 21-residue endothelin-1 is essential for expression of full vasoconstrictor activity: Structure-activity relationships of big endothelin-1. *J. Cardiovasc. Pharmacol.*, **13 (Suppl 5)**, S5–S7.
3. Kashiwabara, T., Inagaki, Y., Ohta, H., Iwamatsu, A., Nomizu, M., Morita, A. and Nishikori, K. (1989) Putative precursors of endothelin have less vasoconstrictor activity *in vitro* but a potent pressor effect *in vivo*. *FEBS Lett.*, **247**, 73–76.
4. Emori, T., Hirata, Y., Ohta, K., Shichiri, M., Shimokado, K. and Marumo, F. (1989) Concomitant secretion of big endothelin and its C-terminal fragment from human and bovine endothelin cells. *Bi chem. Biophys. Res. Commun.*, **162**, 217–223.
5. Sawamura, T., Kimura, S., Shinmi, O., Sugita, Y., Yanagisawa, M. and Masaki, T. (1989) Analysis of endothelin related peptides in culture supernatant of porcine aortic endothelial cells. *Biochem. Biophys. Res. Commun.*, **162**, 1287–1294.
6. McMahon, E. G., Fok, K. F., Moore, W. M., Smith, C. E., Siegel, N. R. and Trapani, A. J. (1989) *In vitro* and *in vivo* activity of chymotrypsin-activated big endothelin (porcine 1–40). *Biochem. Biophys. Res. Commun.*, **161**, 406–413.
7. Takaoka, M., Miyata, Y., Takenobu, Y., Ikegawa, R., Matsumura, Y. and Morimoto, S. (1990) Mode of cleavage of pig big endothelin-1 by chymotrypsin: Production and degradation of mature endothelin-1. *Biochem. J.*, **270**, 541–544.
8. Wypij, D. M., Nichols, J. S., Novak, P. J., Stacy, D. L., Berman, J. and Wiseman, J. S. (1992) Role of mast cell chymase in the extracellular processing of big-endothelin-1 to endothelin-1 in the perfused rat lung. *Biochem. Pharmacol.*, **43**, 845–853.
9. Hisaki, K., Matsumura, Y., Maekawa, H., Fujita, K., Takaoka, M. and Morimoto, S. (1994) Functional conversion of big endothelin-1 to endothelin-1 in the isolated perfused rat lung: The role of phosphoramidon-sensitive endothelin-1 converting enzyme. *Am. J. Physiol.*, **266**, H422–H428.
10. Matsumura, Y., Ikegawa, R., Takaoka, M. and Morimoto, S. (1990) Conversion of porcine big endothelin to endothelin by an extract from the porcine aortic endothelial cells. *Biochem. Biophys. Res. Commun.*, **167**, 203–210.
11. Ikegawa, R., Matsumura, Y., Takaoka, M. and Morimoto, S. (1990) Evidence for pepstatin-sensitive conversion of porcine big endothelin-1 to endothelin-1 by the endothelial cell extract. *Biochem. Biophys. Res. Commun.*, **167**, 860–866.
12. Ohnaka, K., Takayanagi, R., Yamauchi, T., Okazaki, H., Ohashi, M., Umeda, F. and Nawata, H. (1990) Identification and characterization of endothelin converting activity in cultured bovine endothelial cells. *Biochem. Bipolys. Res. Commun.*, **168**, 1128–1136.
13. Sawamura, T., Kimura, S., Shinmi, O., Sugita, Y., Kobayashi, M., Mitsui, Y., Yanagisawa, M., Goto, K. and Masaki, T. (1990) Characterization of endothelin converting enzyme activities in soluble fraction of bovine cultured endothelial cells. *Biochem. Biophys. Res. Commun.*, **169**, 1138–1144.
14. Sawamura, T., Kimura, S., Shinmi, O., Sugita, Y., Yanagisawa, M., Goto, K. and Masaki, T. (1990) Purification and characterization of putative endothelin converting enzyme in bovine adrenal medulla: Evidence for a cathepsin D-like enzyme. *Biochem. Biophys. Res. Commun.*, **168**, 1230–1236.
15. Wu-Wong, J. R., Budzik, G. P., Devine, E. M. and Opgenorth, T. J. (1990) Characterization of endothelin converting enzyme in rat lung. *Biochem. Biophys. Res. Commun.*, **171**, 1291–1296.
16. Takaoka, M., Takenobu, Y., Miyata, Y., Ikegawa, R., Matsumura, Y. and Morimoto, S. (1990) Pepsin, An aspartic protease, converts porcine big endothelin to 21-residue endothelin. *Biochem. Biophys. Res. Commun.*, **166**, 436–442.
17. Lees, W. E., Kalinka, S., Meech, J., Capper, S. J., Cook, N. D. and Kay, J. (1990) Generation of human endothelin by cathepsin E. *FEBS Lett.*, **273**, 99–102.
18. Sawamura, T., Shinmi, O., Kishi, N., Sugita, Y., Yanagisawa, M., Goto, K., Masaki, T. and Kimura, S. (1990) Analysis of big endothelin-1 digestion by cathepsin D. *Biochem. Biophys. Res. Commun.*, **172**, 883–889.
19. Takaoka, M., Hukumori, Y., Shiragami, K., Ikegawa, R., Matsumura, Y. and Morimoto, S. (1990) Proteolytic processing of porcine big endothelin-1 catalyzed by cathepsin D. *Biochem. Biophys. Res. Commun.*, **173**, 1218–1223.
20. Shields, P. P., Gonzales, T. A., Charles, D., Gilligan, J. P. and Stern, W. (1991) Accumulation of pepstatin in cultured endothelial cells and its effect on endothelin processing. *Biochem. Biophys. Res. Commun.*, **177**, 1006–1012.

21. Bird, J. E., Waldron, T. L., Little, D. K., Asaad, M. M., Dorso, C. R., DiDonato, G. and Norman, J. A. (1992) The effects of novel cathepsin E inhibitors on the big endothelin pressor response in conscious rats. *Biochem. Biophys. Res. Commun.*, **182**, 224–231.
22. Sasahara, M., Hazama, F., Amano, S., Hayase, Y., Yukioka, N., Kawai, J. and Kataoka, H. (1988) Effect of hypertension on lysosomal enzyme activities in aortic endothelial cells. *Atherosclerosis*, **70**, 53–62.
23. D'Orléans-Juste, P., Lidbury, P. S., Warner, T. D. and Vane, J. R. (1990) Intravascular big endothelin increases circulating levels of endothelin-1 and prostanoids in the rabbit. *Biochem. Pharmacol.*, **39**, R21–R22.
24. Matsumura, Y., Hisaki, K., Takaoka, M. and Morimoto, S. (1990) Phosphoramidon, a metalloproteinase inhibitor, suppresses the hypertensive effect of big endothelin-1. *Eur. J. Pharmacol.*, **185**, 103–106.
25. Fukuroda, T., Noguchi, K., Tsuchida, S., Nishikibe, M., Ikemoto, F., Okada, K. and Yano, M. (1990) Inhibition of biological actions of big endothelin-1 by phosphoramidon. *Biochem. Biophys. Res. Commun.*, **172**, 390–395.
26. McMahon, E. G., Palomo, M. A., Moore, W. M., McDonald, J. F. and Stern, M. K. (1991) Phosphoramidon blocks the pressor activity of porcine big endothelin-1-(1–39) *in vivo* and conversion of big endothelin-1-(1–39) to endothelin-1-(1–21) *in vitro*. *Proc. Natl. Acad Sci.*, **88**, 703–707.
27. Pollock, D. M. and Opgenorth, T. J. (1991) Evidence for metalloprotease involvement in the *in vivo* effects of big endothelin-1. *Am. J. Physiol.*, **261**, R257–R263.
28. Pollock, D. M. and Opgenorth, T. J. (1991) Comparison of the hemodynamic effects of endothelin-1 and big endothelin-1 in the rat. *Biochem. Biophys. Res. Commun.*, **179**, 1122–1126.
29. Gardiner, S. M., Compton, A. M., Kemp, P. A. and Bennett, T. (1991) The effects of phosphoramidon on the regional haemodynamic responses to human proendothelin [1–38] in conscious rats. *Br. J. Pharmacol.*, **103**, 2009–2015.
30. Le Monnier de Gouville, A-C. and Cavero, I. (1991) Cross tachyphylaxis to endothelin isopeptide-induced hypotension: A phenomenon not seen with proendothelin. *Br. J. Pharmacol.*, **104**, 77–84.
31. D'Orléans-Juste, P., Télémaque, S. and Claing, A. (1991) Different pharmacological profiles of big-endothelin-3 and big-endothelin-1 *in vivo* and *in vitro*. *Br. J. Pharmacol.*, **104**, 440–444.
32. Gardiner, S. M., Kemp, P. A. and Bennett, T. (1992) Effects of the neutral endopeptidase inhibitor, SQ28,603, on regional haemodynamic responses to atrial natriuretic peptide or proendothelin-1 [1–38] in conscious rats. *Br. J. Pharmacol.*, **106**, 180–186.
33. Gardiner, S. M., Kemp, P. A., Compton, A. M. and Bennett, T. (1992) Coeliac haemodynamic effects of endothelin-1, endothelin-3, proendothelin-1 [1–38] and proendothelin-3 [1–41] in conscious rats. *Br. J. Pharmacol.*, **106**, 483–488.
34. Salvati, P., Dho, L., Calabresi, M., Rosa, B. and Patrono, C. (1992) Evidence for a direct vasoconstrictor effect of big endothelin-1 in the rat kidney. *Eur. J. Pharmacol.*, **221**, 267–273.
35. Matsumura, Y., Ikegawa, R., Tsukahara, Y., Takaoka, M. and Morimoto, S. (1990) Conversion of big endothelin-1 to endothelin-1 by two types of metalloproteinases derived from porcine aortic endothelial cells. *FEBS Lett.*, **272**, 166–170.
36. Okada, K., Miyazaki, Y., Takada, J., Matsuyama, K., Yamaki, T. and Yano, M. (1990) Conversion of big endothelin-1 by membrane-bound metalloendopeptidase in cultured bovine endothelial cells. *Biochem. Biophys. Res. Commun.*, **171**, 1192–1198.
37. Ikegawa, R., Matsumura, Y., Tsukahara, Y., Takaoka, M. and Morimoto, S. (1990) Phosphoramidon, a metalloproteinase inhibitor, suppresses the secretion of endothelin-1 from cultured endothelin cells by inhibiting a big endothelin-1 converting enzyme. *Biochem. Biophys. Res. Commun.*, **171**, 669–675.
38. Matsumura, Y., Ikegawa, R., Tsukahara, Y., Takaoka, M. and Morimoto, S. (1991) N-Ethylmaleimide differentiates endothelin converting activity by two types of metalloproteinases derived from vascular endothelial cells. *Biochem. Biophys. Res. Commun.*, **178**, 531–538.
39. Okada, K., Takada, J., Arai, Y., Matsuyama, K. and Yano, M. (1991) Importance of the C-terminal region of big endothelin-1 for specific conversion by phosphoramidon-sensitive endothelin converting enzyme. *Biochem. Biophys. Res. Commun.*, **180**, 1019–1023.
40. Ahn, K., Beningo, K., Olds, G. and Hupe, D. (1992) The endothelin-converting enzyme from human umbilical vein is a membrane-bound metalloprotease similar to that from bovine aortic endothelial cells. *Proc. Natl. Acad. Sci.*, **89**, 8606–8610.
41. Warner, T. D., Mitchell, J. A., D'Orléans-Juste, P., Ishi, K., Förstermann, U. and Murad, F. (1992) Characterization of endothelin-converting enzyme from endothelial cells and rat brain: Detection of the formation of biologically active endothelin-1 by rapid bioassay. *Mol. Pharmacol.*, **41**, 399–403.
42. Matsumura, Y., Umekawa, T., Kawamura, H., Takaoka, M., Robinson, P. S., Cook, N. D. and Morimoto, S. (1992) A simple method for measurement of phosphoramidon-sensitive endothelin converting enzyme activity. *Life Sci.*, **51**, 1603–1611.

43. Ohnaka, K., Takayanagi, R., Ohashi, M. and Nawata, H. (1991) Conversion of big endothelin isopeptides to mature endothelin isopeptides by cultured bovine endothelial cells. *J. Cardiovasc. Pharmacol.*, **17 (Suppl 7)**, S17–S19.
44. Hisaki, K., Matsumura, Y., Ikegawa, R., Nishiguchi, S., Hayashi, K., Takaoka, M. and Morimoto, S. (1991) Evidence for phosphoramidon-sensitive conversion of big endothelin-1 to endothelin-1 in isolated rat mesenteric artery. *Biochem. Biophys. Res. Commun.*, **177**, 1127–1132.
45. Hisaki, K., Matsumura, Y., Nishiguchi, S., Fujita, K., Takaoka, M. and Morimoto, S. (1993) Endothelium- independent pressor effect of big endothelin-1 and its inhibition by phosphoramidon in rat mesenteric artery. *Eur. J. Pharmacol.*, **241**, 75–81.
46. Matsumura, Y., Ikegawa, R., Tsukahara, Y., Takaoka, M. and Morimoto, S. (1991) Conversion of big endothelin-1 to endothelin-1 by two-types of metalloproteinases of cultured porcine vascular smooth muscle cells. *Biochem. Biophys. Res. Commun.*, **178**, 899–905.
47. Hioki, Y., Okada, K., Ito, H., Matsuyama, K. and Yano, M. (1991) Endothelin converting enzyme of bovine carotid artery smooth muscles. *Biochem. Biophys. Res. Commun.*, **174**, 446–451.
48. Ikegawa, R., Matsumura, Y., Tsukahara, Y., Takaoka, M. and Morimoto, S. (1991) Phosphoramidon inhibits the generation of endothelin-1 from exogeneously applied big endothelin-1 in cultured vascular endothelial cells and smooth muscle cells. *FEBS Lett.*, **293**, 45–48.
49. Sessa, W. C., Kaw, S., Hecker, M. and Vane, J. R. (1991) The biosynthesis of endothelin-1 by human polymorphonuclear leukocytes. *Biochem. Biophys. Res. Commun.*, **174**, 613–618.
50. Noguchi, K., Fukuroda, T., Ikeno, Y., Hirose, H., Tsukada, Y., Nishikibe, M., Ikemoto, F., Matsuyama, K. and Yano, M. (1991) Local formation and degradation of endothelin-1 in guinea pig airway tissues. *Biochem. Biophys. Res. Commun.*, **179**, 830–835
51. Shinyama, H., Uchida, T., Kido, H., Hayashi, K., Watanabe, M., Matsumura, Y., Ikegawa, R., Takaoka, M. and Morimoto, S. (1991) Phosphoramidon inhibits the conversion of intracisternally administered big endothelin-1 to endothelin-1. *Biochem. Biophys. Res. Commun.*, **178**, 24–30.
52. Hashim, M. A. and Tadepalli, A. S. (1991) Functional evidence for the presence of a phosphoramidon-sensitive enzyme in rat brain that converts big endothelin-1 to endothelin-1. *Life Sci.*, **49**, PL207–PL211.
53. Télémaque, S. and D'Orléans-Juste, P. (1991) Presence of a phosphoramidon-sensitive endothelin-converting enzyme which converts big-endothelin-1, but not big-endothelin-3, in the rat vas deferens. *Naunyn-Schmiedeberg's Arch. Pharmacol.*, **344**, 505–507.
54. Advenier, C., Lagente, V., Zhang, Y. and Naline, E. (1992) Contractile activity of big endothelin-1 on the human isolated bronchus. *Br. J. Pharmacol.*, **106**, 883–887.
55. Takada, J., Hata, M., Okada, K., Matsuyama, K. and Yano, M. (1992) Biochemical properties of endothelin converting enzyme in renal epithelial cell lines. *Biochem. Biophys. Res. Commun.*, **182**, 1383–1388.
56. Kundu, G. C. and Wilson, I. B. (1992) Identification of endothelin converting enzyme in bovine lung membranes using a new fluorogenic substrate. *Life Sci.*, **50**, 965–970.
57. Takada, J., Okada, K., Ikenaga, T., Matsuyama, K. and Yano, M. (1991) Phosphoramidon-sensitive endothelin-converting enzyme in the cytosol of cultured bovine endothelial cells. *Biochem. Biophys. Res. Commun.*, **176**, 860–865.
58. Takaoka, M., Shiragami, K., Fujino, K., Miki, K., Miyake, Y., Yasuda, M., Wang, G-F., Hisaki, K., Matsumura, Y. and Morimoto, S. (1991) Phosphoramidon-sensitive endothelin converting enzyme in rat lung. *Biochem. Int.*, **25**, 697–704.
59. Sawamura, T., Shinmi, O., Kishi, N., Sugita, Y., Yanagisawa, M., Goto, K., Masaki, T. and Kimura, S. (1993) Characterization of phosphoramidon-sensitive metalloproteinases with endothelin-converting enzyme activity in porcine lung membrane. *Biochim. Biophys. Acta*, **1161**, 295–302.
60. Matsumura, Y., Tsukahara, Y., Kuninobu, K., Takaoka, M., and Morimoto, S. (1992) Phosphoramidon-sensitive endothelin-converting enzyme in vascular endothelial cells converts big endothelin-1 and big endothelin-3 to their mature form. *FEBS Lett.*, **305**, 86–90.
61. Takaoka, M., Fujino, K., Miki, K., Matsumura, Y. and Morimoto, S. A phosphoramidon-sensitive endothelin-converting enzyme in rat lung membrane recognizes both big endothelin-1 and -3 as substrate. (submitted).
62. Ohnaka, K., Nishikawa, M., Takayanagi, R., Haji, M. and Nawata, H. (1992) Partial purification of phosphoramidon-sensitive endothelin converting enzyme in porcine aortic endothelial cells: High affinity for *ricinus communis* agglutinin. *Biochem. Biophys. Res. Commun.*, **185**, 611–616.
63. Inoue, A., Yanagisawa, M., Kimura, S., Kasuya, Y., Miyauchi, T., Goto, K. and Masaki, T. (1989) The human endothelin family: Three structurally and pharmacologically distinct isopeptides predicted by three separate genes. *Proc. Natl. Acad. Sci.*, **86**, 2863–2867.
64. Matsumoto, H., Suzuki, N., Onda, H. and Fujino, M. (1989) Abundance of endothelin-3 in rat intestine, pituitary gland and brain. *Biochem. Biophys. Res. Commun.*, **164**, 74–80.

65. Shinmi, O., Kimura, S., Sawamura, T., Sugita, Y., Yoshizawa, T., Uchiyama, Y., Yanagisawa, M., Goto, K., Masaki, T. and Kanazawa, I. (1989) Endothelin-3 is a novel neuropeptide: Isolation and sequence determination of endothelin-1 and endothelin-3 in porcine brain. *Biochem. Biophys. Res. Commun.*, **164**, 587–593.
66. Kosaka, T., Suzuki, N., Matsumoto, H., Itoh, Y., Yasuhara, T., Onda, H. and Fujino, M. (1989) Synthesis of the vasoconstrictor peptide endothelin in kidney cells. *FEBS Lett.*, **249**, 42–46.
67. Bloch, K. D., Eddy, R. L., Shows, T. B. and Quertermous, T. (1989) cDNA cloning and chromosomal assignment of the gene encoding endothelin-3. *J. Biol. Chem.*, **264**, 18156–18161.
68. Onda, H., Ohkubo, S., Ogi, K., Kosaka, T., Kimura, C., Matsumoto, H., Suzuki, N. and Fujino, M. (1990) One of the endothelin gene family, endothelin 3 gene, is expressed in the placenta. *FEBS Lett.*, **261**, 327–330.
69. Bloch, K. B., Hong, C. C., Eddy, R. L., Shows, T. B. and Quertermous, T. (1991) cDNA cloning and chromosomal assignment of the endothelin 2 gene: Vasoactive intestinal contractor peptide is rat endothelin 2. *Genomics*, **10**, 236–242.
70. Ohnaka, K., Takayanagi, T., Yamauchi, T., Umeda, F. and Nawata, H. (1991) Cultured bovine endothelial cells convert big endothelin isopeptides to mature endothelin isopeptides. *Biochem. Int.*, **23**, 499–506.
71. Gardiner, S. M., Kemp, P. A. and Bennett, T. (1992) Inhibition by phosphoramidon of the regional haemodynamic effects of proendothelin-2 and -3 in conscious rats. *Br. J. Pharmacol.*, **107**, 584–590.
72. Matsumura, Y., Fujita, K., Takaoka, M. and Morimoto, S. (1993) Big endothelin-3-induced hypertension and its inhibition by phosphoramidon in anaesthetized rats. *Eur. J. Pharmacol.*, **230**, 89–93.
73. Pollock, D. M., Divish, B. J., Milicic, I., Novosad, E. I., Burres, N. S. and Opgenorth, T. J. (1993) *In vivo* characterization of a phosphoramidon-sensitive endothelin-converting enzyme in the rat. *Eur. J. Pharmacol.*, **231**, 459–464.
74. Yorimitsu, K., Shinmi, O., Nishiyama, M., Moroi, K., Sugita, Y., Saito, T., Inagaki, Y., Masaki, T. and Kimura, S. (1992) Effect of phosphoramidon on big endothelin-2 conversion into endothelin-2 in human renal adenocarcinoma (ACHN) cells. *FEBS Lett.*, **314**, 395–398.
75. Masaki, T., Kimura, S., Yanagisawa, M. and Goto, K. (1991) Molecular and cellular mechanism of endothelin regulation: Implications for vascular function. *Circulation*, **84**, 1457–1468.
76. Rubanyi, G. M. and Botelho, L. H. P. (1991) Endothelins. *FASEB J.*, **5**, 2713–2720.
77. Matsumura, Y., Ikegawa, R., Suzuki, Y., Takaoka, M., Uchida, T., Kido, H., Shinyama, H., Hayashi, K., Watanabe, M. and Morimot, S. (1991) Phosphoramidon prevents cerebral vasospasm following subarachnoid hemorrhage in dogs: The relationship to endothelin-1 levels in the cerebrospinal fluid. *Life Sci.*, **49**, 841–848.
78. Clozel, M. and Watanabe, H. (1993) BQ-123, a peptidic endothelin ET_A receptor antagonist, prevents the early cerebral vasospasm following subarachnoid hemorrhage after intracisternal but not intravenous injection. *Life Sci.*, **52**, 825–834.
79. Watanabe, T., Suzuki, N., Shimamoto, N., Fujino, M. and Imada, A. (1991) Contribution of endogenous endothelin to the extension of myocardial infarct size in rats. *Circ. Res.*, **69**, 370–377.
80. Grover, G. J., Sleph, P. G., Fox, M. and Trippodo, N. C. (1992) Role of endothelin-1 and big endothelin-1 in modulating coronary vascular tone, contractile function and severity of ischemia in rat hearts. *J. Pharmacol. Exp. Ther.*, **263**, 1074–1082.
81. Vemulapalli, S., Rivelli, M., Chiu, P. J. S., Prado, M. and Hey, J. A. (1992) Phosphoramidon abolishes the increases in endothelin-1 release induced by ischemia-hypoxia in isolated perfused guinea pig lungs. *J. Pharmacol. Exp. Ther.*, **262**, 1062–1069.

6 Pharmacological Interactions of Endothelin with Various Regulatory Agents

Sam Rebello and Anil Gulati

Department of Pharmaceutics & Pharmacodynamics, University of Illinois at Chicago, 833 S. Wood Street, Chicago, IL 60612, USA

INTRODUCTION

Endothelins (ETs) are a family of peptides which have been implicated in the regulation of a complex array of cellular functions through a multitude of interactions. The direct action of ET via activation of its receptors, and its interactions with various regulatory agents, all occurring simultaneously, governs the final response of ET. During the past few years, investigations in many laboratories have shown that these interactions are involved in a variety of physiological functions, involving the cardiovascular, renal, pulmonary, endocrine and central nervous system. Considering this fact, it was thought necessary to review these interactions in a separate chapter.

ENDOTHELIN INTERACTIONS WITH VASOACTIVE AGENTS

EDRF (Endothelium derived relaxing factor)

The endothelial cell has a unique intrinsic feature; it produces the most potent vasoconstrictor peptide (ET-1), and yet it also releases an equally potent vasodilator substance, endothelium-derived relaxing factor (EDRF/NO). It is apparent that under normal physiological conditions there exists a delicate balance between endothelium-derived contracting and relaxing factors. ET is known to cause an initial and transient vasodilation followed by a sustained vasoconstriction. The vasodilation is thought to be via the activation of ET_B receptor which causes release of vasodilators, one of which is the EDRF[1-4]. ET-3 is more potent in releasing NO[1], and it is known that NO mediates the vasoactive effects of ET-3 in rat mesenteric microvascular beds[5]. Acetylcholine[6-9] and bradykinin[6,7,10] antagonize the contractile actions of ET by receptor mediated release of EDRF. In contrast to arteries, the effect of ET is particularly pronounced in the veins because in veins the potency of EDRF to antagonize ET-induced contractions is less marked[6,7,11]. ET-1 produces a marked change in the membrane-depolarization of canine veins as compared to that of arteries[11]. This strong depolarization produced by ET may blunt the hyperpolarization produced by EDRF, thereby dominating the effects of the latter. Thus, in human forearm microcirculation, ET-1 dominates the actions of NO[12]. It appears that ET may be interfering with the cGMP-dependent mechanisms of EDRF to relax the vasculature.

EDRF has also been reported to modulate the actions of ET. EDRF suppresses the release of ET from endothelial cells[13] and it mediates the antiaggregatory action of ET on platelets[14]. cGMP, a second messenger for EDRF, has been shown to inhibit inositol phosphate formation in rat aorta and bovine aortic smooth muscle cells[15]. cGMP also inhibited the activation of protein kinase C (PKC) by ET[16]. By these mechanisms, cGMP can interfere with the signal transduction of ET. Therefore, EDRF appears to be one of the physiological modulators of ET[17] which can prevent excessive vasoconstriction and thrombotic occlusion of the vascular bed. Impaired production of EDRF, as in hyperlipidemia, hypertension, or atherosclerosis could result in an unopposed release of ET and pathological constriction of diseased blood vessels.

Thrombin

Thrombin exhibits a variety of interactions with ET. The expression of ET gene is stimulated by thrombin in endothelial cells[18] and mesangial cells[19]. It releases ET-1 and big-ET-1 from porcine aortic strips with endothelium[20], ET-1 from isolated rat glomeruli and mesangial cells[21], rabbit tracheal epithelial cells[22] and astrocytes[23], by a mechanism that probably involves intracellular calcium mobilization and activation of PKC[24]. In intact porcine aorta, L-NMMA augments the thrombin-induced release of ET. Moreover, nitroglycerin (a substance which produces EDRF), superoxide dismutase (an enzyme which inhibits the breakdown of EDRF by superoxide ions), and 8-bromo-cGMP (a nonhydrolyzable analog of cGMP) significantly inhibits the thrombin-induced ET production by intact porcine aorta[13,25]. These observations suggest that thrombin may have a modulatory effect on ET production via EDRF's cGMP dependent mechanism. Thrombin also stimulates ET-1 release by affecting the *de novo* synthesis since it was shown that cycloheximide, a protein synthesis inhibitor, blocked its effect in human umbilical vein endothelial cells[26]. Inhibition of phosphorylation of myosin light chain kinase (MLCK) blocked thrombin-stimulated ET release, indicating that myosin light chain phosphorylation elicited by MLCK may facilitate the formation of filamentous myosin and actin, which are probably involved in ET-1 secretion[27].

Since thrombin is generated during clotting of blood, an increased production and release of ET-1 from endothelial cells may be of importance in the pathogenesis of vasospasm associated with activation of the coagulation cascade. Activation of the coagulation cascade with concomitant formation of thrombin is a known event in unstable angina and myocardial infarction. Thrombin stimulates platelet aggregation, whereas ET inhibits it[28,29]. ET-1 inhibits the release of plasminogen activator inhibitor (PAI-1) antigen[30], and has a suppressive effect on thrombin-stimulated release of both tissue plasminogen activator (t-PA) and plasminogen activator inhibitor (PAI-1) from endothelial cells[31]. This suggests that ET-1 has an antifibrinolytic action on thrombin-induced fibrinolysis. When local blood flow decreases, the coagulation cascade is activated, and during such circumstances thrombin-induced ET release may contribute to the vasospasm. However, since thrombin can also release TXA_2 and EDRF there can be a close interplay between thrombin induced ET synthesis and modulation of ET-induced vasoconstriction by EDRF and TXA_2. Since ET-1 can potentiate the thrombin-induced DNA synthesis in vascular smooth muscle cells[32], these interactions may be of significant importance during vascular injury.

Atrial Natriuretic Peptide (ANP)

Human ANP is a 28 amino acid peptide derived from cardiac myocytes, which is secreted in response to atrial tension (after volume expansion, hypertension, or salt overload) and it causes natriuresis and diuresis. ET-1 has been be shown to stimulate ANP secretion in atrial[33] or ventricular[34] myocytes of newborn rats. Low doses of ET-1 exert a short acting and prostanoid mediated inhibitory action, whereas high doses cause a long-lasting stimulation of ANP[35]. ET-1 induced rise in blood pressure in newborn calves[36], or left atrial pressure in dogs[37], or right atrial pressure in pigs[38] was positively correlated with ANP levels. This increase was seen even at subpressor doses where no change in the blood pressure was observed[36], indicating that ET affects ANP release not only via changes in the hemodynamic parameters, but it may also exert direct action on the cardiac myocytes[39,40]. Therefore, apart from stretch stimulus, the endothelium may serve as an additional sensor and facilitate ANP release via ET-1. This is evident from increased levels of ANP in co-cultures of bovine aortic endothelial cells and neonatal rat atrial myocytes[41]. Moreover, it has been proposed that ANP and ET-1 signalling systems coexist in the endothelial cells and that the ET-1 signal negates the ANP-dependent guanylyl cyclase activation and cGMP formation[42]. The possibility of ET-1 as a physiological modulator of both basal and stimulated ANP release also exists[43]. In anesthetized dogs, ANP (26 pmol/kg/min) alone decreased the blood pressure, cardiac output, plasma aldosterone and plasma renin activity, whereas ET-1 (12 pmol/kg/min) attenuated the ANP response by increasing the blood pressure and renin activity without changing the aldosterone levels. ET-1 further potentiated the decrease in cardiac output and increase in total peripheral resistance induced by ANP[44]. ANP inhibited angiotensin-II (A-II) or thrombin stimulated release of ET-1 from human umbilical vein endothelial cells[45,46] and arginine-vasopressin-stimulated ET-1 secretion from mesangial cells[47]. Therefore, circulating ANP may suppress excess secretion of ET-1 caused by activation of the renin-angiotensin system and the coagulation cascade. It appears that there may be a reciprocal paracrine interaction between ANP and ET-1 in regulation of vascular tonus and fluid homeostasis.

Arginine-vasopressin (AVP)

Both ET and AVP are co-localized within freshly isolated endothelial cells of the rabbit thoracic aorta[48]. AVP has been shown to stimulate the gene expression of ET-1 in endothelial cells[49], rat mesenteric arterial beds[50] and human VSMC[51]. The mitogenic actions of AVP on human mesangial cells is mediated, at least in part, via ET-1 production[52]. During the infusion of vasopressin (VP), the increase in mean pressure was accompanied by an 85% increase in plasma ET-1[53], whereas ET-1 infusion increased plasma VP[54,55]. Centrally administered ET-1 can also produce an increase in plasma VP[56]. Increased VP may potentiate the atrial stretching mediated by ANP release. This is because peripheral administration of VP has been reported to release ANP via V_1-receptor, under expansion of extracellular fluid volume accompanied by increase in blood pressure or right atrial pressure[57,58].

Locally synthesized ET has been shown to interact with the regulatory mechanisms of the inner medullary collecting ducts (IMCD) to influence renal water handling. Despite the decrease in glomerular filtration rate (GFR) and renal blood flow due to its vasoconstrictor action, ET has a diuretic effect, suggesting a direct tubular action. The water diuresis induced by ET-1 can be antagonized by antidiuretic hormone (ADH) infusion[59]. The IMCD appears to be an important site where ET exerts its actions. In the IMCD, ET-1 inhibits AVP-induced cAMP accumulation[60] and water permeability[61]. ET-1 causes a rapid, dose-dependent and reversible fall in AVP- but not cAMP-stimulated water permeability[62,63]. The ET-1 effect on AVP-stimulated water permeability is completely blocked by PKC inhibitor (calphostin) or pertussis toxin, but not by indomethacin[63]. These results suggest that ET-1 interacts with AVP signal prior to cAMP formation via PKC, and pertussis toxin-sensitive mechanisms. It is also possible that ET-stimulated ANP release might have inhibited the action of VP on the renal collecting ducts. A local ADH-antagonistic action of endogenous ET-1 is also possible because ET receptors are present in the renal inner medulla[64]. Furthermore, the demonstration of preproET mRNA in IMCD cells[65], the presence of immunoreactive ET in the medullary tissue[66], and the magnitude of ET release from the collecting duct epithelium suggests that ET-1 may serve as an autocrine regulator of AVP action in the IMCD.

Calcitonin-Gene Related Peptide (CGRP)

CGRP is a potent vasodilator is sensory nerve fibers which is released in the ocular area following trigeminal stimulation, and causes dilation of cerebral and ocular vessels. It is colocalized with ET-1 in the neuroepithelial bodies of intrapulmonary airways and alveolar parenchyma of newborn mammals[67]. Co-infusion of ET and CGRP in rats inhibited the ET-induced hypertension and reversed hindquarter vasoconstriction, but did not change the ET-induced vasoconstriction in the renal and mesenteric beds[68]. This indicates that the ability of CGRP to counteract ET effects may be dependent on the vascular bed. CGRP decreases ET-1-induced contractions and ET-1 decreases CGRP-induced relaxations[69]. The similar time courses of their effect and high potencies indicate that the two peptides regulate or even counteract each other *in vivo*. This interaction can be of pathophysiological significance because increased levels of CGRP[70] and ET[71] have been reported in subarachnoid hemorrhage.

ENDOTHELIN AND RENIN-ANGIOTENSIN SYSTEM

The renin-angiotensin system acts as a principal regulator of the extracellular fluid volume. ET-1 has actions similar to angiotensin-II (A-II), in that it can also cause a net reabsorption of Na^+ from the proximal tubules. ET-1 and A-II exhibit a synergistic effect on the systolic pressure when given at subthreshold doses[72]. A-II stimulates ET gene expression in endothelial cells[73–75], vascular smooth muscle cells (VSMC)[51,76] and cardiomyocytes[77]. It also increases the production of ET-1 in human endothelial[78], VSMC[51] and mesangial[79] cells. In spontaneously hypertensive rat mesenteric resistance arteries with intact endothelium, stimulation of ET-1 production by A-II augments the contractile responses to norepinephrine. This effect could be antagonized by phosphoramidon[80]. Moreover, ET receptors are subjected to heterologous regulation by A-II. Rat aortic smooth muscle cells, incubated with A-II for 18 h at 37°C, exhibited dose-dependent down-regulation of ET-1 binding sites without affecting the affinity. This effect was simulated by phorbol-12,13-dibutyrate, a PKC activator, and blocked by Sar1-Ile8-A-II, an A-II receptor antagonist, showing that A-II selectively down-regulated ET binding sites in vascular smooth muscle cells by a mechanism involving protein kinase C[81]. In cultured neonatal rat cardiomyocytes, A-II selectively upregulates ET_B receptors via AT_1 receptors[82]. On the other hand, in rat aortic smooth muscle cells, ET-1 treatment decreased AT_2 binding sites by 45%[83], and in cultured pulmonary artery endothelial cells ET-1 stimulated the conversion of A-I to A-II[84]. The physiological significance of this interaction needs further investigation.

Systemic infusions of ET-1 dramatically elevate the plasma renin activity as well as aldosterone levels[54,55]. The increase in aldosterone can be indirect via renin activation, or due to direct action of ET-1 on the adrenal glomerulosa cells[85]. It was also shown that ET-1 exerts a direct stimulation of aldosterone secretion[86] in a Ca^{+2}-dependent manner, and it potentiates A-II mediated aldosterone stimulation through a mechanism involving PKC[87]. ET-1 can also activate the vascular renin-angiotensin system which might lead to increase in plasma levels of renin[88]. However, *in vitro* studies employing superfused juxtaglomerular cells[89–91], renal cortical slices[89,92] and isolated glomeruli[93] show that ET-1 inhibits renin. These results indicate that ET can modulate renin release depending upon whether it is acting as a locally produced, or as a circulating peptide. When secreted locally it may inhibit renin and aldosterone release, thereby reducing Na^+ reabsorption and increasing Na^+ excretion. The effect of locally produced ET can be further modulated by EDRF which has been shown to inhibit renin release *in vitro*[94], and by PGI_2 and PGE_2 which are renin secretagogues[95,96]. Thus the renin-ET interaction can be further complicated by diverse signals from the renal endothelium which lies adjacent to the renin-producing juxtaglomerular cells. On the other hand, high levels of circulating ET can increase renin release either by direct action on the adrenal glomerulosa cells, or indirectly by producing renal vasoconstriction. Renin can further increase ET-stimulated aldosterone release and thereby enhance reabsorption and decrease excretion of sodium.

ENDOTHELIN INTERACTIONS WITH THE MEDIATORS OF INFLAMMATION

Prostaglandins

In addition to EDRF, eicosanoids (PGI$_2$, PGE$_2$, PGD$_2$ and TXA$_2$) are other products released due to activation of ET$_B$ receptors on the endothelial cells[97-99]. This may be another compensatory mechanism for the control of ET-induced vasoconstriction[100,101]. Indomethacin potentiates the pressor response obtained during intravenous infusion of ET-1[102], suggesting that prostanoids can blunt the pressor response of ET *in vivo*. ET releases prostacyclin (PGI$_2$) in human umbilical vein endothelial cells[103], rat and guinea-pig lungs[102,104], rabbit kidney[105,106], heart[107] and spleen[105]. PGI$_2$ has also been proposed to inhibit endothelial production of ET via cAMP[108] and to mediate the antiaggregatory action of ET[28,29] on platelets. Although ET may stimulate the release of arachidonic acid in all vascular smooth muscles, the specific eicosanoid formed in response to ET may vary considerably among different vascular beds. ET-1-induced contractions were reversed by PGI$_2$ in isolated human internal mammary artery, whereas, in human saphenous vein, PGI$_2$ was less effective in reversing ET-1-induced contractions[7]. PGI$_2$ was more effective than NO in blocking the constrictor effects of ET-1 in human veins[109]. ET increases, whereas PGI$_2$ decreases DNA synthesis of VSMC[110]. It appears that ET-1 and PGI$_2$ have opposing actions, and that PGI$_2$ can act as an modulator of ET-1 in certain vascular beds. ET-1 stimulated PGE$_2$-accumulation in the inner medullary collecting duct plays a role in ET-1-mediated inhibition of Na$^+$-K$^+$-ATPase[111,112]. ET-1 can also release PGE$_2$ in human monocytes[113], rabbit spleen and kidneys[105], and TXA$_2$ in liver[114]. In kidneys, ET-stimulated production of PGF$_{2\alpha}$[115] may be partly responsible for the renal arteriolar constriction. Endothelin-prostaglandin interactions are prominent in the pulmonary system, where ET causes bronchoconstriction and pulmonary hypertension. ET-1 stimulated the production or release of TXA$_2$[102,116-120] and histamine[121] in pulmonary mast cells, TXB$_2$[122] and PGD$_2$[123,124] in rat and guinea-pig lungs. ET-1 also releases PGE$_2$ and PGF$_{2\alpha}$ from primary cultures of feline tracheal epithelial cells[125]. Although ET-1 elicits potent bronchoconstrictor response, the significance of prostaglandin mechanisms in its effect is unknown.

Bradykinin

Bradykinin has been shown to stimulate the expression of preproET-1 mRNA in bovine glomerular endothelial cells[126], but it also causes a concentration-dependent suppression of ET release from cultured human endothelial cells[127]. Bradykinin can activate B$_1$- and/or B$_2$-receptors. The activation of B$_1$-receptors increases production of ET-1, whereas B$_2$-receptor stimulation decreases ET-1 production via NO synthesis[128]. Since only a few studies have been reported, it is difficult to speculate at present the importance of this interaction.

Platelet activating factor (PAF)

PAF is a phospholipid with a wide range of biological activities and plays a pivotal role in inflammation. It is also a key molecule in the activation of polymorphonuclear leukocytes (PMN), causing chemotaxis, aggregation, superoxide release and degranulation. A single bolus dose of ET-1 to conscious rats induced a rapid decrease in the number of circulating PMN[129]. ET-1 can stimulate the production of PAF in human PMN[130]. PAF produced as a result of ET-1 stimulation was detected mainly in the incubation buffer, whereas, PAF produced as a result of a chemotactic peptide, N-formyl-methionyl-leucyl-phenylalanine (fMLP), stimulation was detected mainly in the cell fraction. Further, ET-1 induced PMN aggregation was via calcium-dependent PAF production. This shows that fMLP stimulates the PAF synthesis but not its release, but ET-1 stimulates both. ET-1 is also known to increase the vascular permeability. ET-1 increased vascular permeability in specific vascular beds including the upper and lower bronchi, stomach and kidney of rats, which was partly mediated and/or modulated by the secondary release of TXA_2[131]. It has been shown that PAF mediates ET-1-induced vascular permeability. Since ET-1 can activate PLA_2, which if present in human PMN, may provide substrates for acetyltransferase and subsequently for PAF synthesis. ET-1 and PAF interact in vascular smooth muscle cells to enhance TXA_2 production[132]. The stimulation of TXA_2 biosynthesis may be a result of PLA_2 activation by ET-1 and also by PAF. ET-1 can stimulate the production of PAF, and PAF may stimulate the PLA_2 through the receptor mediated mechanism, and subsequently activate arachidonic acid cascade leading to increased production of TXA_2. The aggregation of PMN to endothelial cells are early steps of inflammation. This followed by increase in vascular permeability may cause influx of protein and other inflammatory mediators. Furthermore, endothelial cells exposed to inflammatory mediators, such as thrombin, TNF and IL-1, react by synthesizing PAF and ET-1[133]. Therefore, there can be a close interplay between ET and other regulatory agents during inflammation.

Cytokines

The endothelium is responsive to cytokines which induce changes in the endothelial cell structure and function by a process called endothelial cell activation. Once activated the endothelial cells express numerous constitutive and inducible effector functions. Cytokines have been shown to modulate the endothelial phenotype by altering the production of vasoactive mediators released by the endothelium. Studies indicate that ET gene expression can be stimulated by IL-1[134,135], TNF_α[136,137] and TGF_β[19,51,138] in various cell types. IL-1[134,139], IL-2[134], TGF_β[140,141], TNF_α[136,140,141], IFN_τ[140,141] and GMCSF[142] increase the production of ET in endothelial cells from different blood vessels. Among the cytokines, TGF_β is the most potent in releasing ET. Cytokines can also increase ET production in non-endothelial cells. For example, ET production was increased by $IL-1_\beta$, TNF_α and IL-6 in amnion cells[143], TGF_β in human thyroid follicular cells[144], $IL-1_\alpha$ and $IL-1_\beta$ in human kerotinocytes[145], TGF_β, TNF_α, and $IL-1_\beta$ in renal epithelial cells[146], TNF in mesangial cells[137], and IL-8, TNF_α and TGF_β in guinea-pig tracheal epithelial cells[147]. In bovine aortic endothelial cells, IFN_τ alone failed to exert a significant effect on endothelial expression of NO and ET-1. It exerts a potent inhibitory action on TNF_α-stimulated induction of NO synthase activity and NO release, whereas it potentiates TNF_α-stimulated ET-1 expression when added concurrently[148]. Generally,

TGF$_\beta$ and TNF$_\alpha$ have antagonistic effects on various endothelial cell functions, but they both increase ET[140]. ET also modulates the action of cytokines. In human umbilical vein endothelial cells, ET-1 enhanced the suppression of t-PA antigen release and reduced the stimulation of PAI-1 antigen release induced by either IL-1$_\beta$ or TNF$_\alpha$[149], suggesting that ET-1 may be a regulatory factor for these cytokines in endothelial cell-mediated fibrinolysis. These interactions indicate the existence of a cytokine-endothelium axis. During the process of inflammation cytokines may increase the production of ET, which may participate in or synergize with other agents in modulating cell growth, vascular tone and fibrinolysis under conditions such as vasculitis, glomerulonephritis, etc. Since immune mechanisms play an important role in the etiology of atherosclerosis, thrombosis and inflammation, the interaction between ET and cytokines, particularly interleukins, TNF$_\alpha$ and IFN$_\tau$ can be significant.

Lipoproteins

Native LDL had no effect whereas, oxidatively modified LDL (O-LDL) suppressed production of ET-1 and also thrombin-stimulated production of ET-1 in porcine aortic endothelial cells and human umbilical vein endothelial cells[150]. On the contrary, in human umbilical vein endothelial cells, O-LDL dose-dependently stimulated secretion of ET-1[151]. Modified LDLs have also been shown to induce secretion of ET-1 by human macrophages[152]. O-LDL can induce expression of ET mRNA and increase ET-1 release in porcine and human aortic endothelial cells in culture, and this ET-1 production can not be modulated by NO[153]. O-LDL is more atherogenic than LDL because it can cause accumulation of cholesterol esters in the cells of the macrophage system more rapidly than the native LDL[154], and induce toxicity in the endothelial cells[155,156]. O-LDL accumulates in atherosclerosis[157], and there has been increasing evidence that O-LDL inhibits vasorelaxation by inactivating NO[158,159] and exerts a direct vasoconstrictor action[160,161]. Since ET-1 levels are increased in patients with symptomatic atherosclerotic vascular disease[162] and hyperlipoproteinemia[163], O-LDL mediated increase in ET-1 can be of functional significance *in vivo*.

MITOGENIC INTERACTIONS OF ENDOTHELIN

In addition to being a potent vasoconstrictor, ET also serves as a growth promoting factor for many cell types. It is known to stimulate c-fos and c-myc expression and proliferation of vascular smooth muscle cells in a dose-dependent manner[164,165]. It also influences DNA synthesis, expression of protooncogenes, cell proliferation and causes hypertrophy. The mitogenic potency of ETs is low as compared to other known mitogens, but in concert, it can exert significant mitogenic actions in a variety of cell types. Polypeptide mitogens, including platelet-derived growth factor (PDGF), epidermal growth factor (EGF), transforming growth factors (TGF$_\alpha$ and TGF$_\beta$), basic fibroblast growth factor (bFGF), insulin and insulin-like growth factors (IGF-1) are known to cause migration and proliferation of vascular smooth muscle cells. ET-1 acts as a comitogen with these growth factors to increase DNA synthesis and cell proliferation (Table 6.1). On the other hand, prostacyclin[110], EDRF and ANP[167] inhibit mitogenic action of ET-1. The comitogenic effect of ET-2 is similar to ET-1, whereas ET-3 is less potent[168]. Interestingly, some of the growth factors also increase the gene expression and subsequent production of ET-1 (Table 6.2). It was observed that ET-1 promoted the expression of transcripts for PDGF-A chain, TGF_β and thrombospondin[76], and down-regulated the transcripts encoding $PDGF_\alpha$ type receptor[51] in the VSMC of SHR. Although specific mechanisms underlying these mitogenic interactions are unknown, these growth factors may bind to distinct

Table 6.1 Mitogenic interactions of ET with growth factors in various cell types

Factor	Cell type	Species	[ET] + [Factor]	% Increase [ET + Factor]/Factor	Ref.
TGF_α	aortic VSMC	rat	1 nM + 100 ng/ml	1048/371	[169]
	fibroblasts	rat kidney	1 ng/ml + 1 ng/ml	45–50/15–20*¶	[170]
TGF_β	fibroblasts	Swiss 3T3	3 nm + 0.3 ng/ml	2052/578	[171]
	fibroblasts	rat kidney	1 ng/ml + 1 ng/ml	400–500/300¶	[170]
EGF	aortic VSMC	rat	1 nm + 10 ng/ml	679/274	[169]
	fibroblasts	Swiss 3T3	3 nM + 30 ng/ml	3497/402	[171]
	fibroblasts	rat	10 nM + 10 ng/ml	2800/1400	[172]
	fibroblasts	rat kidney	1 ng/ml + 1 ng/ml	400–500/300¶	[170]
	breast stromal	human	10 nM + 10 ng/ml	143/85	[173]
bFGF	fibroblasts	Swiss 3T3	10 nM + 0.63 nM	1900/900	[174]
	fibroblasts	Swiss 3T3	3 nM + 0.03 ng/ml	2655/131	[171]
	fibroblasts	rat kidney	1 ng/ml + 1 ng/ml	170/100¶	[170]
	melanocytes	human	10 nM + 10 nM	138/77	[175]
Insulin	fibroblasts	Swiss 3T3	10 nM + 1.7 µM	1500/300	[174]
	fibroblasts	Swiss 3T3	3 nM + 1 µg/ml	441/141	[171]
	fibroblasts	Swiss 3T3	10 nM + 1 µg/ml	400/0	[176]
	fibroblasts	rat kidney	1 ng/ml + 1 ng/ml	260/80¶	[170]
	mesangial	rat	0.1 µM + 0.1 µg/ml	158/46	[177]
IGF-1	fibroblasts	Swiss 3T3	10 nM + 1 ng/ml	1229/64	[178]
	fibroblasts	rat kidney	1 ng/ml + 2 ng/ml	280/120¶	[170]
	breast stromal	human	10 nM + 10 ng/ml	905/71	[173]
	thyroid	rat	10 ng/ml + 1 ng/ml	100/25	[179]
	thyroid	rat	100 nM + 10 ng/ml	198/40	[179]
	fibroblasts	placenta	250 ng/ml + 100 ng/ml	~1050/250†	[180]
PDGF	aortic VSMC	rat	1 nM + 5 ng/ml	321/102	[169]
	aortic VSMC	rat	100 nM + 50 ng/ml	1067/750	[168]
	aortic VSMC	rat	100 nM + 50 ng/ml	1167/750**	[168]
	aortic VSMC	rat	100 nM + 50 ng/ml	1000/750***	[168]
	fibroblasts	Swiss 3T3	10 nM + 0.33 nM	2400/80	[174]
	fibroblasts	Swiss 3T3	3 nM + 1 ng/ml	2729/307	[171]
	fibroblasts	rat kidney	1 ng/ml + 1 ng/ml	240/110¶	[170]
	osteoblasts	murine	10 nM + 3 ng/ml	2900/1700	[181]
Bombesin	fibroblasts	Swiss 3T3	3 nM + 0.3 nM	604/184	[171]
	breast stromal	human	10 nM + 100 nM	68/31	[173]

Synergistic effect of ET-1 with other mitogens was quantified by measuring [³H]thymidine incorporation as an index of DNA synthesis, or increase in cell number.
*value represents $G_1 \to S$ transition
**ET-2
***ET-3
†Basal thymidine uptake was determined in the presence of serum free medium and 0.1% BSA
¶in presence of 0.1% newborn calf serum

Table 6.2 Effect of growth modulators on gene expression and production of ETs

Modulator	Cell type	Species	ET Gene expression	ET Production	Ref.
TGF$_\alpha$	renal adenocarcinoma	human	?	+	[185]
TGF$_\beta$	renal adenocarcinoma	human	?	+	[185]
	endothelial	porcine	?	+	[186]
	endothelial	bovine	+	?	[187]
	endothelial stromal	human	+	?	[188]
	VSMC	SHR	+	+	[76]
	mesangial	human	+	+	[19]
	VSMC	human	+	+	[51]
	MDCK	dog	+	?	[138]
	MDCK	dog	?	+	[189]
EGF	amnion	human	+	?	[135]
	VSMC	human	+	+	[51]
	renal adenocarcinoma	human	?	+	[185]
bFGF	renal adenocarcinoma	human	?	+	[185]
Insulin	endothelial	bovine	+	?	[190]
	endothelial	bovine	+	+	[191]
	mesangial	human	?	+	[52]
	endothelial	porcine	?	+	[192]
IGF-1	endothelial	porcine	?	+	[192]
PDGF	VSMC	human	+	+	[51]
	VSMC	SHR	+	+	[76]
	renal adenocarcinoma	human	?	+	[185]
Thrombin	endothelial	bovine	+	+	[18]
	endothelial	bovine	+	+	[187]
	mesangial	human	+	+	[19]
	endothelial	porcine	+	?	[193]
A-II	endothelial	SHR	+	?	[74]
	VSMC	human	+	+	[51]
	VSMC	SHR	+	+	[76]
	endothelial	bovine	+	?	[49]
	endothelial	human	?	+	[78]
	mesangial	human	?	+	[79]
NGF	renal adenocarcinoma	human	?	+	[185]
Bombesin	breast stromal (T47D)	human	?	+	[173]
Heparin	endothelial	bovine	−	−	[194]
Oxyhemoglobin	endothelial	bovine	?	+	[195]
	endothelial	bovine	+	+	[196]
	VSMC	rat	?	+	[196]
Hemoglobin	endothelial	bovine	?	+	[197]

Gene expression was assessed by measuring the levels of mRNA transcripts for preproET-1 and production was quantified by radioimmunoassay for ET-1

receptors and generate multiple intracellular signals by causing activation of PKC, stimulation of Na^+/H^+ exchange and/or increasing intracellular calcium, which converge to interact synergistically to initiate a proliferative response. ET-1 may thereby act as a competence factor in these interactions and prime the cells to respond to progression factors.

During local vascular injuries, many active substances are released from the platelets and endothelial cells. PDGF from platelets is a potent mitogenic and pro-atherogenic vasoconstrictor protein. ET-1 stimulates PDGF secretion from cultured human mesangial cells[182], and this can regulate growth of mesangial and perhaps smooth muscle cells, since both cell types express PDGF receptors. ET and PDGF together, may be involved in vasoconstriction, mitogenesis, wound healing and pathogenesis of atherosclerosis. Furthermore, it is speculated that ET in concert with TFG_α, TGF_β, PDGF and EGF, can participate in angiogenesis and extracellular matrix deposition during the process of vascular remodelling after injury. In humans there exists a direct correlation between the plasma levels of ET and insulin[183]. Insulin upregulates the ET_A receptors in vascular smooth muscle cells *in vitro*, and it shows synergy with ET-1 in stimulating cell proliferation[184]. Interaction of insulin and ET may therefore represent a link between hyperinsulinemia and hypertension. Therefore, it is possible that ET may synergize with one or more of the above growth factors to regulate the vascular growth under various conditions.

ENDOTHELIN INTERACTIONS IN THE ENDOCRINE SYSTEM

The presence of ET and its receptors in the various endocrine organs, raise the possibility that locally produced ETs may serve as important pleiotropic peptide regulators of the production, secretion, or actions of endocrinal hormones. Although intravenous ET does not cross the blood brain barrier, it has several neuroendocrine actions[198]. It has been hypothesized that circulating ET may be acting via the subfornical organ (SFO). The SFO lacks the blood brain barrier, and has two major efferent projections to the anteroventral third ventricular area of the preoptic region and the hypothalamus. Locally released or circulating ET could therefore activate the peptidergic neurons of the SFO to exert its excitatory effects on the release of neurohypophyseal hormones and/or on the sympathetic system[199-201]. Table 6.3 illustrates the *in vitro* actions of ETs on various endocrinal organs. In the neurohypophysis, ET shows a similar distribution pattern like oxytocin (OT) and VP, suggesting co-localization[202-204]. This indicates that neurohypophyseal ET may act locally to modulate the secretion of OT and AVP, and/or as a classic circulating hormone like OT and AVP. In the adenohypophysis, ET has stimulatory action on the release of ACTH, FSH, LH, TSH and GH, whereas, it exerts inhibitory action on PRL release. ET-1 has a biphasic effect on PRL release; initial transient stimulation followed by long lasting inhibition[205,206]. Since many hormones exhibit cell-cell interactions in the pituitary, it is possible that ET may induce stimulation of one cell type, which in turn may influence the secretion of PRL from another cell type, causing inhibition at a lower concentration and stimulation at a higher concentration. The inhibition of PRL secretion by ET-3 is via a PTX-sensitive G protein, probably G_k and/or G_i which mediates an increase in K^+ conductance and a decrease in adenylyl cyclase activity, respectively[207]. Since these pathways are used by DA, it is important to investigate whether ET modulates the actions of DA. This interaction also raises an intriguing question whether the pituitary ET serves as paracrine peptidergic prolactin inhibiting factor in the absence of DA.

Some agents such as OT, CGRP, A-II, ACTH and histamine are less effective in steroid secretion capacity when tested in collagenase-dispersed adrenocortical cell preparations, as compared to their efficacy in intact adrenal gland preparations[238]. When steroidogenesis or blood flow are stimulated by ACTH or histamine, the secretion of ET in the adrenal vein is increased[238]. This observation suggests that the increase in perfusate flow following vasodilation, and the consequent increase in corticosterone secretion may be linked to the release of ET from the vascular endothelium. Therefore, ACTH and possibly other hormones, may produce a direct and indirect action through ET on the intact gland, and this effect may explain the differences in responsiveness of the intact adrenal gland and *in vitro* preparations. In glomerulosa cells of the adrenal gland, ET-1 enhanced ACTH-[223] and A-II-stimulated[224] aldosterone secretion. Since cAMP is thought to mediate the effects of ACTH, and ET-1 potentiated the steroidogenic effect of 8-bromo-cAMP, it appears that action of ET-1 on ACTH-induced steroidogenesis was at least in part to events distal to the binding of ACTH to its receptors. ET stimulated aldosterone secretion was quantitatively similar to that produced by VP but smaller as compared to A-II[226]. In addition to this, intravenous ET can increase plasma renin level which can indirectly contribute to the increase aldosterone levels[55]. ET possessing dual effects, stimulation of aldosterone and cell proliferation, may have a role in the pathogenesis of idiopathic hyperaldosteronism. Malignant hypertension is associated with an increased secretion of aldosterone in a significant number of cases. On treatment, the aldosterone

Table 6.3 Modulation of endocrine hormones by endothelin peptides

Endocrine Gland	System	Species	[ET]	Effect	Ref.
HYPOTHALAMUS					
GnRH	hypothalamic neurons	rat	100 nM ET-1, ET-3	↑	[208]
LHRH	arcuate nucleus-median eminence fragments	rat	10 nM-1 µM ET-3	↑	[209]
PITUITARY					
Arginine vasopression	perifused hypothalamus	rat	0.1–10 nM ET-1	↑	[210]
	hypothamamic slices	rat	10 pM µM ET-1, ET-3	↓	[211]
	explants of hypothalamo-neurohypophyseal complex	rat	0.01–10 nM ET-3	↑	[212]
ACTH	pituitary cells	rat	100 nM ET-1	↑	[213]
FSH	pituitary cells	rat	100 nM ET-1	↑	[214]
	pituitary cells	rat	100 nM ET-1	↑	[213]
	ant. pituitary cells	rat	0.01 pM-1, µM ET-3	↑	[215]
LH	pituitary cells	rat	100 nM ET-1	↑	[214]
	pituitary cells	rat	100 nM ET-1	↑	[213]
	anterior pituitary cells	rat	1,10,100 nM ET-1, ET-3	↑	[216]
	ant. pituitary cells	rat	10 pM-1 µM ET-3	↑	[215]
	ant. pituitary cells	rat	10 pM-1 µM ET-3	↔	[205]
	ant. pituitary cells	rat	1 µM ET-1, 2, 3	↑	[217]
TSH	pituitary cells	rat	100 nM ET-1	↑	[213]
	ant. pituitary cells	rat	0.01 pM-1 µM ET-3	↑	[215]
	ant. pituitary cells	rat	10 pM-1 µM ET-3	↔	[205]
GH	pituitary cells	rat	100 nM ET-1	↑	[213]
	ant. pituitary cells	rat	10 pM-1 µM ET-3	↔	[205]
PRL	ant. pituitary slices	rat	0.01-1 µM ET-1, ET-3	↑	[218]
	decidual cells	human	10 nM ET-1*, ET-2, ET-3	↓	[219]
	ant. pituitary cells	rat	100 nM ET-1	↓	[207]
	ant. pituitary cells	rat	0.01 pM-1 µM ET-3	↓	[215]
	cultured pituitary cells	rat	0.05 µM ET-3	↓#	[205]
	ant. pituitary cells	rat	1–10³ pM ET-1, ET-2, ET-3	↓	[220]
	anterior pituitary cells	rat	1 pM ET-1 1 nM ET-2, 0.1 nM ET-3	↓	[221]
	anterior pituitary cells	rat	0.1, 10 nM ET-1, ET-3	↓#	[206]
ADRENALS					
Aldosterone	aderno-capsular cells	rabbit	10 pM ET-1	↑	[222]
	zona glomerulosa cells	bovine	0.1, 1, 10 nM ET-1, ET-3	↑	[85]

Pharmacological interactions

Table 6.3 (Continued)

Endocrine Gland	System	Species	[ET]	Effect	Ref.
	glomerulosa cells	bovine	0.1 nM ET-1	↑¶	[223]
	zona glomerulosa cells	bovine	0.1 nM ET-1 1 nM ET-2, 10 nM ET-3	↑§	[224]
	adrenal tissue slices	human	0.01–100 nM ET-1	↑	[225]
	zona glomerulosa cells	rat	10 nM ET-1	↑	[226]
	zona glomerulosa cells	bovine	01, 1, 10 nM ET-1	↑	[227]
	adrenocortical cells	human	10, 100 fM ET-1, ET-3	↑	[228]
	zona glomerulosa cells	rat	100, 10 fM ET-1, ET-3	↑	[229]
	zona glomerulosa cells	rat	0.1 pM ET-1 0.01 pM ET-2, ET-3	↑	[229]
Cortisol	zona fasiculata cells	bovine	10 nM ET-1	↔	[230]
	glomerulosa cells	bovine	0.1 nM ET-1	↔¶	[223]
	adrenocortical cells	human	10 fM ET-1, ET-3	↑	[228]
	adrenal tissue slices	human	0.01–100 nM ET-1	↔	[225]
Corticosterone	adrenocapsular cells	rabbit	0.01–10 pM ET-1	↔	[222]
	adrenocortical cells	rat	100, 10 fM ET-1, ET-3	↑	[229]
	fasciculata/reticulata cells	rat	0.1 pM ET-1 0.1 nM ET-2, 0.1 µM ET-3	↑	[229]
TESTES					
Testosterone	leydig cells	rat	1, 100 nM ET-1, ET-3	↑	[231]**
	leydig cells MA-10	murine	1 pM–1 µM ET-1	↑	[232]
OVARIES					
Progesterone	ovarian follicles@	rat	40 pM–40 µM ET-1, ET-3	↑	[233]
	granulosa cells	porcine	0.1 M ET-1	↑†	[234]
	granulosa cells	porcine	100 nM ET-1	↓†ff	[235]
	granulosa cells	porcine	10–100 nM ET-1	↑	[236]
	granulosa cells	porcine	50 nM ET-1, ET-2, ET-3	↓‡	[237]
Estradiol	ovarain follicles@	rat	40 pM–40 µM ET-1, ET-3	↑	[233]
	granulosa cells	porcine	10–100 nM ET-1	↔	[236]
Testosterone	ovarian follicles@	rat	40 pM–40 µM ET-1, ET-3	↑	[233]

↑ = stimulation, ↓ = inhibition and ↔ = no significant change
* inhibited insulin and IGF-1 stimulated PRL release.
Aldosterone/Cortisol production was stimulated by ACTH (¶), or A-II (§)
Progesterone production was stimulated by FSH (†), LH (‡), or human chorionic gonadotrophin (ff)
initial transient stimulation followed by long-lasting inhibition
@ follicular development was followed by administration of pregnant mare's serum gonadotrophin
** Additive effect was seen between ET-1 and human chorionic gonadtrophin (hcG)

secretion normalizes much later than the renin-angiotensin system, the main stimulator of aldosterone secretion, suggesting the action of an additional aldosterone stimulator(s), one of which might be ET-1. Significant endothelial changes and damage occur in malignant hypertension, which might lead to increased secretion of ET-1. The role of ET-1 in the acceleration of disease process in malignant hypertension is speculative at this time, but if ET-1 does have a role, then aldosterone overproduction induced by ET-1 is a reasonable hypothesis. Most studies show that ET-1 did not affect the basal[223,230] or ACTH-stimulated release of cortisol from the zona fasiculata cells[223]. However, cortisol caused a 2- to 5-fold increase in ET-1 release from rat and rabbit aortic vascular smooth muscle cells but no such response was observed in the endothelial cells of bovine aorta[239]. Glucocorticoid excess in Cushing's disease is associated with hypertension. Glucocorticoid stimulated ET release in this condition may be responsible for the increased vascular tone.

Sex hormones have been shown to modulate the plasma levels and actions of ET. In humans, administration of male hormones elevated, whereas, administration of female hormones lowered ET levels[240]. In rabbit myometrium, the density, but not the affinity, of ET receptors were up-regulated by estrogen and down-regulated by progesterone[241,242]. This is consistent with the finding that in rabbits, estrogen causes increase in uterine contractility, whereas, progesterone has an inhibitory effect. 17$_\beta$-estradiol dose-dependently increased the density of ET receptors in the myometrium with an ED$_{50}$ of 0.7 µg/kg/4 days[241,242], a value that is compatible with the ovarian production rate (0.85 µg/day) of this hormone in rabbits[243]. This was corroborated by the observation that during pregnancy, a progressive decline in the myometrial ET receptor density was seen with concomitant increase in the progesterone/17$_\beta$-estradiol ratio. At parturition, when the progesterone block was removed, the ET receptor density returned to that of non-pregnant concentration[244]. These studies support the view that sex steroid regulate ET receptors. This also raises the question as to how ET and sex steroids regulate the uterine tone. Uterine strips from rats treated with estrogen & progesterone (2 mg, s.c.) were less sensitive to the stimulatory effects of ET than were the strips from estrogen (1 µg, s.c.) treated animals[245], suggesting that progesterone can diminish the contractile response to the stimulatory effects of ET. Progesterone may reduce sensitivity to ET by directly interfering with the calcium fluxes, or by decreasing ET receptor density or binding affinity. The decreased responsiveness to ET after progesterone treatment complements the finding[246] that, first and second trimester pregnant women have ET levels in peripheral plasma lower than those in nonpregnant controls. Also the uterine vascular responses to ET-1 were blunted in pregnant ewes. These results explain the normal lack of uterine contractility during early pregnancy, when uterine growth (and presumably stretching) is more marked.

Relaxin is a peptide hormone produced by the corpus luteum, which is detectable during the late luteal phase and throughout pregnancy. It is a known inhibitor of uterine contractility and may play an important role in the maintenance of uterine quiescence during pregnancy. ET-1 stimulated contractility in rat uterine horn segments previously inhibited by relaxin, and relaxin reduced the increased contractility produced by earlier exposure to ET[245]. ET-1 can release PGF$_{2\alpha}$ from proliferative human endometrial explants[248], and OT receptors mediate the release of ET-1 from rabbit endometrial cells[249]. It is possible that during induction of labor OT may cause contractions of the myometrium directly via myometrial OT receptors, or indirectly by releasing ET. These interactions can be of physiological importance, especially during labor.

ENDOTHELIN-NEUROTRANSMITTER/NEUROMODULATOR INTERACTIONS

Both peripherally and centrally produced ETs have emerged as important vasoconstrictor peptides, which have been shown to have a myriad of interactions with classic neurotransmitters in the peripheral and the central nervous system.

Norepinephrine

Catecholamines can stimulate ET gene expression in VSMC[193]. Cultured porcine endothelial cells derived from the aorta, spontaneously released immunoreactive ET which could be potentiated by epinephrine via α-adrenoceptor[250]. In rat vas deferens[251,252], mesenteric arteries[253,254], guinea-pig pulmonary[255] and femoral[256] artery, the nerve stimulation-evoked release of [^{3}H]NE was reduced by ET-1 but not by ET-3[252]. ET-1 also suppressed renal nerve-stimulated NE efflux in dog kidney *in vivo*[257]. Infusion of ET-1 (1 ng/kg/min) in the renal artery of anesthetized dogs caused suppression of low frequency renal nerve stimulation-induced release of NE. This effect was specific for ET and was not due to the reduction in renal blood flow induced by ET-1 *per se* because Bay K 8644, a calcium agonist, caused a similar reduction in renal blood flow but had no effect on NE release[258]. The mechanism of ET-induced suppression of NE release is not mediated through prostaglandins[253], although PGs are known to inhibit adrenergic neurotransmitter release. Since neural release of NE is regulated by presynaptic α_2-adrenoceptors and adenosine receptors, it is possible that ET interacts with these regulatory mechanisms or acts directly on some pathways of NE release. Centrally administered ET-1 has been shown to elicit a pressor response by activating the sympathetic nervous system[56,259,260]. In addition to the effect on neural release, ET also modulates the catecholamine release from other storage sites. ET-1 has been shown to enhance the efflux of epinephrine and norepinephrine from the adrenal chromaffin cells[261]. ET-1 also enhances the contractile response to exogenously applied NE in the guinea-pig pulmonary artery[255], rabbit aorta[262], human mammary artery rings[263], rat mesenteric[253,254] and tail[264] arteries. This potentiating effect of ET appears to be through the sensitization of α-adrenoceptors. UK-14,304, an α_2-adrenoceptor agonist, was virtually inactive in exerting vasoconstriction of isolated rat tail artery, but in the presence of ET-1 it caused dose-dependent pressor response[265]. Further evidence for this proposal comes from the observation that, ET-1 pretreatment antagonized the hypotensive and potentiated the hypertensive effect of clonidine[266,267], a centrally acting hypotensive agent and α_2-adrenoceptor agonist. It is therefore evident that ET has a differential effect on the neuroeffector junction, presynaptic inhibition and postsynaptic potentiation. This differential response may result in the conservation of neurotransmitters, or provide a compensatory mechanism for neurotransmitter depletion.

Acetylcholine

It is thought that ET synthesized by the smooth muscle cells can act as a paracrine modulator of cholinergic neurotransmission. In guinea-pig ileum, ET-1 and ET-3 inhibited the [^{3}H]Ach release[252]. ET-3 has been suggested to inhibit sympathetic ganglionic transmission at presynaptic sites by reducing Ach release via TXA_2 stimulation[268]. In the rabbit bladder strips[269], transmural electrical stimulation elicited contractions that were attenuated by the muscarinic receptor blocker, atropine, and completely blocked in the presence of atropine and α, β-methylene ATP, a compound which desensitizes purinoceptors. ET-1 reduced these contractions by 20%, and this attenuation was seen even after blocking the purinergic component with α, β-methylene ATP. However, when the bladder strips were treated with atropine, the remaining non-cholinergic component of the electrically-induced contraction was not sensitive to ET-1. Further, ET-1 did not affect the contractions produced by exogenous Ach or ATP. This suggests that ET interferes with Ach action through a prejunctional mechanism.

Dopamine

ET-3 evoked the release of DA/NE from the cortical slices and DA from the striatal slices, in a concentration-dependent manner along with calcium release[270]. Similarly, ET-1 has been shown to release DA in the neostriatum[271]. Intrastriatal infusion of ET-3 as such did not change the basal release of DA, but after perfusion of DA releasing agent (ouabain or KCl) it could increase the DA levels. This effect of ET-3 was attenuated by calcium-free conditions[272]. These results indicate that ET could be modifying the exocytosis to enhance DA release after depolarization.

Serotonin

ET is co-localized with 5-HT in endothelial cells of rabbit aorta[273], and in the neuroepithelial bodies of intrapulmonary airways and alveolar parenchyma of newborn mammals[67]. ET-1 interacts with serotonin-mediated platelet aggregation. Concomitant addition of ET-1 and 5-HT causes an increased reponse, whereas, preincubation of platelet suspension with ET-1 resulted in a concentration-dependent inhibition of serotonin-mediated platelet aggregation[274]. This discrepancy is due to the time of activation of PKC. It is known that activation of PKC prior to the addition of an agonist, suppresses signal transduction between receptor and PLC and inhibits platelet aggregation, but when activated during the stimulation of platelet activation, it produces a maximal platelet response and inhibits by negative feedback, the coupling between receptor activation and PLC[275]. Moreover, ET-1 inhibited serotonergic amplification of epinephrine-induced platelet aggregation[274]. It is possible that ETs modify the platelet response to serotonin, by a noncompetitive interaction with the serotonin receptors and stimulation of PKC. 5-HT induces vasoconstriction at lower doses, and vasodilation at higher doses. ET-1 blocked the vasodilator response[276], and amplified contractions to 5-HT in mammary and coronary arteries[263,277], and rabbit ear arteries[278]. This indicates that pretreatment with ET-1 increases the arterial sensitivity to 5-HT. Therefore, ET-1 and 5-HT may act in concert, in dynamic arterial contraction leading to reduction of blood flow to the affected tissues. Since 5-HT does not produce endothelium-dependent relaxation in human coronary and internal mammary arteries[7,279], ET-1 may importantly contribute to vascular mechanisms involved in acute ischemic syndromes. At present the neuromodulatory interactions between ET and 5-HT are unknown.

ATP

The vas deferens which has predominantly sympathetic innervation, has been studied extensively for the neuromodulatory influences of ET. Transmural field stimulation of rat and guinea-pig vas deferens causes a phasic and tonic contraction, "twitch and hump". The twitch response is thought to be due to the release of ATP or a similar substance, and the hump response is partly due to NE release[280-284]. ET-1 enhanced

Pharmacological interactions 85

the putatively purinergic twitch response[251] as well as the contractile responses to exogenous ATP[251,252,285,286]. In the presence of α_1-adrenoceptor blockade, ET could greatly increase electrically-induced contractions, but this effect was abolished after desensitization of purinoceptors by α, β-methylene ATP[287]. Moreover, the potentiation of ATP response by ET-1 could not be blocked by denervation[286]. ET-1 enhanced the vasoconstrictor response to ATP in rabbit ear artery, and it also potentiated the ATP-mediated component of the vasconstrictor response to perivascular nerve stimulation in the rabbit jejunal artery[288]. From these results, it can be postulated that the interaction between ET and ATP may be a postjunctional phenomenon, where the purinoceptors are sensitized.

Substance P

Substance P is one of the peptides found in the sensory neurons of the dorsal root ganglia. It is also present in hypothalamus, and is transported to the anterior pituitary via portal vessels. It can influence the release of anterior pituitary hormones like ET. In a dynamic perfusion system, it was observed that ET-1 increased SP release from rat hypothalamus and anterior pituitary[289]. It was also shown that ET-1 actions in the spinal cord were inhibited by substance P antagonist[290], implying that the actions of ET might be partially mediated by substance P. The presence of substance P and ET binding sites in the pituitary and spinal neurons raise the possibility of further neuromodulatory interactions between these two peptides.

Brain natriuretic peptide

Brain natriuretic peptide (BNP) shows high structural and functional homology with atrial natriuretic peptide (ANP), and has been reported to have the same antagonistic actions against A-II as ANP has in the CNS. Moreover, BNP has been shown to share its receptor with ANP in the brain. ET-1 administered icv evoked a pressor response accompanied by increase in catecholamines, ACTH and AVP, and this was attenuated by central administration of BNP[199,291]. Binding sites for ET[292] and BNP[293] exist in the SFO. Furthermore, there is a neural network between SFO and hypothalamic nuclei (paraventricular nucleus, PVN). Therefore, there is a possibility that icv administered ET-1 and BNP may interact in the SFO, and that their effect may be transmitted to the PVN neurons which regulate the sympathetic nervous system and ACTH secretion. The neuronal projections from the SFO to the PVN also contain angiotensinergic fibers. If centrally administered ET acts in the SFO to activate angiotensinergic fibers, then BNP may have a modulatory influence on these aminergic pathways. Therefore, there can be a close interplay between these and other neuromodulators in activation of the sympathetic nervous system.

CONCLUSION

Since the discovery of ET by Yanagisawa, the first phase of research has elapsed. This phase has yielded constructive data suggesting the modulatory role of ET in many physiological systems. It appears that in the complex network of the human system, ETs serve as delicate sensors in the endothelium and neurons to respond to pathological challenges. Their action in concert with other regulators is more significant than their individual effects. Their role in the modulation of the endocrine and central nervous system functions appears to be of immense clinical significance. Further detailed studies are required to dissect the interactive influences of ETs, and to fully justify their presence. With the development of selective agonists and antagonists, we can unfold the regulatory functions of ETs. This would mark the second phase of the "endothelin explosion". The interaction of ET with numerous regulatory agents clearly indicates that in any physiological system the final response of ET is governed, not only by its direct actions, but also by other agents. Therefore, the knowledge gained by investigating these interactions in detail, will be useful in designing strategies for the successful treatment of pathophysiological states, wherein ETs are implicated.

Acknowledgements

The authors are grateful to Baxter Healthcare Corporation, Miles Incorporated and the National Institute of Health for providing research funds to our laboratory.

References

1. Warner, T. D., Mitchell, J. A., de Nucci, G. & Vane, J. R. (1989) Endothelin-1 and endothelin-3 release EDRF from isolated perfused arterial vessels of the rat and rabbit. *J Cardiovasc Pharmacol*, **13 (Suppl 5)**, S85–S88.
2. Fukuda, N., Izumi, Y., Soma, M., Watanabe, Y., Watanabe, M., Hatano, M. & Sakuma, I. (1990) L-N^G-monomethyl arginine inhibits the vasodilating effects of low dose of endothelin-3 on rat mesenteric arteries. *Biochem Biophys Res Commun*, **167**, 739–745.
3. Moritoki, H., Miyano, H., Takeuchi, S., Yamaguchi, M., Hisayama, T. & Kondoh, W. (1993) Endothelin-3-induced relaxation of rat thoracic aorta: a role for nitric oxide formation. *Br J Pharmacol*, **108**, 1125–1130.
4. Hirata, Y., Emori, T., Eguchi, S., Kanno, K., Imai, T., Ohta, K. & Marumo, F. (1993) Endothelin receptor subtype B mediates synthesis of nitric oxide by cultured bovine endothelial cells. *J. Clin Invest*, **91**, 1367–1373.
5. Kurose, I., Fukumura, D., Miura, S., Sekizuka, E., Nagata, H., Suematsu, M. & Tsuchiya, M. (1993) Nitric oxide mediates vasoactive effects of endothelin-3 on rat mesenteric microvascular beds *in vivo*. *Angiology*, **44**, 483–490.
6. Luscher, T. F., Yang, Z., Tschudi, M., von Segesser, L., Stulz, P., Boulanger, C., Turina, M. & Buhler, F. R. (1990) Interaction between endothelin-1 and endothelium-derived relaxing factor in human arteries and veins. *Circ Res*, **66**, 1088–1094.
7. Yang, Z. H., Buhler, F. R., Diederich, D. & Luscher, T. F. (1989) Different effects of endothelin-1 on cAMP- and cGMP-mediated vascular relaxation in human arteries and veins: comparison with norepinephrine. *J Cardiovasc Pharmacol*, **13 (Suppl 5)**, S129–S131.
8. Dohi, Y. & Luscher, T. F. (1990) Aging differentially affects direct and indirect actions of endothelin-1 in perfused mesenteric arteries of the rat. *Br J Pharmacol*, **100**, 889–893.
9. Luscher, T. F., Diederich, D., Yang, Z. & Buhler, F. R. (1989) Endothelin overrides endothelium-derived relaxing factor in hypertensive resistance arteries. *Kidney Int*, **35(1)**, 331.
10. Ohde, H., Morimoto, S. & Ogihara, T. (1991) Bradykinin suppresses endothelin-induced contraction of coronary artery through its B2-receptor on the endothelium. *Biochem Int*, **23**, 1127–1132.
11. Miller, V. M., Komori, K., Burnett, J. C., Jr. & Vanhoutte, P. M. (1989) Differential sensitivity of endothelin in canine arteries and veins. *Am J Physiol*, **257**, H1127–H1131.
12. Kiowski, W., Linder, L., Luscher, T. F. & Buhler, F. R. (1990) Endothelin-1 induced vasocontriction in man: reversal by a calcium channel blockade, but not by nitrovasodilators or endothelium-derived relaxing factor. *Circulation*, **83**, 469–475.

13. Boulanger, C. & Luscher, T. F. (1990) Release of endothelin from the porcine aorta. Inhibition by endothelium-derived nitric oxide. *J Clin Invest*, **85**, 587–590.
14. Kato, K., Sawada, S., Toyoda, T., Kobayashi, K., Shirai, K., Yamamoto, K., Tamagaki, T., Yamagami, M., Yoneda, M., Takada, O. et al. (1992) Influence of endothelin on human platelet aggregation and prostacyclin generation from human vascular endothelial cells in culture. *Jpn Circ J*, **56**, 422–431.
15. Hirata, M., Kohse, K. P., Chang, C. H., Ikebe, T. & Murad, F. (1990) Mechanism of cyclic GMP inhibition of inositol phosphate formation in rat aorta segments and cultured bovine aortic smooth muscle cells. *J Biol Chem*, **265**, 1268–1273.
16. Lang, D. & Lewis, M. J. (1991) Endothelium-derived relaxing factor inhibits the endothelin-1-induced increase in protein kinase C activity in rat aorta. *Br J Pharmacol*, **104**, 139–144.
17. Miller, W. L., Cavero, P. G., Aarhus, L. L., Heublein, D. M. & Burnett, J. C., Jr. (1993) Endothelin-mediated cardiorenal hemodynamic and neuroendocrine effects are attenuated by nitroglycerin *in vivo*. *Am J Hypertens*, **6**, 156–163.
18. Emori, T., Hirata, Y., Imai, T., Ohta, K., Kanno, K., Eguchi, S. & Marumo, F. (1992) Cellular mechanism of thrombin on endothelin-1 biosynthesis and release in bovine endothelial cells. *Biochem Pharmacol*, **44(12)**, 2409–2411.
19. Zoja, C., Orisio, C., Perico, N., Benigni, A., Morigi, M., Benatti, L., Rambaldi, A. & Remuzzi, G. (1991) Constitutive expression of endothelin gene in cultured human mesangial cells and its modulation by transforming growth factor-beta, thrombin, and a thromboxane A2 analogue. *Lab Invest*, **64(1)**, 16–20.
20. Kohno, M., Yasunari, K., Murakawa, K., Yokokawa, K., Horio, T., Fukui, T. & Takeda, T. (1990) Release of immunoreactive endothelin from porcine aortic strips. *Hypertension*, **15**, 718–723.
21. Fukunaga, M., Fujiwara, Y., Ochi, S., Yokoyama, K., Fujibayashi, M., Orita, Y., Fukuhara, Y., Ueda, N. & Kamada, T. (1991) Stimulatory effect of thrombin on endothelin-1 production in isolated glomeruli and cultured mesangial cells of rats. *J Cardiovasc Pharmacol*, **17 (Suppl 7)**, S411–S413.
22. Rennick, R. E., Milner, P. & Burnstock, G. (1993) Thrombin stimulates release of endothelin and vasopressin, but not substance P, from isolated rabbit tracheal epithelial cells. *Eur J Pharmacol*, **230**, 367–370.
23. Ehrenreich, H., Costa, T., Clouse, K. A., Pluta, R. M., Ogino, Y., Coligan, J. E. & Burd, P. R. (1993) Thrombin is a regulator of astrocytic endothelin-1. *Brain Res*, **600(2)**, 201–207.
24. Kohno, M., Yokokawa, K., Horio, T., Yasunari, K., Murakawa, K., Ikeda, M. & Takeda, T. (1992) Release mechanism of endothelin-1 and big endothelin-1 after stimulation with thrombin in cultured porcine endothelial cells. *J Vasc Res*, **29**, 56–63.
25. Boulanger, C. M. & Luscher, T. F. (1991) Hirudin and nitrates inhibit the thrombin-induced release of endothelin from the intact porcine aorta. *Circ Res*, **68**, 1768–1772.
26. Kohno, M., Yasunari, K., Yokokawa, K., Murakawa, K., Horio, T., Kanayama, Y., Fuzisawa, M., Inoue, T. & Takeda, T. (1990) Thrombin stimulates the production of immunoreactive endothelin-1 in cultured human umbilical vein endothelial cells. *Metabolism*, **39**, 1003–1005.
27. Kitazumi, K. & Tasaka, K. (1992) Thrombin-stimulated phosphorylation of myosin light chain and its possible involvement in endothelin-1 secretion from porcine aortic endothelial cells. *Biochem Pharmacol*, **43**, 1701–1709.
28. Lidbury, P. S., Thiemermann, C., Thomas, G. R. & Vane, J. R. (1989) Endothelin-3: selectivity as an anti-aggregatory peptide *in vivo*. *Eur J Pharmacol*, **166**, 335–338.
29. Herman, F., Magyar, K., Chabrier, P. E., Braquet, P. & Filep, J. (1989) Prostacyclin mediates antiaggregatory and hypotensive actions of endothelin in anaesthetized beagle dogs. *Br J Pharmacol*, **98**, 38–40.
30. Kaji, T., Yamamoto, C., Sakamoto, M. & Koizumi, F. (1992) Endothelin modulation of tissue plasminogen activator release from human vascular endothelial cells in culture. *Blood Coagul Fibrinolysis*, **3**, 5–10.
31. Yamamoto, C., Kaji, T., Sakamoto, M. & Koizumi, F. (1992) Effect of endothelin on the release of tissue plasminogen activator and plasminogen activator inhibitor-1 from cultured human endothelial cells and interaction with thrombin. *Thromb Res*, **67**, 619–624.
32. Kanthou, C., Parry, G., Wijelath, E., Kakkar, V. V. & Demoliou Mason, C. (1992) Thrombin-induced proliferation and expression of platelet-derived growth factor-A chain gene in human vascular smooth muscle cells. *FEBS Lett*, **314**, 143–148.
33. Muir, T. M., Hair, J., Inglis, G. C., Dow, J. W., Lindop, G. B. & Leckie, B. J. (1993) Hormonal control of atrial natriuretic peptide synthesis and secretion from cultured atrial myocytes. *J Mol Cell Cardiol*, **25**, 509–518.
34. Irons, C. E., Murray, S. F. & Glembotski, C. C. (1993) Identification of the receptor subtype responsible for endothelin-mediated protein kinase C activation and atrial natriuretic factor secretion from atrial myocytes. *J Biol Chem*, **268**, 23417–23421.

35. Shirakami, G., Nakao, K., Saito, Y., Magaribuchi, T., Mukoyama, M., Arai, H., Hosoda, K., Suga, S., Mori, K. & Imura, H. (1993) Low doses of endothelin-1 inhibit atrial natriuretic peptide secretion. *Endocrinology*, **132**, 1905–1912.
36. Amadieu-Farmakis, M., Davicco, M. J., Giry, J. & Barlet, J. P. (1991) Effects of angiotensin II, arginine-vasopressin, endothelin and catecholamines on plasma atrial natriuretic peptide concentrations in the conscious newborn calf. *J Dev Physiol*, **16(1)**, 51–56.
37. Donckier, J., Hanet, C., Galanti, L., Stoleru, L., Van Mechelen, H., Robert, A., Ketelslegers, J. M. & Pouleur, H. (1992) Low-dose endothelin-1 potentiates volume-induced secretion of atrial natriuretic factor. *Am J Physiol*, **263**, H939–H944.
38. Tsuchiya, H., Otsuka, A., Mikami, H., Katahira, K., Tsunetoshi, T., Kohara, K., Higaki, J., Nugent, C. A. & Ogihara, T. (1990) Increased atrial natriuretic factor secretion after endothelin injection in dogs. *Methods Find Exp Clin Pharmacol*, **12**, 379–383.
39. Horio, T., Kohno, M. & Takeda, T. (1993) Cosecretion of atrial and brain natriuretic peptides stimulated by endothelin-1 from cultured rat atrial and ventricular cardiocytes. *Metabolism*, **42**, 94–96.
40. Schiebinger, R. J. & Greening, K. M. (1992) Interaction between stretch and hormonally stimulated atrial natriuretic peptide secretion. *Am J Physiol*, **262**, H78–H83.
41. Lew, R. A. & Baertschi, A. J. (1989) Endothelial cells stimulate ANF secretion from atrial myocytes in co-culture. *Biochem Biophys Res Commun*, **163**, 701–709.
42. Marala, R. B., Duda, T. & Sharma, R. K. (1993) Interaction of atrial natriuretic factor and endothelin-1 signals through receptor guanylate cyclase in pulmonary artery endothelial cells. *Mol Cell Biochem*, **120**, 69–80.
43. Fyhrquist, F., Sirvio, M. L., Helin, K., Saijonmaa, O., Metsarinne, K., Paakkari, I., Jarvinen, A. & Tikkanen, I. (1993) Endothelin antiserum decreases volume-stimulated and basal plasma concentration of atrial natriuretic peptide. *Circulation*, **88**, 1172–1176.
44. Ota, K., Kimura, T., Shoji, M., Inoue, M., Sato, K., Ohta, M., Yamamoto, T., Tsunoda, K., Abe, K. & Yoshinaga, K. (1992) Interaction of ANP with endothelin on cardiovascular, renal, and endocrine function. *Am J Physiol*, **262**, E135–E141.
45. Kohno, M., Yasunari, K., Yokokawa, K., Murakawa, K., Horio, T. & Takeda, T. (1991) Inhibition by atrial and brain natriuretic peptides of endothelin-1 secretion after stimulation with angiotensin II and thrombin of cultured human endothelial cells. *J Clin Invest*, **87**, 1999–2004.
46. Kohno, M., Horio, T., Yokokawa, K., Kurihara, N. & Takeda, T. (1992) C-type natriuretic peptide inhibits thrombin- and angiotensin II-stimulated endothelin release via cyclic guanosine 3′,5′-monophosphate. *Hypertension*, **19**, 320–325.
47. Kohno, M., Horio, T., Ikeda, M., Yokokawa, K., Fukui, T., Yasunari, K., Murakawa, K., Kurihara, N. & Takeda, T. (1993) Natriuretic peptides inhibit mesangial cell production of endothelin induced by arginine vasopressin. *Am J Physiol*, **264**, F678–F683.
48. Milner, P., Bodin, P., Loesch, A. & Burnstock, G. (1990) Rapid release of endothelin and ATP from isolated aortic endothelial cells exposed to increased flow. *Biochem Biophys Res Commun*, **170**, 649–656.
49. Imai, T., Hirata, Y., Emori, T., Yanagisawa, M., Masaki, T. & Marumo, F. (1992) Induction of endothelin-1 gene by angiotensin and vasopressin in endothelial cells. *Hypertension*, **19**, 753–757.
50. Tomobe, Y., Yanagisawa, M., Fujimori, A., Masaki, T. & Goto, K. (1993) Arginine-vasopressin increases the release of ET-1 into perfusate of rat mesenteric artery. *Biochem Biophys Res Commun*, **191**, 654–661.
51. Resink, T. J., Hahn, A. W., Scott Burden, T., Powell, J., Weber, E. & Buhler, F. R. (1990) Inducible endothelin mRNA expression and peptide secretion in cultured human vascular smooth muscle cells. *Biochem Biophys Res Commun*, **168**, 1303–1310.
52. Bakris, G. L., Fairbanks, R. & Traish, A. M. (1991) Arginine vasopressin stimulates human mesangial cell production of endothelin. *J Clin Invest*, **87(4)**, 1158–1164.
53. Emmeluth, C. & Bie, P. (1992) Effects, release and disposal of endothelin-1 in conscious dogs. *Acta Physiol Scand*, **146**, 197–204.
54. Miller, W. L., Redfield, M. M. & Burnett, J. C. J. (1989) Integrated cardiac, renal, and endocrine actions of endothelin. *J Clin Invest*, **83**, 317–320.
55. Goetz, K. L., Wang, B. C., Madwed, J. B., Zhu, J. L. & Leadley, R. J. J. (1988) Cardiovascular, renal, and endocrine responses to intravenous endothelin in conscious dogs. *Am J Physiol*, **255**, R1064–R1068.
56. Matsumura, K., Abe, I., Tsuchihashi, T., Tominaga, M. & Kobayashi, K. (1991) Central effect of endothelin on neurohormonal responses in conscious rabbits. *Hypertension*, **17**, 1192–1196.
57. Inoue, M., Kimura, T. & Ota, K. (1988) Effect of vasopressin on atrial natriuretic peptide release and renal function in dogs. *Am J Physiol*, **255** (4pt. 1), E449–E455.

58. Ruskoaho, T., Toth, M. & Lang, M. (1985) Atrial natriuretic peptide secretion: synergistic effect of phorbol ester and A23187. *Biochem Biophys Res Commun*, **133**, 581–588.
59. Schnermann, J., Lorenz, J. N., Briggs, J. P. & Keiser, J. A. (1992) Induction of water diuresis by endothelin in rats. *Am J Physiol*, **263**, F516–F526.
60. Kohan, D. E. & Hughes, A. K. (1993) Autocrine role of endothelin in rat IMCD: inhibition of AVP-induced cAMP accumulation. *Am J Physiol*, **265**, F126–F129.
61. Edwards, R. M., Stack, E. J., Pullen, M. & Nambi, P. (1993) Endothelin inhibits vasopressin action in rat inner medullary collecting duct via the ET_B receptor. *J Pharmacol Exp Ther*, **267(3)**, 1028–1033.
62. Oishi, R., Nonoguchi, H., Tomita, K. & Marumo, F. (1991) Endothelin-1 inhibits AVP-stimulated osmotic water permeability in rat inner medullary collecting duct. *Am J Physiol*, **261**, F951–F956.
63. Nadler, S. P., Zimpelmann, J. A. & Hebert, R. L. (1992) Endothelin inhibits vasopressin-stimulated water permeability in rat terminal inner medullary collecting duct. *J Clin Invest*, **90**, 1458–1466.
64. Kohzuki, M., Johnston, C. I., Chai, S. Y., Casley, D. & Mendelsohn, F. A. O. (1989) Localization of endothelin receptors in rat kidney. *Eur J Pharmacol*, **160**, 193–194.
65. MacCumber, M. W., Ross, C. A., Glaser, B. M. & Snyder, S. H. (1989) Endothelin: visualization of mRNAs by *in situ* hybridization provides evidence for local action. *Proc Natl Acad Sci USA*, **86**, 7285–7289.
66. Kitamura, K., Tanaka, T., Ogawa, T., Eto, T. & Tanaka, K. (1989) Immunoreactive endothelin in rat kidney inner medulla: marked decrease in spontaneously hypertensive rats. *Biochem Biophys Res Commun*, **162**, 38–44.
67. Seldeslagh, K. A. & Lauweryns, J. M. (1993) Endothelin in normal lung tissue of newborn mammals: immunocytochemical distribution and co-localization with serotonin and calcitonin gene-related peptide. *J Histochem Cytochem*, **41(10)**, 1495–1502.
68. Gardiner, S. M., Compton, A. M., Kemp, P. A., Bennett, T., Foulkes, R. & Hughes, B. (1991) Haemodynamic effects of human alpha-calcitonin gene-related peptide following administration of endothelin-1 or N^G-nitro-L-arginine methyl ester in conscious rats. *Br J Pharmacol*, **103**, 1256–1262.
69. Bakken, I. J., Vincent, M. B., White, L. R., Juul, R., Edvinsson, L. & Sjaastad, O. (1992) Mutual modification of vasoactivity by calcitonin gene-related peptide and endothelin-1 in isolated porcine ophthalmic artery. *Neuropeptides*, **23**, 209–214.
70. Juul, R., Edvisson, L., Gisvold, S. E., Ekman, R., Brubakk, A. O. & Fredriksen, T. A. (1990) Calcitonin gene-related peptide-LI in subarachnoid hemorrhage in man. Signs of activation of the trigemino-cerebrovascular system? *Br J Neurosurg*, **4(3)**, 171–179.
71. Suzuki, H., Sato, S., Suzuki, Y., Takekoshi, K., Ishihara, N. & Shimoda, S. (1990) Increased endothelin concentration in CSF from patients with subarachnoid hemorrhage. *Acta Neurol Scand*, **81**, 553–554.
72. Yoshida, K., Yasujima, M., Kohzuki, M., Kanazawa, M. & Yoshinaga, K. (1992) Endothelin-1 augments pressor response to angiotensin II infusion in rats. *Hypertension*, **20**, 292–297.
73. Imai, T., Hirata, Y., Eguchi, S., Kanno, K., Ohta, K., Emori, T., Sakamoto, A., Yanagisawa, M., Masaki, T. & Marumo, F. (1992) Concomitant expression of receptor subtype and isopeptide of endothelin by human adrenal gland. *Biochem Biophys Res Commun*, **182**, 1115–1121.
74. Dohi, Y., Hahn, A. W., Boulanger, C. M., Buhler, F. R. & Luscher, T. F. (1992) Endothelin stimulated by angiotensin II augments contractility of spontaneously hypertensive rat resistance arteries. *Hypertension*, **19**, 131–137.
75. Chua, B. H., Chua, C. C., Diglio, C. A. & Siu, B. B. (1993) Regulation of endothelin-1 mRNA by angiotensin II in rat heart endothelial cells. *Biochim Biophys Acta*, **1178**, 201–206.
76. Hahn, A. W., Resink, T. J., Scott-Burden, T., Powell, J., Dohi, Y. & Buhler, F. R. (1990) Stimulation of endothelin mRNA and secretion in rat vascular smooth muscle cells: a novel autocrine function. *Cell Regul*, **1**, 649–659.
77. Ito, H., Hirata, Y., Adachi, S., Tanaka, M., Tsujino, M., Koike, A., Nogami, A., Murumo, F. & Hiroe, M. (1993) Endothelin-1 is an autocrine/paracrine factor in the mechanism of angiotensin II-induced hypertrophy in cultured rat cardiomyocytes. *J Clin Invest*, **92**, 398–403.
78. Ciafre, S. A., D'Armiento, F. P., Di Gregorio, F., Colasanti, P., Di Benedetto, A., Langella, A., Di Ieso, N., Liguori, A., Colasanti, R., Napoli, C. et al. (1993) Angiotensin II stimulates endothelin-1 release from human endothelial cells. *Recenti Prog Med*, **84**, 248–253.
79. Bakris, G. L. & Re, R. N. (1993) Endothelin modulates angiotensin II-induced mitogenesis of human mesangial cells. *Am J Physiol*, **264**, F937–F942.
80. Sawamura, T., Kasuya, Y., Matsushita, Y., Suzuki, N., Shinmi, O., Kishi, N., Sugita, Y., Yanagisawa, M., Goto, K. & Masaki, T. (1991) Phosphoramidon inhibits the intracellular conversion of big endothelin-1 to endothelin-1 in cultured endothelial cells. *Biochem Biophys Res Commun*, **174**, 779–784.
81. Roubert, P., Gillard, V., Plas, P., Guillon, J. M., Chabrier, P. E. & Braquet, P. (1989) Angiotensin II

and phorbol-esters potently down-regulate endothelin (ET-1) binding sites in vascular smooth muscle cells. *Biochem Biophys Res Commun*, **164**, 809–815.
82. Kanno, K., Hirata, Y., Tsujino, M., Imai, T., Shichiri, M., Ito, H. & Marumo, F. (1993) Up-regulation of ET_B receptor subtype mRNA by angiotensin II in rat cardiomyocytes. *Biochem Biophys Res Commun*, **194**, 1282–1287.
83. Kambayashi, Y., Bardhan, S. & Inagami, T. (1993) Peptide growth factors markedly decrease the ligand binding of angiotensin II type 2 receptor in rat cultured vascular smooth muscle cells. *Biochem Biophys Res Commun*, **194**, 478–482.
84. Kawaguchi, H., Sawa, H. & Yasuda, H. (1991) Effect of endothelin on angiotensin coverting enzyme activity in cultured pulmonary artery endothelial cells. *J Hypertens*, **9**, 171–174.
85. Cozza, E. N., Gomez Sanchez, C. E., Foecking, M. F. & Chiou, S. (1989) Endothelin binding to cultured calf adrenal zona glomerulosa cells and stimulation of aldosterone secretion. *J Clin Invest*, **84**, 1032–1035.
86. Pecci, A., Gomez Sanchez, C. E., de Bedners, M. E., Lantos, C. P. & Cozza, E. N. (1993) *In vivo* stimulation of aldosterone biosynthesis by endothelin: loci of action and effects of doses and infusion rate. *J Steroid Biochem Mol Biol*, **45**, 555–561.
87. Cozza, E. N. & Gomez Sanchez, C. E. (1993) Mechanisms of ET-1 potentiation of angiotensin II stimulation of aldosterone production. *Am J Physiol*, **265**, E179–E183.
88. Rakugi, H., Tabuchi, Y., Nakamaru, M., Nagano, M., Higashimori, K., Mikami, H. & Ogihara, T. (1990) Endothelin activates the vascular renin-angiotensin system in rat mesenteric arteries. *Biochem Int*, **21**, 867–872.
89. Moe, O., Tejedor, A., Campbell, W. B., Alpern, R. J. & Henrich, W. L. (1991) Effects of endothelin on *in vivo* renin secretion. *Am J Physiol*, **260** (4pt. 1), E521–E535.
90. Takagi, M., Matsuoka, H., Atarashi, K. & Yagi, S. (1988) Endothelin: a new inhibitor of renin release. *Biochem Biophys Res Commun*, **157**, 1164–1168.
91. Takagi, M., Tsukada, H., Matsuoka, H. & Yagi, S. (1989) Inhibitory effect of endothelin on renin release *in vitro*. *Am J Physiol*, **257**, E833–E838.
92. Matsumura, Y., Nakase, K., Ikegawa, R., Hayashi, K., Ohyama, T. & Morimoto, S. (1989) The endothelium-derived vasoconstrictor peptide endothelin inhibits renin release *in vitro*. *Life Sci*, **44**, 149–157.
93. Rakugi, H., Nakamaru, M., Saito, H.., Higaki, J. & Ogihara, T. (1988) Endothelin inhibits renin release from isolated rat glomeruli. *Biochem Biophys Res Commun*, **155**, 1244–1247.
94. Beierwaltes, W. H. & Carretero, O. A. (1992) Nonprostanoid endothelium-derived factors inhibit renin release. *Hypertension*, **19**, II68–II73.
95. Beierwlates, W. H., Schryver, S., Sanders, E., Strand, J. & Romero, J. C. (1982) Renin release selectively stimulated by prostglandin I_2 in isolated rat glomeruli. *Am J Physiol*, **243**, F276–F283.
96. Beierwaltes, W. H. (1990) Possible endothelial modulation of prostaglandin-stimulated renin release. *Am J Physiol*, **258**, F1363–F1371.
97. Rakugi, H., Nakamaru, M., Tabuchi, Y., Nagano, M., Mikami, H. & Ogihara, T. (1989) Endothelin stimulates the release of prostacyclin from rat mesenteric arteries. *Biochem Biophys Res Commun*, **160**, 924–928.
98. Filep, J. G., Battistini, B., Côté, Y. P., Beaudoin, A. R. & Sirois, P. (1991) Endothelin-1 induces prostacyclin release from bovine aortic endothelial cells. *Biochem Biophys Res Commun*, **177**, 171–176.
99. Spatz, M., Stanimirovic, D., Uematsu, S. & Roberts, L. J. (1993) Prostaglandin D2 and endothelin-1 induce the production of prostaglandin $F_{2\alpha}$, 9α, 11β-prostaglandin F2, prostaglandin E2, and thromboxane in capillary endothelium of human brain. *Prostaglandins Leukot Essent Fatty Acids*, **49(4)**, 789–793.
100. Chou, S. Y., Dahhan, A. & Porush, J. G. (1990) Renal actions of endothelin: interaction with prostacyclin. *Am J Physiol*, **259**, F645–F652.
101. Kohan, D. E. & Padilla, E. (1993) Osmolar regulation of endothelin-1 production by rat inner medullary collecting duct. *J Clin Invest*, **91**, 1235–1240.
102. de Nucci, G., Thomas, R., D'Orleans Juste, P., Antunes, E., Walder, C., Warner, T. D. & Vane, J. R. (1988) Pressor effects of circulating endothelin are limited by its removal in the pulmonary circulation and by the release of prostacyclin and endothelium-derived relaxing factor. *Proc Natl Acad Sci USA*, **85**, 9797–9800.
103. Muck, A. O., Seeger, H., Korte, K. & Lippert, T. H. (1993) The effect of 17 β-estradiol and endothelin-1 on prostacyclin and thromboxane production in human endothelial cell cultures. *Clin Exp Obstet Gynecol*, **20(4)**, 203–206.
104. D'Orleans Juste, P., Telemaque, S., Claing, A., Ihara, M. & Yano, M. (1992) Human big-endothelin-1 and endothelin-1 release prostacyclin via the activation of ET1 receptors in the rat perfused lung. *Br J Pharmacol*, **105**, 773–775.

105. Rae, G. A., Trybulec, M., de Nucci, G. & Vane, J. R. (1989) Endothelin-1 releases eicosanoids from rabbit isolated perfused kidney and spleen. *J Cardiovasc Pharmacol*, **13 (Suppl 5)**, S89–S92.
106. Telemaque, S., Gratton, J. P., Claing, A. & D'Orleans Juste, P. (1993) Endothelin-1 induces vasoconstriction and prostacyclin release via the activation of endothelin ETA receptors in the perfused rabbit kidney. *Eur J Pharmacol*, **237**, 275–281.
107. Karwatowska-Prokopczuk, E. & Wennmalm, A. (1990) Effects of endothelin on coronary flow, mechanical performance, oxygen uptake, and formation of purines and on outflow of prostacyclin in the isolated rabbit heart. *Circ Res*, **6(1)**, 46–54.
108. Yokokawa, K., Kohno, M., Yasunari, K., Murakawa, K. & Takeda, T. (1991) Endothelin-3 regulates endothelin-1 production in cultured human endothelial cells. *Hypertension*, **18**, 304–15.
109. Haynes, W. G. & Webb, D. J. (1993) Venoconstriction to endothelin-1 in humans: role of calcium and potassium channels. *Am J Physiol*, **265**, H1676–H1681.
110. Nakaki, T., Ohta, M. & Kato, R. (1991) Inhibition of endothelin-1 induced DNA synthesis by prostacyclin and its stable analogues in vascular smooth muscle cells. *J Cardiovasc Pharmacol*, **17 (Suppl 7)**, S177–S178.
111. Zeidel, M. L., Brady, H. R., Kone, B. C., Gullans, S. R. & Brenner, B. M. (1989) Endothelin, a peptide inhibitor of Na(+)-K(+)-ATPase in intact renal tubular epithelial cells. *Am J Physiol*, **257**, C1101–C1107.
112. Kohan, D. E., Padilla, E. & Hughes, A. K. (1993) Endothelin B receptor mediates ET-1 effects on cAMP and PGE2 accumulation in rat IMCD. *Am J Physiol*, **265**, F670–F676.
113. McMillen, M. A., Huribal, M., Kumar, R. & Sumpio, B. E. (1993) Endothelin-stimulated human monocytes produce prostaglandin E2 but not leukotriene B4. *J Surg Res*, **54**, 331–335.
114. Kurihara, T., Akimoto, M., Kurokawa, K., Ishiguro, H., Niimi, A., Maeda, A., Sigemoto, M., Yamashita, K., Yokoyama, I., Hirayama, Y. *et al.* (1992) Relationship between endothelin and thromboxane A2 in rat liver microcirculation. *Life Sci*, **51**, PL281–PL285.
115. Munger, K. A., Takahashi, K., Awazu, M., Frazer, M., Falk, S. A., Conger, J. D. & Badr, K. F. (1993) Maintenance of endothelin-induced renal arteriolar constriction in rats is cyclooxygenase dependent. *Am J Physiol*, **264**, F637–F644.
116. Battistini, B., Filep, J. & Sirois, P. (1990) Potent thromboxane-mediated *in vitro* bronchoconstrictor effect of endothelin in the guinea-pig. *Eur J Pharmacol*, **178**, 141–142.
117. Pons, F., Touvay, C., Lagente, V., Mencia Huerta, J. M. & Braquet, P. (1991) Comparison of the effects of intra-arterial and aerosol administration of endothelin-1 (ET-1) in the guinea-pig isolated lung. *Br J Pharmacol*, **102**, 791–796.
118. Nambu, F., Yube, N., Omawari, M., Okegawa, T., Kawaski, A. & Ikeda, S. (1990) Inhibition of endothelin-induced bronchoconstriction by OKY-046, a selective thromboxane A2 synthetase inhibitor, in guinea-pigs. *Adv in prostaglandins, thromboxane, and leukotriene res*, **21**, 453–456.
119. Filep, J. G., Battistini, B. & Sirois, P. (1990) Endothelin induces thromboxane release and contraction of isolated guinea-pig airways. *Life Sci*, **47**, 1845–1850.
120. Filep, J. G., Battistini, B. & Sirois, P. (1991) Pharmacological modulation of endothelin-induced contraction of guinea-pig isolated airways and thromboxane release. *Br J Pharmacol*, **103**, 1633–1640.
121. Uchida, Y., Ninomiya, H., Sakamoto, T., Lee, J. Y., Endo, T., Nomura, A., Hasegawa, S. & Hirata, F. (1992) ET-1 released histamine from guinea-pig pulmonary but not peritoneal mast cells. *Biochem Biophys Res Commun*, **189**, 1196–1201.
122. Lueddeckens, G., Bigl, H., Sperling, J., Becker, K., Braquet, P. & Forster, W. (1993) Importance of secondary TXA_2 release in mediating of endothelin-1 induced bronchoconstriction and vasopressin in the guinea-pig. *Prostaglandins Leukot Essent Fatty Acids*, **48**, 261–263.
123. Ninomiya, H., Yu, X. Y., Hasegawa, S. & Spannhake, E. W. (1992) Endothelin-1 induces stimulation of prostaglandin synthesis in cells obtained from canine airways by bronchoalveolar lavage. *Prostaglandins*, **43**, 401–411.
124. Millul, V., Lagente, V., Gillardeaux, O., Boichot, E., Dugas, B., Mencia Huerta, J. M., Bereziat, G., Braquet, P. & Masliah, J. (1991) Activation of guinea pig alveolar macrophages by endothelin-1. *J Cardiovasc Pharmacol*, **17 (Suppl 7)**, S233–S235.
125. Wu, J. M., Cheng, T., Sun, S. D., Niu, D. D., Zhang, J. X., Wang, S. H., Tang, J. & Tang, C. S. (1993) Effect of endothelin, angiotensin II and ANP on proliferation of vascular smooth muscle cells and cardiomyocytes. *Sci China B*, **36**, 948–953.
126. Marsden, P. A., Dorfman, D. M., Collins, T., Brenner, B. M., Orkin, S. H. & Ballerman, B. J. (1991) Regulated expression of endothelin-1 in glomerular capillary endothelial cells. *Am J Physiol*, **261** (1 pt 2), F117–F125.
127. Yoshida, H. & Nakamura, M. (1992) Inhibition by angiotensin converting enzyme inhibitors of endothelin secretion from cultured human endothelial cells. *Life Sci*, **50**, PL195–PL200.

128. Momose, N., Fukuno, K., Morimoto, S. & Ogihara, T. (1993) Captopril inhibits endothelin-1 secretion from endothelial cells through bradykinin. *Hypertension*, **21**, 921–924.
129. Lopez Farre, A., Riesco, A., Moliz, M., Egido, J., Casado, S., Hernando, L. & Caramelo, C. (1991) Inhibition by L-arginine of the endothelin-mediated increase in cytosolic calcium in human neutrophils. *Biochem Biophys Res Commun*, **178**, 884–891.
130. Gomez Garre, D., Guerra, M., Gonzalez, E., Lopez Farre, A., Riesco, A., Caramelo, C., Escanero, J. & Egido, J. (1992) Aggregation of human polymorphonuclear leukocytes by endothelin: role of platelet-activating factor. *Eur J Pharmacol*, **224**, 167–172.
131. Sirois, M. G., Filep, J. G., Rousseau, A., Fournier, A. & Plante, G. E. (1992) Endothelin-1 enhances vascular permeability in conscious rats: role of thromboxane A2. *Eur J Pharmacol*, **214**, 119–125.
132. Takayasu Okishio, M., Terashita, Z. & Kondo, K. (1990) Endothelin-1 and platelet activating factor stimulate thromboxane A2 biosynthesis in rat vascular smooth muscle cells. *Biochem Pharmacol*, **40**, 2713–2717.
133. Kon, V. & Badr, K. F. (1991) Biological actions and pathophysiologic significance of endothelin in the kidney. *Kidney Int*, **40**, 1–12.
134. Yoshizumi, M., Kurihara, H., Morita, T., Yamashita, T., Oh hashi, Y., Sugiyama, T., Yanagisawa, M., Masaki, T. & Yazaki, Y. (1990) Interleukin 1 increases the production of endothelin-1 by cultured endothelial cells. *Biochem Biophys Res Commun*, **166**, 324–329.
135. Sunnergren, K. P., Word, R. A., Sambrook, J. F., MacDonald, P. C. & Casey, M. L. (1990) Expression and regulation of endothelin precursor mRNA in a vascular human amnion. *Mol Cell Endocrinol*, **68**, R7–14.
136. Marsden, P. A. & Brenner, B. M. (1992) Transcriptional regulation of the endothelin-1 gene by TNFα. *Am J Physiol*, **262**, C854–C861.
137. Kohan, D. E. (1992) Production of endothelin-1 by rat mesangial cells: regulation by tumor necrosis factor. *J Lab Clin Med*, **119**, 477–484.
138. Horie, M., Uchida, S., Yanagisawa, M., Matsushita, Y., Kurokawa, K. & Ogata, E. (1991) Mechanisms of endothelin-1 mRNA and peptides induction by TGFβ and TPA in MDCK cells. *J Cardiovasc Pharmacol*, **17 (Suppl 7)**, S222–S225.
139. Katabami, T., Shimizu, M., Okano, K., Yano, Y., Nemoto, K., Ogura, M., Tsukamoto, T., Suzuki, S., Ohira, K., Yamada, Y. et al. (1992) Intracellular signal transduction for interleukin-1β-induced endothelin production in human umbilical vein endothelial cells. *Biochem Biophys Res Commun*, **188**, 565–570.
140. Kense, S. M., Takahashi, K., Lam, H. C., Rees, A., Warren, J. B., Porta, M., Molinatti, P., Ghatei, M. & Bloom, S. R. (1991) Cytokine stimulated endothelin release from endothelial cells. *Life Sci*, **48**, 1379–1384.
141. Brown, M. R., Vaughan, J., Jimenez, L. L., Vale, W. & Baird, A. (1991) Transforming growth factor β: role in mediating serum-induced endothelin production by vascular endothelial cells. *Endocrinology*, **129**, 2355–2360.
142. Namiki, A., Hirata, Y., Fukazawa, M., Ishikawa, M., Moroi, M., Aikawa, J., Yamaguchi, T. & Machii, K. (1992) Granulocyte-colony stimulating factor stimulates immunoreactive endothelin-1 release from cultured bovine endothelial cells. *Eur J Pharmacol*, **227**, 339–341.
143. Mitchell, M. D., Lundin, S. S. & Edwin, S. S. (1991) Endothelin production by amnion and its regulation by cytokines. *Am J Obstet Gynecol*, **165(1)**, 120–124.
144. Tseng, Y. C., Lahiri, S., Jackson, S., Burman, K. D. & Wartofsky, L. (1993) Endothelin binding to receptors and endothelin production by human thyroid follicular cells: effects of transforming growth factor β and thyrotropin. *J Clin Endocrinol Metab*, **76**, 156–161.
145. Imokawa, G., Yada, Y. & Miyagishi, M. (1992) Endothelins secreted from human keratinocytes are intrinsic mitogens for human melanocytes. *J Biol Chem*, **267**, 24675–24680.
146. Ohta, K., Hirata, Y., Imai, T., Kanno, K., Emori, T., Shichiri, M. & Marumo, F. (1990) Cytokine-induced release of endothelin-1 from porcine renal epithelial cell line. *Biochem Biophys Res Commun*, **169**, 578–584.
147. Endo, T., Uchida, Y., Matsumoto, H., Suzuki, N., Nomura, A., Hirata, F. & Hasegawa, S. (1992) Regulation of endothelin-1 synthesis in cultured guinea pig airway epithelial cells by various cytokines. *Biochem Biophys Res Commun*, **186**, 1594–1599.
148. Lamas, S., Michel, T., Collins, T., Brenner, B. M. & Marsden, P. A. (1992) Effects of interferon-gamma on nitric oxide synthase activity and endothelin-1 production by vascular endothelial cells. *J Clin Invest*, **90**, 879–887.
149. Yamamoto, C., Kaji, T., Sakamoto, M. & Kozuka, H. (1993) Modulation by endothelin-1 of tissue plasminogen activator and plasminogen activator inhibitor-1 release from cultured human vascular endothelial cells: interaction of endothelin-1 with cytokines. *Biol Pharm Bull*, **16**, 714–715.
150. Jougasaki, M., Kugiyama, K., Saito, Y., Nakao, K., Imura, H. & Yasue, H. (1992) Suppression of

endothelin-1 secretion by lysophosphatidylcholine in oxidized low density lipoprotein in cultured vascular endothelial cells. *Circ Res*, **71**, 614–619.
151. Horio, T., Kohno, M., Yasunari, K., Murakawa, K., Yokokawa, K., Ikeda, M., Fukui, T. & Takeda, T. (1993) Stimulation of endothelin-1 release by low density and very low density lipoproteins in cultured human endothelial cells. *Atherosclerosis*, **101**, 185–190.
152. Martin Nizard, F., Houssaini, H. S., Lestavel Delattre, S., Duriez, P. & Fruchart, J. C. (1991) Modified low density lipoproteins activate human macrophages to secrete immunoreactive endothelin. *FEBS Lett*, **293**, 127–130.
153. Boulanger, C. M., Tanner, F. C., Bea, M. L., Hahn, A. W., Werner, A. & Luscher, T. F. (1992) Oxidized low density lipoproteins induce mRNA expression and release of endothelin from human and porcine endothelium. *Circ Res*, **70**, 1191–1197.
154. Henriksen, T., Mahoney, E. M. & Steinberg, D. (1983) Enhanced macrophage degradation of biologically modified low density lipoprotein. *Arteriosclerosis*, **3**, 149–159.
155. Henriksen, T., Evensen, S. A. & Carlander, B. (1979) Injury to human endothelial cells in culture induced by low density lipoproteins. *Scand J Clin Lab Invest*, **39**, 361–368.
156. Hessler, J. R., Robertson, A. L. & Chisolm, G. M. (1979) LDL-induced cytotoxicity and its inhibition by HDL in human vascular smooth muscle and endothelial cells in culture. *Atherosclerosis*, **32**, 213–229.
157. Yla-Hertulla, S., Palinski, W., Rosenfeld, M. E., Parthasarathy, S., Carew, T. E., Butler, S., Witztum, J. L. & Steinberg, D. (1989) Evidence for the presence of oxidatively modified low density lipoprotein in atherosclerotic lesions of rabbit and man. *J Clin Invest*, **84**, 1086–1095.
158. Tanner, F. C., Noll, G., Boulanger, C. M. & Luscher, T. F. (1991) Oxidized low density lipoproteins inhibit relaxations of porcine coronary arteries. *Circulation*, **83**, 2012.
159. Chin, J. H., Azhar, S. & Hoffman, B. B. (1992) Inactivation of endothelium-derived relaxing factor by oxidized lipoproteins. *J Clin Invest*, **89**, 10.
160. Galle, J., Bassenge, E. & Busse, R. (1990) Oxidized low-density lipoproteins potentiate vasoconstrictions to various agonists by direct interaction with vascular smooth muscle. *Cir Res*, **66**, 1287–1293.
161. Simon, B. C., Cunningham, L. D. & Cohen, R. A. (1990) Oxidized low-density lipoproteins cause contraction and inhibit endothelium-dependent relaxation in the pig coronary artery. *J Clin Invest*, **86**, 75.
162. Lerman, A., Edwards, B. S., Hallett, J. W., Heublein, D. M., Sandberg, S. M. & Burnett, J. C. L. (1991) Circulating and tissue endothelin immunoreactivity in advanced atherosclerosis. *N Engl J Med*, **325**, 997–1001.
163. Arendt, R. M., Wilbert-Lampen, U. & Heucke, L. (1990) Increased plasma endothelin in patients with hyperlipoproteinemia and stable or unstable angina. *Circulation*, **82**, III–248.
164. Komuro, I., Kurihara, H., Sugiyama, T., Yoshizumi, M., Takaku, F. & Yazaki, Y. (1988) Endothelin stimulates c-fos and c-myc expression and proliferation of vascular smooth muscle cells. *FEBS Lett*, **238**, 249–252.
165. Nakaki, T., Nakayama, M., Yamamoto, S. & Kato, R. (1989) Endothelin-mediated stimulation of DNA synthesis in vascular smooth muscle cells. *Biochem Biophys Res Commun*, **158**, 880–883.
166. Nakaki, T., Nakayama, M. & Kato, R. (1990) Inhibition by nitric oxide and nitric oxide-producing vasodilators of DNA synthesis in vascular smooth muscle cells. *Eur J Pharmacol*, **189**, 347–353.
167. Neuser, D., Knorr, A., Stasch, J. P. & Kazda, S. (1990) Mitogenic activity of endothelin-1 and -3 on vascular smooth muscle cells is inhibited by atrial natriuretic peptides. *Artery*, **17**, 311–324.
168. Weissberg, P. L., Witchell, C., Davenport, A. P., Hesketh, T. R. & Metcalfe, J. C. (1990) The endothelin peptides ET-1, ET-2, ET-3 and sarafotoxin S6b are co-mitogenic with platelet-derived growth factor for vascular smooth muscle cells. *Atherosclerosis*, **85**, 257–262.
169. Hirata, Y., Takagi, Y., Fukuda, Y. & Marumo, F. (1989) ET is a potent mitogen for rat vascular smooth muscle cells. *Atherosclerosis*, **78**, 225–228.
170. Yeh, Y. C., Burns, E. R., Yeh, J. & Yeh, H. W. (1991) Synergistic effects of endothelin-1 (ET-1) and transforming growth factor alpha (TGFα) or epidermal growth factor (EGF) on DNA replication and G1 to S phase transition. *Biosci Rep*, **11**, 171–180.
171. Brown, K. D. & Littlewood, C. J. (1989) Endothelin stimulates DNA synthesis in Swiss 3T3 cells. Synergy with polypeptide growth factors. *Biochem J*, **263**, 977–980.
172. Muldoon, L. L., Pribnow, D., Rodland, K. D. & Magun, B. E. (1990) Endothelin-1 stimulates DNA synthesis and anchorage-independent growth of Rat-1 fibroblasts through a protein kinase C-dependent mechanism. *Cell Regul*, **1**, 379–390.
173. Schrey, M. P., Patel, K. V. & Tezapsidis, N. (1992) Bombesin and glucocorticoids stimulate human breast cancer cells to produce endothelin, a paracrine mitogen for breast stromal cells. *Cancer Res*, **52**, 1786–1790.

174. Kusuhara, M., Yamaguchi, K., Nagasaki, K., Hayashi, C., Suzaki, A., Hori, S., Handa, S. & Abe, K. (1990) Production of endothelin in human cancer cell lines. *Cancer Res*, **50**, 3257–3261.
175. Yada, Y., Higuchi, K. & Imokawa, G. (1991) Effects of endothelins on signal transduction and proliferation in human melanocytes. *J Biol Chem*, **266**, 18352–18357.
176. Fabregat, I. & Rozengurt, E. (1990) Vasoactive intenstinal contractor, a novel peptide, shares a common receptor with endothelin-1 and stimulates Ca^{2+} mobilization and DNA synthesis in Swiss 3T3 cells. *Biochem Biophys Res Commun*, **167**, 161–167.
177. Badr, K. F., Murray, J. J., Breyer, M. D., Takahashi, K., Inagami, T. & Harris, R. C. (1989) Mesangial cell, glomerular and renal vascular responses to endothelin in rat kidney. *J Clin Invest*, **83**, 336–342.
178. Takuwa, N., Takuwa, Y., Yanagisawa, M., Yamashita, K. & Masaki, T. (1989) A novel vasoactive peptide stimulates mitogenesis through inositol lipid turnover in swiss 3T3 cells. *J Biol Chem*, **264**, 7856–7861.
179. Miyakawa, M., Tsushima, T., Isozaki, O., Demura, H., Shizume, K. & Arai, M. (1992) Endothelin-1 stimulates c-fos mRNA expression and acts as a modulator on cell proliferation of rat FRTL5 thyroid cells. *Biochem Biophys Res Commun*, **184**, 231–238.
180. Fant, M. E., Nanu, L. & Word, R. A. (1992) A potential role for endothelin-1 in human placental growth: interactions with the insulin-like growth factor family of peptides. *J Clin Endocrinol Metab*, **74**, 1158–1163.
181. Schvartz, I., Ittoop, O., Davidai, G. & Hazum, E. (1992) Endothelin rapidly stimulates tyrosine phosphorylation in osteoblast-like cells. *Peptides*, **13**, 159–163.
182. Jaffer, F. E., Knauss, T. C., Poptic, E. & Abboud, H. E. (1990) Endothelin stimulates PDGF secretion in cultured human mesangial cells. *Kidney Int*, **38**, 1193–1198.
183. Wolpert, H. A., Steen, S. N., Istfan, N. W. & Simonson, D. C. (1993) Insulin modulates circulating endothelin-1 levels in humans. *Metabolism*, **42**, 1027–1030.
184. Frank, H. J., Levin, E. R., Hu, R. M. & Pedram, A. (1993) Insulin stimulates endothelin binding and action on cultured vascular smooth muscle cells. *Endocrinology*, **133**, 1092–1097.
185. Tokito, F., Suzuki, N., Hosoya, M., Matsumoto, H., Ohkubo, S. & Fujino, M. (1991) Epidermal growth factor (EGF) decreased endothelin-2 (ET-2) production in human renal adenocarcinoma cells. *FEBS Lett*, **295**, 17–21.
186. Hassoun, P. M., Thappa, V., Landman, M. J. & Fanburg, B. L. (1992) Endothelin 1: mitogenic activity on pulmonary artery smooth muscle cells and release from hypoxic endothelial cells. *Proc Soc Exp Biol Med*, **199**, 165–170.
187. Ohlstein, E. H., Storer, B. L., Butcher, J. A., Debouck, C. & Feuerstein, G. (1991) Platelets stimulate expression of endothelin mRNA and endothelin biosynthesis in cultured endothelial cells. *Circ Res*, **69**, 832–841.
188. Economos, K., MacDonald, P. C. & Casey, M. L. (1992) Endothelin-1 gene expression and biosynthesis in human endometrial HEC-1A cancer cells. *Cancer Res*, **52**, 554–557.
189. Uchida, Y., Saotome, M., Nonura, A., Ninomiya, H., Ohse, H., Hirata, F. & Hasegawa, S. (1991) Endothelin-1-induced relaxation of guinea pig trachealis muscles. *J Cardiovasc Pharmacol*, **17 (Suppl 7)**, S210–S212.
190. Oliver, F. J., de la Rubia, G., Feener, E. P., Lee, M. E., Loeken, M. R., Shiba, T., Quertermous, T. & King, G. L. (1991) Stimulation of endothelin-1 gene expression by insulin in endothelial cells. *J Biol Chem*, **266**, 23251–23256.
191. Hu, R. M., Levin, E. R., Pedram, A. & Frank, H. J. (1993) Insulin stimulates production and secretion of endothelin from bovine endothelial cells. *Diabetes*, **42**, 351–358.
192. Hattori, Y., Kasai, K., Nakamura, T., Emoto, T. & Shimoda, S. (1991) Effect of glucose and insulin on immunoreactive endothelin-1 release from cultured porcine aortic endothelial cells. *Metabolism*, **40(2)**, 165–169.
193. Yanagisawa, M., Kurihara, H., Kimura, S., Tomobe, Y., Kobayashi, M., Mitsui, Y., Yazaki, Y., Goto, K. & Masaki, T. (1988) A novel potent vasoconstrictor peptide produced by vascular endothelial cells. *Nature*, **332**, 411–415.
194. Imai, T., Hirata, Y., Emori, T. & Marumo, F. (1993) Heparin has an inhibitory effect on endothelin-1 synthesis and release by endothelial cells. *Hypertension*, **21**, 353–358.
195. Cocks, T. M., Malta, E., King, S. J., Woods, R. L. & Angus, J. A. (1991) Oxyhaemoglobin increases the production of endothelin-1 by endothelial cells in culture. *Eur J Pharmacol*, **196**, 177–182.
196. Kasuya, H., Weir, B. K., White, D. M. & Stefansson, K. (1993) Mechanism of oxyhemoglobin-induced release of endothelin-1 from cultured vascular endothelial cells and smooth muscle cells. *J Neurosurg*, **79(6)**, 892–898.
197. Fuwa, I., Mayberg, M., Gadjusek, C., Harada, T. & Luo, Z. (1993) Enhanced secretion of endothelin by endothelial cells in response to hemoglobin. *Neurol Med Chir*, **33(11)**, 739–743.
198. Vierhapper, H., Hollenstein, U., Roden, M. & Nowotny, P. (1993) Effect of endothelin-1 in

man-impact on basal and stimulated concentrations of luteinizing hormone, follicle-stimulating hormone, thyrotropin, growth hormone, corticotropin, and prolactin. *Metabolism*, **42**, 902–906.
199. Makino, S., Hashimoto, K., Hirasawa, R., Hattori, T., Kageyama, J. & Ota, Z. (1990) Central interaction between endothelin and brain natriuretic peptide on pressor and hormonal responses. *Brain Res*, **534**, 117–121.
200. Wall, K. M., Nasr, M. & Ferguson, A. V. (1992) Actions of endothelin at the subfornical organ. *Brain Res*, **570**, 180–187.
201. Wall, K. M. & Ferguson, A. V. (1992) Endothelin acts at the subfornical organ to influence the activity of putative vasopressin and oxytocin-secreting neurons. *Brain Res*, **586**, 111–116.
202. Yoshizawa, T., Shinmi, O., Giaid, A., Yanagisawa, M., Gibson, S. J., Kimura, S., Uchiyama, Y., Masaki, T. & Kanazawa, I. (1990) Endothelin: a novel peptide in the posterior pituitary system. *Science*, **247**, 462–464.
203. Nakamura, S., Naruse, M., Naruse, K., Shioda, S., Nakai, Y. & Uemura, H. (1993) Colocalization of immunoreactive endothelin-1 and neuropophysial hormones in the axons of the neural lobe of the rat pituitary. *Endocrinology*, **132**, 530–533.
204. Ritz, M. F., Stuenkel, E. L., Dayanithi, G., Jones, R. & Nordmann, J. J. (1992) Endothelin regulation of neuropeptide release from nerve endings of the posterior pituitary. *Proc Natl Acad Sci USA*, **89**, 8371–8375.
205. Samson, W. K., Skala, K. D., Alexander, B. D. & Huang, F. L. (1990) Pituitary site of action of endothelin: selective inhibition of prolactin release *in vitro*. *Biochem Biophys Res Commun*, **169**, 737–743.
206. Dymshitz, J., Laudon, M. & Ben Jonathan, N. (1992) Endothelin-induced biphasic response of lactotrophs cultured under different conditions. *Neuroendocrinology*, **55**, 724–729.
207. Burris, T. P., Kanyicska, B. & Freeman, M. E. (1991) Inhibition of prolactin secretion by endothelin-3 is pertussis toxin-sensitive. *Eur J Pharmacol*, **198**, 223–225.
208. Krsmanovic, L. Z., Stojilkovic, S. S., Bhalla, T., Al Damluji, S., Weiner, R. I. & Catt, K. J. (1991) Receptors and neurosecretory actions of endothelin in hypothalamic neurons. *Proc Natl Acad Sci*, **88**, 11124–11128.
209. Moretto, M., Lopez, F. J. & Negro Vilar, A. (1993) Endothelin-3 stimulates luteinizing hormone-releasing hormone (LHRH) secretion from LHRH neurons by a prostaglandin-dependent mechanism. *Endocrinology*, **132**, 789–794.
210. Shichiri, M., Hirata, Y., Kanno, K., Ohta, K., Emori, T. & Marumo, F. (1989) Effect of endothelin-1 on release of arginine-vasopressin from perifused rat hypothalamus. *Biochem Biophys Res Commun*, **163**, 1332–1337.
211. Yamamoto, S., Morimoto, I., Yamashita, H. & Eto, S. (1992) Inhibitory effects of endothelin-3 on vasopressin release from rat supraoptic neucleus *in vitro*. *Neurosci Lett*, **141**, 147–150.
212. Rossi, N. F. (1993) Effect of endothelin-3 on vasopressin release *in vitro* and water excretion *in vivo* in Long-Evans rats. *J Physiol Lond*, **461**, 501–511.
213. Stojilkovic, S. S., Iida, T., Merelli, F. & Catt, K. J. (1991) Calcium signaling and secretory responses in endothelin-stimulated anterior pituitary cells. *Mol Pharmacol*, **39**, 762–770.
214. Stojilkovic, S. S., Merelli, F., Iida, T., Krsmanovic, L. Z. & Catt, K. J. (1990) Endothelin stimulation of cytosolic calcium and gonadotropin secretion in anterior pituitary cells. *Science*, **248**, 1663–1666.
215. Kanyicska, B., Burris, T. P. & Freeman, M. E. (1991) Endothelin-3 inhibits prolactin and stimulates LH, FSH and TSH secretion from pituitary cell culture. *Biochem Biophys Res Commun*, **174**, 338–343.
216. Stojilkovic, S. S., Balla, T., Fukuda, S., Cesnjaj, M., Merelli, F., Krsmanovic, L. Z. & Catt, K. J. (1992) Endothelin ETA receptors mediate the signaling and secretory actions of endothelins in pituitary gonadotrophs. *Endocrinology*, **130**, 465–474.
217. Samson, W. K. (1992) The endothelin-A receptor subtype transduces the effects of the endothelins in the anterior pituitary gland. *Biochem Biophys Res Commun*, **187**, 590–595.
218. Domae, M., Yamada, K., Hanabusa, Y. & Furukawa, T. (1992) Inhibitory effects of endothelin-1 and endothelin-3 on prolactin release: possible involvement of endogenous endothelin isopeptides in the rat anterior pituitary. *Life Sci*, **50**, 715–722.
219. Chao, H. S., Myers, S. E. & Handwerger, S. (1993) Endothelin inhibits basal and stimulated release of prolactin by human dicidual cells. *Endocrinology*, **133**, 505–510.
220. Samson, W. K., Skala, K. D., Alexander, B. D., Huang, F. L. & Gomez Sanchez, C. (1992) A prolactin release inhibiting activity isolated from neurointermediate lobe extracts is an endothelin-like peptide. *Regul Pept*, **39**, 103–112.
221. Samson, W. K. & Skala, K. D. (1992) Comparison of the pituitary effects of the mammalian endothelins: vasoactive intestinal contractor (endothelinβ, rat endothelin-2) is a potent inhibitor of prolactin secretion. *Endocrinology*, **130**, 2964–2970.

222. Morishita, R., Higaki, J. & Ogihara, T. (1989) Endothelin stimulates aldosterone biosynthesis by dispersed rabbit adreno-capsular cells. *Biochem Biophys Res Commun*, **160**, 628–632.
223. Rosolowsky, L. J. & Campbell, W. B. (1990) Endothelin enhances adrenocorticotropin-stimulated aldosterone release from cultured bovine adrenal cells. *Endocrinology*, **126**, 1860–1866.
224. Cozza, E. N., Chiou, S. & Gomez Sanchez, C. E. (1992) Endothelin-1 potentiation of angiotensin II stimulation of aldosterone production. *Am J Physiol*, **262**, R85–R89.
225. Zeng, Z. P., Naruse, M., Guan, B. J., Naruse, K., Sun, M. L., Zang, M. F., Demura, H. & Shi, Y. F. (1992) Endothelin stimulates aldosterone secretion *in vitro* from normal adrenocortical tissue, but no adenoma tissue, in primary aldosteronism. *J Clin Endocrinol Metab*, **74**, 874–878.
226. Woodcock, E. A., Tanner, J. K., Caroccia, L. M. & Little, P. J. (1990) Mechanisms involved in the stimulation of aldosterone production by angiotensin II, vasopressin and endothelin. *Clin Exp Pharmacol Physiol*, **17**, 263–267.
227. Sanchez Ferrer, C. F. & Marin, J. (1990) Endothelium-derived contractile factors. *Gen Pharmacol*, **21**, 589–603.
228. Hinson, J. P., Vinson, G. P., Kapas, S. & Teja, R. (1991) The role of endothelin in the control of adrenocortical function: stimulation of endothelin release by ACTH and the effects of endothelin-1 and endothelin-3 on steroidogenesis in rat and human adrenocortical cells. *J Endocrinol*, **128**(2), 275–280.
229. Hinson, J. P., Kapas, S., Teja, R. & Vinson, G. P. (1991) Effect of the endothelins on aldosterone secretion by rat zona glomerulosa cells *in vitro*. *J Steroid Biochem Mol Biol*, **40**, 437–439.
230. Cozza, E. N. & Gomez Sanchez, C. E. (1990) Effects of endothelin-1 on its receptor concentration and thymidine incorporation in calf adrenal zona glomerulosa cells: a comparative study with phorbol esters. *Endocrinology*, **127**, 549–554.
231. Conte, D., Questino, P., Fillo, S., Nordio, M., Isidori, A. & Romanelli, F. (1993) Endothelin stimulates testosterone secretion by rat Leydig cells. *J Endocrinol*, **136**, R1–R4.
232. Ergul, A., Glassberg, M. K., Majercik, M. H. & Puett, D. (1993) Endothelin-1 promotes steroidogenesis and stimulates protooncogene expression in transformed murine Leydig cells. *Endocrinology*, **132**, 598–603.
233. Usuki, S., Saitoh, T., Suzuki, N., Kitada, C., Goto, K. & Masaki, T. (1991) Endothelin-1 and endothelin-3 stimulate ovarian steroidogenesis. *J Cardiovasc Pharmacol*, **17** (Suppl 7), S256–S259.
234. Flores, J. A., Quyyumi, S., Leong, D. A. & Veldhuis, J. D. (1992) Actions of endothelin-1 on swine ovarian (granulosa) cells. *Endocrinology*, **131**, 1350–1358.
235. Kamada, S., Kubota, T., Hirata, Y., Imai, T., Ohta, K., Taguchi, M., Marumo, F. & Aso, T. (1993) Endothelin-1 is an autocrine/paracrine regulator of porcine granulosa cells. *J Endocrinol Invest*, **16**, 425–431.
236. Kamada, S., Kubota, T., Hirata, Y., Taguchi, M., Eguchi, S., Marumo, F. & Aso, T. (1992) Direct effect of endothelin-1 on the granuloma cells of the porcine ovary. *J Endocrinol*, **134**, 59–66.
237. Iwai, M., Hasegawa, M., Taii, S., Sagawa, N., Nakao, K., Imura, H., Nakanishi, S. & Mori, T. (1991) Endothelins inhibit luteinization of cultured porcine granulosa cells. *Endocrinology*, **129**, 1909–1914.
238. Hinson, J. P., Vinson, G. P., Kapas, S. & Teja, R. (1991) The relationship between adrenal vascular events and steroid secretion: the role of mast cells and endothelin. *J Steroid Biochem Mol Biol*, **40**, 381–389.
239. Kanse, S. M., Takahashi, K., Warren, J. B., Ghatei, M. & Bloom, S. R. (1991) Glucocorticoids induce endothelin release from vascular smooth muscle cells but not endothelial cells. *Eur J Pharmacol*, **199**(1), 99–101.
240. Polderman, K. H., Stehouwer, C. D., van Kamp, G. J., Dekker, G. A., Verheugt, F. W. & Gooren, L. J. (1993) Influence of sex hormones on plasma endothelin levels. *Ann Intern Med*, **118**, 429–432.
241. Maggi, M., Fantoni, G., Peri, A., Giannini, S., Brandi, M. L., Orlando, C. & Serio, M. (1991) Steroid modulation of oxytocin/vasopressin receptors in the uterus. *J Steroid Biochem Mol Biol*, **40**, 481–491.
242. Maggi, M., Vannelli, G. B., Peri, A., Brandi, M. L., Fantoni, G., Giannini, S., Torrisi, C., Guardabasso, V., Barni, T., Toscano, V. *et al.* (1991) Immunolocalization, binding, and biological activity of endothelin in rabbit uterus: effect of ovarian steroids. *Am J Physiol*, **260**, E292–E305.
243. Eaton, L. W. M. & Hilliard, J. (1971) Estradiol-17β, progesterone and 20α-hydroxypregn-4-en-3-one in rabbit ovaries venous plasma. I. Steroid secretion from paired ovaries with an without corpora luteal effect of LH. *Endocrinology*, **89**, 105–111.
244. Peri, A., Vannelli, G. B., Fantoni, G., Giannini, S., Barni, T., Orlando, C., Serio, M. & Maggi, M. (1992) Endothelin in rabbit uterus during pregnancy. *Am J Physiol*, **263**, E158–E167.
245. McGovern, P. G., Goldsmith, L. T., Schmidt, C. L., Von Hagen, S., Linden, M. & Weiss, G. (1992) Effects of endothelin and relaxin on rat uterine segment contractility. *Biol Reprod*, **46**, 680–685.
246. Usuki, S., Saitoh, T., Sawamura, T., Suzuki, N., Shigemitsu, S., Yanagisawa, M., Goto, K., Fujino, M. & Masaki, T. (1990) Increased maternal plasma concentration of endothelin-1 during labor pain or on

delivery and the existence of a large amount of endothelin-1 in amniotic fluid. *Gynecol Endocrinol*, **4**, 85–97.
247. Yang, D. & Clark, K. E. (1992) Effect of endothelin-1 on the uterine vasculature of the pregnant and estrogen-treated nonpregnant sheep. *Am J Obstet Gynecol*, **167**, 1642–1650.
248. Cameron, I. T., Davenport, A. P., Brown, M. J. & Smith, S. K. (1991) Endothelin-1 stimulates prostaglandin $F_{2\alpha}$ release from human endometrium. *Prostagl Leukotr Essent Fatty Acids*, **42**, 155–157.
249. Orlando, C., Brandi, M. L., Peri, A., Giannini, S., Fantoni, G., Calabresi, E., Serio, M. & Maggi, M. (1990) Neurohypophyseal hormone regulation of endothelin secretion from rabbit endometrial cells in primary culture. *Endocrinology*, **126**, 1780–1783.
250. Kohno, M., Murakawa, K., Yokokawa, K., Yasunari, K., Horio, T., Kurihara, N. & Takeda, T. (1989) Production of endothelin by cultured porcine endothelial cells: modulation by adrenaline. *J Hypertens Suppl*, **7**, S130–S131.
251. Wiklund, N. P., Ohlén, A., Wiklund, C. U., Hedqvist, P. & Gustafsson, L. E. (1990) Endothelin modulation of neuroeffector transmission in rat and guinea pig vas deferens. *Eur J Pharmacol*, **185**, 25–33.
252. Wiklund, N. P., Wiklund, C. U., Cederqvist, B., Ohlen, A., Hedqvist, P. & Gustafsson, L. E. (1991) Endothelin modulation of neuroeffector transmission in smooth muscle. *J Cardiovasc Pharmacol*, **17 (Suppl 7)**, S335–S339.
253. Tabuchi, Y., Nakamaru, M., Rakugi, H., Nagano, M. & Ogihara, T. (1989) Endothelin enhances adrenergic vasoconstriction in perfused rat mesenteric arteries. *Biochem Biophys Res Commun*, **159**, 1304–1308.
254. Nakamaru, M., Tabuchi, Y., Rakugi, H., Nagano, M. & Ogihara, T. (1989) Actions of endothelin on adrenergic neuroeffector junction. *J Hypertens Suppl*, **7**, S132–S133.
255. Wiklund, N. P., Ohlen, A. & Cederqvist, B. (1989) Adrenergic neuromodulation by endothelin in guinea pig pulmonary artery. *Neurosci Lett*, **101**, 269–273.
256. Wiklund, N. P., Ohlen, A. & Cederqvist, B. (1988) Inhibition of adrenergic neuroeffector transmission by endothelin in the guinea-pig femoral artery. *Acta Physiol Scand*, **134**, 311–312.
257. Takagi, H., Hisa, H. & Satoh, S. (1991) Effects of endothelin on adrenergic neurotransmission in the dog kidney. *Eur J Pharmacol*, **203**, 291–294.
258. Suzuki, Y., Matsumura, Y., Umekawa, T., Hayashi, K., Takaoka, M. & Morimoto, S. (1992) Effects of endothelin-1 on antidiuresis and norepinephrine overflow induced by stimulation of renal nerves in anesthetized dogs. *J Cardiovasc Pharmacol*, **19**, 905–910.
259. Nishimura, M., Takahashi, H., Matsusawa, M., Ikegaki, I., Sakamoto, M., Nakanishi, T., Hirabayashi, M. & Yoshimura, M. (1991) Chronic intracerebroventricular infusions of endothelin elevate arterial pressure in rats. *J Hypertens*, **9**, 71–76.
260. Yamamoto, T., Kimura, T., Ota, K., Shoji, M., Inoue, M., Sato, K., Ohta, M. & Yoshinaga, K. (1991) Central effects of endothelin-1 on vasopressin and atrial natriuretic peptide release and cardiovascular and renal function in conscious rats. *J Cardiovasc Pharmacol*, **17 (Suppl 7)**, S316–S318.
261. Boarder, M. R. & Marriott, D. B. (1991) Endothelin-1 stimulation of noradrenaline and adrenaline release from adrenal chromaffin cells. *Biochem Pharmacol*, **41(4)**, 521–526.
262. Henrion, D. & Laher, I. (1993) Potentiation of norepinephrine-induced contractions by endothelin-1 in the rabbit aorta. *Hypertension*, **22**, 78–83.
263. Yang, Z. H., Richard, V., von Segesser, L., Bauer, E., Stulz, P., Turina, M. & Luscher, T. F. (1990) Threshold concentrations of endothelin-1 potentiate contractions to norepinephrine and serotonin in human arteries. A new mechanism of vasospasm? *Circulation*, **82**, 188–195.
264. Reid, J. J., Vo, P. A., Lieu, A. T., Wong Dusting, H. K. & Rand, M. J. (1991) Modulation of norepinephrine-induced vasoconstriction by endothelin-1 and nitric oxide in rat tail artery. *J Cardiovasc Pharmacol*, **17 (Suppl 7)**, S272–S275.
265. MacLean, M. R. & McGrath, J. C. (1990) Effects of pre-contraction with endothelin-1 on α_2-adrenoceptor- and (endothelium-dependent) neuropeptide Y-mediated contractions in the isolated vascular bed of the rat tail. *Br J Pharmacol*, **101**, 205–211.
266. Gulati, A. & Srimal, R. C. (1993) Endothelin antagonizes the hypotension and potentiates the hypertension induced by clonidine. *Eur J Pharmacol*, **230**, 293–300.
267. Gulati, A. (1992) Evidence for antagonistic activity of endothelin for clonidine induced hypotension and bradycardia. *Life Sci*, **50**, 153–160.
268. Kushiku, K., Ohjimi, H., Yamada, H., Tokunaga, R. & Furukawa, T. (1991) Endothelin-3 inhibits ganglionic transmission at preganglionic sites through activation of endogenous thromboxane A_2 production in dog cardiac sympathetic ganglia. *J Cardiovasc Pharmacol*, **17 (Suppl 7)**, S197–S199.
269. Saenz De Tejada, I., Mueller, J. D., De Las Morenas, A., Machado, M., Moreland, R. B., Krane, R. J., Wolfe, H, J. & Traish, A. M. (1992) Endothelin in the urinary bladder. I. Synthesis of endothelin-1

by epithelia, smooth muscle and fibroblasts suggest autocrine and paracrine cellular regulation. *The J Urology*, **148**, 1290–1298.
270. Koizumi, S., Kataoka, Y., Niwa, M. & Kumakura, K. (1992) Endothelin-3 stimulates the release of catecholamine from cortical and striatal slices of the rat. *Neurosci Lett*, **134**, 219–222.
271. Fuxe, K., Kurosawa, N., Cintra, A., Hallstrom, A., Goiny, M., Rosen, L., Agnati, L. F. & Ungerstedt, U. (1992) Involvement of local ischemia in endothelin-1 induced lesions of the neostriatum of the anaesthetized rat. *Exp Brain Res*, **88**, 131–139.
272. Konya, H., Nagai, K., Masuda, H. & Kakishita, E. (1992) Endothelin-3 modification of dopamine release in anaesthetised rate striatum; an *in vivo* microdialysis study. *Life Sci*, **51**, 499–506.
273. Loesch, A., Bodin, P. & Burnstock, G. (1991) Colocalization of endothelin, vasopressin and serotonin in cultured endothelial cells of rabbit aorta. *Peptides*, **12**, 1095–1103.
274. Pietraszek, M. H., Takada, Y. & Takada, A. (1992) Endothelins inhibit serotonin-induced platelet aggregation via a mechanism involving protein kinase C. *Eur J Pharmacol*, **219**, 289–293.
275. Seiss, W. (1991) Multiple signal-transduction pathways synergize in platelet activation. *NIPS*, **6**, 51.
276. Li, T., Croce, K. & Winquist, R. J. (1992) Vasoconstrictor and vasodilator effects of serotonin in the isolated rabbit kidney. *J Pharmacol Exp Ther*, **263**, 928–932.
277. Nakayama, K., Ishigai, Y., Uchida, H. & Tanaka, Y. (1991) Potentiation by endothelin-1 of 5-hydroxytrypatamine-induced contraction in coronary artery of the pig. *Br J Pharmacol*, **104**, 978–986.
278. Wong Dusting, H. K., La, M. & Rand, M. J. (1991) Effect of endothelin-1 on responses of isolated blood vessels to vasoconstrictor agonists. *J Cardiovasc Pharmacol*, **17 (Suppl 7)**, S236–S238.
279. Forstermann, U., Mugge, A., Bode, S. M. & Frolich, J. C. (1988) Response of human coronary arteries to aggregating plateles: Importance of endothelium-derived relaxing factor and prostanoids. *Circ Res*, **63**, 306–312.
280. Feldan, J. S., Hogaboom, G. K., Westfall, D. P. & O'Donell, J. P. (1982) Comparisons of contractions of the smooth muscle of the guinea-pig vas deferens induced by ATP and related nucleotides. *Eur J Pharmacol*, **81**, 193.
281. Sneddon, P., Westfall, D. P. & Fedan, J. S. (1982) Co-transmitters in the motor nerves the guinea-pig vas deferens. *Science*, **218**, 693.
282. Meldrum, L. A. & Burnstock, G. (1983) Evidence that ATP acts as a co-transmitter with noradrenaline in sympathetic nerves supplying the guinea-pig vas deferens. *Eur J Pharmacol*, **92**, 161.
283. Stjarne, L. & Astrand, P. (1985) Relative pre- and postjunctional roles of noradrenaline and adenosine 5′-triphosphate as neurotransmitters of sympathetic nerves of guinea-pig and mouse vas deferens. *Neuroscience*, **14**, 929.
284. Friel, D. D. (1988) An ATP-sensitive conductance in single smooth muscle cells from the rat vas deferens. *J Physiol*, **401**, 361.
285. Wiklund, N. P., Ohlen, A., Wiklund, C. U., Cederqvist, B., Hedqvist, P. & Gustafsson, L. E. (1989) Neuromuscular actions of endothelin on smooth, cardiac and skeletal muscle from guinea-pig, rat and rabbit. *Acta Physiol Scand*, **137**, 399–407.
286. Donoso, M. V., Montes, C. G., Lewin, J., Fournier, A., Calixto, J. B. & Huidobro Toro, J. P. (1992) Endothelin-1 (ET)-induced mobilization of intracellular Ca^{2+} stores from the smooth muscle facilitates sympathetic cotransmission by potentiation of adenosine 5′-triphosphate (ATP) motor activity: studies in the rat vas deferens. *Peptides*, **13**, 831–840.
287. Mutafova Yambolieva, V. & Radomirov, R. (1993) Effects of endothelin-1 on postjunctionally-mediated purinergic and adrenergic components of rat vas deferens contractile responses. *Neuropeptides*, **24**, 35–42.
288. La, M. & Rand, M. J. (1993) Endothelin-1 enhances vasoconstrictor responses to exogenously administered and neurogenically released ATP in rabbit isolated perfused arteries. *Eur J Pharmacol*, **249**(2), 133–139.
289. Calvo, J. J., Gonzalez, R., De Carvalho, L. F., Takahashi, K., Kanse, S. M., Hart, G. R., Ghatei, M. A. & Bloom, S. R. (1990) Release of substance P from rat hypothalamus and pituitary by endothelin. *Endocrinology*, **126**, 2288–2295.
290. Yoshizawa, T., Kimura, S., Kanazawa, I., Uchiyama, Y., Yanagisawa, M. & Masaki, T. (1989) Endothelin localizes in the dorsal horn and acts on the spinal neurons: possible involvement of dihydropyridine-sensitive calcium channels and substance P release. *Neurosci Lett*, **102**, 179–184.
291. Makino, S., Hashimoto, K., Hirasawa, R., Hattori, T. & Ota, Z. (1992) Central interaction between endothelin and brain natriuretic peptide on vasopressin secretion. *J Hypertens*, **10**, 25–28.
292. Koseki, C., Imai, M., Hirata, Y., Yanagisawa, M. & Masaki, T. (1989) Autoradiographic localization of [^{125}I]-endothelin-1 binding sites in rat brain. *Neurosci Res*, **6**, 581–585.
293. Brown, J. & Czarnecki, A. (1990) Autoradiographic localization of atrial and brain natriuretic peptide receptors in rat brain. *Am J Physiol*, **258**, R57–R63.

7 Biological Activities of Endothelin and their Clinical Significance

Govind Singh, Avadhesh C. Sharma, Sam Rebello and Anil Gulati

Department of Pharmaceutics and Pharmacodynamics (M/C 865), The University of Illinois at Chicago, 833 South Wood Street, Chicago, Illinois 60612-7231, USA

INTRODUCTION

It is now well recognized that vascular endothelium plays an important role in regulation of vascular tone. Endothelial cells produce not only vasodilators, such as endothelium derived relaxing factor (EDRF) and prostacyclin (PGI$_2$), but also vasoconstrictors, like thromboxane (TXA$_2$) and endothelin (ET). ET was initially isolated from a conditioned medium of the cultured porcine aortic endothelial cells[1]. Autoradiographic studies demonstrated that ET-1 binding sites are distributed not only in the vascular system but also in other organs including brain, lung, adrenal gland, kidney, gastrointestinal tract, etc[2,3]. These findings indicate that ET exists in vascular endothelium and also in numerous other tissues, and therefore it can mediate multiple functions depending on the tissues and organs. Numerous reports are now available showing a wide variety of biological actions of ET. A number of clinical studies have been conducted in which ET levels were measured in plasma and cerebrospinal fluid. These studies suggest that ET may be involved in the pathophysiological processes of several diseases.

BIOLOGICAL ACTIONS OF ET

The biological actions of ET have been summarized in Table 7.1. Majority of the proposed actions of ET are based on the data obtained with exogenously administered ET agonists and antagonists, and by detection of local changes in the production of ET. The relevance of these data is unclear at present since it is not known whether ET acts as a local regulatory peptide or as a circulatory hormone[4] or both.

Cardiovascular system

ET has many functions in a vascular system. ET has been demonstrated to induce hypertrophy of myocardial cells[32-34]. ET possesses positive chronotropic[35,36] and

Table 7.1 Biological actions attributed to ET related peptides

Biological actions	References
Systemic hemodynamics Biphasic response on blood pressure; initial hypotension followed by sustained hypertension. Increase in total peripheral resistance.	Clarke et al.[5], Dohi et al.[6], Gardiner et al.[7]

Regional Circulation
  Vasodilation followed by vasoconstriction in different vascular beds.
  Contracts arterioles, venules and some larger arteries. Venules are more sensitive than arterioles.
	Hof et al.[8], Anggard et al.[9], Boric et al.[10]

Heart
  Positive inotropic and chronotropic effects on heart.
  Intense vasoconstriction of coronary vasculature.
  Hypertrophy of cardiac myocytes
	Garcia et al.[11], Hirata et al.[12], Kremer et al.[13], Galron et al.[14], Suzuki et al.[15]

Endocrine System
  Neuropeptide activity.
  Hypothalamic-pituitary axis: stimulation of gonadotrophin secretion from anterior pituitary, and arginine vasopressin and oxytocin release from posterior pituitary.
  Regulation of parathyroid function
  Melanization
  Increases secretion of atrial natriuretic factor, renin, aldosterone, prostaglandins, tissue plasminogen activator and catecholamines.
	Calvo et al.[16], Kanyicska et al.[17], Yoshizawa et al.[18], Fujii et al.[19], Yada et al.[20]
	
	Nakamoto et al.[21]

Renovascular System
  Severe increase in renal vascular resistance, decreases glomerular filteration rate (GFR), renal blood flow and ultrafiltration coefficient.
  Inhibits sodium and water reabsorption
	Cairns et al.[22], Goetz et al.[23], King et al.[24], Garcia et al.[11]

Gastrointestinal tract (GIT)
  Hepatic vasoconstriction and increase in glucose output. Decreases GIT blood flow
  Regulation of sinusoidal blood flow via constriction of fat-storing cells.
  Enhances ethanol-induced ulceration
	Gandhi et al.[25], Takahashi et al.[26], Pinzani et al.[27], Wallace et al.[28], Morales et al.[29]

Pulmonary System
  Bronchial constrictor
  Releases thromboxane from pulmonary mast cells
	Filep et al.[30]

Promitogenic actions Stimulates growth of vascular smooth muscle cells, Swiss 3T3 fibroblasts, mesangial cells, glial cells, melanocytes and tumor cells.	Kester et al.[31], Yada et al.[20]

inotropic[37] effect. The positive inotropic effect on the myocardium results in a transient increase in cardiac output[38-40]. The inotropic action of ET appears to be mediated directly through its receptor, because it could not be blocked by α-adrenergic, β-adrenergic, serotonergic and histaminergic receptor antagonists. ETs elicit a long lasting vasoconstriction in almost all arteries and veins[41]. ET seems to be produced in peripheral vascular beds. Probably the released ET-1 acts on the underlying smooth muscle, resulting in a significant increase in peripheral vascular resistance[42]. Intravenous administration of ET-1 induced a sustained increase in arterial blood pressure in both conscious[1,43,44] and anesthetized animals[45-47]. In a typical experiment measuring the changes in mean arterial pressure after a bolus injection of ET, a depressor response was observed due to the release of vasodilators like prostacyclin and endothelium derived relaxing factors[48-50]. After 5-10 minutes, mean arterial pressure increases due

Biological activities 101

to a sustained increase in the total peripheral resistance and a transient increase in cardiac output. In contrast, infusions of low doses of ET-1 and ET-3 have elicited only a vasodilatory action[51]. Several reports are available demonstrating the initial transient but potent vasodilation of ET that appears to be selective for certain arterial beds[52,53].

Central nervous system (CNS)

Central ET mechanism has been implicated in several biological functions including the regulation of blood pressure[54], respiration[55], fluid and electrolyte homeostasis[56] and behavioral functions[57,58]. ET binding sites are highly concentrated in the choroid plexus, subfornical organ, hippocampus and cerebellum[59]. High density of ET-1 binding sites was also observed in human postmortem brain samples using autoradiography[60]. The presence of ET-1 and ET-3 has been demonstrated in the CNS of rat[61,62], porcine[63] and human[64]. ET-1 mRNA has also been shown to be present in the CNS using in situ hybridization[18,65,66]. Lee et al.[67] have provided convincing evidence that ET can be synthesized in the neurons.

Intracerebroventricular injection of ET in conscious rabbits provoked an increase in arterial blood pressure and renal sympathetic nerve activity accompanied by an increase in plasma norepinephrine, epinephrine, and vasopressin[68]. These findings suggest that ET produced in CNS may modulate the cardiovascular functions. Systemic administration of ET has minimal effects on cerebral blood flow (CBF) or cerebral vessel caliber[69,70] despite occasional claims to the contrary[71] presumably because the blood-brain barrier restricts the access of intraluminal polypeptides to smooth muscle of cerebral resistance vessels[72]. Administration of ET by routes that circumvent the blood brain barrier, such as intracisternal injections[73], intrastriatal injections[74], and onto the adventitial surface of the exposed middle cerebral artery[75,76], invariably produces marked reductions in CBF and leads to ischemic damage of the cerebral tissue[74,76].

Neuroendocrine system

ET has a wide variety of actions on the endocrine system. Functions of virtually all endocrine tissues are shown to be influenced by ETs. Endocrine tissues have a capability to synthesize and secrete ETs. The presence of immunoreactive ETs was found in the paraventricular and supraoptic nuclei of the hypothalamus, the anterior and posterior lobes of pituitary gland[77], in the adrenals[78], ovaries[79], thyroid[80] and parathyroid cells[19]. Investigators have considered ET to be an endocrine or paracrine hormone or a trophic factor[81,82]. In 1990, Yoshizawa et al.[81] proposed two possible roles of ET in this system. Firstly, ET might act locally to modulate the secretion of posterior pituitary hormones, oxytocin and vasopressin. Secondly, ET might be released from the nerve terminals in the posterior pituitary and act as a circulating hormone.

ETs are as potent as gonadotropin releasing hormone (GnRH) in stimulating release of luteinizing hormone, and as important as dopamine in modulating secretion of prolactin from pituitary cells in culture[56]. Secretion of vasopressin and oxytocin from pituitary is enhanced by ETs[83]. Aldosterone secretion is stimulated by ET-1 in rabbit[84] and human zona glomerulosa cells in culture[85]. Physiological role of ET is suggested by its involvement in regulation of ovarian steroidogenesis and development of the follicle[86]. In male and female reproductive tracts ET contracts smooth muscle for sperm transport. Since ET_A has been found in smooth muscle and testicular myoid cells[87], the role of ET in sperm transport seems plausible.

There are conflicting reports that ET influences the secretion of thyrotropin. Kanyicska et al.[17] found that ET-3 increases the release of thyrotropin from anterior pituitary cell culture. On the other hand, Samson et al.[82] found that ET-1 had no effect on the release of thyrotropin from cultured anterior pituitary cells. In another study, ET-1 inhibited thyroglobulin release from human thyroid cell culture after 6 days of incubation[88] and also inhibited thyroid stimulating hormone induced iodine metabolism in porcine thyroid cells in culture via interaction with ET receptor[89]. It appears that ET mechanisms are involved in the regulation of thyroid function or vice versa. *In vivo* studies have suggested that in hyperthyroid rats ET-1 production was increased leading to higher plasma ET-1 and pituitary ET-1 levels[90] which in turn produced down regulation of ET receptors in the pituitary[91]. Renal ET mechanisms have also been found to be altered in the hypo- and hyper-thyroid rats[92].

ET is involved in accelerated atherosclerosis in patients with diabetes[93]. Insulin stimulates ET-1 gene expression in endothelial cells[94]. Therefore, ET as endocrine or paracrine factor may potentially contribute to the complications of diabetes.

Reproductive and fetoplacental system

ET may play an important role in the growth and development of placental tissues. The action of ET has been studied in umbilical cord and chorionic plate vessels. A five fold increase in ET-like immunoreactivity in amniotic fluid was observed at term in comparison to mid trimester values, suggesting a possible role in the constriction of umbilical vessels during delivery[95]. Isolated umbilical arteries and veins were also constricted by ET-1[96]. ET may regulate utero-placental blood flow. ET produced vasoconstrictor effects in small uterine arteries from pregnant women *in vitro*[97]. Uterine smooth muscle is also affected by ET. It stimulates contractile effects in myometrial strips from pregnant women with a similar force and frequency to that produced by oxytocin[98]. Autoradiographic studies have revealed high densities of ET-1, ET-2 and ET-3 in the human uterus, localized to glandular epithelial cells and blood vessels, suggesting a possible role in the control of menstruation[99]. These findings implicate that ET may be involved during labor and in the regulation of vascular tone[100].

Respiratory system

The most often described cause of human asthma is bronchial obstruction, which involves airway smooth muscle contractions. Intravenous infusion of ET-1 to rats increased microvascular permeability in the trachea and bronchi, but not the lung parenchyma[101]. ET-1 also increased rabbit tracheal smooth muscle cell proliferation[102]. It may also act as paracrine hormone in the airways, being synthesized and released from the epithelium and diffusing to underlying smooth muscles. ET-1 is one of the most potent contractile agonists known in human isolated bronchus and pulmonary artery[103].

Human bronchial smooth muscle cells possess specific binding sites for ET-1 and the human bronchial epithelial cells have been shown to secrete ET like substance[66]. ET immunoreactivity has been localized to pulmonary endocrine cells, especially in the fetal lung and in carcinomas of the lung. It is postulated that the mitogenic activity of ET plays a role in embryological development of the lung and in the pathology of pulmonary tumors.

Renal function

Growing number of evidences suggest that ET plays a role in several renal functions. ET is produced in the kidney both by endothelial and non endothelial cells[104]. The renal vasculature is highly sensitive to the vasoconstrictive effects of infused ET. Infusion of ET-1 causes a profound increase in renal vascular resistance and a marked decrease in renal plasma flow[105–107]. Experiments in the isolated perfused rat or rabbit kidney also support a direct effect of ET on renal vasculature[22,108]. These findings suggest the role of ET in local control of blood flow in the kidney and perhaps in autoregulation. GFR is also affected by ET. Administration of intravenous ET-1 to rats and dogs produces a dose-dependent and sustained decrease in GFR[23,24,107,109]. Reduction of GFR by ET-1 is also observed during direct intrarenal infusion[110–112].

The effects of ET on renin secretion depends on whether ET acts as a circulating or local peptide. When ET is secreted locally, it is likely to inhibit renin release[113–115]. On the other hand, high levels of circulating ET would increase renin secretion as a result of renal vasoconstriction.

The precise role of ET on renal sodium excretion is unclear. In some studies, systemic infusion of ET-1 decrease Na^+ excretion[116]. In contrast, studies in the isolated perfused kidney have consistently shown an increase in Na^+ excretion despite a dramatic decline in GFR[108,117]. Some of the studies have demonstrated that ET increase urine flow rate though it decreases renal blood flow and GFR[23,118].

CLINICAL SIGNIFICANCE OF ET

ET peptide family is involved in almost every system of the body. Plasma concentrations of ET have been reported to be elevated in several cardiovascular and non cardiovascular disorders. However, many of the reported elevations are marginal and there are several conflicting results from different groups. ET may be involved in some of the disorders described below although it should be reemphasized that elevated circulatory levels certainly do not prove a causal relationship. It would be premature to speculate in which disease ET will eventually be proven to play a significant role.

Cardiovascular disorders

Due to the anatomical position of endothelium, it is exposed to the circulating blood and the mechanical forces generated by the disturbed homeostasis. Endothelium is

Hypertension

The endothelium has been established as a target and mediator of hypertension. Morphological and functional changes in the endothelium occur both in experimental and human hypertension. However, severity of the defect and mechanisms involved among vascular beds and models of hypertension are heterogenous. Endothelium-dependent relaxations are impaired in the aorta, carotid artery and cerebral and mesenteric arterioles in hypertension. The potentiating effects of threshold concentrations of ET on the vasoconstrictor response to noradrenaline are enhanced in hypertension. Thus, subtle and distinct endothelial defects occur in various vascular beds and other mechanisms including adrenergic mechanism may contribute to the development of hypertension. Evidence suggests increase in plasma ET levels in genetic model of hypertensive rats[120]. Chronic hypertension produced by infusion of ET-1 in rats is prevented by captopril, indicating that ET-induced hypertension involves stimulation of the renin-angiotensin system, though it did not increase angiotensin II levels[121]. In normotensive male subjects, and sex- and age-matched patients with mild essential hypertension, who did not receive antihypertensive drugs for more than 6 months, exhibited a decrease in responsiveness to ET-1 in small subcutaneous resistance arteries[122].

The role of ET in hypertension is controversial; circulating levels appear unaltered except in the presence of renal failure or atherosclerosis. The local vascular production of ET, however, may still be increased. Furthermore, Hughes et al.[123] demonstrated that renal ET-1 levels are altered in spontaneously hypertensive (SHR) rats. The level of ET-1 mRNA was only reduced in inner medulla and inner medullary collecting duct cells of 8–9 week old SHR. ET-1 production is reduced in renal medulla, and terminal collecting duct of SHR subsequent to the development of hypertension. Such decreases in inner medullary collecting duct ET-1 production may contribute to the hypertensive state in SHR. However, hypertensive patients with chronic renal failure or on regular hemodialysis and hypertensive renal graft recipients did not differ from the corresponding normotensive population with regard to the plasma level of ET, demonstrating that an increased plasma level of ET does not play a major role in the pathogenesis of renal hypertension[124].

In clinical studies conducted by Barnard et al.[125] and Chang et al.[126], plasma ET levels were found to be significantly greater than the normal group indicating that ET-1 functions as a reactive mediator during vasoconstriction in case of pulmonary hypertension. The expression of ET has also been detected in several pulmonary tumors and is postulated to play a role in the growth and/or differentiation of these tumors[127]. However, there is no direct evidence that there is a link between the effects of the ETs and the pathophysiology of asthma. Nevertheless, ETs are known to be synthesized and released from respiratory epithelial cells, and have potent effects in non-vascular components of the respiratory tract, indicating the possible involvement of ET in this disease[128]. Elevation in the levels of immunoreactive ET in bronchoalveolar lavage have been detected in asthmatic patients[129,130].

Besides role in pulmonary and renal hypertension, ET mechanisms have also been demonstrated in pregnancy-induced hypertension. Relation between concentrations of ET and atrial natriuretic peptide (ANP) in maternal plasma, and vasospasm in the uterine and umbilical arteries of hypertensive pregnancies were observed. ET released from the vascular endothelium might cause vasospasm in pregnancy induced hypertension. However, this does not seem to increase the concentration of ET in the maternal plasma, probably because of its rapid disappearance from the blood circulation. Since ANP dilates the blood vessels, increase in the release of ANP in hypertensive pregnancies may be a compensatory mechanism against vasospasm[131]. In another study, where circulating ET-1 levels were measured in pregnant women suffering from pregnancy-induced preeclamptic toxemia, increased ET-1 levels have been demonstrated to play a role in the pathogenesis of preeclampsia[132].

Myocardial infarction and ischemia

Several studies are available demonstrating increased levels of ET-1 following myocardial infarction. Elevated plasma levels of ET-1 were found to be a consistent feature in patients with well-tolerated infarction, uncomplicated by heart failure, hypotension, arrhythmias or ischemia[133]. In coronary occluded rats myocardial ET-1 levels were found to be elevated. Similarly ET-1 levels were also found to be elevated 24 hours after the inset of acute myocardial infarction[134]. Though, plasma ET-1 levels correlated well with the wall motion abnormality index, thrombin-antithrombin II complex and β-thromboglobulin[135], it was not found to correlate well with increased creatinine kinase levels, suggesting that it might reflect myocardial ischemia rather than infarction[133,136]. In another study, Naruse et al.[137] found that only ET-1 levels but not thrombomodulin, were found to be elevated in acute myocardial infarction patients, indicating that plasma ET-1 is not due to simple injury of the endothelium. The extent of ventricular damage following myocardial infarction in rats is reduced by ET antibodies thus provides strong evidence for the role of ETs in the pathogenesis of myocardial infarction. However, in patients with stable angina or unstable angina, the systemic or coronary venous blood ET-1 levels were not found to be different than normal subjects[137]. Although these studies clearly indicate that ET levels are elevated in early phase of myocardial infarction, the exact role of ET in the pathogenesis or myocardial ischemia leading to infarction and other related cardiovascular complication remains unclear.

Congestive heart failure

ET may play a role as a neurohumoral factor leading to severe vasoconstriction during congestive heart failure. Increased circulating plasma ET may be particularly relevant to the pulmonary vasoconstriction encountered in congestive heart failure, with a correlation that the greatest increase of plasma ET occurs in patients with marked pulmonary hypertension with congestive heart failure. Elevated ET-1 specifically correlated with the extent of pulmonary hypertension in congestive heart failure patients[138]. Mechanisms contributing to increase of ET in CHF may include hemodynamic factors like increased atrial and venous pressures, reduced perfusion pressure and shear stress. It is evident that ET may participate in the adaptation to acute reduction in perfusion pressure in CHF. However, in the progression of CHF, ET may cause severe systemic vasoconstriction and cardiovascular remodelling leading to severe CHF. It has been suggested that ET receptor antagonists or ET-converting enzyme inhibitors might have a beneficial role in the treatment of heart failure[139].

Vascular diseases

There are number of vascular diseases associated with increased circulating levels of ET such as atherosclerosis[140], Takayasu's arteritis and Raynaud's disease[141]. Kauffmann et al.[142] examined the plasma levels of ET-1 during upright tilt in healthy subjects and in the patients with multiple system atrophy who showed the impairment of baroreceptor reflex. They found that the arterial blood pressure did not change and plasma ET-1 significantly increased during upright tilt in normal subjects. In patients with multiple system atrophy, plasma ET-1 remained unchanged while the arterial blood pressure fell considerably during tilt[142].

Endocrine disorders

ETs are produced in almost all endocrine organs, and act through specific receptors which are also widely distributed in the endocrine system. ET interacts with various endocrine hormones to elicit a large number of physiologic secretory responses. However, since few clinical studies have documented the involvement of ET-1 in endocrine disorders, at present the role of ET in the pathophysiology of these diseases is highly speculative.

Elevated ET levels were reported in the plasma of patients with diabetes mellitus (DM)[143], type II DM (non insulin-dependent diabetes mellitus) with associated retinopathy[144] and type I DM (insulin-dependent diabetes mellitus) with microalbuminuria[145]. In contrast, ET levels were found to be similar in type II DM patients and healthy subjects[146]. In another study, increased ET concentrations were obtained in patients wih type I and type II DM. The elevation of ET depends on the duration of the disease, at least in patients with type I DM, and correlates with the occurrence of arterial hypertension, reduced renal function and age[147]. In addition, it has been proposed that the activity of ET-converting enzyme may be suppressed in DM[148] giving rise to increased levels of big-ET-1 as compared to ET-1. DM is primarily associated with endothelial damage or dysfunction, which may give rise to high levels of ET via activation by other humoral factors released by the endothelium. Moreover, this may also facilitate the access of ET to the underlying vascular smooth muscles causing vasoconstriction. The finding of increased ET in type II DM with simple retinopathy[144] suggests the initial stage of the disease, since retinopathy is often the early manifestation of DM. mRNA levels for ET-1 in glomeruli of diabetic rats are also increased with the progression of diabetic nephropathy[149]. Further studies are needed to explore the causal role of ET in the genesis of DM and the associated cardiovascular problems.

ET-1 immunoreactivity was increased in the intestinal tissue samples obtained from patients with Crohn's disease and ulcerative colitis[150]. Since these condition are characterized by immunologic hypersensitivity and vascular abnormalities, it could be possible that immune mediators such as cytokines and macrophages may cause ET production which may contribute to the intestinal ischemia through vasoconstriction.

It has been suggested that ET may be acting as a circulating hormone during pregnancy and labor in both fetal and maternal circulation. High levels of ET-1 were found in the amniotic fluid during pregnancy[151]. ET-1 levels in the umbilical vein and artery were higher than those in the maternal vein[152-154] after delivery, suggesting some role during the induction of labor. Advancing gestational age and spontaneous term labor did not alter the amniotic fluid concentrations of ET-1 and ET-2, whereas women with preterm labor and positive amniotic fluid cultures for microorganisms had higher amniotic fluid concentrations of ET-1 and ET-2 than did those without microbial invasion of the amniotic cavity[155]. This suggests the role of ET in the mechanism responsible for preterm delivery associated with intraamniotic infections. Increased amniotic levels of ET are also seen in cases of intrauterine growth retardation[156]. In addition to this, studies indicate that ET may be involved in fetal asphyxia[157,158] and fetal hypoxia[154,159] due to its potent vasoconstrictor activity. It is well recognized that hypoxia and acidemia during the fetal life lead to potent vasoconstriction and increased blood pressure. Augmented circulating levels of ET-1, possibly triggered by birth stress, may play a role in redistribution of blood volume to vital organs and/or it can influence constriction of placental vessels/uterus during labor.

The key role of endothelium in modulating cardiovascular homeostasis during normal pregnancy and the importance of endothelial cell damage in the pathophysiologic characteristics of preeclampsia have been recognized. Preeclampsia is a state of hypertension accompanied by arterial vasospasm, proteinuria and edema during pregnancy. The plasma ET levels were increased in preeclampsia as compared to that in normotensive pregnancy[132,152,153,160-164]. The ET concentration was positively correlated with uric acid levels and inversely related to the creatinine clearance[162] indicating renal dysfunction, but it could not be attributed to the increase in arterial pressure seen in these patients[132]. ET levels were also elevated in patients with preeclampsia and HLLP (hemolysis, elevated liver functions and low platelet count) syndrome as compared to those with only preeclampsia[161]. Increased ET levels although not responsible for its cause, can exacerbate the cardiovascular effects observed in this state, and may increase the chances of maternal and fetal morbidity.

Neurological disorders

A number of clinical studies have been conducted in which ET-1 and ET-3 levels have been measured in plasma and cerebrospinal fluid. Kraus et al.[165] measured cerebrospinal fluid ET-1 and ET-3 levels in patients with subarachnoid hemorrhage (SAH), cerebral vasospasm, and compared with normal controls. ET-3 and not ET-1 levels were significantly elevated in patients with SAH indicating that ETs may participate in cerebral vasospasm and subsequent neurologic deterioration. Suzuki et al.[166] reported the increased concentration of ET-1 in cerebrospinal fluid in patients with SAH. In addition to this, Hamann et al.[167] reported that there was a significant elevation of big ET-1 in the early stages of SAH. To evaluate the role of ET and particularly ET_A receptors in the early cerebral vasoconstriction following SAH in the rat, Clozel and Watanabe[168] demonstrated that ET acting on ET_A receptor plays a role in the pathogenesis of cerebral vasoconstriction.

Ziv et al.[169] measured the plasma levels of ET-1 and ET-3 in patients with acute ischemic stroke (cerebral infarction) within the first 72 hours after the onset, and found a marked increase in plasma ET-1 levels as compared to those in the control subjects, suggesting a possible role in cerebral ischemia. In another study, Hoffman et al.[170] reported seven fold higher level of ET-1 in CSF than plasma of normal subjects. The levels of ET-1 in CSF of patients suffering from depression were decreased, suggesting the role of ET-1 in psychiatric disorders. Presence of ET receptors in brain areas[171] and decreased ET-1 levels in CSF of depressed patients implicate ET mechanisms in the pathophysiology of depression. Increased circulatory levels of the ET peptides have also been reported during migraine attacks[172].

Renal disorders

Evidence suggests the role of ET in the development of several renal diseases including cyclosporine nephrotoxicity, acute renal failure and glomerular inflammation[4,173,174]. Severe renal vasoconstriction is central to the pathogenesis of renal failure in the hepatorenal syndrome. Moore et al.[175] found significantly higher plasma ET-1 but not ET-3 concentrations in subjects with hepatorenal syndrome than in the normal subjects indicating a role of ETs in the pathogenesis of this syndrome. In another study, the plasma ET concentration was significantly higher in patients with cirrhosis and endotoxemia than normal subjects. These results indicate that elevated plasma ET, may play a contributory role in kidney dysfunction in patients with cirrhosis[176]. Mujauchi et al.[177] reported the increasing levels of ET-1, ET-3 and big ET-1 in plasma of patients undergoing chronic hemodialysis compared to those with age matched normal healthy volunteers.

Hepatic disorders

There are many reports regarding elevation of ET levels in patients with hepatic disorders specially in liver cirrhosis[176,178,179]. On the other hand, no elevation or a decrease in liver cirrhosis has been reported by others[180,181]. The reasons for this discrepancy is not known. The increase in plasma ET concentration during the first week after orthotopic liver transplantation has also been observed[182,183].

Other diseases

ET-1 concentration was measured in tissue extracts from human breast cancers, benign breast tumors and normal breast tissues. ET-1 concentration was significantly higher in tissue extracts from breast cancer than in those from benign breast cancer cells[184]. ET is also involved in gastric muscosal damage and producing ulcerogenic actions[28,185].

CONCLUSION AND FUTURE PROSPECTS

The discovery of ET has gained widespread interest in the scientific community because of its potent and concerted actions on the heart, smooth muscles, kidneys, brain and other organs and its ability to act as paracrine and endocrine hormone. ET has been shown to possess numerous biological actions and may be involved in the pathophysiology of several clinical conditions. Current advances leading to the development of ET modulators including specific ET receptor agonists and antagonists are likely to have some therapeutic utility in disorders like CHF, pulmonary and renal hypertension and related disorders.

Acknowledgements

The authors are grateful to Baxter Healthcare Corporation, Miles Incorporated and National Institutes of Health for providing research funds to our laboratory.

References

1. Yanagisawa, M., Kurihara, H., Kimura, S., Tomobe, Y., Kobayashi, M., Mitsui, Y., Yazaki, Y., Goto, K. & Masaki, T. (1988) A novel potent vasoconstrictor peptide produced by vascular endothelial cells. *Nature*, **332**, 411–415.
2. Koseki, C., Imai, M., Hirata, Y., Yanagisawa, M. & Masaki, T. (1989) Autoradiographic distribution in rat tissues of binding sites for endothelin: a neuropeptide? *Am J Physiol*, **256**, R858–866.
3. Masaki, T. (1993) Biochemical characteristics of endothelin. *Seikagaku*, **65**, 1289–1298.
4. Simonson, M. S. (1993) Endothelins: multifunctional renal peptides. *Physiol Rev*, **73**, 375–411.
5. Clarke, J. G., Larkin, S. W., Benjamin, N., Keogh, B. E., Chester, A., Davies, G. J., Taylor, K. M. & Maseri, A. (1989) Endothelin-1 is a potent long-lasting vasoconstrictor in dog peripheral vasculature in vito. *J Cardiovasc Pharmacol*, **13(Suppl 5)**, S211–S212.
6. Dohi, Y. & Luscher, T. F. (1990) Aging differentially affects direct and indirect actions of endothelin-1 in perfused mesenteric arteries of the rat. *Br J Pharmacol*, **100**, 889–893.
7. Gardiner, S. M., Compton, A. M., Kemp, P. A. & Bennett, T. (1990) Cardiac output effects of endothelin-1, -2 and -3 and sarafotoxin S6b in conscious rats. *J Auton Nerv Syst*, **30**, 143–147.
8. Hof, R. P., Hof, A. & Takiguchi, Y. (1989) Massive regional differences in the vascular effects of endothelin. *J Hypertens Suppl*, **7**, S274–S275.
9. Anggard, E. E., Botting, R. M. & Vane, J. R. (1990) Endothelins. *Blood Vessels*, **27**, 269–281.
10. Boric, M. P., Donoso, V., Fournier, A., St.Pierre, S. & Huidobro Toro, J. P. (1990) Endothelin reduces microvascular blood flow by acting on arterioles and venules of the hamster cheek pouch. *Eur J Pharmacol*, **190**, 123–133.
11. Garcia, R., Lachance, D. & Thibault, G. (1990) Positive inotropic action, natriuresis and atrial natriuretic factor release induced by endothelin in the conscious rat. *J Hypertens*, **8**, 725–731.
12. Hirata, Y. (1989) Endothelin-1 receptors in cultured vascular smooth muscle cells and cardiocytes of rats. *J Cardiovasc Pharmacol*, **13(Suppl 5)**, S157–S158.
13. Kremer, S. G., Zeng, W. & Skorecki, K. L. (1992) Simultaneous fluorescence measurement of calcium and membrane potential responses to endothelin. *Am J Physiol*, **263**, C1302–C1309.
14. Galron, R., Kloog, Y., Bdolah, A. & Sokolovsky, M. (1989) Functional endothelin/sarafotoxin receptors in rat heart myocytes: structure-activity relationships and receptor subtypes. *Biochem Biophys Res Commun*, **163**, 936–943.
15. Suzuki, T., Hoshi, H. & Mitsui, Y. (1990) Endothelin stimulates hypertrophy and contractility of neonatal rat cardiac myocytes in a serum-free medium. *FEBS Lett*, **268**, 149–151.
16. Calvo, J. J., Gonzalez, R., De Carvalho, L. F., Takahashi, K., Kanse, S. M., Hart, G. R., Ghatei, M. A. & Bloom, S. R. (1990) Release of substance P from rat hypothalamus and pituitary by endothelin. *Endocrinology*, **126**, 2288–2295.
17. Kanyicska, B., Burris, T. P. & Freeman, M. E. (1991) Endothelin-3 inhibits prolactin and stimulates LH, FSH and TSH secretion from pituitary cell culture. *Biochem Biophys Res Commun*, **174**, 338–343.

18. Yoshizawa, T., Shinmi, O., Giaid, A., Yanagisawa, M., Gibson, S. J., Kimura, S., Uchiyama, Y., Polak, J. M., Masaki, T. & Kanazawa, I. (1990) Endothelin: a novel peptide in the posterior pituitary system. *Science*, **247**, 462–464.
19. Fujii, Y., Moreira, J. E., Orlando, C., Maggi, M., Aurbach, G. D., Brandi, M. L. & Sakaguchi, K. (1991) Endothelin as an autocrine factor in the regulation of parathyroid cells. *Proc Natl Acad Sci USA*, **88**, 4235–4239.
20. Yada, Y., Higuchi, K. & Imokawa, G. (1991) Effects of endothelins on signal transduction and proliferation in human melanocytes. *J Biol Chem*, **266**, 18352–18357.
21. Nakamoto, H., Suzuki, H., Murakami, M., Kageyama, Y., Ohishi, A., Fukuda, K., Hori, S. & Saruta, T. (1989) Effects of endothelin on systemic and renal haemodynamics and neuroendocrine hormones in conscious dogs. *Clin Sci*, **77**, 567–572.
22. Cairns, H. S., Rogerson, M. E., Fairbanks, L. D., Neild, G. H. & Westwick, J. (1989) Endothelin induces an increase in renal vascular resistance and a fall in glomerular filtration rate in the rabbit isolated perfused kidney. *Br J Pharmacol*, **98**, 155–160.
23. Goetz, K. L., Wang, B. C., Madwed, J. B., Zhu, J. L. & Leadley, R. J. J. (1988) Cardiovascular, renal, and endocrine responses to intravenous endothelin in conscious dogs. *Am J Physiol*, **255**, R1064–R1068.
24. King, A. J., Brenner, B. M. & Anderson, S. (1989) Endothelin: a potent renal and systemic vasoconstrictor peptide. *Am J Physiol*, **256**, F1051–F1058.
25. Gandhi, C. R., Stephenson, K. & Olson, M. S. (1990) Endothelin, a potent peptide agonist in the liver. *J Biol Chem*, **265**, 17432–17435.
26. Takahashi, K., Jones, P. M., Kanse, S. M., Lam, H. C., Spokes, R. A., Ghatei, M. A. & Bloom, S. R. (1990) Endothelin in the gastrointestinal tract. Presence of endothelin-like immunoreactivity, endothelin-1 messenger RNA, endothelin receptors, and pharmacological effect. *Gastroenterology*, **99**, 1660–1667.
27. Pinzani, M., Failli, P., Ruocco, C., Casini, A., Milani, S., Baldi, E., Giotti, A. & Gentilini, P. (1992) Fat-storing cells as liver-specific pericytes. Spatial dynamics of agonist-stimulated intracellular calcium transients. *J Clin Invest*, **90**, 642–646.
28. Wallace, J. L., Cirino, G., de Nucci, G., McKnight, W. & MacNaughton, W. K. (1989) Endothelin has potent ulcerogenic and vasoconstrictor actions in the stomach. *Am J Physiol*, **256**, G661–G666.
29. Morales, R. E., Johnson, B. R. & Szabo, S. (1992) Endothelin induces vascular and mucosal lesions, enhances the injury by HCl/ethanol, and the antibody exerts gastroprotection. *FASEB J*, **6**, 2354–2360.
30. Filep, J. G., Battistini, B. & Sirois, P. (1990) Endothelin induces thromboxane release and contraction of isolated guinea-pig airways. *Life Sci*, **47**, 1845–1850.
31. Kester, M., Simonson, M. S., McDermott, R. G., Baldi, E. & Dunn, M. J. (1992) Endothelin stimulates phosphatidic acid formation in cultured rat mesangial cells: role of a protein kinase C-regulated phospholipase D. *J Cell Physiol*, **150**, 578–585.
32. Ito, K., Goseki, N., Endo, M., Hirata, Y. & Marumo, F. (1991) Postoperative changes in immunoreactive plasma endothelin concentrations. *Nippon Geka Gakkai Zasshi*, **92**, 1571–1576.
33. Shubeita, H. E., McDonough, P. M., Harris, A. N., Knowlton, K. U., Glembotski, C. C., Brown, J. H. & Chien, K. R. (1990) Endothelin induction of inositol phospholipid hydrolysis, sarcomere assembly, and cardiac gene expression in ventricular myocytes. A paracrine mechanism for myocardial cell hypertrophy. *J Biol Chem*, **265**, 20555–20562.
34. Sugden, P. H., Fuller, S. J., Mynett, J. R., Hatchett, R. J., Bogoyevitch, M. A. & Sugden, M. C. (1993) Stimulation of adult rat ventricular myocyte protein synthesis and phosphoinositide hydrolysis by the endothelins. *Biochim Biophys Acta*, **1175**, 327–332.
35. Ishikawa, T., Yanagisawa, M., Kimura, S., Goto, K. & Masaki, T. (1988) Positive chronotropic effects of endothelin, a novel endothelium-derived vasoconstrictor peptide. *Pflugers Arch*, **413**, 108–110.
36. Reid, J. J., Wong Dusting, H. K. & Rand, M. J. (1989) The effect of endothelin on noradrenergic transmission in rat and guinea-pig atria. *Eur J Pharmacol*, **168**, 93–96.
37. Hu, J. R., Von Harsdorf, R. & Lang, R. E. (1988) Endothelin has potent inotropic effects in rat atria. *Eur J Pharmacol*, **158**, 275–278.
38. Vigne, P., Lazdunski, M. & Frelin, C. (1989) The inotropic effect of endothelin-1 on rat atria involves hydrolysis of phosphatidylinositol. *FEBS Lett*, **249**, 143–146.
39. Baydoun, A. R., Peers, S. H., Cirino, G. & Woodward, B. (1990) Vasodilator action of endothelin-1 in the perfused rat heart, *J Cardiovasc Pharmacol*, **15**, 759–763.
40. Gardiner, S. M., Compton, A. M., Kemp, P. A. & Bennett, T. (1990) Regional and cardiac haemodynamic responses to glyceryl trinitrate, acetylcholine, bradykinin and endothelin-1 in conscious rats: effects of N^G-nitro-L-arginine methyl ester. *Br J Pharmacol*, **101**, 632–639.
41. Miyauchi, T., Tomobe, Y., Shiba, R., Ishikawa, T., Yanagisawa, M., Kimura, S., Sugishita, Y., Ito, I., Goto, K & Masaki, T. (1990) Involvement of endothelin in the regulation of human vascular tonus. Potent vasoconstrictor effect and existence in endothelial cells. *Circulation*, **81**, 1874–1880.

42. Onizuka, M., Miyauchi, T., Mitsui, K., Suzuki, N., Ueno, H., Goto, K., Masaki, T. & Hori, M. (1993) Plasma levels of endothelin-1 and thrombin-antithrombin III complex in patients undergoing open chest operations. *J Thorac Cardiovasc Surg*, **105**, 559–560.
43. Given, M. B., Lowe, R. F., Lippton, H., Hyman, A. L., Sander, G. E. & Giles, T. D. (1989) Hemodynamic actions of endothelin in conscious and anesthetized dogs. *Peptides*, **10**, 41–44.
44. Watanabe, T., Kusumoto, K., Kitayoshi, T. & Shimamoto, N. (1989) Positive inotropic and vasoconstrictive effects of endothelin-1 in *in vivo* and *in vitro* experiments: characteristics and the role of L-type calcium channels. *J Cardiovasc Pharmacol*, **13(Suppl 5)**, S108–11.
45. Minkes, R. K., Coy, D. H., Murphy, W. A., McNamara, D. B. & Kadowitz, P. J. (1989) Effects of porcine and rat endothelin and an analog on blood pressure in the anesthetized cat. *Eur J Pharmacol*, **164**, 571–575.
46. Minkes, R. K. & Kadowitz, P. J. (1989) Differential effects of rat endothelin on regional blood flow in the cat. *Eur J Pharmacol*, **165**, 161–164.
47. Tippins, J. R., Antoniw, J. W. & Maseri, A. (1989) Endothelin-1 is a potent constrictor in conductive and resistive coronary arteries. *J Cardiovasc Pharmacol*, **13(Suppl 5)**, S177–S179.
48. de Nucci, G., Thomas, R., D'Orleans Juste, P., Antunes, E., Walder, C., Warner, T. D. & Vane, J. R. (1988) Pressor effects of circulating endothelin are limited by its removal in the pulmonary circulation and by the release of prostacyclin and endothelium-derived relaxing factor. *Proc Natl Acad Sci USA*, **85**, 9797–9800.
49. Gardiner, S. M., Compton, A. M. & Bennett, T. (1990) Regional haemodynamic effects of endothelin-1 and endothelin-3 in conscious Long Evans and Brattleboro rats. *Br J Pharmacol*, **99**, 107–112.
50. Luscher, T. F., Yang, Z., Tschudi, M., von Segesser, L., Stulz, P., Boulanger, C., Siebenmann, R., Turina, M. & Buhler, F. R. (1990) Interaction between endothelin-1 and endothelium-derived relaxing factor in human arteries and veins. *Circ Res*, **66**, 1088–1094.
51. Nakamoto, H., Suzuki, H., Murakami, M., Kageyama, Y., Naitoh, M., Sakamaki, Y., Ohishi, A. & Saruta, T. (1991) Different effects of low and high doses of endothelin on haemodynamics and hormones in the normotensive conscious dog. *J Hypertens*, **9**, 337–344.
52. Wright, C. E. & Fozard, J. R. (1988) Regional vasodilation is a prominent feature of the haemodynamic response to endothelin in anaesthetized, spontaneously hypertensive rats. *Eur J Pharmacol*, **155**, 201–203.
53. Hoffman, A., Grossman, E., Ohman, K. P., Marks, E. & Keiser, H. R. (1990) The initial vasodilation and the later vasoconstriction of endothelin-1 are selective to specific vascular beds. *Am J Hypertens*, **3**, 789–791.
54. Gulati, A. & Rebello, S. (1992) Characteristics of endothelin receptors in the central nervous system of spontaneously hypertensive rats. *Neuropharmacology*, **31**, 243–250.
55. Fuxe, K., Andbjer, B., Kalia, M. & Agnati, L. F. (1989) Centrally administered endothelin-1 produces apnoea in the alpha-chloralose-anaesthetized male rat. *Acta Physiol Scand*, **137**, 157–158.
56. Samson, W. K., Skala, K. D., Alexander, B. D. & Huang, F. L. (1991) Hypothalamid endothelin: presence and effects related to fluid and electrolyte homeostasis. *J Cardiovasc Pharmacol*, **17(Suppl 7)**, S346–S349.
57. Lecci, A., Maggi, C. A., Rovero, P., Giachetti, A. & Meli, A. (1990) Effect of endothelin-1, endothelin-3 and C-terminal hexapeptide, endothelin (16–21) on motor activity in rats. *Neuropeptides*, **16**, 21–24.
58. Moser, P. C. & Pelton, J. T. (1989) Behavioral effects of centrally administered endothelin in the rat. *Br J Pharmacol*, **96**, 347.
59. Niwa, M., Kawaguchi, T., Fujimoto, M., Kataoka, Y. & Taniyama, K. (1991) Receptors for endothelin in the central nervous system. *J Cardiovasc Pharmacol*, **17(Suppl 7)**, S137–S139.
60. Jones, C. R., Hiley, C. R., Pelton, J. T. & Mohr, M. (1989) Autoradiographic visualization of the binding sites for [^{125}I]endothelin in rat and human brain. *Neurosci Lett*, **97**, 276–279.
61. Matsumoto, H., Suzuki, N., Onda, H. & Fujino, M. (1989) Abundance of endothelin-3 in rat intestine, pituitary gland and brain. *Biochem Biophys Res Commun*, **164**, 74–80.
62. Yoshimi, H., Hirata, Y., Fukuda, Y., Kawano, Y., Emori, T., Kuramochi, M., Omae, T. & Marumo, F. (1989) Regional distribution of immunoreactive endothelin in rats. *Peptides*, **10**, 805–808.
63. Shinmi, O., Kimura, S., Yoshizawa, T., Sawamura, T., Uchiyama, Y., Sugita, Y., Kanazawa, I., Yanagisawa, M., Goto, K. & Masaki, T. (1989) Presence of endothelin-1 in porcine spinal cord: isolation and sequence determination. *Biochem Biophys Res Commun*, **162**, 340–346.
64. Takahashi, K., Ghatei, M. A., Jones, P. M., Murphy, J. K., Lam, H. C., O'Halloran, D. J. & Bloom, S. R. (1991) Endothelin in human brain and pituitary gland: presence of immunoreactive endothelin, endothelin messenger ribonucleic acid, and endothelin receptors. *J Clin Endocrinol Metab*, **72**, 693–699.
65. MacCumber, M. W., Ross, C. A. & Snyder, S. H. (1990) Endothelin in brain: receptors, mitogenesis, and biosynthesis in glial cells. *Proc Natl Acad Sci USA*, **87**, 2359–2363.

66. Giaid, A., Masaki, T., Ouimet, T., Yanagisawa, M., Gaspar, L., Cantin, M., Kimura, S. & Castellucci, V. F. (1991) Expression of endothelin-like peptide in the nervous system of the marine mollusk Aplysia. *J Cardiovasc Pharmacol*, **17(Suppl 7)**, S449–S451.
67. Lee, M. E., de la Monte, S. M., Ng, S. C., Bloch, K. D. & Quertermous, T. (1990) Expression of the potent vasoconstrictor endothelin in the human central nervous system. *J Clin Invest*, **86**, 141–147.
68. Matsumura, K., Abe, I., Tsuchisashi, T., Tominaga, M., Kobayashi, K. & Fujishima, M. (1991) Central effects of endothelin on neurohormonal responses in conscious rabbits. *Hypertension*, **17**, 1192–1196.
69. Clozel, M. & Clozel, J. P. (1989) Effects of endothelin on regional blood flows in squirrel monkeys. *J Pharmacol Exp Ther*, **250**, 1125–1131.
70. Kadel, K. A., Heistad, D. D. & Faraci, F. M. (1990) Effects of endothelin in blood vessels of the brain and choroid plexus. *Brain Res*, **518**, 78–82.
71. Willette, R. N. & Sauermelch, C. F. (1990) Abluminal effects of endothelin in cerebral microvasculature assessed by laser-Doppler flowmetry. *Am J Physiol*, **259**, H1688–H1693.
72. Koseki, C., Imai, M., Hirata, Y., Yanagisawa, M. & Masaki, Y. (1989) Autoradiographic distribution in rat tissues of binding sites for endothelin: A neuropeptide? *Am J Physiol*, **256**, R858–R866.
73. Macrae, I., Robinson, M., McAuley, M., Reid, J. & McCulloch, J. (1991) Effects of intracisternal endothelin-1 injection on blood flow to the lower brain stem. *Eur J Pharmacol*, **203**, 85–91.
74. Fuxe, K., Kurosawa, N., Cintra, A., Hallstrom, A., Goiny, M., Rosen, L., Agnati, L. F. & Ungerstedt, U. (1992) Involvement of local ischemia in endothelin-1 induced lesions of the neostriatum of the anaesthetized rat. *Exp Brain Res*, **88**, 131–139.
75. Robinson, M. J., Macrae, I. M., Todd, M., Reid, J. L. & McCulloch, J. (1990) Reduction of local cerebral blood flow to pathological levels by endothelin-1 applied to the middle cerebral artery in the rat. *Neurosci Lett*, **118**, 269–272.
76. Macrae, I. M., Robinson, M. J., Graham, D. I., Reid, J. L. & McCulloch, J. (1993) Endothelin-1-induced reductions in cerebral blood flow: dose dependency, time course, and neuropathological consequences. *J Cereb Blood Flow Metab*, **13**, 276–284.
77. Stojilkovic, S. S. & Catt, K. J. (1992) Neuroendocrine actions of endothelins. *Trends Pharmacol Sci*, **13**, 385–391.
78. Imai, T., Hirata, Y., Eguchi, S., Kanno, K., Ohta, K., Emori, T., Sakamoto, A., Yanagisawa, M., Masaki, T. & Marumo, F. (1992) Concomitant expression of receptor subtype and isopeptide of endothelin by human adrenal gland. *Biochem Biophys Res Commun*, **182**, 1115–1121.
79. Iwai, M., Hasegawa, M., Taii, S., Sagawa, N., Nakao, K., Imura, H., Nakanishi, S. & Mori, T. (1991) Endothelins inhibit luteinization of cultured porcine granulosa cells. *Endocrinology*, **129**, 1909–1914.
80. Colin, I., Berbinschi, A., Denef, J. F. & Ketelslegers, J. M. (1992) Detection and identification of endothelin-1 immunoreactivity in rat and porcine thyroid follicular cells. *Endocrinology*, **130**, 544–546.
81. Yue, T. L., Gleason, M. M., Lysko, P. G. & Feuerstein, G. (1990) Effect of endothelins on cytosolic free calcium concentration in neuroblastoma NG108-15 and NCB-20 cells. *Neuropeptidss*, **17**, 7–12.
82. Samson, W. K., Skala, K. D., Alexander, B. D. & Huang, F. L. (1990) Pituitary site of action of endothelin: selective inhibition of prolactin release *in vitro*. *Biochem Biophys Res Commun*, **169**, 737–743.
83. Samson, W. K. & Skala, K. D. (1992) Comparison of the pituitary effects of the mammalian endothelins: vasoactive intestinal contractor (endothelin-beta, rat endothelin-2) is a potent inhibitor of prolactin secretion. *Endocrinology*, **130**, 2964–2970.
84. Morishita, R., Higaki, J. & Ogihara, T. (1989) Endothelin stimulates aldosterone biosynthesis by dispersed rabbit adreno-capsular cells. *Biochem Biophys Res Commun*, **160**, 628–632.
85. Zeng, Z. P., Naruse, M., Guan, B. J., Naruse, K., Sun, M. L., Zang, M. F., Demura, H. & Shi, Y. F. (1992) Endothelin stimulates aldosterone secretion *in vitro* from normal adrenocortical tissue, but not adenoma tissue, in primary aldosteronism. *J Clin Endocrinol Metab*, **74**, 874–878.
86. Flores, J. A., Quyyumi, S., Leong, D. A. & Veldhuis, J. D. (1992) Actions of endothelin-1 on swine ovarian (granulosa) cells. *Endocrinology*, **131**, 1350–1358.
87. Sakaguchi, H., Kozuka, M., Hirose, S., Ito, T. & Hagiwara, H. (1992) Properties and localization of endothelin-1-specific receptors in rat testicles. *Am J Physiol*, **263**, R15–R18.
88. Jackson, S., Tseng, Y. C., Lahiri, S., Burman, K. D. & Wartofsky, L. (1992) Receptors for endothelin in cultured human thyroid cells and inhibition by endothelin of thyroglobulin secretion. *J Clin Endocrinol Metab*, **75**, 388–392.
89. Miyakawa, M., Tsushima, T., Isozaki, O., Demura, H., Shizume, K. & Arai, M. (1992) Endothelin-1 stimulates c-fos mRNA expression and acts as a modulator on cell proliferation of rat FRTL5 thyroid cells. *Biochem Biophys Res Commun*, **184**, 231–238.
90. Singh, G., Thompson, E. B. & Gulati, A. (1994) Altered endothelin-1 concentration in brain, peripheral regions during thyroid dysfunction. *Pharmacology*, **49**, 184–191.

91. Rebello, S., Thompson, E. B. & Gulati, A. (1993) Endothelin mechanisms in altered thyroid states in the rat. *Eur J Pharmacol*, **237**, 9–16.
92. Singh, G., Sharma, A. C., Thompson, E. B. & Gulati, A. (1994) Renal endothelin mechanism in altered thyroid states. *Life Sci*, **54**, 1901–1908.
93. Yamauchi, T. Ohnaka, K., Takayanagi, R., Umeda, F. & Nawata, H. (1990) Enhanced secretion of endothelin-1 by elevated glucose levels from cultured bovine aortic endothelial cells. *FEBS Lett*, **267**, 16–18.
94. Oliver, F. J., de la Rubia, G., Feener, E. P., Lee, M. E., Loeken, M. R., Shiba, T., Quertermous, T. & King, G. L. (1991) Stimulation of endothelin-1 gene expression by insulin in endothelial cells. *J Biol Chem*, **266**, 23251–23256.
95. Benigni, A., Perico, N., Gaspari, F., Zoja, C., Bellizzi, L., Gabanelli, M. & Remuzzi, G. (1991) Increased renal endothelin production in rats with reduced renal mass. *Am J Physiol*, **260**, F331–F339.
96. Hemsen, A. & Lundberg, J. M. (1992) Free haemoglobin interferes with detection of endothelin peptides. *Biochem Biophys Res Commun*, **189**, 777–781.
97. Lindblom, B., Lundberg, J. M., Lunell, N. O., Nisell, H., Noren, H. & Wolff, K. (1991) Endothelin —a potent constrictor of small myometrial arteries of term pregnant women. *Acta Obstet Gynecol Scand*, **70**, 267–270.
98. Wood, J. G., Yan, Z. Y. & Cheung, L. Y. (1992) Relative potency of endothelin analogues on changes in gastric vascular resistance. *Am J Physiol*, **262**, G977–G982.
99. Davenport, A. P., Cameron, I. T., Smith, S. K. & Brown, M. J. (1991) Binding sites for iodinated endothelin-1, endothelin-2 and endothelin-3 demonstrated on human uterine glandular epithelial cells by quantitative high resolution autoradiography. *J Endocrinol*, **129**, 149–154.
100. Svane, D., Larsson, B., Alm, P., Andersson, K. E. & Forman, A. (1993) Endothelin-1: immunocytochemistry, localization of binding sites, and contractile effects in human uteroplacental smooth muscle. *Am J Obstet Gynecol*, **168**, 233–241.
101. Filep, J. G., Sirois, M. G., Rousseau, A., Fournier, A. & Sirois, P. (1991) Effects of endothelin-1 on vascular permeability in the conscious rat: interactions with platelet-activating factor. *Br J Pharmacol*, **104**, 797–804.
102. Nomura, A., Ninomiya, H., Saotome, M., Ohse, H., Ishii, Y., Uchida, Y., Hirata, F. & Hasegawa, S. (1991) Multiple mechanisms of bronchoconstrictive responses to endothelin-1. *J Cardiovas Pharmacol*, **17(Suppl 7)**, S213–S215.
103. Lagente, V., Boichot, E., Mencia Huerta, J. & Braquet, P. (1990) Failure of aerosolized endothelin (ET-1) to induce bronchial hyperreactivity in the guinea pig. *Fundam Clin Pharmacol*, **4**, 275–280.
104. Nord, E. P. (1993) Renal actions of endothelin. *Kidney Int*, **44**, 451–463.
105. Hoyer, D., Waeber, C. & Palacios, J. M. (1989) [^{125}I]endothelin-1 binding sites: autoradiographic studies in the brain and periphery of various species including humans. *J Cardiovasc Pharmacol*, **13(Suppl 5)**, S162–S165.
106. Badr, K. F., Munger, K. A., Sugiura, M., Snajdar, R. M., Schwartzberg, M. & Inagami, T. (1989) High and low affinity binding sites for endothelin on cultured rat glomerular mesangial cells. *Biochem Biophys Res Commun*, **161**, 776–781.
107. Chou, S. Y., Dahhan, A. & Porush, J. G. (1990) Renal actions of endothelin: interaction with prostacyclin. *Am J Physiol*, **259**, F645–F652.
108. Ferrario, R. G., Foulkes, R., Salvati, P. & Patrono, C. (1989) Hemodynamic and tubular effects of endothelin and thromboxane in the isolated perfused rat kidney. *Eur J Pharmacol*, **171**, 127–134.
109. Hirata, Y., Matsuoka, H., Kimura, K., Fukui, K., Hayakawa, H., Suzuki, E., Sugimoto, T., Yanagisawa, M. & Masaki, T. (1989) Renal vasoconstriction by the endothelial cell-derived peptide endothelin in spontaneously hypertensive rats. *Circ Res*, **65**, 1370–1379.
110. Banks, R. O. (1990) Effects of endothelin on renal function in dogs and rats. *Am J Physiol*, **258**,F775–F780.
111. Katoh, T., Chang, H., Uchida, S., Okuda, T. & Kurokawa, K. (1990) Direct effects of endothelin in the rat kidney. *Am J Physiol*, **258**, F397–F402.
112. Kon, V., Yoshioka, T., Fogo, A. & Ichikawa, I. (1989) Glomerular actions of endothelin *in vivo*. *J Clin Invest*, **83**, 1762–1767.
113. Takagi, M., Matsuoka, H., Atarashi, K. & Yagi, S. (1988) Endothelin: a new inhibitor of renin release. *Biochem Biophys Res Commun*, **157**, 1164–1168.
114. Rakugi, H., Nakamaru, M., Saito, H., Higaki, J. & Ogihara, T. (1988) Endothelin inhibits renin release from isolated rat glomeruli. *Biochem Biophys Res Commun*, **155**, 1244–1247.
115. Moe, O., Tejedor, A., Campbell, W. B., Alpern, R. J. & Henrich, W. L. (1991) Effects of endothelin on *in vitro* renin secretion. *Am J Phisol*, **260**, E521–E525.
116. Miller, W. L., Redfield, M. M. & Burnett, J. C. J. (1989) Integrated cardiac, renal, and endocrine actions of endothelin. *J Clin Invest*, **83**, 317–320.

117. Nitta, K., Naruse, M., Sanaka, T., Tsuchiya, K., Naruse, K., Zeng, Z., Demura, H. & Sugino, N. (1990) Natriuretic and diuretic effects of endothelin in perfused rat kidney. *Endocrinol Japan*, **36**, 887–890.
118. Badr, K. F., Murray, J. J., Breyer, M. D., Takahashi, K., Inagami, T. & Harris, R. C. (1989) Mesangial cell, glomerular and renal vascular responses to endothelin in the rat kidney. Elucidation of signal transduction pathways. *J Clin Invest*, **83**, 336–342.
119. Luscher, T. F. (1992) Endogeneous and exogenous nitrates and their role in myocardial ischaemia. *Br J Clin Pharmacol*, **34(Suppl 1)**, 29S–35S.
120. Khraibi, A. A., Heublein, D. M., Knox, F. G. & Burnett, J. C. (1993) Increased plasma levels of endothelin-1 in the Okamoto spontaneously hypertensive rat. *Mayo Clin Proc*, **68**, 42–46.
121. Mortensen, L. H. & Fink, G. D. (1992) Captopril prevents chronic hypertension produced by infusion of endothelin-1 in rats. *Hypertension*, **19**, 676–680.
122. Schiffrin, E. L., Deng, L. Y. & Larochelle, P. (1992) Blunted effects of endothelin upon small subcutaneous resistance arteries of mild essential hypertensive patients. *J Hypertens*, **10**, 437–444.
123. Hughes, A. K., Cline, R. C. & Kohan, D. E. (1992) Alterations in renal endothelin-1 production in the spontaneously hypertensive rat. *Hypertension*, **20**, 666–673.
124. Stockenhuber, F., Gottsauner Wolf, M., Marosi, L., Liebisch, B., Kurz, R. W. & Balcke, P. (1992) Plasma levels of endothelin in chronic renal failure and after renal transplantation: impact on hypertension and cyclosporin A associated nephrotoxicity. *Clin Sci*, **82**, 255–258.
125. Barnard, J. W., Barman, S. A., Adkins, W. K., Longenecker, G. I. & Taylor, A. E. (1991) Sustained effects of endothelin-1 on rabbit, dog and rat pulmonary circulation. *Am J Physiol*, **261**, H479–H486.
126. Chang, H., Wu, G. J., Wang, S. M. & Hung, C. R. (1993) Plasma endothelin levels and surgically correctable pulmonary hypertension. *Ann Thorac Surg*, **55**, 450–458.
127. Giaid, A., Hamid, Q. A., Springall, D. R., Yanagisawa, M., Shinmi, O., Sawamura, T., Masaki, T., Kimura, S., Corrin, B. & Polak, J. M. (1990) Detection of endothelin immunoreactivity and mRNA in pulmonary tumors. *J Pathol*, **162**, 15–22.
128. Hay, D. W., Henry, P. J. & Goldie, R. G. (1993) Endothelin and the respiratory system. *Trends Pharmacol Sci*, **14**, 29–32.
129. Nomura, A., Uchida, Y., Kameyana, M., Saotome, M., Oki, K. & Hasegawa, S. (1989) Endothelin and bronchial asthma. *Lancet*, **2**, 747–748.
130. Mattoli, S., Soloperto, M., Marini, M. & Fasoli, A. (1991) Levels of endothelin in the bronchoalveolar lavage fluid of patients with symptomatic asthma and reversible airflow obstruction. *J Allergy Clin Immunol*, **88**, 376–384.
131. Lumme, R., Laatikainen, T., Vuolteenaho, O. & Leppaluoto, J. (1992) Plasma endothelin, atrial natriuretic peptide (ANP) and uterine and umbilical artery flow velocity waveforms in hypertensive pregnancies. *Br J Obstet Gynaecol*, **99**, 761–764.
132. Schiff, E., Ben Baruch, G., Peleg, E., Rosenthal, T., Alcalay, M., Devir, M. & Mashiach, S. (1992) Immunoreactive circulating endothelin-1 in normal and hypertensive pregnancies. *Am J Obstet Gynecol*, **166**, 624–628.
133. Stewart, D. J., Cernacek, P., Costello, K. B. & Rouleau, J. L. (1992) Elevated endothelin-1 in heart failure and loss of normal response to postural change. *Circulation*, **85**, 510–517.
134. Miyauchi, T., Yanagisawa, M., Tomizawa, T., Sugishita, Y., Suzuki, N., Fujino, M., Ajisaka, R., Goto, K. & Masaki, T. (1989) Increased plasma concentrations of endothelin-1 and big endothelin-1 in acute myocardial infarction. *Lancet*, **2**, 53–54.
135. Yasuda, M., Kohno, M., Tahara, A., Itagane, H., Toda, I., Akioka, K., Teragaki, M., Oku, H., Takeuchi, K. & Takeda, T. (1990) Circulating immunoreactive endothelin in ischemic heart disease. *Am Heart J*, **119**, 801–806.
136. Kubac, G. Cernacek, P., Mohamed, F. & Stewart, D. J. (1990) Plasma endothelin (ET) is elevated in the early hours following myocardial infarction (MI): possible diagnostic and prognostic implications. *J Hypertens*, **8(Suppl 3)**, S4
137. Stewart, D. J. (1991) Role of EDRF and endothelin in coronary vasomotor control. *Basic Res Cardiol*, **86(Suppl 2)**, 77–87.
138. Cody, R. J., Haas, G. J., Binkley, P. F., Capers, Q. & Kelley, R. (1992) Plasma endothelin correlates with the extent of pulmonary hypertension in patients with chronic congestive heart failure. *Circulation*, **85**, 504–509.
139. Clavell, A., Stingo, A., Margulies, K., Lerman, A., Underwood, D. & Burnett Jr, J.C. (1993) Physiological significance of endothelin: Its role in congestive heart failure. *Circulation (Suppl)*, **87**, V45–V50.
140. Lerman, A., Edwards, B. S., Hallett, J. W., Heublein, D. M., Sandberg, S. M. & Burnett, J. C. J. (1991) Circulating and tissue endothelin immunoreactivity in advanced atherosclerosis. *N Engl J Med*, **325**, 997–1001.

141. Zamora, M. R., O'Brien, R. F., Rutherford, R. B. & Weil, J. V. (1990) Serum endothelin-1 concentrations and cold provocation in primary Raynaud's phenomenon. *Lancet*, **336**, 1144–1147.
142. Kaufmann, H., Oribe, E. & Oliver, J. A. (1991) Plasma endothelin during upright tilt: relevance for orthostatic hypotension? *Lancet*, **338**, 1542–1545.
143. Takahashi, K., Ghatei, M. A., Lam, H. C., O'Halloran, D. J. & Bloom, S. R. (1990) Elevated plasma endothelin in patients with diabetes mellitus. *Diabetologia*, **33**, 306–310.
144. Kawamura, M., Ohgawara, H., Naruse, M., Suzuki, N., Iwasaki, N., Naruse, K., Hori, S., Demura, H. & Omori, Y. (1992) Increased plasma endothelin in NIDDM patients with retinopathy. *Diabetes Care*, **15**, 1396–1397.
145. Collier, A., Leach, J. P., McLellan, A., Jardine, A., Morton, J. J. & Small, M. (1992) Plasma endothelinlike immunoreactivity levels in IDDM patients with micro albuminuria. *Diabetes Care*, **15**, 1038–1040.
146. Kanno, K., Hirata, Y., Shichiri, M. & Marumo, F. (1991) Plasma endothelin-1 levels in patients with diabetes mellitus with or without vascular complication. *J Cardiovasc Pharmacol*, **17(Suppl 7)**, S475–S476.
147. Haak, T., Jungmann, E., Felber, A., Hillmann, U. & Usadel, K. H. (1992) Increased plasma levels of endothelin in diabetic patients with hypertension. *Am J Hypertens*, **5**, 161–166.
148. Tsunoda, K., Abe, K., Sato, T., Yokosawa, S. & Yoshinaga, K. (1991) Decreased conversion of big endothelin-1 to endothelin-1 in patients with diabetes mellitus. *Clin Exp Pharmacol Physiol*, **18**, 731–732.
149. Fukui, M., Nakamura, T., Ebihara, I., Osada, S., Tomino, Y., Masaki, T., Goto, K., Furuichi, Y. & Koide, H. (1993) Gene expression for endothelins and their receptors in glomeruli of diabetic rats. *J Lab Clin Med*, **122**, 149–156.
150. Murch, S. H., Braegger, C. P., Sessa, W. C. & MacDonald, T. T. (1992) High endothelin-1 immunoreactivity in Crohn's disease and ulcerative colitis. *Lancet*, **339**, 381–385.
151. Nisell, H., Hemsen, A., Lunell, N. O., Wolff, K. & Lundberg, M. J. (1990) Maternal and fetal levels of a novel polypeptide, endothelin: evidence for release during pregnancy and delivery. *Gynecol Obstet Invest*, **30**, 129–132.
152. Ihara, Y., Sagawa, N., Hasegawa, M., Okagaki, A., Li, X. M., Inamori, K., Itoh, H., Mori, T., Saito, Y., Shirakami, G. et al. (1991) Concentrations of endothelin-1 in material and umbilical cord blood at various stages of pregnancy. *J Cardiovasc Pharmacol*, **17(Suppl 7)**, S443–S445.
153. Mastrogiannis, D. S., O'Brien, W. F., Krammer, J. & Benoit, R. (1991) Potential role of endothelin-1 in normal and hypertensive pregnancies. *Am J Obstet Gynecol*, **165**, 1711–1716.
154. Isozaki Fukuda, Y., Kojima, T., Hirata, Y., Ono, A., Sawaragi, S., Sawaragi, I. & Kobayashi, Y. (1991) Plasma immunoreactive endothelin-1 concentration in human fetal blood: its relation to asphyxia. *Pediatr Res*, **30**, 244–247.
155. Romero, R., Avila, C., Edwin, S. S. & Mitchell, M. D. (1992) Endothelin-1,2 levels are increased in the amniotic fluid of women with preterm labor and microbial invasion of the amniotic cavity. *Am J Obstet Gynecol*, **166**, 95–99.
156. Raboni, S., Folli, M., Bresciani, D., Modena, A., Merialdi, A., Berbinschi, A. & Ketelslegers, J. (1991) Amniotic endothelin increase during pregnancy. *Am J Obstet Gynecol*, **164**, 237.
157. Rosenberg, A. A., Kennaugh, J., Koppenhafer, S. L., Loomis, M., Chatfield, B. A. & Abman, S. H. (1993) Elevated immunoreactive endothelin-1 levels in newborn infants with persistent pulmonary hypertension. *J Pediatr*, **123**, 109–114.
158. Kojima, T., Isozaki Fukuda, Y., Takedatsu, M., Hirata, Y. & Kobayashi, Y. (1992) Circulating levels of endothelin and atrial natriuretic factor during postnatal life. *Acta Paediatr*, **81**, 676–677.
159. Hashiguchi, K., Takagi, K., Nakabayashi, M., Takeda, S., Sakamoto, S., Naruse, M., Naruse, K. & Demura, H. (1991) Relationship between fetal hypoxia and endothelin-1 in fetal circulation. *J Cardiovasc Pharmacol*, **17(Suppl 7)**, S509–S510.
160. Taylor, R. N., Varma, M., Teng, N. N. & Roberts, J. M. (1990) Women with preeclampsia have higher plasma endothelin levels than women with normal pregnancies. *J Clin Endocrinol Metab*, **71**, 1675–1677.
161. Nova, A., Sibai, B. M., Barton, J. R., Mercer, B. M. & Mitchell, M. D. (1991) Maternal plasma level of endothelin is increased in preeclampsia. *Am J Obstet Gynecol*, **165**, 724–727.
162. Clark, B. A., Halvorson, L., Sachs, B. & Epstein, F. H. (1992) Plasma endothelin levels in preeclampsia: elevation and correlation with uric acid levels and renal impairment. *Am J Obstet Gynecol*, **166**, 962–968.
163. Kraayenbrink, A. A., Dekker, G. A., van Kamp, G. J & van Geijn, H. P. (1993) Endothelial vasoactive mediators in preeclampsia. *Am J Obstet Gynecol*, **169**, 160–165.
164. Samuels, P., Steinfeld, J. D., Braitman, L. E., Rhoa, M. F., Cines, D. B. & McCrae, K. R. (1993) Plasma concentration of endothelin-1 in women with cocaine-associated pregnancy complications. *Am J Obstet Gynecol*, **168**, 528–533.

165. Kraus, G. E., Bucholz, R. D., Yoon, K. W., Kneuepfer, M. M. & Smith, K. R. J. (1991) Cerebrospinal fluid endothelin-1 and endothelin-3 levels in normal and neurological patients: A clinical study and literature review. *Surg Neurol*, **35**, 20–29.
166. Suzuki, H., Sato, S., Suzuki, Y., Takekoshi, K., Ishihara, N. & Shimoda, S. (1990) Increased endothelin concentration in CSF from patients with subarachnoid hemorrhage. *Acta Neurol Scand*, **81**, 553–554.
167. Hamann, G., Isenberg, E., Strittmatter, M. & Schimrigk, K. (1993) Absence of elevation of big endothelin in subarachnoid hemorrhage. *Stroke*, **24**, 383–386.
168. Clozel, M. & Watanabe, H. (1993) BQ-123, a peptidic endothelin ET_A receptor antagonist, prevents in early cerebral vasospasm following subarachnoid hemorrhage after intracisternal but not intravenous injection. *Life Sci*, **52**, 825–834.
169. Ziv, I., Fleminger, G., Djaldetti, R., Achiron, A., Melamed, E. & Sokolovsky, M. (1992) Increased plasma endothelin-1 in acute ischemic stroke. *Stroke*, **23**, 1014–1016.
170. Hoffman, A., Keiser, H. R., Grossman, E., Goldstein, D. S., Gold, P. W. & Kling, M. (1989) Endothelin concentrations in cerebrospinal fluid in depressive patients. *Lancet*, **2**, 1519.
171. Koseki, C., Imai, M., Hirata, Y., Yanagisawa, M. & Masaki, T. (1989) Autoradiographic localization of [^{125}I]-endothelin-1 binding sites in rat brain. *Neurosci Res*, **6**, 581–585.
172. Farkkila, M., Palo, J., Saijonmaa, O. & Fyhrquist, F. (1992) Raised plasma endothelin during acute migraine attack. *Cephalalgia*, **12**, 383–384.
173. Kon, V. & Badr, K. F. (1991) Biological actions and pathophysiologic significance of endothelin in the kidney. *Kidney Int*, **40**, 1–12.
174. Simonson, M., Osanai, T., Wann, S., Baldi, E., Mene, P., Nakazato, Y., Kester, M., Thomas, C. & Dunn, M. (1991) Effects of endothelin on cultured human and rat glomerular mesangial cells. *Contrib Nephrol*, **95**, 1–11.
175. Moore, K., Wendon, J., Frazer, M., Karani, J., Williams, R. & Badr, K. (1992) Plasma endothelin immunoreactivity in liver disease and the hepatorenal syndrome. *N Engl J Med*, **327**, 1774–1778.
176. Uchihara, M., Izumi, N., Sato, C. & Marumo, F. (1992) Clinical significance of elevated plasma endothelin concentration in patients with cirrhosis. *Hepatology*, **16**, 95–99.
177. Miyauchi, T., Sugishita, Y., Yamaguchi, I., Ajisaka, R., Tomizawa, T., Onizuka, M., Matsuda, M., Kono, I., Yanagisawa, M., Goto, K. & et al. (1991) Plasma concentrations of endothelin-1 and endothelin-3 are altered differently in various pathophysiological conditions in humans. *J Cardiovasc Pharmacol*, **17(Suppl 7)**, S394–S397.
178. Gulberg, V., Gerbes, A. L., Vollmar, A. M. & Paumgartner, G. (1992) Endothelin-3 like immunoreactivity in plasma of patients with cirrhosis of the liver. *Life Sci*, **51**, 1165–1169.
179. Uemasu, J., Matsumoto, H. & Kawasaki, H. (1992) Increased plasma endothelin levels in patients with liver cirrhosis. *Nephron*, **60**, 380.
180. Adachi, M., Yang, Y. Y., Trzeciak, A., Furuichi, Y. & Miyamoto, C. (1992) Identification of a domain of ET_A receptor required for ligand binding. *FEBS Lett*, **311**, 179–183.
181. Veglio, F., Pinna, G., Melchio, R., Rabbia, F., Panarelli, M., Gagliardi, B. & Chiandussi, L. (1992) Plasma endothelin levels in cirrhotic subjects. *J Hepatol*, **15**, 85–87.
182. Lerman, A., Click, R. L., Narr, B. J., Wiesner, R. H., Krom, R. A., Textor, S. C. & Burnett, J. C. J. (1991) Elevation of plasma endothelin associated with systemic hypertension in humans following orthotopic liver transplantation. *Transplantation*, **51**, 646–650.
183. Textor, S. C., Wilson, D. J., Lerman, A., Romero, J. C., Burnett, J. C., Jr., Wiesner, R., Dickson, E. R. & Krom, R. A. (1992) Renal hemodynamics, urinary eicosanoids, and endothelin after liver transplantation. *Transplantation*, **54**, 74–80.
184. Yamashita, J., Ogawa, M., Inada, K., Yamashita, S., Matsuo, S. & Takano, S. (1991) A large amount of endothelin-1 is present in human breast cancer tissues. *Res Commun Chem Pathol Pharmacol*, **74**, 363–369.
185. Whittle, B. J., Payne, A. N. & Esplugues, J. V. (1989) Cardiopulmonary and gastric ulcerogenic actions of endothelin-1 in the guinea pig and rat. *J Cardiovasic Pharmacol*, **13(Suppl 5)**, S103–S107.

8 Endothelin Mechanisms in the Central Nervous System: Role in Pathophysiology

Anil Gulati

Department of Pharmaceutics and Pharmacodynamics (m/c 865), The University of Illinois at Chicago, 833 South Wood Street, Chicago, IL60612, USA

INTRODUCTION

Endothelin (ET), a vasoconstrictor peptide[1], contains 21 amino acids with a molecular weight of 2492 and shows little homology with other known vasoactive peptides. It is synthesized as a prepropeptide whose gene expression is induced by several vasoactive substances. The presence of mRNA encoding for the preproform of ET has been shown[1,2]. There are at least three forms of ET, all possessing two intrachain disulfide bridges – a feature shared by two other peptide groups, sarafotoxin and murine vasoactive intestinal constrictor[3]. Recently, the genes encoding three isopeptides for ET have been found to co-exist in the human genome: ET-1, the first isolated ET; ET-2, in which Leu^6-Met^7 of ET-1 are replaced by Trp^6-Leu^7, and ET-3 in which Ser^2-Ser^4-Ser^5-Leu^6-Met^7 are replaced by Thr^2-Phe^4-Thr^5-Tyr^6-Lys^7 of ET-1[4,5]. The strong sequence similarities, including the perfectly conserved four Cys residues and the C-terminal Trp residue, convincingly suggest that ET and SRT 6b have a common evolutionary origin[6]. The structure of ET-1 has been configured by means of NMR-Spectroscopy and exact distance geometry and molecular dynamics have been calculated[7,8]. Arai et al.[9] cloned receptors for ET and found that these were highly specific for ET-1 binding. The values of inhibition constant for ET-1, ET-2, ET-3 and SRT 6b were found to be 0.92, 7.2, 52 and 900 nM respectively. Sakurai et al.[10] also cloned an ET receptor and found that these receptors were non-selective and could not distinguish between ET-1, ET-2 and ET-3 in displacing ET-1. ET is the expression product of prepro ET gene. The prepro ET gene produces prepro ET mRNA which in turn produces an approximately 200 residue precursor peptide prepro ET. The prepro ETs are large polypeptides and demonstrate species specific differences in aminoacid sequence. The prepro ET is proteolytically cleaved to form pro ET also known as big ET[1,2,6]. A protease enzyme putatively called "endothelin converting enzyme" cleaves Trp^{21}-Val^{22} of pro ET to form the mature ET peptide. This conversion is essential for full biological activity[11]. It has been suggested that several intracellular signaling pathways are coupled to ET-1 receptors. Some of the likely mechanisms are:

stimulation of phospholipase C; initiation of Ca^{++} fluxes and inhibition of adenyl cyclase[12,13].

ET mechanisms in the central nervous system (CNS) have been found to play an important regulatory role in the control of cardiovascular system[14-17], respiration[18,19], behavior[20,21] and fluid and electrolyte balance[22]. ET has also been implicated in several pathological conditions of cerebrovascular and cardiovascular systems. The role of central ET mechanisms in biological functions and in clinical disorders have been reviewed[13,23] but significant progress has been made since the publication of those reviews.

ENDOTHELIN AS A NEUROMODULATOR/NEUROTRANSMITTER

ET-1 and ET-3 have been demonstrated in rat[24-26], porcine[27-30] and human brain including pituitary gland[31]. ET-immunoreactive neurons and nerve fibers have also been demonstrated in porcine paraventricular and supraoptic nuclei and posterior pituitary lobe[28] and ET-1 like immunoreactivity has been found in porcine spinal cord[32]. Immunoreactive ET and ETmRNA have also been shown in the neurons of spinal cord and dorsal root ganglia[33]. In the CNS of pig the highest concentration of ET like immunoreactivity was found in the choroid plexus, while ET was also found to be present in the hypothalamus[30]. The localization of ET like immunoreactivity in both glial and neuronal cells of hippocampus has been shown[34]. ETmRNA has been demonstrated, using *in situ* hybridization, in porcine paraventricular nucleus[28], cultured rat cerebellar astrogila[35] and in human brain[36]. In rats the distribution of ET like immunoreactivity was found in the cerebral cortex, diencephalon, midbrain, pons-medulla, cerebellum and pituitary[24]. The regional distribution of ET-1 in human brain has been reported, where high concentration of ET was found in the cerebral cortex, spinal cord, hippocampus, hypothalamus, cerebellum, medulla oblongata while smaller amounts were observed in other regions of the brain[37]. The presence of both ET-1[38] and ET-3 have been demonstrated to be present in the cerebrospinal fluid (CSF) of humans[39-41]. The concentration of ET-3 was found to be 1.5 times greater than ET-1 in CSF[39]. In another study, it was found that big-ET-1 was the major molecular form of ET present in human CSF. RNA blot and *in situ* hybridization confirmed the widespread pattern of ET transcription and indicated that the highest density of cells containing ETmRNA is in the hypothalamus. Immunocytochemical studies detected ET immunoreactivity in neurons, providing evidence of the synthesis of ET in neurons[42]. The diffuse distribution of ET containing neurons suggests that it may be functioning as an intracellular messenger, either directly as a neurotransmitter or as a neuromodulator. Enzymes required to convert big-ET to ET have been shown to be present in the CNS. Phosphoramidon and EDTA inhibitable ET converting enzymes are present in brain and the localization of this enzyme correlates with the presence of immunoreactivity of ET-1, ET-1 binding sites and mRNA for ET-1 in the rat brain[43]. Human brain has also been shown to contain a metalloprotease enzyme that converts big-ET-1 to ET-1[44].

ET receptors have been shown to be widely distributed in the CNS[45-48]. Specific [^{125}I] ET-1 binding sites in the CNS have been reported. They are highly concentrated in the choroid plexus, subfornical organ, hippocampus and cerebellum[49,50]. Jones et al.[47] found high density of ET-1 binding sites in human postmortem brain using autoradiography. Specific binding of ET-1 to NG108-15 cells revealed the presence of single class of high affinity binding sites[51]. ET-1 bound to a single site in homogenates of rat cerebellum, the structural requirements for binding do not require the presence of the disufide bridges characteristic of the ET/SRT family. Rather, the binding may be more sensitive to the presence of bulky side chain substituents[52]. Molecular cloning and characterization of ET receptor has been done and it was found that the ET receptor is of ET_B type in porcine cerebellum[53]. Rat cerebral astrocytes also showed a very high level of expression of ET_B type of receptors[54]. Explant cultures of rat cerebellum, brain stem and spinal cord showed the existence of ET receptors on astrocytes using either autoradiographic or electrophysiological techniques[55,56]. The existence of multiple types of ET receptors on neuronal cells appear to exist. Specific binding sites for synthetic ET isoforms were studied on intact cells of the SK-N-MC cell line, derived from human neuroblastoma and it was found that the binding was characteristic of ET_A type of receptor[57]. On the other hand, specific ET binding sites in human cerebral cortices using binding assay and cross-linking analysis were found to be of ET_B type[58].

ET-1 has been shown to induce an increase in intracellular Ca^{2+} and formation of inositol 1,4,5-trisphosphate formation in cultured rat and human glioma cells.[59] The stimulation of the breakdown of phosphoinositide by ET-1 and ET-3 in rat and guinea pig brain has also been demonstrated[60,61]. ET receptors in the NG108-15 cells are coupled to G protein, ET stimulated phosphoinositide metabolism in a dose-dependent manner leading to an increase in free intracellular Ca^{2+}. Neither ET induced phosphoinositide hydrolysis nor ET induced increase in intracellular free Ca^{2+} were affected by pertussis toxin suggesting that G protein coupled to ET receptors in these cells was not sensitive to pertusis toxin[51]. Besides, ET in a dose dependent (1–30 nM) manner stimulated the release of preloaded aspartate from cultured cerebellar granule cells[62]. ET causes a biphasic increase in intracellular Ca^{++} in cultured glial cells[63]. The effect of ET on calcium channels also supports the role of ET in neuronal functions. ET activates the L-type or dihydropyridine-sensitive, voltage-dependent calcium channels in vascular smooth muscle cells thereby inducing a positive inward movement of calcium ion, leading to smooth muscle contraction[64]. Neurons have similar L type of calcium channels and the results of Yoshizawa et al.[27] support the possibility that ET may be functioning as a neuromodulator through the dihydropyridine sensitive L type of calcium channels to release neurohormones like atrial natriuretic peptide (ANP), substance P etc. ET mediated Ca^{++} signaling has been studied in NG108-15 neuroblastoma x glioma cells, and it has been demonstrated that peak intracellular Ca^{++} responses to ET-1 involve mobilization of Ca^{++} from inositol phosphate-sensitive intracellular stores and influx of extracellular Ca^{++} through nonclassical Ca^{++} channels, while the plateau responses are mediated by Ca^{++} influx through dihydropyridine-sensitive, voltage gated channels[65]. Using single cell video imaging of intracellular Ca^{2+} it has been demonstrated that binding of ET to its receptors modulates the intracellular Ca^{2+} of both neurons and glial cells in primary cultures of rat cerebellum[66].

ONTOGENY OF CENTRAL ET SYSTEM

The influence of age on the binding characteristics of ET receptors was studied in preterm (18 days of gestation), term (21 days of gestation) and 1 week post term rats. ET-1 binding showed a significantly greater density in 1 week post term rats as compared to preterm and term animals. The affinity of ET-1 binding was not affected. Similarly, SRT 6b binding was significantly higher in 1 week post term rats as compared to preterm and term rats. The increased binding was due to an increase in ET receptor density while the affinity was not affected during aging[67]. ET receptors at different ages were studied in male Fischer 344 rats. In rats aged 4, 15 and 25 months, [^{125}I] ET-1 binding showed high affinity, single binding sites in cerebral cortex and spinal cord membranes. The density and affinity of ET binding sites in cerebral cortex and spinal cord were found to be similar in rats of various age groups. Another ligand [^{125}I] SRT 6b, which also binds to ET receptors, showed similar binding in rats of various age groups. The IC_{50} and K_i values of ET-1 and ET-2 in the cerebral cortex and spinal cord were similar in rats of different age groups. However, the K_i and IC_{50} values of ET-3 for [^{125}I] SRT 6b binding sites in spinal cord of 24 month old rats were found to be significantly lower than in 4 and 15 months old rats[68].

In order to determine the role of central ET mechanisms in the development of hypertensive state ET like immunoreactivity and the characteristics of ET receptors were studied in spontaneously hypertensive (SHR) rats of different age before and subsequent to the development of hypertension. It was found that the concentration of endogenous ET-1 was very low at 1 week of age and it gradually increased and a maximum level was reached at 6 weeks of age and this is the time when SHR rats show a clear hypertensive state. In the hypothalamus of normotensive Wistar-Kyoto (WKY) rats ET-1 levels were found to be 96.79 ± 6.85 pg/g tissue. The levels increased wth age at 6 and 8 weeks of age ET-1 like immunoreactivity was found to be 416.38 ± 25.97 pg/g tissue and 348.72 ± 24.10 pg/g tissue, respectively. In SHR rats ET-1 levels in the hypothalamus were found to be similar to WKY rats at one week but were significantly lower at 6 and 8 weeks of age. Receptor binding studies indicate that ET receptors are down-regulated in the cardiovascular active areas, hypothalamus and ventrolateral medulla of SHR rats[16]. It is possible that central ET mechanisms are contributing towards the development of hypertension in SHR rats.

CENTRAL ET AND HYPOTHALAMO-NEUROHYPOPHYSEAL SYSTEM

High density of ET binding sites in the anterior pituitary[45-47,68] indicate that ET might be involved in the control of release of anterior pituitary hormones. The presence of ET like immunoreactivity in magnocellular neurons of the hypothalamus and the demonstration of binding sites in the median eminence[28,45,46] and in gonadotrophs of the anterior pituitary[70] suggest the delivery of ET to the pituitary gland through the long portal vessels and potential trophic effect of ET on pituitary hormone secretion. The presence of ET like immunoreactivity in the hypothalamo-neurohypophyseal system led Yoshizawa et al.[28] to propose that there are two roles of ET in this system.

Firstly, ET might act locally to modulate the secretion of posterior pituitary hormones, oxytocin (OX) and arginine vasopressin (AVP) and secondly, ET might be released from the nerve terminals in the posterior pituitary and act as a circulating hormone. A third role of ET has also been proposed, that it acts as a trophic factor in the anterior pituitary[71].

Gross et al.[72]. found that peripheral infusion as well as icv administration of ET-1 produced stimulation of glucose metabolism of rat pituitary lobes, which was mediated via L type of Ca^{++} channels. Shichiri et al.[73] have shown the release of VP by ET-1 from perfused rat hypothalamus. This release could be inhibited by nicardipine suggesting that it is mediated by Ca^{++} influx through DHP-sensitive Ca^{++} channels. High level of ET-3 like immunoreactivity greater than that of ET-1/ET-2 like immunoreactivity has been found in pituitary gland[25]. ET-3, when administered intravenously, produced a significant increase in plasma adrenocorticotropic hormone (ACTH) and corticosterone levels which could be abolished by pretreatment of corticotropin releasing hormone (CRH) antagonist, alpha-helical CRH[74]. It has been shown that ET-3 but not ET-1 inhibits the release of prolactin (PRL) from cultured anterior pituitary cells in a concentration-related manner, while the release of luteinizing hormone (LH), growth hormone (GH) or thyroid stimulating hormone (TSH) was not affected[71]. The release of prolactin by ET-3 was not dependent on calcium channels[75]. However, intracerebroventricular injection of ET-3 (6 or 60 ng) or intravenous infusion of ET-3 (10, 30 or 300 ng) failed to alter the release of PRL or LH[75]. Subsequently, Samson[76] found that the rank order for the prolactin inhibiting effect of ET is ET-1 = ET-2 ≪ ET-3 and that BQ-123, a selective ET_A receptor antagonist, antagonized the effects of ET. ET-3 has been found to inhibit spontaneous release of PRL with an almost identical dose-response relationship as ET-1. These inhibitory effects were not affected by application of a dopamine D_2 receptor antagonist, YM-09151-1 (10^{-7} M)[77]. The signal transduction mechanism in ET induced inhibition of PRL release appears to be stimulation of phosphoinositide turnover[78].

Stojilkovic et al.[79-81] found that ET-1 stimulated the release of GH, LH and FSH from the perfused pituitary cells as efficiently as the gonadotropin-releasing hormone (GnRH). ET receptors were identified in two GnRH neuronal cell lines (GT1-1 and GT1-7) and ET produced a stimulation of the breakdown of inositol phosphates and the secretion of GnRH[82]. ET-3 stimulates LH secretion from anterior pituitary cells cultured in vitro and also produced a stimulation of the release of LHRH from arcuate nucleus-median eminence fragments and LHRH-secreting neuronal cell line in vitro[83]. It appears that prostaglandin mechanism is involved in the action of ET-3 or ET-1 on the median eminence[84] and in ET-3 evoked LHRH secretion[83]. ET-3 elicited a concentration-dependent inhibition of PRL but stimulated the release of LH, FSH and TSH from anterior pituitary cell culture[85]. ET-1 bound specifically to pituitary cells, induced rapid formation of IP_3 and DAG and also mobilized intracellular Ca^{++} through dihydropyridine sensitive Ca^{++} channels. The secretory response of ET appeared to be similar to, but independent of GnRH, the signal transduction mechanism appeared to be similar to, but independent of GnRH, the signal transduction mechanism appears to be common[79,81]. These findings suggest that locally produced ET may act as a neuroendocrine or paracine factor in pituitary functions and that ET has the capacity of regulate neurosecretion and participate in the hypothalamic control of anterior pituitary functions.

Centrally administered ET dose-dependently evoked the elevation of plasma AVP which could be attenuated by centrally administered brain natriuretic peptide (BNP)[86]. Administration of ET-1 (0.35 ng/kg/min) in the third ventricle of conscious rats slightly stimulated the AVP release but did not affect the release of atrial natriuretic peptide (ANP), higher dose of ET-1 (3.5 ng/kg/min) increased plasma levels of AVP and ANP[87]. In fetal diencephalic cultures of neurons ET produced a concentration related increase in the secretion of ANP[88]. ET has been shown to influence the activity of putative AVP and OX secreting neurons at the subfornical organ[89,90]. Calvo et al.[91] further demonstrated that perfusion of rat hypothalamus and posterior pituitary with ET-1 stimulated the release of substance P but did not affect the release of vasoactive intestinal peptide (VIP), 7B2 and somatostatin (SM) from the hypothalamus or ACTH, 7B2 and VIP from the pituitary. The release of sustance P from hypothalamus or pituitary due to stimulation by ET-1 was not blocked when a calcium free medium was used, indicating that this release was not dependent upon extracellular calcium. The physiological significance of substance P release following ET-1 stimulation is not known. Substance P is known to influence the release of pituitary hormones including PRL[92-94]. It is possible that ET-1 stimulation releases substance P which in turn regulates the release of some pituitary hormones.

Most of the studies conducted have demonstrated that ET affects the secretion of several hormones; we have conducted some studies to determine the effect of hormonal imbalance on the central ET mechanisms. Altered thyroid state was produced by chornic administration of thyroxine or methimazole and a state of hyper- or hypo-thyroidism was produced in rats. It was found that ET concentration and receptor characteristics in the cerebral cortex and hypothalamus were not altered during hyper- or hypo-thyroidism. ET concentrations were significantly increased in the plasma and pituitary of hyperthyroid rats and ET receptors were found to be down-regulated in the pituitary of hyperthyroid rats[95,96].

CENTRAL ET AND RESPIRATORY SYSTEM

Intracisternal administration of ET-1 in rats produced expiratory apnea, which developed within 2–3 min and was preceded by a significant increase in relative tidal volume[97]. Centrally administered ET-1 also induced apnea in adult cats and in 2–18 days old piglets. Since acute central hypoxia is known to induce respiratory depression and to increase sympathetic activity and blood pressure, it is possible that ET may be involved in mediating hypoxic cardiorespiratory responses[19]. Somatostatin also produces apnea but the dose of ET-1 required to produce apnea is 10 times lower than the dose of somatostatin needed for similar effect. The existence of ET-1 binding sites in brain stem[17,45,46] suggests that centrally administred ET-1 produces apnea via an effect on the neuronal networks controlling respiration[97]. Another possibility is that a local effect on cerebral blood flow may also contribute to the production of apnea. Since angiotensin II, a vasoconstrictor peptide, upon central administration, failed to produce apnea[98] the possibility of direct action of ET on neurons is more likely. The role of central ET in sudden infant death has been speculated[97]. It has been demonstrated that cerebral microvessel endothelia produce less ET under low oxygen pressure and more under low carbondioxide pressure[99]. ET induced apnea could lead to a decrease in the release of ET as a part of compensatory mechanism. Administration of ET in the cisterna magna produced a biphasic effect on the phrenic nerve activity an initial increase and subsequent decrease in the burst activity and then phrenic nerve activity often disappeared[100]. Intracisternal ET-3 has also been shown to produce an inhibition of phrenic nerve activity[10].

CENTRAL ET AND CARDIOVASCULAR SYSTEM

Administration of ET into the lateral or the third cerebral ventricle of conscious rats has been reported to produce complex changes in blood pressure consisting of increases of a brief decrease followed by an increase. Ferguson and Smith[15] found that microinjection of ET in urethane-anesthetized rats produced dose-dependent biphasic effect, increase in blood pressure followed by a decrease. On the other hand, Minamisawa et al.[102] found a decrease followed by an increase of blood pressure after icv administration of ET in conscious rat. ET administered in the cisterna magna produced an immediate rise in the blood pressure, renal nerve activity and heart rate [101,103]. Similar changes were obtained when ET was applied to the ventral surface of medulla. Microinjection of ET in nucleus tractus solitarius (NTS) increased the blood pressure and the renal nerve activity while intrathecal injection decreased both of them[101,103]. ET administered icv dose-dependently increased blood pressure, plasma catecholamines and ACTH. These responses were attenuated by brain natriuretic peptide[104]. ET-1 (3 to 10 pmol) applied to the fourth ventricle of anesthetized ventilated rats decreased blood pressure, heart and renal blood flow. Micropneumophoresis of ET-1 (100–300 fmol) into discrete glutamate-responsive cardiovascular loci within the NTS, produced depressor and bradycardic responses. ET-1 was ineffective in evoked swallowing responses when microinjected in glutamate sensitive deglutitive sites in the NTS[105]. It appears that low doses of centrally administered ET evokes hypotension and bradycardia by a specific neuronal action in the CNS.

Administration of ET in the lateral cerebral ventricle (icv) of conscious[14] as well as anesthetized[106] rats increased the blood pressure and the heart rate in a dose-related manner[14]. Similar findings have been reported in rabbit[107]. ET-1 (30 pmol/kg icv) administered to conscious rats produced a profound pressor and vasoconstrictor response which was followed by cardiovascular collapse and death within 20 min after the administration of the peptide[108]. Chronic intracerebroventricular infusions of ET (10 pmol/h for 7 days) increased the arterial pressure on days 5, 6 and 7 of the infusion, this was accompanied by an increase in the urinary excretion of vasopressin[109]. Administration of ET-1 (0.35 ng/kg/min for 45 min, icv) produced an increase in blood pressure without any change in heart rate, plasma AVP and ANP and renal solute excretion but administration of higher dose of ET-1 (3.5 ng/kg/min, icv) produced a marked increase in blood pressure along with increases in plasma AVP and ANP, but urine flow, urinary osmolality and urinary Na$^+$ and K$^+$ excretion decreased. These responses could be attenuated by [1-(β-mercapto-β, β-cyclopentamethylenepropionic acid), 2-O-methyltyrosine] arginine vasopressin (TMeAVP), a V_1 blocker and by prazosin[110].

ET in the CNS is a potent stimulator for the sympathetic drive and this might be responsible for the increase in blood pressure and vasoconstriction. It is possible that in SHR rats elevated ET levels in the CNS may lead to the increase in blood pressure and down-regulation of its receptors. The binding of [^{125}I] SRT 6b and [^{125}I] ET-1 in the cerebral cortex, dorsomedial medulla and spinal cord membranes was found to be similar in 8 week old SHR and WKY rats. However, in hypothalamus and ventrolateral medulla the binding of [^{125}I] ET-1 and [^{125}I] SRT 6b was decreased in SHR as compared to WKY rats. Thus, down-regulation of ET receptors in the hypothalamus and ventrolateral medulla of SHR rats might be contributing to the regulation of blood pressure[16,17,111]. Banasik et al.[112] have suggested a role for brain ET receptors in cardiovascular regulation but found no differences in the affinity or density of the binding of ET receptors in the hypothalamus of WKY and SHR rats. In view of this report, experiments were performed again and a decreased density of ET-1 receptors in the hypothalamus of SHR rats, as compared to WKY rats was observed[17]. The differences in results could be attributed to the age of rat[13,17]. The plasma ET levels are significantly elevated in patients with severe hypertension[113] as well as in patients of essential hypertension[114]. Further, ET-1 produced a dose-dependent (3.0 to 7.5 pmol/kg/min for 7 days) increase in blood pressure, when infused intravenously into normal rats[115]. Repeated administration of ET produced a larger pressor response with each repetition suggesting that abnormally high ET production could play a role in the development of hypertension[116].

Han et al.[117] found that intrathecal ET-1 as well as ET-3, at all doses (1 to 100 pmol), produced a dose-dependent depressor effect. The role of ET in spinal cord was studied in WKY and SHR rats. Concentration-dependent inhibition of [^{125}I] ET-1 or [^{125}I] SRT 6b binding to spinal cord membranes by unlabelled ET-1, ET-2 and ET-3 was performed. The K_i and IC_{50} values of ET-1 and ET-2 were found to be similar in WKY and SHR rats. However, the K_i and IC_{50} values of ET-3 were found to be significantly lower in SHR as compared to WKY rats[118]. Thus, in spinal cord of SHR rats, ET receptors were more sensitive to ET-3 as compared to WKY rats.

Intracisternal administration of ET (0.01 to 0.03 nmol) gave rise to an increase in mean arterial pressure with minimal effects on heart rate and significant elevation of plasma norepinephrine and epinephrine. Autoradiographic measurement of cerebral blood flow revealed a widespread and profound ischemia throughout the caudal brain stem. The levels of flow in the caudal brainstem were below the ischemic threshold[119,120] and would result in irreversible deterioration and derangement of neuronal function[121]. Since ischemia in the medullary region is known to activate compensatory circulatory reflexes in the medulla oblongata that result in increased sympathetic and vagal outflow[122] which could be responsible for the increase in blood pressure due to centrally administered ET. However, a recent study shows that intracisternal ET-1 altered the firing pattern of vasomotor neurons in the rostral ventrolateral medulla[123] indicating a selective action of ET on the central cardiovascular active areas. The presence of endothelin binding sites in carotid body, nodose ganglia, superior cervical ganglia and NTS strongly suggest the involvement of this peptide in arterial chemoreceptor reflex regulating blood pressure[124]. In addition, the interaction of central ET with vasodilator factors viz nitric oxide and prostacyclin, α adrenoceptors and renin peripherally and the report of decreased density of ET-1 binding sites in the brain of spontaneously hypertensive rats[16,17] point to its physiological and pathological role in the regulation of blood pressure.

ET MECHANISMS AND CEREBROVASCULAR SYSTEM

ET has been shown to produce contraction of the cerebral blood vessels of rats[125-128], dog[129-131], goat[127,128], cats[131,132] and human[133,134]. Intracisternal administration of ET-1 has been found to produce a sustained contraction of the basilar artery[131,132,135,136] and reduction in blood flow particularly to the lower brain stem[126]. Willette et al.[137] found that intravenous ET-1 (10–300 pmol) reduced arterial blood pressure and microvascular resistance and increased microvascular perfusion, while intracarotid administration of lower doses of ET-1 increased microvascular perfusion, reduced microvascular resistance and arterial blood pressure but higher doses (>300 pmol) of ET-1 reduced microvascular perfusion and increased microvascular resistance and arterial blood pressure in rats. The contractile activity of ET in canine basilar arteries was studied *in vitro* and *in vivo*. ET produced dose-dependent contractions of basilar arteries *in vitro* which could be reversed by nicardipine or papverine. Intracisternal injection of ET produced biphasic contraction of the basilar artery lasting for more than 24 hours[130,138]. Other ETs have also been found to constrict the cerebral vasculature. ET-1, ET-2 and ET-3 produced concentration-dependent decrease in lumen diameter with EC_{50} values of 0.7, 1.5 and 58 nmol/l, respectively[139]. The effect of ET-1 on the internal maxillary artery of unanesthetized goats was a dose-dependent sustained decreases in blood flow. This decrease was more marked during hypotension[140]. Similar effect has also been reported in rabbits[141]. Robinson et al.[142]. applied ET-1 topically to the middle cerebral artery in the rat and measured the blood flow using [^{14}C] iodoantipyrine and quantitative autoradiography. The blood flow was markedly reduced in areas supplied by the middle cerebral artery while other areas remained unaffected. Perivascular subarachnoid microapplication of ET-1 induced marked vasoconstriction of pial arterioles and veins in cat. The pial veins were more sensitive to ET-1 than pial arterioles[143]. A recent study using cats shows that low doses of intravascular ET-1 constricts while high doses of ET-1 dilates the cerebral microvessels through the induction of nitric oxide[144]. It could be argued that ET induced contraction of cerebral blood vessels is due to a secondary effect of altered tissue metabolism. However, it was found that ET causes cerebral vasoconstriction even in the presence of substantial increases in glucose metabolism[145].

The vasoconstricting action of ET is manifested most strongly if either the endothelium is damaged or it is applied from the adventitial side[131,146,147]. Intracarotid or intravertebral arterial injection of ET-1 did not produce any effect on cerebral blood flow or basilar artery caliber but when it was given in a lateral ventricle or in the cisterna magna it produced marked cerebral vasoconstriction providing further evidence that ET does not cross the BBB readily and acts mainly from the adventitial side[131]. The existence of BBB in the form of tight junctions between the endothelial cells could explain the basilar artery vasoconstriction from the adventitial but not from the luminal side. Laser-Doppler flowmetry has been used to assess the intraparenchymal effects of ET-1 on cortical microvascular perfusion in anesthetized rats. Intraparenchymal microinjection of ET-1 elicited monophasic dose-related reduction in microvascular perfusion, suggesting that abluminal actions of ET-1 mediate cerebral vasoconstriction and hypoperfusion[148]. Ogura et al.[149] further studied the problem of intra- and extra-luminal actions of ET in isolated cerebral arteries. They found that extra-luminal application of ET was more effective in causing vasoconstriction and for a longer duration than intraluminal application. The constrictor effect was attenuated by Ca^{++} free solution and nimodipine. The differential effect of ET may either reflect the efficacy of barrier function of cerebrovascular endothelium or may be due to physiological antagonism to endogenous vasodilator factors[150]. There are reports indicating that ET-1 has no effect on the permeability of BBB to either a small molecule like sodium fluorescein[125] or to the permeability of hamster cheek pouch to a large molecule like dextran[151]. However, a recent report clearly indicates that ET can induce an increase in the release of ^{51}Cr from human cultured microvascular endothelium through a receptor specific activation of protein kinase C and intracellular calcium mobilization[152].

It appears that ET-1 induced contractions are dependent on either mobilization of intracellular Ca^{++} or the influx of extracellular Ca^{++} through dihydropyridine insensitive Ca^{++} channels[139]. Noncompetitive antagonism of ET-1 induced contraction with calcium channel blockers has been observed in feline cerebral arteries[147]. Salom et al.[153] analyzed the effect of ET-1 on the cerebral vasculature of goat and found that Ca^{++} free medium and nicardipine inhibited and Bay K 8644 potentiated ET-1 induced contractions. ET-1 also increased $^{45}Ca^{++}$ uptake in isolated arteries. ET-1 and ET-2 were found to be more potent in inducing elevation of cytosolic free Ca^{++}, inhibiting [^{125}I] ET-1 binding and stimulating [^3H]thymidine incorporation as compared to ET-3 in cultured porcine basilar arterial smooth muscle cells[154]. These results suggest that ET-1 induced contraction of cerebral arteries depends upon activation of Ca^{++} influx through dihydropyridine sensitive channels. Besides, additional mechanisms may also be involved[155] and ET have been shown to activate Na^+/H^+ exchange in brain capillary endothelial cells through a high affinity ET-3 receptor that is not coupled to phospholipase C^{156}. Incubation of blood vessels with indomethacin potentiated the response in intact blood vessels[157] suggesting that ET may have a direct effect on the cerebral vasculature and the sensitivity of these vessels may be modulated by cyclooxygenase products released from the endothelium. ET-1 stimulates the production of prostaglandin D_2 (PGD_2) in the endothelial cells derived from human brain capillaries. PGD_2 was found to be converted to potent vasoconstrictors ($PGF_{2\alpha}$, $11\beta PGF_2$ and TXB_2) and vasodilator (PGE_2), indicating that ET may be producing its effect through prostaglandin system[158]. Protein kinase C inhibitors, sphingosine and H-7 ([1-(5-isoquinolinylsulfonyl)-2-methyl-piperazine]), attenuated vasoconstriction of rat basilar artery in response to ET-1[159].

ET MECHANISMS IN SUBARACHNOID HEMORRHAGE

The properties of ET in producing a contractile response of isolated human cerebral arteries[133] is strikingly similar to those of a vasoconstrictor peptide found in CSF of patients with cerebral vasospasm following subarachnoid hemorrhage[160-162]. ET elicited slow, potent, dose-dependent and long lasting contractions of rat basilar artery segments. These contractions were much stronger in rats subjected to a prior subarachnoid hemorrhage as compared to control[163]. In another study, an increased sensitivity of cerebral vessels to ET after subarachnoid hemorrhage has been demonstrated in rats[164]. Intracisternal injection of ET-1 produced 34.6% reduction in the diameter of basilar artery of dogs, similar reduction (43%) was also observed in dogs receiving double injection of blood in the cisterna magna[165]. Moreover, ET levels in the CSF of patients with subarachnoid hemorrhage were raised from 0.4 ± 0.2 pmol/L at day 0–1 to 2.2 ± 0.6 pmol/L at day 6 and then decreased gradually[166]. Fujimori et al.[167] found significantly elevated ET-1 levels in patients of subarachnoid hemorrhage with cerebral vasospasm. The increase was observed more in plasma than in CSF. ET-1 and ET-3 concentrations were measured in patients of subarachnoid hemorrhage with and without cerebrovasospasm. A distinct peak of both ET-1 and ET-3 in CSF of patients with subarachnoid hemorrhage coincided documented signs of cerebrovasospasm[168]. Suzuki et al.,[169] has also shown that ET-3 is also increased in the CSF of patients with subarachnoid hemorrhage Kraus et al.[170] reported significantly raised CSF level of ET-3 and not of ET-1 in patients suffering from subarachnoid hemorrhage with cerebral vasospasm. They did not find statistically significant difference in CSF level of ET-3 from the control group even though the levels of ET-1 as well as ET-3 were raised with wide variation in different patients. The ET-3 level in CSF was also found to be raised in patients who had undergone temporal lobectomy or got spinal cord injury. It is difficult to say whether these raised levels were the result of pathological conditions or they were reaction of the CNS to injury in an effort to reduce the damage or they in fact aggravated the damage.

The effect of ET converting enzyme inhibitor, phosphoramidon on cerebral vasospasm due to subarachnoid hemorrhage was studied in dogs. Intracisternal pretreatment of phosphoramidon potently suppressed the decrease in diameter of the basilar artery after subarachnoid hemorrhage[171]. Actinomycin D, a ribonucleic acid synthesis inhibitor, when administered intravenously for 5 days beginning on the day of subarachnoid hemorrhage in dogs completely inhibited the development of vasospasm[172]. Several studies have also been performed to determine the preventive effect of ET antagonists on the development of vasospasm following subarachnoid hemorrhage. Intracisternal administration of FR 139317, a potent ET_A receptor antagonist did not affect the basal diameter of the basilar artery per se but significantly reduced the vasoconstriction of the basilar artery at day 7 of subarachnoid hemorrhage in dogs[173]. Clozel and Watanabe[174] also found that BQ-123, a specific ET_A receptor antagonist, when given intracisternally completely prevented the decrease in cerebral blood flow at 60 and 120 min after subarachnoid hemorrhage. In another study, the subarachnoid hemorrhage induced constriction of rabbit basilar artery could be reversed by ET receptor antagonist[175]. The preventive effect of another ET_A receptor antagonist, BQ-485, on vasospasm due to subarachnoid hemorrhage in dogs was studied. Systemic continuous infusion of 120 mg/day of BQ-485 inhibited the narrowing of basilar artery on day 7 of subarachnoid hemorrhage[176]. In animal model of subarachnoid hemorrhage levels of immunoreactive ET-1 in the basilar artery increased significantly on day 2 and vasospasm due to subarachnoid hemorrhage could be reversed by monoclonal antibody against ET-1[137]. In contrast, a study reports that ET levels in plasma and CSF of dogs were not affected by vasospasm due to subarachnoid hemorrhage and intracisternal injection of BQ-123 or phosphoramidon did not prevent the subarachnoid hemorrhage induced cerebral vasospasm[178].

Ehrenreich et al.[179] have shown the synthesis and release of ET-3 by rat brain glial cells which could be the extravascular source of intracerebral vasoregulation capable of influencing regional cerebral blood flow. The presence of ET in the same cells was earlier shown by Marsault et al.[180]. Thus glial cells may be playing a crucial role in regulating regional cerebral blood flow through ET secretion. It is believed that ETs are produced by astrocytes and this production can be potentiated by ET stimulants as thrombin which accumulates locally during the course of cerebral bleeding[168,181]. It may also be triggered due to the infiltration of ET producing cells like macrophages in the CNS[182]. Brain endothelial cells and choroid plexus cells could also contribute to the increase in production of ET in the CNS following subarachnoid hemorrhage[99,172,182,183].

ET MECHANISMS IN CEREBRAL ISCHEMIA

Transient unilateral forebrain ischemia was produced in Mongolian gerbils by temporary ligation of common carotid artery on one side. Significantly darker immunostaining was observed in most animals for ET, CGRP and ANP in forebrain of the ischemic cerebral hemisphere. NPY immunoreactivity was not affected by cerebral ischemia. In animals that survived 12 h after reopening of common carotid artery areas of degenerating tissue was observed along with exclusive concentration of ET in these areas[184]. Transient forebrain ischemia in the gerbils was found to produce a marked motor deficit, an acute reduction in ET receptor density and increases in ET-like immunoreactivity in the brain[185]. Permanent occlusion of the middle cerebral artery of rats was accompanied by marked elevation of ET-1 on the ipsilateral side, while transient ischemia followed by recirculation led to only a slight increase in ET-1[186]. ET levels were found to be elevated in focal and global ischemia in rats. The increase was found to be more than 100% in the ischemic zone[187]. Plasma ET-1 and ET-3 concentrations were measured in 16 patients within the first 72 hours after the onset of nonhemorrhagic cerebral infarction. A four fold elevation in plasma ET-1 levels in patients of cerebral infarction was observed as compared to healthy control subjects. ET-3 levels in the plasma were not affected[188]. Hamann et al.[189] measured big-ET in 12 patients with acute severe ischemic stroke. A marked elevation of big-ET was observed during the first 2 weeks after the initial stroke. Patients with a poor outcome showed significantly higher levels of big-ET in contrast to patients with a better prognosis.

All the above studies demonstrate that ET-1 levels are increased during cerebral ischemia. The mechanism responsible for the increase could be due to tissue hypoxia. Studies indicate that tissue hypoxia causes release of ET like immunoreactivity[190-192]. The concentration of ET in CNS is much higher than in the peripheral circulation and cerebral blood vessels are very sensitive to ET. Abluminal application of ET produces severe vasoconstriction of cerebral blood vessels[131,148]. Several studies indicate that ET-1 when administered directly in the CNS or applied to the cerebral blood vessels produces severe reduction of local cerebral blood flow to pathological levels leading to ischemia[142,183,194].

The use of local injection of ET-1 in the brain was proposed as model of focal ischemia in rats[18]. Local injection of ET-1 was utilized to induce ischemia in rat striatum which was accompanied by a marked increase of lactate and dopamine but not glutamate[195]. Intrastriatal administration of ET-1 (0.043 to 0.43 nmol) produced dose-dependent striatal lesions with a peak lesion volume after 24–48 hours. ET-3 was less potent in producing striatal lesions compared to ET-1[194]. ET-1 induced ischemia of the striatum could be attenuated by dihydralazine[194], siagoside[195] and by a vigilance promoting drug, modafinil[196]. Application of ET-1 (1 nmol) to the exposed middle cerebral artery of anesthetized rats reduced the blood flow in the brain areas supplied by middle cerebral artery. The local cerebral blood flow was reduced beyond the threshold for ischemic damage[142]. Neuropathological evidence of tissue damage was evident 4 hours after the application of ET-1 to the middle cerebral artery. At 10^{-4} M concentration ET-1 produced similar volume of ischemia as reported for permanent middle cerebral occlusion[197]. In another study, perivascular application of ET-1 using a stereotoxically placed cannula positioned just above the left middle cerebral artery of conscious rats produced up to 92% reduction in local cerebral blood flow in the areas supplied by the artery[198]. In addition significant increase in blood flow was observed in some brain areas ipsilateral to the insult. Twenty four hours following the application of ET-1 the pattern and extent of ischemic damage was found to be similar to that observed with permanent occlusion of the rat middle cerebral artery[193]. Intracisternal injection of ET-1 (5 and 10 pmol/mouse) significantly increased the area of infarction by 15.5% and 23.5%, respectively. However, ET-1 (0.01, 1 and 100 nmol/l) added to the primary neuronal cultures of chick embryo cerebral hemispheres for 1 h and 24 h did not influence the viability of the neurons or the protein content of the cultures[199] indicating that ET is not a direct neurotoxin but produces cerebral ischemia due to its vasoconstrictor action. This is supported by a study where epineural application of ET-1 increased the microvascular resistance and decreased the endoneurial blood flow in a dose-dependent manner along with a temporary ischemic conduction of sciatic motor fibers of rats. The vasoconstrictor effect could be attenuated by a calium channel blocker, nimodipine but not by an α-adrenoceptor blocker, phentolamine[200]. There is only one report which concludes that a protection of hypoxia/ischemia occurs by centrally administered ET-1[201]. The model used in the study i.e. measurement of the duration of gasping movements of isolated heads after decapitation is not a reliable method and does not account for several other factors which affect the gasping movement of isolated heads.

ET MECHANISMS AND BEHAVIOR

Significant behavioral effects are produced upon central administration of ET. The effects include marked ataxia, decreased movement, a flat body posture and a tendency to direct movements to one side with low doses. Higher doses induce longitudinal rolling of the body (barrel-rolling)[163]. These results were confirmed by Lecci et al.[20]. They found that ET-3 also produces similar behavioral effects. The loss of righting reflex was more marked with ET-1 as compared to ET-3. The C-terminal fragment ET (16–21) (a full agonist in guinea-pig bronchus) did not have any effect on the behavior of rat when administered by intracerebroventricular route[20]. Dose-dependent barrel-rolling was produced by ET-1 injection in the lateral caudal periaqueductal gray matter of freely moving rats, which could be blocked by NMDA receptor antagonist, D, L-2-amino-5-phosphonovalerate[202]. Injection of ET-1 (9 pmol) into lateral cerebral ventricle of rats produced barrel-rolling and other signs of convulsions along with a high rate of glucose utilization. The behavioral and cerebral metabolic activation due to centrally administered ET-1 could be blocked by MK-801, nimodipine and methylene blue given in the lateral cerebral ventricle[203]. Intrathecal administration of ET also produced marked behavioral responses which consisted of a complete paresis of the hind limbs. There was extensive damage of motoneurons as evidenced by the loss of calcitonin gene-related peptide (CGRP) like immunoreactivity in the ventral horns following ET administration[204].

ET-3, when administered in the third cerebral ventricle, has been found to produce a dose-related inhibitory effect on water intake. The peptide attenuated water drinking behavior in response to both endogenous and exogenous stimuli, including osmotic stimulus indicating a direct neuronal action unrelated to any changes in local blood flow. Moreover, passive immunoneutralization of endogenous ET by pretreatment with an antiserum accentuated water drinking in response to angiotensin II[205]. ET-3 like immunoreactivity in the extracts of rat hypothalamic median eminence and in the anterior and intermediate lobes of the pituitary exceeded those present in extracts of abdominal aorta, while ET-1 was found to be abundant in abdominal aorta and cerebral cortex and was in lower concentration in the hypothalamus and anterior pituitary. Since ET-3 elevated plasma levels of vasopressin the authors concluded that ET-3 and not ET-1 plays a role in drinking behavior and fluid and electrolyte homeostasis[22], and dipsogenic actions of ET are mediated through ET_A receptors in the brain[206]. ET-3 microinjection into the third ventricle of conscious, water-loaded male rats evoked a dose-related natriuresis[207]. ET reduces the production of CSF in rabbit and this reduction was found to be more marked in animals treated with indomethacin[208] indicating that ET may play a role in regulation of the brain fluid balance.

Administration of ET-1 and ET-3 in the lateral cerebral ventricle of rats, inhibited the supraspinal micturition reflex. The bladder motility was inhibited, while contraction of the isolated urinary bladder was induced. Intravenous administration of ET-1 and ET-3 inhibiting the supraspinal micturition reflex was also observed[209]. Intraperitoneal injection of ET-1, ET-2, ET-3 or big-ET (1–38) to mice produced an abdominal constriction which could not be blocked by atropine or cromakalim. Thus ET-1 induced abdominal constrictor response was not secondary to the release of acetylcholine or due to direct vasoconstrictor action[210]. This response could be blocked by intrathecal or intracerebroventricular administration of morphine. Further, the effect of morphine was reversed by naloxone or β-funaltrexamine[211,212] indicating the interaction of μ opioid receptors with ET-mediated abdominal constrictor response. Intrathecal administration of ET-1 produced dose-dependent antinociceptive effects in the tail flick test, which could be attenuated by pretreatment with naloxone and the δ receptor selective antagonist, naltrindole[213]. Intracerebroventricular administration of ET-1 produced a dose-dependent (0.313, 0.625, 1.25 and 5 pmol/mouse) Ca^{2+} mediated antinociception in mice[214,215]. It was found that centrally administered ET-1 and ET-3 produced an increase in hot plate and tail flick latencies. The antinociception due to ET-1 and ET-3 was not antagonized by naloxone and thus appears to be independent of endogenous opioid mechanisms.

OCULAR EFFECTS OF ENDOTHELIN

Intravitreal injection of ET-1 induced a 34% reduction in retinal blood flow but the blood flow to ciliary body, iris and choroid remained unaffected. Intracameral injection of ET-1 produced a reduction in the pupil size, an increase in the protein concentration in the aqueous humor and an increase in the concentration of PGE_2 in the aqueous humor of cats. The effect of ET-1 on pupil size could be blocked by pretreatment with indomethacin indicating that these effects are mediated through arachidonic acid metabolites[216].

ET MECHANISM IN DEPRESSION, ALZHEIMER'S DISEASE AND MIGRAINE

Hoffman et al.[217] determined the concentration of ET-1 in CSF and plasma of normal subjects and of patients suffering from depression. They found that ET-1 is present in higher (7 times) concentrations in CSF as compared to plasma of normal volunteers. In patients suffering from depression the level of ET in CSF was significantly lower compared to normal volunteers. The study suggested the role of ET in psychiatric disorders particularly due to the presence of ET receptors in the hypothalamus and limbic system[45,46]. These brain areas have been implicated in the pathophysiology of depression. Yoshizawa et al.[218] measured ET-1 concentrations in the CSF of patients with Alzheimer's disease, senile dementia of Alzheimer type and disease control non-demented patients. CSF ET-1 levels were significantly lower in Alzheimer's disease and their was no correlation between CSF ET-1 and other factors such as age, duration of onset, blood pressure, CSF proteins or plasma ET-1 concentrations. ET-CGRP interactions have been predicted to be of importance in vascular beds putatively involved in pain development in the head. CGRP decreased ET induced contractions of the porcine ophthalmic arteries and ET decreased CGRP induced relaxations indicating a possible role of ET in migraine[219,220].

CONCLUSIONS

The presence of ET in the neurons, the location of ET receptors, the ability of ET to initiate second messenger systems and multiple central actions involving not only cerebral vasculature but also other cerebral functions strongly implicate it as a neuromodulator. It is perhaps premature to speculate that it centrally regulates the blood pressure and its dysfunction may be one of the causative factors of hypertension but it can certainly regulate the local cerebral blood flow and may be involved in conditions like cerebral ischemia, subarachnoid hemorrhage and migraine where alteration in local cerebral blood flow may be the responsible factor. Further studies are needed to clarify and define its role in various pathological conditions. Specific agonists and antagonists are vital to the understanding of the role of any endogenous substance and recent studies using ET antagonists and ET converting enzyme inhibitors have provided some lead in understanding the pathophysiology of diseases like subarachnoid hemorrhage. It is almost certain that in near future ET related drugs are likely to be introduced as a new armamentarium for the treatment of at least some of the disease conditions.

Acknowledgements

The author is grateful to Baxter Healthcare Corporation, Miles Incorporated and National Institutes of Health for providing research funds to our laboratory.

References

1. Yanagisawa, M., Kurihara, H., Kimura, S., Tomobe, Y., Kobayashi, M., Mitsui, Y., Yazaki, Y., Goto, K. & Masaki, T. (1988) A novel potent vasoconstrictor peptide produced by vascular endothelial cells. *Nature*, **332**, 411–415.
2. Itoh, Y., Yanagisawa, M., Ohkubo, S., Kimura, C., Kosaka, T., Inoue, A., Ishida, N., Mitsui, Y., Onda, H., Fujino, M. *et al.* (1988) Cloning and sequence analysis of cDNA encoding the precursor of a human endothelium-derived vasoconstrictor peptide, endothelin: identity of human and porcine endothelin. *FEBS Lett*, **231**, 440–444.
3. Ishikawa, N., Tsujioka, K., Tomoi, M., Saida, K. & Mitsui, Y. (1989) Differential activities of two distinct endothelin family peptides of ileum and coronary artery. *FEBS Lett*, **247**, 337–340.
4. Yanagisawa, M., Inoue, A., Ishikawa, T., Kasuya, Y., Kimura, S., Kumagaye, S., Nakajima, K., Watanabe, T. X., Sakakibara, S., Goto, K. *et al.* (1988) Primary structure, synthesis, and biological activity of rat endothelin, an endothelium-derived vasoconstrictor peptide. *Proc Natl Acad Sci USA*, **85**, 6964–6967.
5. Inoue, A., Yanagisawa, M., Kimura, S., Kasuya, Y., Miyauchi, T., Goto, K. & Masaki, T. (1989) The human endothelin family: three structurally and pharmacologically distinct isopeptides predicted by three separate genes. *Proc Natl Acad Sci USA*, **86**, 2863–2867.
6. Yanagisawa, M. & Masaki, T. (1989) Endothelin, a novel endothelium-derived peptide. Pharmacological activities, regulation and possible roles in cardiovascular control. *Biochem Pharmacol*, **38**, 1877–1883.
7. Tamaoki, H., Kobayashi, Y., Nishimura, S., Ohkubo, T., Kyogoku, Y., Nakajima, K., Kumagaye, S., Kimura, T. & Sakakibara, S. (1991) Solution conformation of endothelin determined by means of 1H-NMR spectroscopy and distance geometry calculations. *Protein Eng*, **4**, 509–518.
8. Reily, M. D. & Dunbar, J. B. (1991) The conformation of endothelin-1 in aqueous solution: NMR-derived constraints combined with distance geometry and molecular dynamics calculations. *Biochem Biophys Res Commun*, **178**, 570–577.
9. Arai, H., Hori, S., Aramori, I., Ohkubo, H. & Nakanishi, S. (1990) Cloning and expression of a cDNA encoding an endothelin receptor. *Nature*, **348**, 730–732.
10. Sakurai, T., Yanagisawa, M., Takuwa, Y., Miyazaki, H., Kimura, S., Goto, K. & Masaki, T. (1990) Cloning of a cDNA encoding a non-isopeptide-selective subtype of the endothelin receptor. *Nature*, **348**, 732–735.
11. Matsumura, Y., Hisaki, K., Takaoka, M. & Morimoto, S. (1990) Phosphoramidon, a metalloproteinase inhibitor, suppresses the hypertensive effect of big endothelin-1. *Eur J Pharmacol*, **185**, 103–106.
12. Couraud, P. O., Durieu Trautmann, O., Mahe, E., Marin, P., Le Nguyen, D. & Strosberg, A. D. (1991) Comparison of binding characteristics of endothelin receptors on subpopulations of astrocytes. *Life Sci*, **49**, 1471–1476.
13. Gulati, A. & Srimal, R. C. (1992) Endothelin mechanisms in the central nervous system: A target for drug development. *Drug Development Research*, **26**, 361–387.

monitoring of immunoreactive endothelin-1 and endothelin-3 in ventricular cerebrospinal fluid, plasma, and 24-h urine of patients with subarachnoid hemorrhage. *Res Exp Med (Berl)*, **192**, 257–268.
54. Fujimori, A., Yanagisawa, M., Saito, A., Goto, K. Masaki, T., Mima, T. (1990) Endothelin in plasma and cerebrospinal fluid of patients with subarachnoid hemorrhage. *Lancet*, **336**, 633.
55. Kraus, G. E., Bucholz, R. D., Yoon, K., Knuepfer, M. M., Smith, K. R. (1991) Cerebrospinal fluid endothelin-1 and endothelin-3 levels in normal and neurosurgical patients, a clinical study and literature review. *Surg Neurol*, **35**, 20–29.
56. Hamann, G., Isenberg, E., Strittmatter, M., Schimrigk, K. (1993) Abscence of elevation of big endothelin in subarachnoid hemorrhage. *Stroke*, **24**, 383–386.
57. Hirata, Y., Matsunaga, T., Ando, K., Furukawa, H. Tsukagoshi, H., Marumo, F. (1990) Presence of endothelin-like immunoactivity in human cerebrospinal fluid. *Biochem Biophys Res Commun*, **166**, 1274–1278.
58. Ando, K., Hirata, Y., Takei, Y., Kawakami, M., Marumo, F. (1991) Endothelin-1-Like immunoreactivity in human urine. *Nephron*, **57**, 36–39.
59. Matsumoto, H., Suzuki, N., Onda, H., Fujino, M. (1989) Abundance of endothelin-3 in rat intestine, pituitary gland and brain. *Biochem Biophys Res Commun*, **164**, 74–80.
60. Beckman, J. S. Beckman, T. W., Chen, J., Marshell, P. S., Freeman, B. S. (1990) Apparent hydroxyl radical production by peroxynitrite: implications for endothelial injury from nitric oxide and superoxide. *Proc Natl Acad Sci USA*, **87**, 1620–1624.
61. Mathiesen, T., Andersson, B., Loftenius, A., Holst, H. (1993) Increased interleukin-6 levels in cerebrospinal fluid following subarachnoid hemorrhage. *J Neurosurg*, **78**, 562–567.
62. Ohlstein, E. H., Storer, B. L. (1992) Oxyhemoglobin stimulation of endothelin production in cultured endothelial cells. *J Neurosurg*, **77**, 274–278.
63. Peterson, J. W., Kwun, B.-D., Hackett, J. D., Zervas, N. T. (1990) The role of inflammation in experimental cerebral vasospasm. *J Neurosurg*, **72**, 767–774.
64. Yoshizumi, M., Kurihara, H., Morita, T., Yamashita, T. Oh-hashi, Y., Sugiyama, T. et al. (1990) Interleukin 1 increases the production of endothelin-1 by cultured endothelial cells. *Biochem Biophys Res Commun*, **166**, 324–329.
65. Macdonald, R. L., Weir, B. K. A. (1991) A review of hemoglobin and the pathogenesis of cerebral vasospasm. *Stroke*, **22**, 971–982.
66. Sasaki, T., Asano, T., Sano, K. (1980) Cerebral vasospasm and free radical reactions. *Neurol Med Chir (Tokyo)*, **20**, 145–153.
67. Shishido, T., Suzuki, R., Qian, L., Hirakawa, K. (1994) The role of superoxide anions in the pathogenesis of cerebral vasospasm. *Stroke*, **25**, 864–868.
68. Rubanyi, G. M., Vanhoutte, P. M. (1986). Oxygen-derived free radicals, endothelium, and respon- siveness of vascular smooth muscle. *Am J Physiol*, **250**, H815–H821.
69. Gryglewski, R. J., Palmer, R. M. J., Moncada, S. (1986) Superoxide anion is involved in the breakdown of endothelium-derived vascular relaxing factor. *Nature*, **320**, 454–456.
70. Rubanyi, G. M., Vanhoutte, P. M. (1986) Superoxide anions and hyperoxia inactivate endothelium-derived relaxing factor. *Am J Physiol*, **250**, H822–H827.
71. Yoshizumi, M., Kurihara, H., Sugiyama, T., Takaku, F., Yanagisawa, M., Masaki, T., Yazaki, Y. (1989) Hemodynamic shear stimulates endothelin production by cultured endothelial cells. *Biochem Biophys Res Commun*, **161**, 1859–864.
72. Kourembana, S., Marsden, P. A., McQuillan, L. P., Faller, D. V. (1991) Hypoxia induces endothelin gene expression and secretion in cultured human endothelium, *J Clin Invest*, **88**, 1054–1057.
73. Lerman, A., Bernett, J. C. Jr (1992) Intact and altered endothelium in regulation of vasomotion. *Circulation*, **86** (Suppl III), 12–19.
74. Lerman, A., Sandok, E., Hildebrand, F. J., Burnett, J. C. Jr. (1992) Inhibition of endothelium derived relaxing factor enhances endothelin-mediated vasoconstriction. *Circulation*, **85**, 1894–1898.
75. Ohkuma, H., Suzuki, S., Kimura, M., Sobata, E. (1991) Role of platelet function in symptomatic cerebral vasospasm following aneurysmal subarachnoid hemorrhage. *Stroke*, **22**, 854–859.
76. Sasaki, T., Murota, S., Wakai, S., Asano, T. Sano, K. (1981) Evaluation of prostaglandin biosynthetic activity in canine basilar artery following subarachnoid injection of blood. *J Neurosurg*, **55**, 771–778.
77. Radomski, M. W., Palmer, R. M. J., Moncada, S. (1987) Endogenous nitric oxide inhibits human platelet adhesion to vascular endothelium. *Lancet*, **2**, 1057–1058.
78. Takeuchi, A., Kimura, T., Satoh, S. (1992) Enhancement by endothelin-1 of the release of catecholamines from the canine adrenal gland in response to splanchnic nerve stimulation. *Clin Exp Pharmacol Physiol*, **19**, 663–666.
79. Yang, Z. H., Richard, V., von Segesser, L., Bauer, E., Stulz, P., Turina, M., Luscher, T. F. (1990) Threshold concentration of endothelin-1 potentiate contractions to norepinephrine and serotomin in human arteries. A new mechanism of vasospasm. *Circulation*, **82**, 188–195.

80. Kohno, M., Muruakawa, K., Horio, T., Kurihara, N., Yokokawa, K., Yasunari, K., et al. (1990) Endothelin stimulates release of arterial natriuretic factor in anesthetized rats. *Metabolism*, **391**, 557–559.
81. Shichiri, M., Hirata, Y., Kanno, K. (1989) Effect of endothelin-1 on release of arginin-vasopressin from perfused rat hypothalamus. *Biochem Biophys Res. Commun*, **163**: 1332–1337.
82. Luscher, T. F. (1992) Endothelin: systemic arterial and pulmonary effects of a new peptide with potent biologic properties. *Am Rev Respir Dis*, **146**, S56–S60.

12 Neurological and Psychiatric Aspects of Endothelin Research

Toshihiro Yoshizawa and *Ichiro Kanazawa

Department of Neurology, Institute of Clinical Medicine, University of Tsukuba, Tsukuba City, 305, Japan

*Department of Neurology, Institute of Brain Research, Faculty of Medicine, University of Tokyo, Tokyo, 113, Japan

INTRODUCTION

Endothelin-1 (ET-1) is a 21-amino acid vasoconstrictor peptide, originally isolated from vascular endothelium[1]. Biological activity of ET-1 is not confined to vascular constriction. Recent studies indicated that ET-1 has a wide spectrum of pharmacological effects including the effects on the central nervous system (CNS)[2]. Screening of genomic DNA library disclosed the presence of other isoforms of endothelin, i.e., endothelin-2 (ET-2) and endothelin-3 (ET-3)[3]. Northern blot analysis showed the different patterns of tissue expression of these endothelin isopeptides[4]. In addition, different classes of endothelin receptors were recently identified and were present in various tissues including the CNS, which corresponded with the former studies of endothelin binding[5]. All of these data suggest the essential role of endothelin in the CNS as well as in other tissues.

In this chapter, I briefly summarize the basic aspect of endothelin research in the CNS and review the studies directed to elucidating the relationships between endothelin and the CNS diseases.

ENDOTHELIN IN THE CENTRAL NERVOUS SYSTEM

Pharmacological effects of endothelin on the spinal cord neurons

Although ET-1 was first isolated from vascular endothelium and was characterized as a vasoconstrictor peptide, we thought that ET-1 would have any function in the CNS since a variety of neuropeptides have physiological roles both in the CNS and the peripheral tissues. Therefore, in 1988, we started to investigate the direct action of ET-1 on the spinal neurons with an *in vitro* spinal cord preparation of the newborn rat[6]. As a result, we found that bath-applied ET-1 produced a ventral root depolarization. The ET-1-induced ventral root depolarization was dose-dependent and was depressed by the dihydropyridine sensitive Ca^{2+} channel blocker, nicardipine or the substance P antagonist, spantide. ET-2 and ET-3 produced similar ventral root depolarization. These results suggested that ET-1 may act directly on the spinal neurons and cause substance P release probably through the activation of dihydropyridine-sensitive Ca^{2+} channels[7].

Presence of endothelin in the spinal cord

Because ET-1 was proved to have a direct action on the spinal cord neurons, we tried to isolate endothelin isopeptides from the porcine spinal cord with high performance liquid chromatography (HPLC) and radioimmunoassay (RIA) with antisera raised against endothelin-related peptides. Both ET-1 and ET-3 were detected based on their chromatographic retention times and characteristics of immunoreactivities to the antisera. The concentrations of immunoreactive ET-1 and immunoreactive ET-3 were estimated to be 0.120 pmol/g tissue and 0.009 pmol/g tissue, respectively. From the peak of immunoreactive ET-1, we isolated a single peptide by successive HPLC and RIA, which was identified as ET-1 itself by a gas phase sequencer.

Next, we investigated the porcine spinal cord immunohistochemically to elucidate the localization of ET-1. We found ET-1-like immunoreactivity in motoneurons, dorsal horn neurons and dot- and fiber-like structures in the dorsal horn as well as in the endothelium of spinal cord vessels[7,8]. Giaid et al. also examined the human spinal cord by in situ hybridization and found the presence of ET-1 mRNA in motoneurons, dorsal horn neurons and in the neurons of dorsal root ganglia[9], which confirmed our data in the porcine spinal cord. The presence of ET-1 mRNA and ET-1-like immunoreactivity in the spinal neurons indicated the actual production of ET-1 in neurons.

Presence of endothelin in the brain

We also isolated both ET-1 and ET-3 from porcine brain by HPLC and RIA[10]. The concentrations of immunoreactive ET-1 and immunoreactive ET-3 were 0.140 pmol/g tissue and 0.005 pmol/g tissue. We could not detect any ET-2-like immunoreactivity in the homogenate of porcine brains.

A general immunohistochemical survey for endothelin in rat and porcine CNS revealed that endothelin-like immunoreactivity was most prominent in the paraventricular and supraoptic nuclear neurons and their terminals in the posterior pituitary. Chemical identification of endothelin in porcine hypothalamus by HPLC and RIA indicated the presence of ET-1. Moreover, in situ hybridization demonstrated ET-1 mRNA in porcine paraventricular nuclear neurons. In the rat, endothelin-like immunoreactivity in posterior pituitary was depleted by water deprivation, suggesting a release of endothelin under physiological conditions[11]. These data indicated that ET-1 is produced by porcine hypothalamic neurons and is released from their terminals and suggested that ET-1 may involve the neurosecretory functions.

We also found weak endothelin-like immunoreactivities in neurons of porcine hippocampus and Purkinje cells in cerebellum[12]. Giaid et al. also demonstrated the wide distribution of endothelin mRNA and peptide immunoreactivity in neurons of the human brain[13]. They found that many neurons were labelled by *in situ* hybridization with cRNA probes specific to ET-1, ET-2 or ET-3. Especially, the labelled neurons were distributed in lamina III-IV of cerebral cortex, hypothalamic nuclei, caudate nucleus, amygdala, hippocampus, basal nucleus of Meynert, substantia nigra, raphe nuclei and Purkinje cell layer of the cerebellum. Immunoreactive neurons to endothelin were reported to the fewer than neurons labelled by *in situ* hybridization. However, the distribution of the neurons with ET-like immunoreactivity was similar to that of endothelin mRNA. A similar result was reported by Lee *et al.* in which the expression of ET-1 mRNA in the human brain was examined[14].

The prominent expression of endothelin in the hypothalamus may suggest a role of endothelin in the neurosecretory function or the central vasoregulatory control. On the other hand, the widespread distribution of endothelin may imply the fundamental role in regulating the neuronal functions. Several reports also described the production of endothelin and its mRNA by cultured astroglial cells[15,16]. These data suggest that the physiological roles of endothelin may not only be related to the neuronal functions, but also to the astroglial functions.

Presence of endothelin in cerebrospinal fluid

A number of neuropeptides exist in cerebrospinal fluid (CSF) and change their content under various states of neurological diseases. Previous studies indicated the production of endothelin in the CNS and suggested a role of endothelin as a novel neuropeptide. Therefore, it is reasonable to imagine that endothelin exists in CSF. The presence of immunoreactive ET-1 and ET-3 in CSF has been shown by several reports[17-23]. The mean concentration of ET-1 in CSF in control subjects varied with the assay system. Our data showed that the mean ET-1 concentration in CSF in control subjects was 0.194 pg/ml which was lower than that in plasma[23].

Endothelin receptors in the central nervous system

Several autoradiographic studies with [^{125}I]ET-1 disclosed the widespread distribution of the binding sites for ET-1 in the CNS[24-27]. Especially, high densities were found in hippocampus, cerebellum, brain stem, choroid plexus and subfornical organ. Subcellular fractionation of whole rat brain showed the enrichment of ET-1 binding sites in the synaptosomal fraction[28]. Because these reported binding sites for ET-1 were not similar to the distribution of vasculature, the specific receptors for endothelin in the CNS seems to be related to the neuronal functions.

The binding sites for endothelin were also found in the endothelial cells from brain microvessels[29] and glial cells[16,30-34]. Physiological roles of endothelin in glial cell functions have not been unclear. However, a few data suggested the trophic effects of endothelin on glial cells[15,33,34].

Recently, cDNAs encoding two classes of endothelin receptor (ET_A and ET_B) were cloned[35,36]. Both of these classes of receptors were reported to be expressed in the brain. The functions of these receptors in the brain should be elucidated in future.

Other pharmacological effects and possible physiological role of endothelin in the central nervous system

Several lines of the pharmacological effects of endothelin in the CNS have been reported, which suggested the physiological roles of endothelin in the CNS. These studies are mainly classified as follows: (1) central cardiovascular control (2) neurosecretory effects. These subjects will be reviewed in other chapters of this book. Therefore, we do not deal with these subjects in this chapter.

POSSIBLE RELATIONSHIP BETWEEN ENDOTHELIN AND NEUROPSYCHIATRIC DISEASES

Cerebrospinal fluid endothelin-1 in Alzheimer's disease and senile dementia of Alzheimer type

Alzheimer's disease (AD) and senile dementia of Alzheimer type (SDAT) are neurodegenerative disorders characterized by progressive dementia which occur in middle and late life. Neuropathological and neurochemical analysis disclosed the degeneration of cerebral cortical neurons and several neurotransmitter systems including neuropeptides which may be involved in the pathogenesis of dementia. Alterations in neurotransmitter markers or neuropeptides in CSF were also reported, which may reflect the degenerations of specific neuronal systems in CNS. However, there is no information for an alteration in the CSF ET-1 level or the CNS ET-1 system in AD and SDAT. Therefore, we determined CSF ET-1 concentrations in patients with AD and SDAT compared with those of disease control[23].

Eleven patients with Alzheimer type dementia (ATD) and seven patients of disease control without dementia admitted were included in this study. All patients diagnosed as ATD met NINCDS/ADRDA diagnostic criteria for probable Alzheimer's disease[37]. ATD patients were divided into the following two groups according to the age of onset: (1) Alzheimer's disease (AD) group; 5 patients (5 women) whose onsets were before the age of 65 years. Mean age of patients ± standard deviation (SD) was 64 ± 8.2. (2) senile dementia of Alzheimer type (SDAT) group; 6 patients (1 man and 5 women) whose onsets were after the age of 65 years. Mean age ± SD was 77.5 ± 4.7. Disease control (DC) group included 7 non-demented patients whose mean age ± SD was 58.9 ± 9.5. The mean age in AD group was not significantly different from that in DC group. However, the mean age in SDAT group was higher than that in DC and AD group ($p < 0.05$, unpaired t test).

CSF samples were obtained by lumbar puncture around noon. Blood samples were obtained from 4 AD patients and 6 SDAT patients before lumbar puncture. Each sample was collected in a polypropylene tube containing 300 KIU/ml of aprotinin and 2 mg/dl of EDTA. After centrifugation at 1000 × g for 10 minutes, supernatant of CSF or plasma was stored at −80°C until assayed.

CSF and plasma ET-1 concentrations were determined with sandwich-enzyme immunoassay (sandwich-EIA) for human ET-1[38]. A value of ET-1 in each group was given as mean ± SD. Statistical analysis was performed using a 2-tailed unpaired Student's t test. Correlation coefficient was calculated by the data analysis software of Stat View II.

The CSF ET-1 concentrations in DC, AD and SDAT were 0.194 ± 0.026 pg/ml (range, 0.15 to 0.22 pg/ml), 0.142 ± 0.030 pg/ml (range, 0.09 to 0.17 pg/ml) and 0.198 ± 0.087 pg/ml (range, 0.12 to 0.31 pg/ml), respectively. The CSF ET-1 level was significantly lower in AD group than in DC group ($p < 0.05$). However, the CSF ET-1 level in SDAT group was not significantly different from that in DC or AD group.

Concerning the correlation coefficients between the CSF ET-1 levels and various factors (age, duration from onset, systolic blood pressure, CSF protein level, plasma ET-1 level), none of these factors had significant correlations with CSF ET-1 levels in AD or SDAT group ($p < 0.05$). On the other hand, in DC group, only the age of patient was negatively correlated with the CSF ET-1 level ($p < 0.05$) (correlation coefficient: -0.928).

Because the age distribution in AD group is not significantly different from that in DC group, it is possible to suppose that the lower level of CSF ET-1 level was not correlated with the plasma ET-1 level in AD or SDAT, it is unlikely that CSF ET-1 is derived from plasma ET-1. There is rather a possibility that CSF ET-1 could be derived from the CNS neurons and could reflect the condition of the CNS ET-1 system. In AD, extensive degeneration of cortical and hypothalamic neurons which was reported to express ET-1 mRNA was recognized. The lower level of CSF ET-1 in AD group may reflect the degeneration of these neurons.

In contrast to AD group, the CSF ET-1 level in SDAT group was not significantly different from that in DC group. Since we could not collect data from disease control patients whose ages were matched with that of SDAT patients, the present data in DC group was not always adequate to the statistical analysis in DC and SDAT groups. In consideration of each level of CSF ET-1 in SDAT group, 4 out of 6 indicated the lower levels than that in DC group. However, 2 out of 6 in SDAT group showed higher levels in CSF ET-1. These two patients were bed-ridden for more than two years. From these relevant informations, other factors might influence the CSF ET-1 levels in these patients.

Plasma endothelin-1 levels during upright tilt in patients with multiple system atrophy presenting orthostatic hypotension

Shichiri et al. reported that the plasma ET-1 concentration increased with upright posture and decreased with volume expansion in healthy volunteers[39]. There results raised the possibility that ET-1 is a circulating hormone involved in the control of arterial blood pressure.

Kaufmann et al. examined the plasma levels of ET-1 during upright tilt in healthy subjects and in the patients with multiple system atrophy who showed the impairment of baroreceptor reflex[40]. They found that the arterial blood pressure did not change and the plasma ET-1 significantly increased during upright tilt in normal subjects. In patients with multiple system atrophy, although the arterial blood pressure fell considerably during tilt, plasma ET-1 remained unchanged. From these results, they considered that the increase in plasma ET-1 induced by upright tilt is mediated by baroreceptor reflex. The failure in increase of ET-1 during upright posture in patients with multiple system atrophy is probably due to the impairment of baroreceptor reflex. The source of increased ET-1 may be the release from posterior pituitary because the patients with diabetes inspidus did not show the increase in ET-1 during upright tilt.

The contribution of the lack of increase in plasma ET-1 during upright tilt to orthostatic hypotension in patients with multiple system atrophy was not clear at present. Since baroreceptor-mediated vasopressin release in normal subjects is important for the postural control of arterial blood pressure, baroreceptor-mediated ET-1 release may also be important for the maintenance of arterial blood pressure during postural change.

Plasma and cerebrospinal endothelin in cerebral vasospasm following subarachnoid hemorrhage

Subarachnoid hemorrhage (SAH) often induces the severe cerebral vasospasm which affects the prognosis of patients suffered from SAH. Although the pathophysiology of cerebral vasospasm following SAH has not been fully elucidated, endothelin isopeptides which produce potent and long-term vasoconstriction are supposed to be important causal factors of vasospasm after SAH. Mima *et al.* reported that intracisternally administered ET-1 produced the long-lasting basilar artery contraction in cats and dogs. On the other hand, infusion of ET-1 into the vertebral artery had no effect on basilar artery caliber[41]. De novo synthesis of ET-1 in endothelial cells may be induced by SAH and may produce the vasospasm.

In fact, Suzuki *et al.* reported the raised concentration of CSF ET-1 in patients with SAH[20]. The highest concentration was observed within 4 to 6 days after the attack of SAH. Kraus *et al.* reported the increase in CSF ET-3 concentration in patients with SAH[22]. These data partly support the hypothesis in which endothelin isopeptides produce delayed vasospasm after the attack of SAH.

However, Fujimori *et al.* did not observe the significant correlation between CSF ET-1 and vasospasm after SAH[18]. Hamann *et al.* reported that there were no elevations of big ET-1 in plasma and CSF obtained from patients with acute SAH[42]. They did not observe the significant differences of big ET-1 between patients with and without vasospasm.

From the above results, we cannot conclude that CSF ET-1 increases after SAH and directly contributes to the production of delayed vasospasm. The vasospasm after SAH is probably seen as a multifactorial development. Since a recent study showed that an intracisternally administered ET_A receptor antagonist prevents the early cerebral vasospasm following experimental SAH in rats, ET-1 may be one of the causal factor of delayed vasospasm after SAH[43].

Acute ischemic stroke and endothelin

Ziv *et al.* measured the plasma levels of ET-1 and ET-3 in patients with acute ischemic stroke (cerebral infarction) within the first 72 hours after the onset and found a marked elevation in plasma ET-1 levels in the patients compared with those in the control subjects[44]. According to their report, plasma ET-1 levels in the patients with more severe neurological impairment tended to be higher than the levels in the patients with milder impairment. However, plasma ET-3 levels were below the detection threshold of the assay in all subjects. They discussed the possibility that the ischemic insult may induce the production and release of ET-1 from injured endothelial cells of the involved cerebral microvessels. In fact, the increasing density of ET-1 immunoreactivity in the ischemic area was recognized by Giuffrida et al. in Mongolian gerbils after the occlusion of the common carotid artery of one side[45]. The denser ET-1 immunoreactivity in the area of neuronal degeneration compared with that in the surrounding area was also recognized twelve hours after the reopening of common carotid artery. These data possibly suggest that the ischemia-induced ET-1 production in the ischemic area may cause the elevation of plasma ET-1 levels and the constriction of collateral vessels which may contribute to the worsening of neurological deficits. The drugs which modify the ischemia-induced ET-1 production or the ET-1 induced vasoconstriction would be beneficial in breaking the vicious circle.

Cerebrospinal fluid endothelin-1 in depressive patients

Hoffman et al. reported that the depressive patients had significantly lower CSF concentrations of ET-1 compared with healthy volunteers[17]. According to their report, the mean concentration of CSF ET-1 in control subjects was 8.0 pg/ml. This value was higher than that reported by other groups[21,23]. Therefore, we cannot simply compare this result with the data obtained by other groups. However, the lower concentration of CSF ET-1 could reflect the disease status in depression.

Glioma and endothelin

Kurihara et al. first demonstrated a single class of high-affinity binding sites for $[^{125}I]$ET-1 in surgical specimens of human astrocytoma and glioblastoma[46]. Although low numbers of $[^{125}I]$ET-1 binding sites were detected in the gray matter of normal human cortex, relatively high numbers of $[^{125}I]$ET-1 binding sites were present in the tissue sections derived from glioma. Several studies demonstrated that ET-1 induced intracellular calcium rise and inositol 1,4,5-triphosphate formation in cultured glioma cells[30]. In conjunction with the data showing the production of ET-1 and its mRNA in cultured glial cells[15,16], ET-1 may act on glial cells autologously and may promote the glial growth which may be related to the increase of the human glioma.

FUTURE ASPECTS OF ENDOTHELIN RESEARCH IN NEURO-PSYCHIATRIC DISORDERS

In this chapter, we summarize the possible relationship between endothelin and the human CNS disease. Previous studies suggest a role of endothelin as a neuropeptide which may be functioning in the specific neuronal system such as in the posterior pituitary system. Recent reports suggest that endothelin may have more broad and fundamental functions in cells other than neurons, for example, vascular endothelium of cerebral vessels and glial cells. In future, antagonists for endothelin receptors may be useful tools for elucidating the pathophysiology of the human CNS disease and may become a novel class of therapeutic drugs.

References

1. Yanagisawa, M., Kurihara, H., Kimura, S., Tomobe, Y., Kobayashi, M., Mitsui, Y., et al. (1988) Endothelin: a novel potent vasoconstrictor peptide produced by vascular endothelial cells. *Nature*, **332**, 411–415.
2. Masaki, T., Yanagisawa, M. and Goto, K. (1992) Physiology and Pharmacology of endothelins. *Med. Res. Rev.*, **12**, 391–421.
3. Inoue, A., Yanagisawa, M., Kimura, S., Kasuya, Y., Miyauchi, T., Goto, K., et al. (1989) The human endothelin family: Three structurally and pharmacologically distinct isopeptides predicted by three separate genes. *Proc. Natl. Acad. Sci. USA*, **86**, 2863–2867.
4. Goto, K., Sakurao, T. and Kasuya, Y. (1992) Molecular pharmacology of endothelin in the cardiovascular system. *Nippon Yakurigaku Zasshi*, **100**, 205–218.
5. Sakurai, T., Yanagisawa, M. and Masaki, T. (1992) Molecular characterization of endothelin receptors. *Trends. Pharmacol. Sci.*, **13**, 103–108.
6. Yoshizawa, T., Kimura, S., Kanazawa, I., Yanagisawa, M. and Masaki, T. (1989) Endothelin-1 depolarizes a ventral root potential in the newborn rat spinal cord. *J. Cardiovasc. Pharmacol.*, **13 (Suppl 5)**, S216–S217.
7. Yoshizawa, T., Kimura, S., Kanazawa, I., Uchiyama, Y., Yanagisawa, M. and Masaki, T. (1989) Endothelin localizes in the dorsal horn and acts on the spinal neurones: possible involvement of dihydropyridine-sensitive calcium channels and substance P release. *Neurosci. Lett.*, **102**, 179–184.
8. Shinmi, O., Kimura, S., Yoshizawa, T., Sawamura, T., Uchiyama, Y., Sugita, Y., et al. (1989) Presence of endothelin-1 in porcine spinal cord: isolation and sequence determination. *Biochem. Biophys. Res. Commun.*, **162**, 340–346.
9. Giaid, A., Gibson, S. J., Ibrahim, N. B. N., Legon, S., Bloom, S. R., Yanagisawa, M., et al. (1989) Endothelin-1, and endothelium-derived peptide, is expressed in neurons of the human spinal cord and dorsal root ganglia. *Proc. Natl. Acad. Sci. USA*, **86**, 7634–7638.
10. Shinni, O., Kimura, S., Sawamura, T., Sugita, Y., Yoshizawa, T., Uchiyama, Y., et al. (1989) Endothelin-3 is a novel neuropeptide: isolation and sequence determination of endothelin-1 and endothelin-3 in porcine brain. *Biochem. Biophys. Res. Commun.*, **164**, 587–593.
11. Yoshizawa, T., Shinmi, O., Giaid, A., Yanagisawa, M., Gibson, S. J., Kimura, S., et al. (1990) Endothelin: a novel peptide in the posterior pituitary system. *Science*, **247**, 462–464.
12. Kanazawa, I., Yoshizawa, T. and Masaki, T. (1991) Localization of endothelin in the posterior pituitary system. *In New Trends in Autonomic Nervous System Research*, edited by M. Yoshikawa, pp. 423–425. Amsterdam: Elsevier Science Publishers B.V.
13. Giaid, A., Gibson, S. J., Herrero, M. T., Gentleman, S., Legon, S., Yanagisawa, M., et al. (1991) Topographical localization of endothelin mRNA and peptide immunoreactivity in neurones of the human brain. *Histochemistry*, **95**, 303–314.
14. Lee, M.-E., de la Monte, S. M., Ng, S.-H., Bloch, K. D. and Quertermous, T. (1990) Expression of the potent vasoconstrictor endothelin in the human central nervous system. *J. Clin. Invest.*, **86**, 141–147.
15. MacCumber, M. W., Ross, C. A. and Snyder, S. H. (1990) Endothelin in brain: receptors, mitogenesis and biosynthesis in glial cells. *Proc. Natl. Acad. Sci. USA*, **87**, 2359–2363.
16. Ehrenreich, H., Kehrl, J. H., Anderson, R. W., Rieckmann, P., Vitkovic, L., Coligan, J. E., et al. (1991) A vasoactive peptide, endothelin-3, is produced by and specifically binds to primary astrocytes. *Brain Res.*, **538**, 54–58.
17. Hoffman, A., Keiser, H. R., Grossman, E., Goldstein, D. S., Gold, P. W. and Kling, M. (1989) Endothelin concentrations in cerebrospinal fluid in depressive patients. *Lancet*, **2**, 1519.
18. Fujimori, A., Yanagisawa, M., Saito, A. Goto, K., Masaki, T., Mima, T., et al. (1990) Endothelin in plasma and cerebrospinal fluid of patients with subarachnoid haemorrhage. *Lancet*, **336**, 633.
19. Hirata, Y., Matsunaga, T., Audo, K., Furukawa, T., Tsukagoshi, H. and Marumo, F. (1990) Presence of endothelin-1-like immunoreactivity in human cerebrospinal fluid. *Biochem. Biophys. Res. Commun.*, **166**, 1274–1278.
20. Suzuki, H., Sato, S., Suzuki, Y., Takekoshi, K., Ishihira, N. and Shimoda, S. (1990) Increased endothelin concentration in CSF from patients with subarachnoid hemorrhage. *Acta Neurol. Scand.*, **81**, 553–554.
21. Yamaji, T., Johshita, H., Ishibashi, M., Takaku, F., Ohno, H., Suzuki, N., Matsumoto, H. and Fujino, M. (1990). Endothelin family in human plasma and cerebrospinal fluid. *J. Clin. Endoclinol. Metab.*, **71**, 1611–1615.
22. Kraus, G. E., Bucholz, R. D., Yoon, K. W., Knuepfer, M. M. and Smith, . R. Jr. (1991) Cerebrospinal fluid endothelin-1 and endothelin-3 levels in normal and neurosurgical patients: a clinical study and literature review. *Surgical Neurology*, **35**, 20–29.
23. Yoshizawa, T., Iwamoto, H., Mizusawa, H., Suzuki, H., Matsumoto, H. and Kanazawa, I. (1992)

Cerebrospinal fluid endothelin-1 in Alzheimer's disease and senile dementia of Alzheimer type. *Neuropeptides*, **22**, 85–88.
24. Koseki, C., Imai, M., Hirata, Y., Yanagisawa, M. and Masaki, T. (1989) Autoradiographic distribution in rat tissues of binding sites for endothelin: a neuropeptide? *Am. J Physiol.* 256, R858–866.
25. Jones, C. R., Hiley, C. R., Pelton, J. T. and Mohr, M. (1989) Autoradiographic visualization of the binding sites for [^{125}I]endothelin in rat and human brain. *Neurosci. Lett.*, **97**, 276–279.
26. Kohzuki, M., Chai, S. Y., Paxinos, G., Karavas, A., Casley, D. J., Johnston, C. I., et al. (1991) Localization and characterization of endothelin receptor binding sites in the rat brain visualized by *in vitro* autoradiography. *Neuroscience*, **42**, 245–260.
27. Niwa, M., Kawaguchi, T., Fujimoto, M., Kataoka, Y. and Taniyama, K. (1991) Receptors of endothelin in the central nervous system. *J. Cardiovasc. Pharmacol.*, **17 (Suppl. 7)**, S173–S179.
28. Bolger, G. T., Berry, R. and Jaramillo, J. (1992) Regional and subcellular distribution of [^{125}I]endothelin binding sites in rat brain. *Brain. Res. Bull.*, **28**, 789–797.
29. Vigne, P., Ladoux, A. and Frelin, C. (1991) Endothelin activates Na+/H+ exchange in brain capillary endothelial cells via a high affinity endothelin-3 receptor that is not coupled to phospholipase. *J. Biol. Chem.*, **266**, 5925–5928.
30. Marsault, R., Vigue, P., Breittmayer, J. P. and Frelin, C. (1990) Astrocytes are target cells for endothelins and sarafotoxin. *J. Neurochem.*, **54**, 2142–2144.
31. Hosli, E. and Hosli, L. (1991) Autoradiographic evidence for endothelin receptors on astrocytes in cultures of rat cerebellum, brainstem and spinal cord. *Neurosci. Lett.*, **129**, 55–58.
32. Hosli, L., Hosli, E., Lefkovitgs, M. and Wagner, S. Electrophysiological evidence for existence of receptors for endothelin and vasopressin on cultured astrocytes of rat spinal cord and brainstem. *Neurosci. Lett.*, **131**, 193–195.
33. Hama, H., Sakurai, T., Kasuya, Y., Fujiki, M., Masaki, T. and Goto, K. (1993) Action of endothelin-1 on rat astrocytes through the ET$_B$ receptor. *Biochem. Biophys. Res. Commun.*, **186**, 355–362.
34. Levin, E. R., Frank, H.J. and Pedram, A. (1992) Endothelin receptors on cultured fetal rat diencephalic glia. *J. Neurochem.*, **58**, 659–666.
35. Arai, H., Hori, S., Aramori, I., Ohkubo, H. and Nakanishi, S. (1990) Cloning and expression of a cDNA encoding an endothelin receptor. *Nature*, **348**, 730–732.
36. Sakurai, T., Yangisawa, M., Takuwa, Y., Miyazaki, H., Kimura, S., Goto, K. et al. (1990) Cloning of a cDNA encoding a non-isopeptide-selective subtype of the endothelin receptor. *Nature*, **348**, 732–735.
37. Mckhann, G., Drachman, D., Flostein, M., Katzman, R., Price, D. and Stadlan, M. (1984) Clinical diagnosis of Alzheimer's disease: report of the NINCDS-ADRDA work group under the auspices of department of health and human services task force on Alzheimer's disease. *Neurology*, **34**, 939–944.
38. Suzuki, N., Matsumoto, H., Kitada, C., Masaki, T. and Fujino, M. (1989) A sensitive sandwich-enzyme immunoassay for human endothelin. *J. Immunol. Methods*, **118**, 245–250.
39. Shichiri, M., Hirata, Y., Ando, K., Kanno, K., Emori, T., Ohta, K., et al. (1990) Postural change and volume expansion affect plasma endothelin levels. *JAMA*, **263**, 661.
40. Kaufmann, H., Oribe, E. and Oliver, J. A. (1991) Plasma endothelin during upright tilt: relevance for orthostatic hypotension? *Lancet*, **338**, 1542–1545.
41. Mima, T., Yanagisawa, M., Shigeno, T., Saito, A., Goto, K., Takakura, K., et al. (1989) Endothelin acts in feline and canine cerebral arteries from the adventitial side. *Stroke*, **20**, 1553–1556.
42. Hamann, G., Isenberg, E., Strittmatter, M. and Schimrigk, K. (1993) Absence of elevation of big endothelin in subarachnoid hemorrhage. *Stroke*, **24**, 383–386.
43. Clozel, M. and Watanabe, H. (1992) BQ-123, a peptidic endothelin ET$_A$ receptor antagonist, prevents the early cerebral vasospasm following subarachnoid hemorrhage after intracisternal but not intravenous injection. *Life Sci.*, **52**, 825–834.
44. Ziv, I., Fleminger, G., Djaldetti, R., Aciron, A., Melamed, E. and Sokolovsky, M. (1992) Increased plasma endothelin-1 in acute ischemic stroke. *Stroke*, **23**, 1014–1016.
45. Giuffrida, R., Bellomo, M., Polizzi, G. and Malatino, L. S. (1992) Ischemia-induced change in the immunoreactivity for endothelin and other vasoactive peptides in the brain of the Mongolian gerbil. *J. Cardiovasc. Pharmacol.*, **Suppl. 12**, S41–S44.
46. Kurihara, M., Ochi, A., Kawaguchi, T., Niwa, M., Kataoka, Y. and Mori, K. (1990) Localization and characterization of endothelin receptors in human gliomas: a growth factor? *Neurosurgery*, **27**, 275–281.

13 Endothelin Mechanisms in the Heart: Role in Pathophysiology

Anil Gulati

Department of Pharmaceutics and Pharmacodynamics (m/c 865), The University of Illinois at Chicago, 833 South Wood Street, Chicago, IL 60612, USA

INTRODUCTION

Endothelin (ET) is widely distributed throughout many tissues. The synthesis of ET is regulated by ET genes and analysis of these genes has revealed that three distinct ET genes exist and encode different mature ET sequences (ET-1, ET-2 and ET-3). There are no species differences among isoforms of human, porcine, rat, bovine or dog[1]. Messenger ribonucleic acid (mRNA) encoding preproET has been shown to be present in the endothelial cells of blood vessels in various mammalian tissues including the heart[2]. Several factors like epinephrine, thrombin and angiotensin II can enhance the production of preproET. PreproET is cleaved by an endopeptidase to form proET (big ET) and finally an ET converting enzyme cleaves proET to form mature ET.

ET exerts its biological actions by acting on specific receptors on the cell membranes. ET binding sites have been identified in the heart[3], lung, kidney, adrenal gland and central nervous system (CNS)[4,5]. The intracellular mechanism of action of ET is linked to increases in inositol triphosphate and diacylglycerol, which is accompanied with the increases in intracellular calcium and activation of protein kinase C.

The major biological action of ET described is vasoconstriction. However, in addition, ET has several important cardiovascular, renal and endocrine functions[5,6]. ET has modulatory actions on the renin-angiotensin-aldosterone system and has antinatriuretic effects[7]. ET has been reported to stimulate the secretion of atrial natriuretic peptide from cultured rat atrial myocytes[8]. Plasma ET-1 level increases in various pathological conditions associated with cardiovascular system[9]. Increases in circulating ET have been documented in states of severe cardiovascular stress, including cardiogenic and septic shock[10,11], acute myocardial infarction[12,13] and pulmonary hypertension[14] implicating it in several disease conditions associated with cardiovascular system. Although the clinical significance of elevated levels of ET in these diseases is not clear, however, studies do indicate that ET has biological actions at pathophysiological concentration[6] implicating a possible role of ET mechanisms in the pathogenesis of cardiovascular disorders.

The functional importance of ET increases because of its mitogenic potential, which could contribute to structural changes within the cardiovascular system. ET-1 has been shown to be a smooth muscle mitogen and its synthesis can be increased by damage to the endothelium. Thus, it may play a role in genesis of atherosclerosis and in forms of hypertension in which smooth muscle proliferation has been implicated[15]. ET has also been reported to stimulate the proliferation of fibroblasts, glomerular mesangial and human carcinoma cells with the expression of proto- oncogenes (c-myc, c-fos) in these cells[16].

ET AND MYOCARDIAL CELL HYPERTROPHY

ET has been demonstrated to induce hypertrophy with concomitant increases in the transcripts of muscle-specific genes and a proto-onco-gene, c-fos, as well as augmenting DNA and protein synthesis in cultured neonatal rat cardiomyocytes[17]. ET-1 (10^{-9} to 10^{-7} M) induced dose dependent increases in the gene expression of myosin light chain 2, α-actin, and troponin I. ET-1 also dose-dependently stimulated accumulation of total inositol phosphates in cardiomyocytes. The surface area of cardiomyocytes was significantly increased without any cell proliferation[17]. In another study, the effect of ET-1 on myocardial cell hypertrophy was studied using neonatal rat myocardial cell model. The hypertrophic response was assessed using several parameters. It was found that ET-1 (0.1 to 10 nM concentrations) showed a dose-dependent increase in the number of cells displaying hypertrophy with organized sarcomeric structures. ET-1 (1 nM) resulted in the rapid and transient expression of an immediate early gene expression of an immediate early gene program. Thus, ET-1 activated the immediate early gene expression and sarcomere assembly. Besides, ET-1 also activated the transcription of cardiac genes[18]. Rat cardiac myocytes culture showed an increase in the rate of protein synthesis, morphological size, contraction rate and Ca^{2+} uptake when ET-1 was added[19]. The effect of ET-1 on cardiac myosin heavy chain gene expression was examined in cultured neonatal rat myocardial cells. ET-1 was found to stimulate both α- and β-myosin heavy chain gene expression. Myocardial cells treated with ET-1 (1 to 100 nM) increased the transcription rate of α- and β-myosin heavy chain genes in a dose-dependent manner[20]. ET-1 was also found to increase the cell surface area, ^{3}H-leucine incorporation and gene expression. The increase in ^{3}H-leucine incorporation by ET-1 could be attenuated by BQ-123[21]. Most of the studies were performed on the cultured neonatal rat ventricular myocytes. Sugden et al.[22] studied the effects of ET-1 on protein synthesis and phosphoinositide hydrolysis in ventricular myocytes obtained from adult rat hearts. ET-1 (10^{-11} to 10^{-7} M) produced a dose-dependent increase in phosphoinositide hydrolysis and the rate of protein synthesis. The above studies clearly indicate that ET can lead to hypertrophy of myocardial cells obtained from neonatal or adult animals. The induction of cardiac hypertrophy by ET-1 appears to be mediated through the enhanced Ca^{2+} entry through the sarcolemmal T-type Ca^{2+} channel, possibly through a pathway involving activation of protein kinase C[23].

Recently, both ET_A and ET_B types of receptors have been shown to be present in cardiac fibroblasts with ET_B predominating[24]. It was also found that ET-1 and ET-3 increased the synthesis of type I and III collagens and ET-1 but not ET-3 reduced collagenase activity. The effect of ET on collagen synthesis in cardiac fibroblasts may be mediated through both ET_A and ET_B types of receptors, whereas their effect on collagenase seems to be mediated through ET_A receptors[25].

EFFECT OF ET ON THE HEART

Positive chronotropic effect of ET

ET-1 has been shown to possess positive chronotropic effect[26,27]. The positive chronotropic effect of ET-1 was not affected by the L-type Ca^{2+} channel antagonist, nicardipine. Reid et al.[27] have reported that ET-1 decreases the chronotropic responses to stimulation of intramural sympathetic nerves by approximately 60% in rat and 10–15% in guinea pig atria, but does not affect the stimulation induced release of norepinephrine. The reduction of stimulation induced chronotropic responses by ET-1 appeared to be dependent on the increase in basal rate and the ability of ET-1 to facilitate the norepinephrine uptake.

Ventricular arrhythmias are generally attributed to severe ischemia, the fact that specific ET receptors have also been identified in cardiac myocytes[28,29] and in the cardiac conducting system[30] raises the possibility that ET might possess electrophysiological properties. ET-1 infused into the left circumflex coronary artery or left anterior descending coronary artery produced a dose dependent decrease in blood flow and ECG changes typical of myocardial ischemia. ET-1 when administered to left anterior descending artery produced fatal arrhythmias even in lower doses and several animals died. In contrast, when ET-1 was administered to left circumflex artery no deaths occurred even though the decrease in flow was comparable[31]. The direct effect of ET-1 on the isolated dog right bundle branch, false tendon, ventricular muscle and atrial muscle preparation was studied. ET-1 prolonged the duration of action potentials in all the tissues except atrial muscle, the spontaneous firing of the right bundle branch was suppressed by ET-1 and the prolongation of action potential duration was far more marked in the right bundle branch than in other tissues and it was followed by the development of early after depolarization[32]. The development of early after depolarization might be responsible for the direct actions of ET on the myocardial cells to cause arrhythmias.

Positive inotropic effect of ET

In the heart ET acts as a positive inotropic agent[33,34]. ET exerts a prominent stimulatory action on the isolated heart preparations from rats[35], guinea pigs[33], humans[36], rabbits[37] and ferrets[38]. However, ET-1 could not elicit any effect on the dog ventricular myocardium[39]. The positive inotropic effect of ET was not affected by adrenergic, muscarinic, histaminergic and serotonergic antagonists[33,35,40]. This indicates that the release of endogenous catecholamines, acetylcholine, histamine or serotonin is not involved in the positive inotropic effect of ET.

ET-1 produced a pronounced positive inotropic effect on the rabbit papillary muscle, intermediate one in the guinea pig and rat and none in dog. The rank order of ET-1 induced positive inotropic effects in these species was found to be consistent with that of the density of ET-1 receptors determined by radioreceptor assay[39]. The isoforms of ET (ET-1, ET-2 and ET-3) were found to be equieffective and equipotent in eliciting a positive inotropic response in rabbit[39] suggesting that the subtype of ET receptors responsible for the inotropic effect may be different from those in vascular smooth muscle cells, where ET-1 produces contraction with a much higher potency than ET-3[41].

The characteristics of ET induced positive inotropic effect on mammalian ventricular myocardium were found to be very similar to those of myocardial α-adrenoceptor stimulation[39,42]. ET has been found to influence adrenergic responses[5,43].

The subcellular mechanism of ET induced positive inotropic effect appears to involve phosphoinositide hydrolysis[39,40,44]. ET-1 catalyzed phosphoinositide hydrolysis in a concentration and time dependent manner in rabbit ventricular myocardium. A striking similarity was noted between the characteristic of ET-1 and myocardial α_1-adrenoceptor mediated acceleration of phosphoinositide hydrolysis and regulation of myocardial contractility[45]. Thapsigargin, an inotropic agent, was found to completely antagonize the positive inotropic effect and Ca^{2+} mobilizing action of 100 nM of ET-1. Thapsigargin had no effect on the basal or ET-1 stimulated production of inositol phosphates[46]. Recently, it has been found that there are two components in the positive inotropic effect of ET-1 in guinea pig atria. ET-1 at concentrations of 10 nM and higher produced an initial increasing phase (early component) and a second greater positive inotropic phase (late component). The two components may be mediated by different mechanisms. Stimulation of phosphoinositide hydrolysis and subsequent activation of protein kinase C seems to play a key role in the late component. However, the early component appears to be independent of the protein kinase C activation but may be due to prolongation of the duration of action potential[47]. The potent positive inotropic effect of ET-1 on the mammalian heart has also been demonstrated to be mediated through the apparent sensitization of cardiac myofilaments to intracellular calcium[48] which is in part due to stimulation of the sarcolemmal Na^+-H^+ exchanger by a protein kinase C mediated pathway[44].

When ET is administered into perfused rat heart preparations, it causes a negative inotropic effect because of its vasoconstrictor effect[49]. In dogs, ET produced a potent vasoconstriction of the resistance coronary vessels producing a redistribution of transmural blood flow and a decrease in myocardial contractility secondary to ischemia[50]. Intracoronary injection of ET-1 in swine at a dose producing an extensive coronary vasoconstriction produced no change in regional or global myocardial contractile function[51]. These authors concluded that in spite of strong *in vitro* evidence of positive inotropic effect due to ET-1 the effect is probably not relevant *in vivo*. However, it could be species related as *in vitro* studies do not show any positive inotropic effect in dog ventricle despite the presence of ET-1 binding sites.

ET AND PULMONARY HYPERTENSION

Pulmonary hypertension is a progressive condition, characterized by an increase in pulmonary vascular resistance. The increase in resistance is so marked that it ultimately bradycardia in response to ET-1, and an interesting hypertensive response to ET-3[2] (the vasoconstrictor phenylephrine was however without effect).

We have also used our electrophysiological techniques to determine whether increased circulating concentrations of ET-1 influence the activity patterns of commissural NTS neurons. Extracellular recordings from a total of 28 cNTS neurons tested with systemic ET-1 demonstrated the activity of 10 of these cells to be inhibited and 2 excited[37]. Although these findings clearly emphasize the potential of NTS neurons to respond to circulating ET-1 they provide no definitive evidence regarding the physiological significance of such actions.

Area postrema

In 1988 we first reported that in anaesthetized rats electrical stimulation (and thus activation of neurons) in area postrema (AP) at physiological frequencies resulted in site specific decreases in BP and HR[38]. In view of the data described above demonstrating ET binding sites in AP we therefore speculated that this CVO represented a CNS site at which either centrally produced, or circulating ET may act to influence cardiovascular control mechanisms. This possibility was examined using both microinjection and electrophysiological single unit recording techniques.

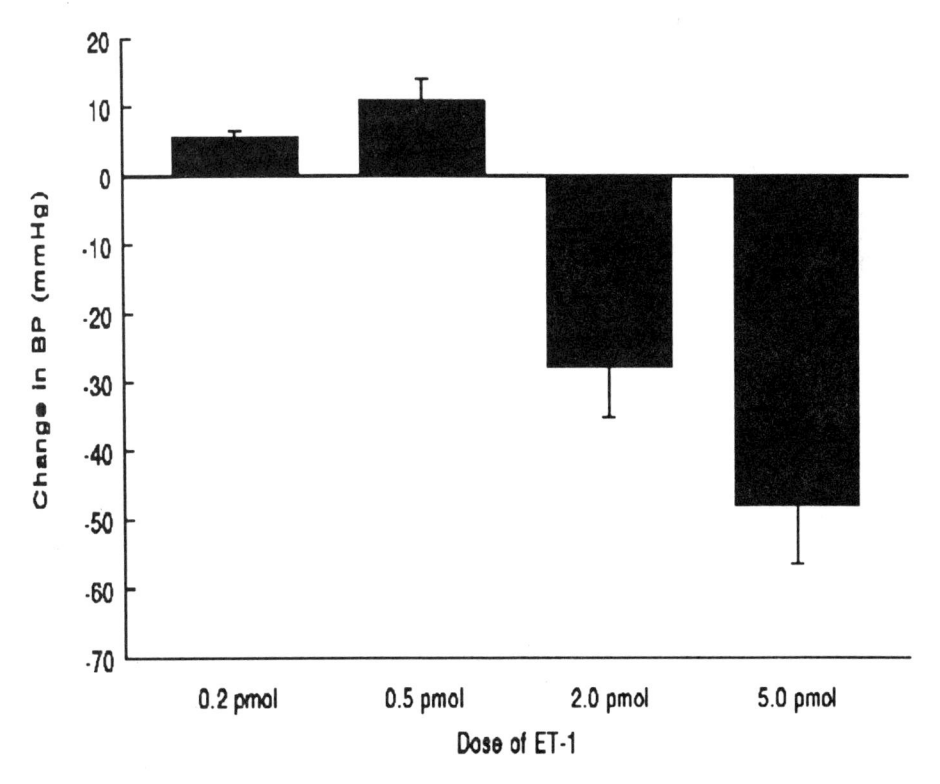

Figure 9.2. This histogram illustrates the mean changes in blood pressure observed in response to microinjection of ET-1 into histologically verified sites within the rat AP.

Microinjections of ET-1 localized in AP were found to elicit dose dependent effects on BP. Low doses of ET (0.2–1.0 pmol) resulted in small, but statistically significant increases in BP, while larger doses (2.0–5.0 pmol), caused large decreases in BP (see Figure 9.2), without consistent changes in HR[36], effects which were not elicited by similar microinjection of the vasoconstrictor methoxamine. Mosqueda-Garcia et al.[2] have also recently reported depressor actions of ET-1 microinjection into AP at similar doses although they do not see the same magnitude of effects which we observed (this difference may be due to the smaller microinjection volume they use which would thus influence fewer AP neurons). In addition this study also reported bradycardia in response to ET-1 microinjection, and found ET-3 to elicit similar effects of greater magnitude.

These data demonstrating depressor and bradycardic actions of ET within AP suggested to us that ET would have to activate AP neurons (electrical stimulation decreases BP and HR), in order to elicit such effects. Our single unit recordings confirmed this speculation. We found that of 60 AP neurons from which we obtained stable extracellular recordings for long enough (usually > 30 min) to evaluate effects of systemic ET-1 administration 27 were activated[37]. These neurons demonstrated rapid, reversible increases in the frequency of action potentials following systemic administration of 0.1–10.0 pmol ET-1, as illustrated in Figure 9.3. The majority of cells being influenced by doses of ET less than 2.0 pmol.

Rostral ventrolateral medulla

The rostral ventrolateral medulla (RVLM) represents another important cardiovascular control centre at which ET may act to influence the cardiovascular system. ET-1 microinjection (0.5 pmol) into this region has been reported to elicit biphasic

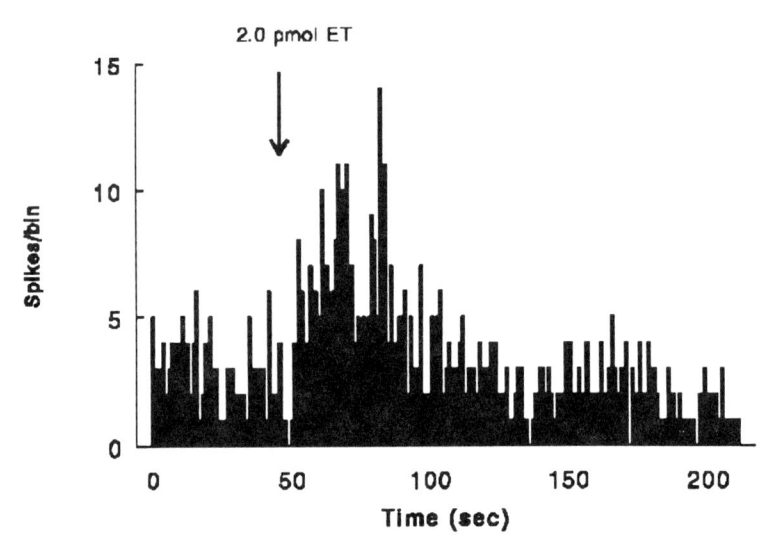

Figure 9.3. This ratemeter record illustrates the effects of systemic administration of ET-1 (time of administration indicated by the arrow) on the activity of an AP neuron.

cardiovascular effects in which an early pressor effect is followed by hypotension and bradycardia[2]. In contrast this study demonstrated that ET-3 elicited only hypertensive and tachycardic effects following administration into RVLM.

The available information regarding the medullary actions of ET in cardiovascular control does thus provide consistent data supporting the following conclusions. Within the NTS ET acts to decrease BP and to inhibit the activity of neurons within the commissural region. However, there has as yet been no systematic evaluation of the effects of ET in the many different anatomical subdivisions of the NTS, an analysis which would lay the essential groundwork from which electrophysiological techniques may ultimately be used to determine the role of ET in controlling the excitability of functionally separate populations of neurons within this region. There also appears to be agreement that pmol doses of ET in the AP elicit decreases in blood pressure, with ET-3 perhaps being more effective in mediating such responses. In accordance with the demonstration that activation of AP neurons decreases BP systemic ET has also been shown to activate AP neurons suggesting potential hormonal actions of the peptide at this CVO. Finally ET-3 has been shown to elicit hypertensive responses after administration into RVLM, an effect which is followed by hypotension following ET-1 microinjection.

SPINAL CORD ACTIONS IN CENTRAL AUTONOMIC CONTROL

A final essential CNS site for cardiovascular regulation is found in the spinal cord, at the location of autonomic preganglionic neurons in the intermediolateral cell column (IML). The demonstration of ET receptors and immunoreactivity in this region (see above) again suggests potential actions of these peptides within IML. However, to date there are few studies evaluating action of ET in the spinal cord. Intrathecal administration of ETs into thoracic (sympathetic preganglionic), or lumbosacral (parasympathetic preganglionic), cord have reported decreases[39], or increases[40], in BP respectively. In accordance with the latter studies there are also data demonstrating that bath applied ET depolarizes dorsal horn neurons *in vitro*, as indicated by the measurement of ventral root potentials with a suction electrode[41]. It would appear that electrophysiological single unit recordings from identified preganglionic neurons of the spinal cord may in the future provide significant information regarding potential actions of ET's in regulation of these essential output neurons.

CONCLUSION

Although the data outlined above indicate some role for central ET in CNS regulation of the cardiovascular system, there is to date little definitive information regarding the precise nature of such involvement. Hopefully, future anatomical studies will provide information regarding the *differential* distribution of ET_A and ET_B receptors, and specific localizations of mRNA'a for the three different isoforms of ET within the CNS. Such data will permit a more focussed approach to determining specific functions of ET's in regions where they are known to be delivered to neuronal tissue. In addition it is unlikely that consistent data will be derived from evaluation of the effects of these peptides into anatomical regions consisting of a variety of different functional groups of neurons. Rather the ability to determine the effects of ET's on specific functional populations of neurons (e.g. VP and OXY secreting neurons in hypothalamus, medullary vagal motor neurons innervating the heart), using anatomical or electrophysiological techniques opens exciting new avenues for the evaluation of the specific functional roles of these peptides in central cardiovascular control.

Acknowledgements

Supported by the Heart and Stroke Foundation of Ontario.

References

1. Kraus, G. E., Bucholz, R. D., Yoon, K. W., Knuepfer, M. M., and Smith, K. R. (1991) Cerebrospinal fluid endothelin-1 and endothelin-3 levels in normal and neurosurgical patients: A clinical study and literature review. *Surgical Neurology*, **35**, 20–29.
2. Mosqueda-Garcia, R., Inagama, T., Appalsamy, M., Sugiura, M., and Robertson, R. M. (1993) Endothelin as a neuropeptide: Cardiovascular effects in the brainstem of normotensive rats. *Circulation Research*, **72**, 21–35.
3. Jones, C. R., Hiley, C. R., Pelton, J. T., and Mohr, M. (1989) Autoradiographic visualization of the binding sites for [^{125}I] endothelin in rat and human brain. *Neuroscience Letters*, **97**, 276–279.
4. Koseki, C., Imai, M., Hirata, Y., Yanagisawa, M., and Masaki, T. (1989) Autoradiographic distribution in rat tissues of binding sites for endothelin: a neuropeptide? *American Journal of Physiology*, **256**, R858–R866.
5. Bolger, G. T., Berry, R., and Jaramillo, J. (1992) Regional and subcellular distribution of [^{125}I]endothelin binding sites in rat brain. *Brain Research Bulletin*, **28**, 789–797.
6. Koseki, C., Imai, M., Hirata, Y., Yanagisawa, M., and Masaki, T. (1989) Binding sites for endothelin-1 in rat tissues: An autoradiographic study. *Journal of Cardiovascular Pharmacology*, **13**, S153–S154.
7. Kohzuki, M., Chai, S. Y., Paxinos, G. *et al.* (1991) Localization and characterization of endothelin receptor binding sites in the rat brain visualized by *in vitro* autoradiography. *Neuroscience*, **42**, 245–260.
8. Banasik, J. L., Hosick, H., Wright, J. W., and Harding, J. W. (1991) Endothelin binding in brain of normotensive and spontaneously hypertensive rats. *The Journal of Pharmacology and Experimental Therapeutics*, **257**, 302–306.
9. Spyer, K. M., McQueen, D. S., Dashwood, M. R., Sykes, R. M., Daly, M. B., and Muddle, J. R. (1991) Localization of [^{125}I]endothelin binding sites in the region of the carotid bifurcation and brainstem of the cat: possible baro- and chemoreceptor involvement. *Journal of Cardiovascular Pharmacology*, **17 (Suppl 7)**, S385–S389.
10. Saper, C. B. and Loewy, A. D. (1980) Efferent connections of the parabrachial nucleus in the rat. *Brain Research*, **197**, 291–317.
11. Voshart, K. and van der Kooy, D. (1981) The organization of the efferent projections of the parabrachial nucleus to the forebrain in the rat: a retrograde fluorescent double-labelling study. *Brain Research*, **212**, 271–286.
12. Hosli, E. and Hosli, L. (1991) Autoradiographic evidence for endothelin receptors on astrocytes in cultures of rat cerebellum, brain stem and spinal cord. *Neuroscience Letters*, **129**, 55–58.
13. Lysko, P. G., Feuerstein, G., Pullen, M., Wu, H. L., and Nambi, P. (1991) Identification of endothelin receptors in cultured cerebellar neurons. *Neuropeptides*, **18**, 83–86.
14. Takahashi, K., Ghatei, M. A., Jones, P. M. *et al.* (1991) Endothelin in human brain and pituitary gland: comparison with rat. *Journal of Cardiovascular Pharmacology*, **17 (Suppl 7)**, S101–S103.
15. Giaid, A., Gibson, S. J., Herrero, M. T. *et al.* (1991) Topographical localization of endothelin mRNA and peptide immunoreactivity in neurons of the human brain. *Histochemistry*, **95**, 303–314.
16. Giaid, A., Gibson, S. J., Ibrahim, N. B. N. *et al.* (1989) Endothelin 1, an endothelium derived peptide, is expressed in neurons of the human spinal cord and dorsal root ganglia. *Proceedings of the National Academy of Science USA*, **86**, 7634–7638.
17. Rebello, S. and Gulati, A. (1991) Endothelin receptor down-regulation in ventrolateral medulla and hypothalamus of spontaneously hypertensive rats. *FASEB Journal*, **5**, 1410.

18. Jeng, A. Y., Savage, P., and Hu, S. (1991) A comparison of the binding of endothelin to various tissues from spontaneously hypertensive and Wistar-Kyoto rats. *Neurochemistry International*, **18**, 541–546.
19. Mendelsohn, F. A. O., Quirion, R., Saavedra, J. M., and Aguilera, G. (1984) Autoradiographic localization of angiotensin II receptors in rat brain. *Proceedings of the National Academy of Science USA*, **81**, 1575–1579.
20. Speth, R. C., Wamsley, J. K., Gehlert, D. R., Chernicky, C. L., Barnes, K. L., and Ferrario, C. M. (1985) Angiotensin II receptor localization in the canine CNS. *Brain Research*, **326**, 137–143.
21. Gehlert, D. R., Speth, R. C., and Wamsley, J. K. (1986) Distribution of [^{125}I] angiotensin II binding sites in the rat brain: a quantitative autoradiographic study. *Neuroscience*, **18**, 837–856.
22. Yamamoto, T., Kimura, T., Ota, K. *et al.* (1992) Central effects of endothelin-1 on vasopressin release, blood pressure, and renal solute excretion. *American Journal of Physiology*, **262**, E856–E862.
23. Samson, W. K., Skala, K. D., Alexander, B. D., and Huang, F. L. (1991) Hypothalamic endothelin: presence and effects related to fluid and electrolyte homeostasis. *Journal of Cardiovascular Pharmacology*, **17 (Suppl 7)**, S346–S349.
24. Makino, S., Hashimoto, K., Hirasawa, R., Hattori, T., and Ota, Z. (1992) Central interaction between endothelin and brain natriuretic peptide on vasopressin secretion. *Journal of Hypertension*, **10**, 25–28.
25. Samson, W. K., Skala, K., Huang, F. L. S., Gluntz, S., Alexander, B., and Gomezsanchez, C. E. (1991) Central nervous system action of endothelin-3 to inhibit water drinking in the rat. *Brain Research*, **539**, 347–351.
26. Wall, K. K., Nasr, M., and Ferguson, A. V. (1992) Actions of endothelin at the subfornical organ. *Brain Research*, **570**, 180–187.
27. Gutman, M. B., Ciriello, J., and Mogenson, G. J. (1985) The effect of paraventricular nucleus lesions on cardiovascular responses elicited by stimulation of the subfornical organ in the rat. *Canadian Journal of Physiology and Pharmacology*, **63**, 816–824.
28. Ferguson, A. V. and Renaud, L. P. (1984) Hypothalamic paraventricular nucleus lesions decrease pressor responses to subfornical organ stimulation. *Brain Research*, **305**, 361–364.
29. Lind, R. W., Van Hoesen, G. W., and Johnson, A. K. (1982) An HRP study of the connections of the subfornical organ of the rat. *The Journal of Comparative Neurology*, **210**, 265–277.
30. Miselis, R. R. (1981) The efferent projections of the subfornical organ of the rat: A circumventricular organ within a neural network subserving water balance. *Brain Research*, **230**, 1–23.
31. Goetz, K. L., Wang, B. C., Madwed, J. B., Zhu, J. L., and Leadley, R. J., Jr. (1988) Cardiovascular, renal, and endocrine responses to intravenous endothelin in conscious dogs. *American Journal of Physiology*, **255**, R1064–R1068.
32. Wall, K. M. and Ferguson, A. V. (1992) Endothelin acts at the subfornical organ to influence the activity of putative vasopressin and oxytocin secreting neurons. *Brain Research*, **586**, 111–116.
33. Kuwaki, T., Koshiya, N., Terui, N., and Kumada, M. (1991) Endothelin-1 modulates cardiorespiratory control by the central nervous system. *Neurochemistry International*, **18**, 519–524.
34. Hashim, M. A. and Tadepalli, A. S. (1991) Functional evidence for the presence of a phosphoramidon-sensitive enzyme in rat brain that converts big endothelin-1 to endothelin-1. *Life Sciences*, **49**, PL207–PL211.
35. Itoh, S. and Vandenbuuse, M. (1991) Sensitization of baroreceptor reflex by central endothelin in conscious rats. *American Journal of Physiology*, **260**, 1106–1112.
36. Ferguson, A. V. and Smith, P. (1990) Cardiovascular responses induced by endothelin microinjection into area postrema. *Regulatory Peptides*, **27**, 75–85.
37. Ferguson, A. V. and Smith, P. (1991) Circulating endothelin influences area postrema neurons. *Regulatory Peptides*, **32**, 11–21.
38. Ferguson, A. V. and Marcus, P. (1988) Area postrema stimulation induced cardiovascular changes in the rat. *American Journal of Physiology*, **255**, R855–R860.
39. Han S. P., Chen, X. L., Westfall, T. C., and Knuepfer, M. M. (1991) Characterization of the depressor effect of intrathecal endothelin in anesthetized rats. *American Journal of Physiology*, **260**, 1685–1691.
40. Giuliani, S., Lecci, A., Maggi, C. A., Rovero, P., and Giachetti, A. (1991) Effect of intrathecal administration of ET-1, ET-3 and ET(16–21) on blood pressure and micturition reflex in anesthetized rats. *Neurochemistry International*, **18**, 565–569.
41. Yoshizawa, T., Kimura, S., Kanazawa, I., Uchiyama, Y., Yanagisawa, M., and Masaki, T. (1989) Endothelin localizes in the dorsal horn and acts on the spinal neurones: possible involvement of dihydropyridine-sensitive calcium channels and substance P release. *Neuroscience Letters*, **102**, 179–184.

10 Endothelin: Cerebrovascular Effects and Potential Role in Cerebral Vasospasm

Robert N. Willette and Eliot H. Ohlstein

Department of Cardiovascular Pharmacology, SmithKline Beecham Pharmaceuticals, 709 Swedeland Road, King of Prussia, PA 19406, USA

INTRODUCTION

The discovery of endothelin (ET) in porcine aortic endothelial cell culture and its description as a potent and long acting vasoconstrictor peptide prompted numerous investigations of the cerebrovascular actions of ET[1,2]. Since these initial studies, ET, its isoforms and its receptor subtypes have been detected in various cell types (neurons, glia, vascular smooth muscle and endothelium) in the brain[3,4]. Thus, ET is no longer viewed strictly as an endothelium-derived peptide. The ability of ET to produce cerebral hypoperfusion, prolonged periods of cerebral vasospasm and brain injury has lead to the suggestion that this peptide may be an important mediator of cerebrovascular sequelae and neuronal injury associated with subarachnoid hemorrhage and ischemic stroke.

The purpose of the present manuscript is to review the laboratory and clinical (where available) evidence for a role of endothelin in cerebral vasospasm. Specifically, the vasoactive and mitogenic properties will be discussed in the context of cerebral vasospasm associated with subarachnoid hemorrhage (SAH).

Cerebrovascular effects of endothelin(s)

ET isoforms (ET-1, ET-2 and ET-3) have complex effects on the cerebrovasculature. In isolated segments of various cerebral arteries, ET-1 potently elicits sustained, concentration-related contraction. In fact, comparative analyses performed using arteries from the pig[5], goat[6], dog (Willette and Ohlstein, unpublished observation) and human[7] indicate that cerebral arteries are among the most sensitive vessels in the body to the contractile effects of ET. The contractile effects of ETs have been observed *in vitro* at all arterial levels of the cerebral circulation including large (basilar and middle cerebral arteries), intermediate (pial arteries) and small (penetrating arteries) cerebral vessels with a rank order potency of ET-1 > ET $\gg$ ET-3[8,9]. In vascular segments, human cerebral veins are less sensitive to the vasoconstrictor effects of ET[7.]

ET also elicits sustained, concentration-related vasoconstriction (Figure 10.1) in a number of species when applied topically to cerebral vessels (large, intermediate and micro) in situ[10-12]. These effects are qualitatively similar to the observations in vitro (above). However, feline pial veins in situ were reported to be more sensitive to the contractile effects of ET than feline pial arteries[13]. In contrast pial viens in the rat are virtually insensitive to ET (see Figure 10.1). At higher doses of ET the prolonged vasoconstriction is of sufficient intensity to override cerebral blood flow autoregulatory mechanisms and cause ischemic brain injury[14-16]. For example, the topical application of ET to the middle cerebral artery results in distal ischemia in the cortical territory of the middle cerebral artery[15]. In addition, ET does not appear to alter the blood-brain-barrier[10].

In contrast to the straightforward effects observed in vitro and in situ, ET has a biphasic effect on the cerebral circulation when administered systemically. In the anesthetized rat, ET caused a transient, dose-related increase in cortical perfusion and a decrease in cortical vascular resistance when administered intravenously[17]. Likewise, the intracarotid administration of ET increased cortical perfusion at low doses. However, high doses (>300 pmol) administrated by this route decreased cortical perfusion and increased cortical vascular resistance. Ischemic changes in the EEG were also evident following high doses. The results suggest that the cerebral vasculature is more sensitive to the vasodilator than the vasoconstrictor effects of circulating ET. A similar response-profile is observed in the hindlimb circulation of the rat[18,19]. The results also suggest that an intraluminal action mediates the vasodilator effect and that ET has only a limited access to the abluminal vasoconstrictor site of action following systemic administration.

Several studies are consistent with an abluminal vasoconstrictor site of endothelin action[20,21]. Mima et al.[22] compared the effects of ET following vetebral and intracisternal administration and observed, angiographically, vasoconstriction of the basilar artery only following intracisternal administration in cats and dogs. Similarly, only dose-related decreases in local microvascular perfusion were observed following parenchymal microinjection of ET-1 in the rat parietal cortex[12]. Finally, ET is a more potent and efficacious vasoconstrictor when applied extraluminally in isolated perfused cerebral microvessels[23]. Based on these results, circulating ET would be expected to dilate cerebral vessels whereas ET released from the cerebral endothelium toward the tunica media may elicit local cerebral vasoconstriction[24]. This scenario may be particularly important during periods of cerebral ischemia and in SAH which are believed to enhance the release of abluminal ET[25,26].

ET mechanisms of vasoconstriction and vasodilation

Based on the rank-order of ET isopeptide potency (ET-1 > ET-2 ≫ ET-3), the vasoconstrictor response is mediated by an irreversible interaction at the ET_A receptor subtype on vascular smooth muscle[27]. Similar to other vasconstrictiors, the vasoconstrictor effects of ET appear to be mediated by multiple intracellular events leading primarily to an increase in intracellular calcium concentrations[28] (for review). The initial increase in intracellular calcium is mediated by a pertussis toxin insensitive G-protein coupled receptor which activates phospholipase C[29,30]. The subsequent

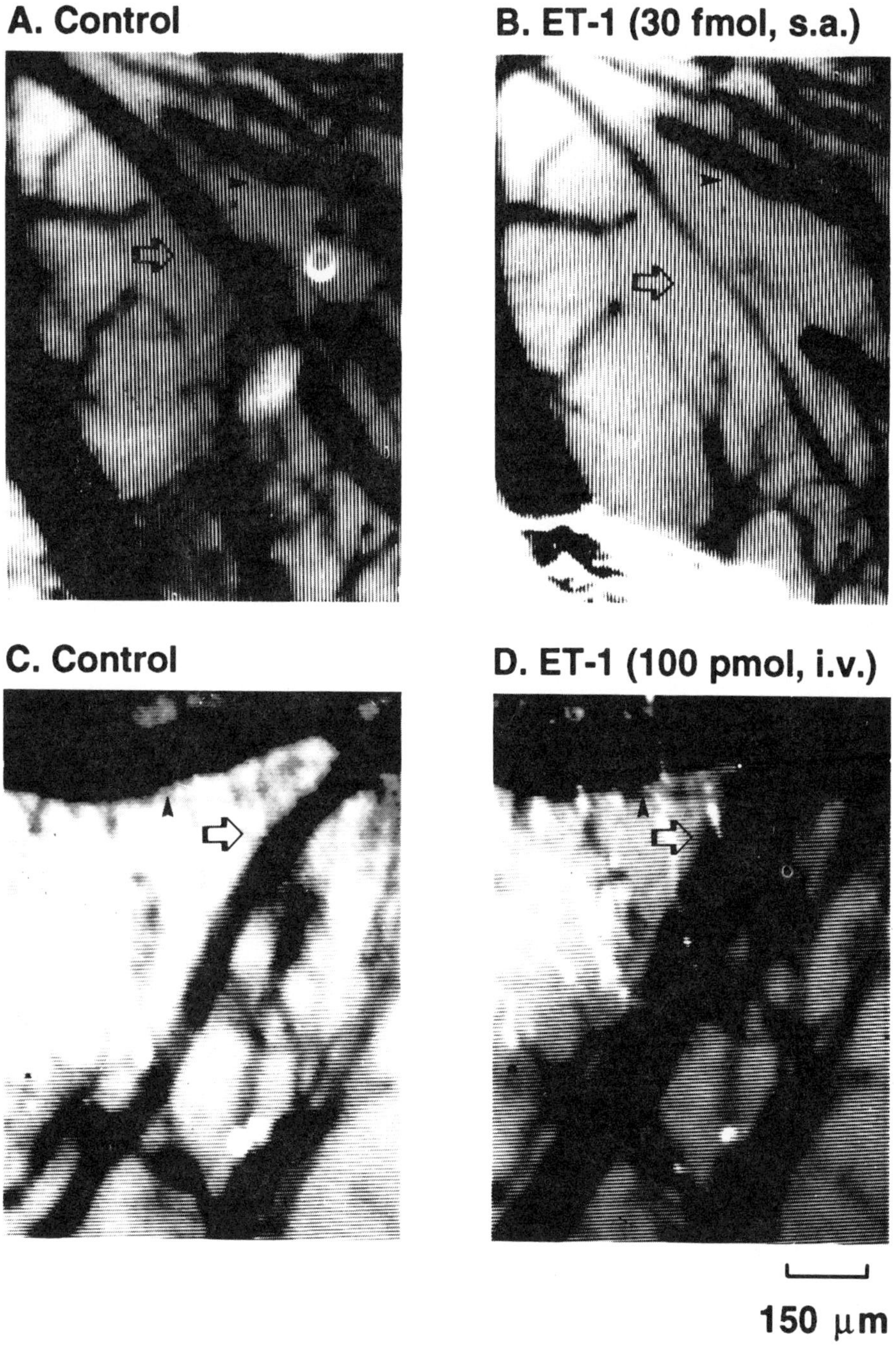

A. Control

B. ET-1 (30 fmol, s.a.)

C. Control

D. ET-1 (100 pmol, i.v.)

150 μm

Figure 10.1. The effects of endothelin-1 (ET) on pial arteries (open arrows) and veins (solid arrowheads) following subarachnoid (s.a.) and intravenous (i.v.) administration in the parietal cortex of the rat. The s.a. administration elicited potent vasoconstriction (A&B) whereas i.v. administration caused vasodilation at low doses (C&D). Note micropipette (M) in A.

production of inositol triphosphate and DAG releases calcium from intracellular stores and sensitizes the contractile process through the activation of protein kinase C, respectively[31]. In addition, ET appears to activate a non-selective cation channel which may depolarize the cell and activate voltage dependent L-type calcium channels in smooth muscle cell culture[32]. However, in segments of the feline middle cerebral artery ET-induced contraction occurred in the absence of depolarization, yet dihydropyridine calcium channel blockers still attenuated the maximum contractile response[33]. The removal of the endothelium from goat and cat cerebral vessels significantly enhanced the contractile effects of ET and strong tachyphylaxis was observed following repeated exposure to endothelin[33,34]. Thus, the activation of phospholipase C and protein kinase C appear to be important events in the initial and sustained contraction mediated by ET in cerebral vessels.

Unlike, the vasoconstrictor effects of ET, the mechanism of the vasodilator effect is unclear. As indicated, the vasodilator effects of systemically administered ET are prominent in the cerebral and hindquarter vascular beds and are mediated within the vessel lumen. Recent evidence suggests that the vasodilator effects are mediated by an interaction with ET_B receptors on the endothelium which have equal affinity for ET-1 and sarafotoxin 6C[35-37]. At this site, several potential mechanisms of action have been suggested. First, nitric oxide may play a role in ET-mediated vasodilation. In this regard, ET has been shown to stimulate nitric oxide generation in cultured endothelial cells[38], however, nitric oxide synthase inhibitors do not attenuate the hypotensive effects of ET[39]. Second, ET may act through the generation of prostacyclin. Indeed, ET increases prostacyclin synthesis in cultured endothelial cells[38], but, cyclo-oxygenase inhibitors do not alter ET-mediated hypotension[40]. Third, ET also elicits platelet activating factor release from endothelial cells which may mediate local vasodilation[41]. Finally, ET may act at a site distant from the endothelium to release a circulating vasodilator. Results from our laboratory would support this contention since ET-induced vasodilation of the hindquarters is not observed when blood is replaced with a nonsanguinous perfusion buffer[19]. This procedure does not alter endothelium-dependent and prostacylin-mediated vasodilation. The relative contribution of these mechanisms to ET-induced vasodilation remains to be determined.

Potential role of endothelin in cerebral vasospasm

Cerebral vasospasm associated with subarachnoid hemorrhage (SAH) is a complex disorder involving endothelial dysfunction and damage, vasoconstriction, vascular proliferation, mural thrombosis and vasonecrosis (Figure 10.2). ET may play a role in some of these processes (i.e., vasoconstriction and proliferation) following synthesis and release from the affected cellular elements, i.e. endothelium, astroglia and neurons.

Asano et al.[42] and Ide et al.[43] were among the first to suggest a potential role for ET in the cerebral vasospasm associated with subarachnoid hemorrhage. These investigators demonstrated a prolonged angiographic spasm (hours to days) of the basilar and anterior spinal arteries following the intracisternal administration of ET in the cat and dog. Subsequent studies demonstrated that the cerebral endotheluim, damaged in spastic arteries, is capable of producing ET[24]. These observations lead to a number of laboratory and clinical studies aimed at the identification and correlation of ET in the

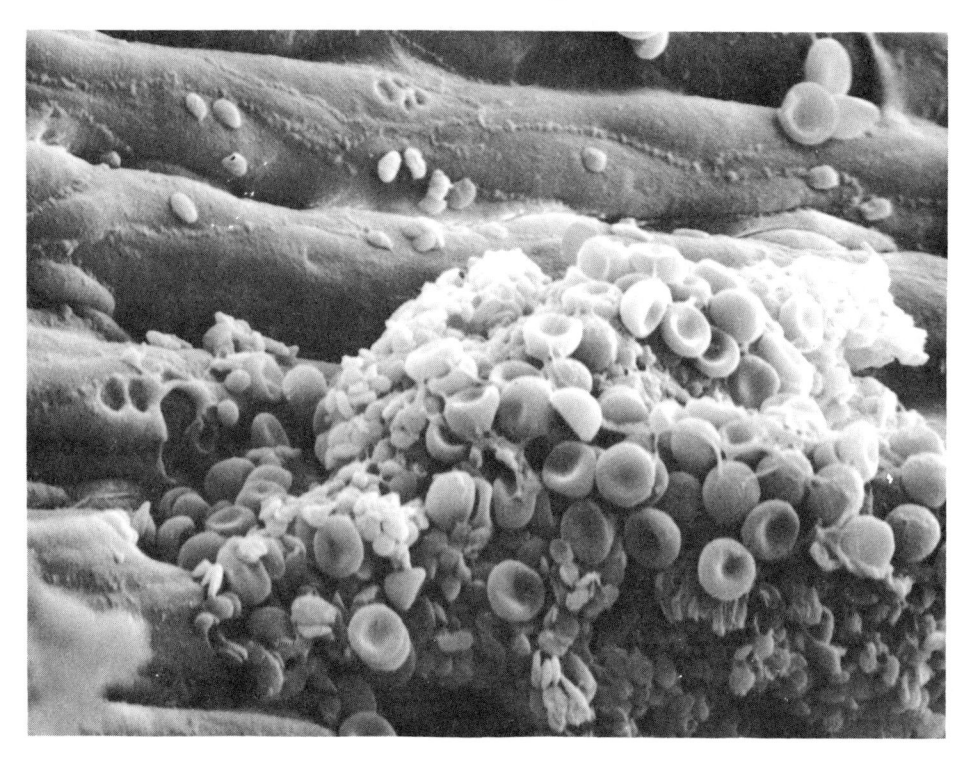

Figure 10.2. Scanning electron micrograph of spastic canine basilar artery perfuse-fixed on day 7 following the intracisternal administration of autologous blood on days 0 and 2 in the canine two-hemorrhage model of cerebral vasospasm associated with SAH. Note that the intima is corrugated, indicative of severe constriction. Also there are small mural thrombi composed of platelets, red blood cells and a fibrin mesh. Focal disruption and "pitting" of the endothelium is also evident (2000x).

cerebrospinal fluid (CSF) and plasma with the symptomatology associated with cerebral vasospasm in subarachnoid hemorrhage (SAH).

In the earliest clinical studies, Masaoka et al.[44] found significantly elevated plasma levels of ET in aneurysmal SAH patients. The highest levels were observed 3–7 days after the onset of SAH. Subsequent studies demonstrated an increase in ET in the CSF following SAH[45]; which reached a peak approximately 4 to 6 days after onset. This time-course suggested that the appearance of ET in the CSF may be related to the onset of delayed cerebral vasospasm. These investigators also demonstrated that both ET-1 and ET-3 were present in the CSF following SAH[46]. The results suggest that ET associated with SAH originates not only from the endothelium, but also derives from neurons and/or glia[47]. In addition, no ET immunoreactivity was observed in CSF obtained following cerebral infarction, subdural hematoma or brain tumor. In yet another study, CSF levels of ET-1 and ET-3 were determined in normal controls, SAH with vasospasm, severe head injury, and temporal lobectomy for intractable epilepsy[48]. These investigators found a significant elevation of ET-3 only in SAH patients with cerebral vasospasm.

Perhaps one of the most convincing demonstrations of ET production in SAH was a small study by Ehrenreich et al.[49]. These investigators performed long-term (up to 19 days) monitoring of ET-1 and ET-3 concentrations in CSF, plasma and 24 h urine obtained from 7 SAH patients. A distinct parallel peak in the CSF levels of ET-1 and ET-3 coincided with clinically documented signs of cerebral vasospasm in these patients. In some patients the CSF levels of ET-1 were 15–25 times greater than the basal values. Similar peaks in urinary ET-1 and ET-3 excretion were also observed in patients with vasospasm. In contrast, the plasma levels of ET-1 and ET-3 remained unchanged in all SAH patients and no peaks were noted in the CSF or urine of SAH patients that did not develop cerebral vasospasm (2 of 7). These clinical findings support a role for ETs in the pathogenesis of cerebral vasospasm associated with SAH.

As might be expected, the limited studies described above are not without controversy and should be interpreted cautiously for the following reasons. First, some studies of SAH patients with cerebral vasospasm have failed to observe any significant increases in CSF levels of ET-1 or big-ET[50,51]. In addition, no significant changes in plasma ET-1 levels were observed. Second, evidence suggests that elevated levels of ETs in the CSF and plasma may result from cerebral disorders associated secondarily with SAH, i.e. depression or infarction[52,53]. Finally, results are difficult to interpret across studies given the considerable variation in control plasma and CSF levels of ETs. For example, control concentrations of ET-1 in CSF may range from <0.1 pmol/l[46] to 11.2 pmol/l[54]. In addition, the predominant molecular form of ET in the CSF has not been established.

In conclusion, many studies suggest that CSF levels of ET(s) are elevated in SAH patients with cerebral vasospasm. However, it is not clear whether ET acts as a mediator of cerebral vasospasm or merely as a marker released as part of the epiphenomena associated with symptomatic cerebral vasospasm.

Factors enhancing endothelin production in SAH

At least two processes may account for the accumulation of ET in the CSF of SAH patients. First, large cerebral vessels enveloped by a thick subarachnoid clot may become anoxic[55]. Anoxia/ischemia has been shown to stimulate ET production and release in the brain under various experimental conditions[25,26,56,57]. Second, the release of oxyhemoglobin from the subarachnoid clot may also act to potently stimulate ET production[58,59]. In our laboratory, the addition of oxyhemoglobin (0.01–100 μM) to cultured bovine endothelial cells produced concentration-dependent increases in immunoreactive ET in the endothelial cell conditioned-medium (Figure 10.3). The EC_{50} concentration for the oxyhemoglobin-induced increase in immunoreactive ET levels was approximately 0.5 μM. The maximal effect of oxyhemoglobin (10 μM) produced approximately a 5-fold increase in immunoreactive ET.

Inhibition of ET and the development of cerebral vasospasm

A variety of laboratory investigations have been performed in an effort to ascertain the role of ET(s) in cerebral vasospasm associated with SAH. In the canine two-hemorrhage model of cerebral vasospasm, ET-1 has been shown to accumulate acutely in the spastic basilar artery[60]. These investigators found that the topical application of and ET-1 monoclonal antibody caused a modest reversal of the spasm observed on day

Cerebrovascular effects

CULTURED BOVINE PULMONARY ARTERY ENDOTHELIAL CELLS

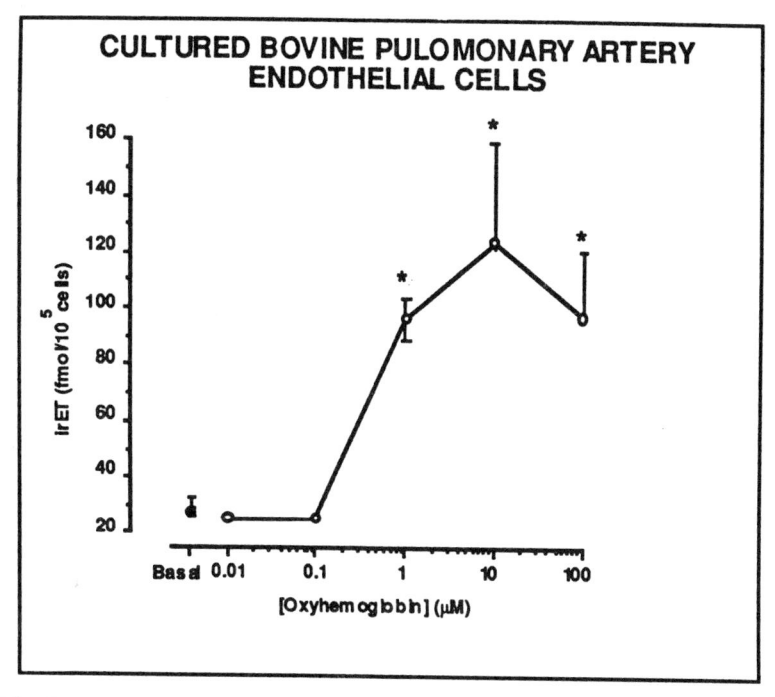

[Graph: y-axis "IrET (fmol/10⁵ cells)" from 20 to 160; x-axis "[Oxyhemoglobin] (μM)" Basal, 0.01, 0.1, 1, 10, 100]

Figure 10.3. Concentration-response curve for oxyhemoglobin-mediated stimulation of immunoreactive ET production in cultured endothelial cells. Solid circle represents basal immunoreactive ET levels in unstimulated endothelial cells. * $p < 0.05$ when compared to basal values (N = 6 per concentration).

2, but had no effect on the delayed cerebral vasospasm observed on day 7. The results suggest that ET-1 may act as a trigger during the early stages of cerebral vasospasm. Similar acute effects were observed following the intracisternal administration of BQ-123, a peptide ET-A receptor antagonist, and the intravenous administration of Ro-46-2005, a nonpeptide ET antagonist, in a rat model of SAH[61,62]. In this model BQ-123 and Ro-46-2005 abolished the reduction in cerebral blood flow observed 60 and 120 min after the intracisternal administration of blood. Another ET-A receptor antagonist, FR139317, was evaluated in the canine chronic model (see above) of delayed cerebral vasospasm[63]. FR13317 was administered intracisternally on days 0, 2, and 4. This antagonist caused a significant reduction in the basilar artery spasm on day 7. More encouraging results were obtained in the canine model of SAH with phosphoramidon, an ET converting enzyme (ECE) inhibitor which prevents the conversion of big-ET to ET-1[64]. Phosphoramidon administered intracisternally on days 0 and 2 reduced the spasm in the basilar artery by approximately 50% on day 7[65]. However, the CSF levels of ET-1 did not differ in the control and phosphoramidon treated dogs on day 7. The results suggest that phosphoramidon may act through and ET-independent mechanism to limit the development of cerebral vasospasm. Perhaps the most impressive results relevent to a potential role of ET in cerebral vasospasm was obtained with actinomycin D, an RNA synthesis inhibitor, in the two-hemorrhage canine model of cerebral vasospasm[66]. Actinomycin D treatment inhibited completely the development of the tenacious basilar vasospasm usually observed on day 7 in this model. The results suggest that some products of protein synthesis, which may include ET, are critical for the development of delayed cerebral vasospasm associated with SAH. Thus, products of protein synthesis, including ET, appear to play a critical role in the development and/or maintenance of delayed cerebral vasospasm.

Mitogenic effects of oxyhemoglobin and ET

The effects of oxyhemoglobin on ET production may also be important in mediating the delayed proliferative lesion in spastic cerebral vessels associated with SAH. In our laboratory, oxyhemoglobin (0.01–100 μM) produced a concentration-dependent increase in vascular smooth muscle cell proliferation in culture (Figure 10.4). The EC_{50} for oxyhemoglobin-mediated mitogenic activity was 0.5 μM and the mitogenic-maximum was 7-fold greater than control.

BQ-123 (1 μM), a selective ET-A receptor antagonist, caused a 65% inhibition of oxyhemoglobin-mediated mitogenesis (Figure 10.5). This was the maximum inhibition and the higher concentrations of BQ-123 did not produce additional inhibition. These data suggest that oxyhemoglobin-elicited mitogenesis is mediated, at least in part, by the stimulation of the ET_A receptors via the generation and liberation of ET-1. Thus, these newly identified properties of oxyhemoglobin suggest that ET may be an important mediator of the proliferative lesion associated with cerebral vasospasm following subarachnoid hemorrhage.

SUMMARY AND CONCLUSION

In summary, the cerebral circulation is extremely sensitive to the vasoactive effects of endothelin (ET). Circulating ET elicits cerebral vasodilation through an interaction

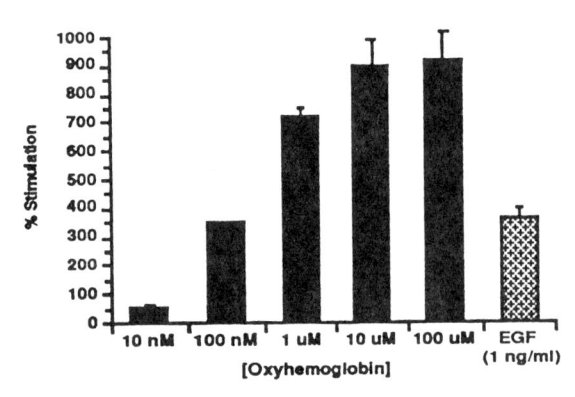

Figure 10.4. Oxyhemoglobin produces concentration-dependent proliferation of rat vascular smooth muscle cells in culture. Epidermal growth factor (EGF) is included as a reference mitogen.

RAT AORTIC VASCULAR SMOOTH MUSCLE

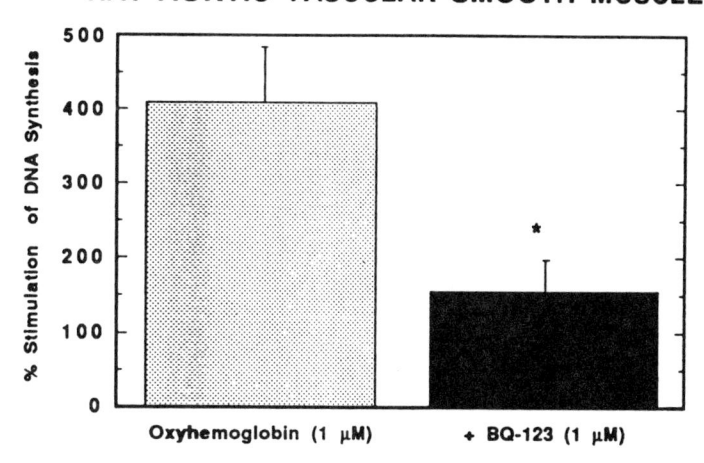

Figure 10.5. BQ-123 (1 µM), an endothelin receptor antagonist, inhibited oxyhemoglobin-mediated proliferation of rat aortic vascular smooth muscle cells in culture. n = 4; * = $p < 0.05$.

with luminal ET-B$_1$ receptors, whereas, subarachnoid ET interacts with abluminal ET-A receptors which mediate prolonged vasoconstriction and ischemia – overriding cerebral blood flow autoregulatory mechanisms. In subarachnoid hemorrhage patients, elevated levels of ET-1 and ET-3 in the CSF appear to correlate with the development of delayed cerebral vasospasm. Under these circumstances, the synthesis and release of ET can be initiated, at least partially, by oxyhemoglobin liberated from the clot. In addition, the mitogenic actions of endothelin, mediated by ET-A receptors, may play a role in the remodelling observed in spastic cerebral vessels. The effects of antagonizing ET mechanisms in models of subarachnoid hemorrhage are still unclear; especially in models of chronic/delayed cerebral vasospasm.

In conclusion, the potent cerebrovascular and mitogenic effects of ET provide compelling evidence for a pathogenic role in cerebrovascular disease, e.g. SAH. However, inhibition of ET action has provided only modest improvement in models of SAH. Thus, further evaluation of novel ET receptor antagonists and/or ECE inhibitors is needed to establish the role of ET in the complex pathologic processes associated with SAH and cerebral ischemia.

Acknowledgements

We would like to thank Dr. Peter Bugelski for the scanning electron microscopy, Mr. Charles Sauermelch for the vascular video microscopy, and Ms. Rose Pimpinella and Ms. Wendy Crowell for their help in preparing this manuscript.

References

1. Yanagisawa, M., Inoue, A., Ishikawa. T., Kasuya, Y. Kimua, S., Kumagaye, S.-I., et al. (1988a) Primary structure, synthesis and biologic activity of rat endothelin, an endothelium-derived vasoconstrictor peptide. *Proc Natl Acad Sci USA*, **85**, 6964–6971.

2. Yanagisawa, M., Kurihara, H., Kimura, S. Tomobe, Y. Kobayashi, M., Mitsui, Y. et al. (1988b) A novel potent vasoconstrictor peptide produced by vascular endothelial cells. *Nature*, **332**, 411–415.
3. MacCumber, M. W., Ross, C. A. and Snyder, S. H. (1990) Endothelin in brain: receptors, mitogensis, and biosynthesis in glial cells. *Proc Natl Acad Sci USA*, **87**, 2359–2363.
4. Gulati, A. and Srimal, R. C. (1992) Endothelin mechanisms in the central nervous system: A target for drug development. *Drug Dev Res*, **26**, 361–387.
5. Fukuda, S., Taga, K. and Shimoji, K. (1991) High sensitivity of porcine cerebral arteries to endothelin. *Experientia*, **47**, 475–477.
6. Vila, J. M. Martin de Aguilera, E., Martinez, M. C. Rodriquez, M. D., Irurzuin, A. and Lluch, S. (1990) Endothelin action on goat cerebral arteries. *J Pharm Pharmacol*, **42**, 370–372.
7. Hardebo, J. E. Kastrom., Owman, C. and Salford, L. G. (1989) Endothelin is a potent constrictor of human intracranial arteries and veins. *Blood Vessels*, **26**, 249–253.
8. Saito, A., Shiba, R., Kimura, S., Yanagisawa, M., Goto, K. and Masaki, T. (1989) Vasoconstrictor response of large cerebral arteries of cats to endothelin, an endothelium-derived vasoactive peptide. *Eur J Pharmacol*, **162**, 353–358.
9. Edwards, R. and Trizna, W. (1990) Response of isolated intracerebral arterioles to endothelins. *Pharmacology*, **41**, 149–152.
10. Faraci, F. M. (1989) Effects of endothelin and vasopressin and cerebral vessels. *Am J Physiol*, **257**, H799–H803.
11. Armstead, W. M. Mirro, R., Leffler, C. W. and Fusija, D. W. (1989) Influence of endothelin on piglet cerebral microcirculation. *Am J Physiol*, **257**, H707–H710.
12. Willette, R. N. and Sauermelch, C. F. (1990) Abluminal effects of endothelin in cerebral microvascular assessed by laser-doppler flowmetry. *Am J Physiol*, **259**, H1688–H1693.
13. Robinson, M. J. and McCulloch, J. (1990) Contractiles response to endothelin in feline cortical vessels *in situ*. *J Cerebral Blood Flow Metab*, **10**, 285–289.
14. Fuxe, K., Cintra, A., Arbjer, B., Anggard, E., Goldstein, M. and Agnati, L. F. (1989) Centrally administered endothelin-1 produces lesions in the brain of the male rat. *Acta Physiol Scand*, **137**, 155–156.
15. Robinson, M. J., Macrae, I. M., Todd, M., Reid, J. L. and McCulloch, J. (1990) Reduction of local cerebral blood flow to pathological levels by endothelin-1 applied to the middle cerebral artery in the rat. *Neurosci Lett*, **118**, 269–272.
16. Fuxe, K., Kurosawa, N., Cintra, A., Hallström, A., Goiny, M., Rosen, L., et al. (1992) Involvement of local ischemia in endothelin-1 induced lesions of the neostriatum of the anesthetized rat. *Exp Brain Res*, **88**, 131–139.
17. Willette, R. N., Sauermelch, C.F., Ezekiel, M., Feuerstein, G. and Ohlstein, E. H. (1990) Effect of endothelin on cortical microvascular perfusion in rats. *Stroke*, **21**, 451–458.
18. Wright, C. E. and Fozzard, J.R. (1988) Regional vasodilation is a prominent feature of the haemodynamic response to endothelin in anesthetized, spontaneously hypertensive rats. *Eur J Pharmacol*, **155**, 201–203.
19. Ohlstein, E. H., Vickery, L., Sauermelch, C. and Willette, R. N. (1990) Vasodilation induced by endothelin: role of EDRF and prostenoids in rat hindquarters. *Am J Physiol*, **259**, H1835–H1841.
20. Polh, U. and Busse, R. (1989) Differential vascular sensitivity to luminally and adventitially applied endothelin-1. *J Cardiovasc Pharmacol*, **13(5)**, S188–S190.
21. Shigeno, T., Mima, T., Takakura, K., Yanagisawa M., Saito, A., Goto K., et al. (1989) Endothelin-1 acts in cerebral arteries from a advential but not from the luminal side. *J Cardiovasc Pharmacol*, **13(5)**, S174–S175.
22. Mima, T., Yanagisawa, M., Shigeno, T., Saito, A., Goto, K., Takakura, K., et al. (1989) Endothelin acts in feline and canine cerebral arteries from the adventitial side. *Stroke*, **20**, 1553–1556.
23. Ogura, K., Takayasu, M. and Dacey, R. G., Jr. (1991) Differential effects of intra- and extraluminal endothelin on cerebral arterioles. *Am J Physiol*, **261**, H531–H537.
24. Yoshimoto, S., Ishizaki, Y., Kurihara, H., Sasaki, T., Yoshizumi M., Yanagisawa, M., et al. (1990) Cerebral microvessel endothelium is producing endothelin. *Brain Res*, **508**, 283–285.
25. Giuffrida, R. and Malatino, L. S. (1992) Endothelin and transient cerebral ischemia: an immunohistochemical study in the mongolian gerbil. *Brain Dysfunct*, **5**, 192–199.
26. Willette, R. N. Ohlstein, E. H., Pullen, M., Sauermelch, C. F., Cohen, A. and Nambi, P. (1993) Transient forebrain ischemia alters acutely endothelin receptor density and immunoreactivity in gerbil brain. *Life Sci*, **52**, 35–40.
27. Arai, H., Hori, S. Aramori, I. Ohkubo, H. and Nakanishi, S. (1990) Cloning and expression of a cDNA encoding an endothelin receptor. *Nature*, **348**, 730–732.
28. Haynes, W. G. and Webb, D. J. (1993) The endothelin family of peptides: local harmones with diverse roles in health and disease? *Clin Sci*, **84**, 585–600.
29. Resink, T. J., Scott-Buden, T. and Buhler, F. R. (1988) Endothelin stimulates phospholipase C in cultured vascular smooth muscle cells. *Biochem Biophys Res Commun*, **157**, 1360–1368.

30. Takuwa, Y., Kasaya, Y., Takuwa, N. et al. (1990) Endothelin receptor is coupled to phospholipase C via a pertussis toxin-insensitive guanine nucleotide-binding regulatory protein in vascular smooth muscle cells. *J Clin Invest*, **85**, 653–658.
31. Griendling, K. K. Tsuda, T. and Alexander, R. W. (1989) Endothelin stimulates diacylglycerol accumulation and activates protein kinase C in cultured vascular smooth muscle cells. *J Biol Chem*, **264**, 8237–8240.
32. Vana Renterghem, C., Vigne, P. Barhanin, J., Schmid-Alliana, A., Frelin, C. and Lazdunski, M. (1988) Molecular mechanism of action of the vasoconstrictor peptide endothelin. *Biochem Biophys Res Commun*, **157**, 977–985.
33. Jansen, L. A., Fallgren, B. and Edvinsson, L. (1989) Mechanism of action of endothelin on isolated feline cerebral arteries: *in vitro* pharmacology and electrophysiology. *J Cereb Flow Metabol*, **9**, 743–748.
34. Salom, J. B., Torregrosa, G., Miranda, F. J., Alabadi, J. A., Alvarez, C. and Alborch, E. (1991) Effects of endothelin-1 on the cerebrovascular bed of the goat. *Eur J Pharmacol*, **192**, 39–45.
35. Warner, T. M., Allcock, G. H., Mickley, E. J., Corder, R. and Vane, J. R. (1993) Comparitive studies with the endothelin receptor antagonists BQ-123 and PD 142893 in indicate at least three endothelin receptors. *J Cardiovas Pharm*, **22 (Suppl 8)** s117–s120.
36. Sakurai, T., Yanagisawa, M. and Masaki, T. (1992) Molecular characterization of endothelin receptors. *Trends Pharmacol Sci*, **13**, 103–106.
37. Karaki, H., Sudjarwo, S. A., Hori, M., Sakata, K., Urade, Y., Takai, M., et al. (1993) ET_B receptor antagonist, IRL 1038, selectivity inhibits the endothelin-induced endothelium-dependent vascular relaxation. *Eur J Pharmacol*, **231**, 371–374.
38. Suzuki, S., Kajikuri, J., Suzuki, A. and Itoh, T. (1991) Effects of endothelin-1 on endothelial cells in the porcine coronary artery. *Circ Res*, **69**, 1361–1368.
39. Gardiner, S. M., Compton, A. M., Kemp, P. A. and Bennett, T. (1990) Regional and cardiac haemodynamic responses to glyceryl trinitrate, acetylcholine, bradykinin and endothelin-1 in conscious rats: effects of N^G-nitro-L-arginine methyl ester. *Br J Pharmacol*, **101**, 632–639.
40. Gardiner, S. M., Compton, A. M., and Bennett, T. (1990) Effects of indomethacin on the regional haemodynamic responses to low doses of endothelins and sarafotoxin. *Br J Pharmacol*, **100**, 158–162.
41. Takayasu, M., Kondo, S. and Terao, S. (1989) Endothelin-induced mobilization of Ca^{2+} and the possible involvement of platelet activating factor and thromboxane A_2. *Biochem Biophys Res Commun*, **160**, 751–757.
42. Asano, T., Ikegaki, L., Suzuki, S. and Shibuya, M. (1989) Endothelin and the production of cerebral vasospasm in dogs. *Biochem Biophys Res. Commun*, **159**, 1345–1351.
43. Ide, K., Yamakawa, K., Nakagomi, T., Sasaki, T., Saito, I., Kurihara, H., et al. (1989) The role of endothelin in the pathogenesis of vasospasm following subarachnoid haemorrhage. *Neurol Res*, **11**, 101–104.
44. Masaoka, H., Suzuki, R., Hitara, Y. et al. (1989) Raised plasma endothelin in aneurysmal subarachnoid haemorrhage. *Lancet* ii, 1402.
45. Suzuki, H., Sato, S., Takekoshi, K., Ishihara, N. and Shimoda, S. (1990) Increased endothelin concentration in CSF from patients with subarachnoid hemorrhage. *Acta Neurol Scand*, **81**, 553–554.
46. Suzuki, H., Sato, S., Suzuki, Y., Oka, M., Tsuchiya, T., Iino, I., et al. (1990) Endothelin immunoreactivity in cerebrospinal fluid of patients with subarachnoid haemorrhage. *Ann Med*, **22**, 233–236.
47. Shinmi, O., Kimura, S., Sawamura, T., Sugita, Y., Yoshizawa, T., Uchiyama, et al. (1989) Endothelin-3 is a novel neuropeptide: isolation and sequence determination of endothelin-1 and endothelin-3 in porcine brain. *Biochem Biophys Res Commun*, **164**, 587–593.
48. Kraus, G. E., Bucholz, R. D., Yook, K.-W., Knuepfer, M. M. and Smith, K. R. (1991) Cerebrospinal endothelin-1 and endothelin-3 levels in normal and neurosurgical patients: a clinial study and literature review. *Surg Neurol*, **35**, 20–29.
49. Ehrenreich, H., Lange, M., Near, K. A., Anneser, F., Schoeller, L. A. C., Schmid, R., et al. (1992) Long term monitoring of immunoreactive endothelin-1 and endothelin-3 in ventricular cerebrospinal fluid, plasma and 24-h urine of patients with subarachnoid hemorrhage. *Res Exp Med*, **192**, 257–268.
50. Yamaji, T., Johshita, H., Ishibashi, M., Takaku, F., Ohno, H., Suzuki, N., et al. (1990) Endothelin family in human plasma and cerebrospinal fluid. *J Clin Endocrinol Metab*, **71**, 1611–1615.
51. Hamann, G., Isenberg, E., Strittmatter, M. and Schimirigk, K. (1993) Absence of elevation of big endothelin in subarachnoid hemorrhage. *Stroke*, **24**, 383–386.
52. Hoffman, A., Keiser, H. R., Grossman, E., Goldstein, D. S., Gold, P. W. and Kling, M. (1989) Endothelin concentrations in cerebrospinal fluid in depressive patients. *Lancet* ii, 1519.
53. Ziv, I., Fleminger, G., Dyaldetti, R., Achiron, A., Melamed. E. and Sokolovsky, M. (1992) Increased plasma endothelin-1 in acute ischemic stroke. *Stroke*, **23**, 1014–1016.
54. Togashi, K., Hirata, Y., Ando, K., Matsunaga, T., Kawakami, M. and Marumo, F. (1990) Abundance of endothelin-3 in human cerebrospinal fluid. *Biochem Res*, **4**, 243–246.

55. Sasaki, T., Kassell, N. F., Colohan, A. R. T. and Nazar, G. B. (1985) Cerebral vasospasm following subarachnoid hemorrhage. In *Cerebrovascular Survey Report for the National Institute of Neurological and Communicative Disorders and Stroke-N.I.H.*, edited by F. H. McDowell and L. R. Caplan, Washington, D. C.: Government Printing Office.
56. Hieda, S. and Gomez-Sanchez, C. E. (1990) Hypoxia increases endothelin release in bovine endothelial cells in culture, but epinephrine, norepinephrine, serotonin, histamine and angiotensin, II, do not. *Life Sci*, **47**, 247–251.
57. Yamashita, K., Kataoka, Y., Niwa, M., Shigematsu, K., Himeno, A., Koizumi, S. *et al.* (1993) Increased production of endothelins in the hippocampus of stroke-prone spontaneously hypertensive rats following transient forebrain ischemia: histochemical evidence. *Cell Mol Neurobiol*, **13**, 15–23.
58. Cocks, T. M., Malta, E., King, E. J., Woods, R. L. and Angus, J. A. (1991) Oxyhemoglobin increases the production of endothelin-1 by endothelial cells in culture. *Eur J Pharmacol*, **196**, 177–182.
59. Ohlstein, E. H. and Storer, B. L. (1992) Oxyhemoglobin stimulation of endothelin production in cultured endothelial cells. *J Neurosurg*, **77**, 274–278.
60. Yamaura, I., Tani, E., Maeda, Y., Minami, N. and Shindo, H. (1992) Endothelin-1 of canine basilar artery in vasospasm. *J Neurosurg*, **76**, 99–105.
61. Clozel, M. and Watanabe, H. (1993) BQ-123, a peptidic endothelin ET (A) receptor antagonist, prevents the early cerebral vasospasm following subarachnoid hemorrhage after intracisternal but not intravenous injection. *Life Sci*, **52**, 825–834.
62. Clozel, M., Breu, V. Burrl, K., Cassal, J. M. Fischll, W., Gray, G. *et al.* (1993) Pathophysiological role of endothelin revealed by the first orally active endothelin receptor antagonist. *Nature*, **365**, 759–761.
63. Nirei, H., Hamada, K., Shoubo, M., Sogabe, K., Notsu, Y. and Ono, T. (1993) An endothelin ET-A receptor antagonist, FR 139317, ameliorates cerebral vasospasm in dogs. *Life Sci*, **52**, 1869–1874.
64. McMahon, E. G., Palomo, M. A. Moore, W. M., McDonald, J. F. and Stern, M.K. (1991) Phosphoramidon blocks the pressor activity of porcine big endothelin- 1-(1-39) *in vivo* and conversion of big endothelin-1-(1-39) to endothelin-1-(1-21) *in vitro*. *Proc Natl Acad Sci USA*, **88**, 703–707.
65. Matsumura, Y., Ikegawa, R., Suzuki, Y, Takaoka, M., Uchida, T., Kido, H., *et al.* (1991) Phosphoramidon prevents cerebral vasospasm following subarachnoid hemorrhage in dogs: the relationship to endothelin-1 levels in the cerebrospinal fluid. *Life Sci*, **49**, 841–848.
66. Shigeno, T., Mima, T., Yanagisawa, M., Saito, A., Goto, K., Yamashita, K. *et al.* (1991) Prevention of cerebral vasospasm by actinomycin D. *J Neurosurg*, **74**, 940–943.

11 The Role of Endothelium and Endothelin in Subarachnoid Hemorrhage

Ryuta Suzuki, Kimiyoshi Hirakawa, and Yukio Hirata*

*Department of Neurosurgery, and *2nd Department of Internal Medicine, Tokyo Medical and Dental University, 1-5-45 Yushima Bunkyo-ku, Tokyo 113, Japan*

BACKGROUND

Subarachnoid hemorrhage accounts for 6-8% of all strokes in North America and 8-10% of all strokes in Japan. Although the mortality from all strokes has declined significantly in recent decades, the incidence of subarachnoid hemorrhage has not changed. The most frequent cause of subarachnoid hemorrhage is rupture of an intracranial aneurysm and accounts for more than 50% of all cases of subarchnoid hemorrhage. Aneurysmal subarachnoid hemorrhage (SAH) is suffered mainly by individuals who are in their prime of life (fifth to seventh decade) and it occurs at the rate of 7–28 cases per 100,000 per year. SAH kills or disables 19,000 individuals in North America[1] or 6300 individuals in Japan per year[2]. Nearly one half of the deaths occur after the initial rupture of the cerebral aneurysm[3]. Therefore, the impact of SAH on public health is significant. It is necessary, therefore, to understand pathophysiology and to establish treatment strategies for SAH.

THE CLINICAL MANIFESTATIONS OF SAH

Only 50 to 75% of patients who survive the initial bleed will be able to resume their previous life style. Even patients who recover suffer from secondary catastrophic changes in the brain and the rest of their body following SAH. Table 11.1 presents the systemic and neurological complications that develop with time after SAH. The pathophysiology of some of the systemic reactions are explained plausibly. It is believed that electrocardiogram changes and cardiac arrhythmias result from increased secretion of catecholamines[4,5]. Neurogenic pulmonary edema may occur as a result of active pulmonary vasoconstriction associated with pulmonary capillary disruption[6]. Hyponatremia is thought to be a cerebral salt wasting syndrome caused by the secretion of natriuretic factors[7]. However, these theories remain to be proven.

Table 11.1 Complications listed according to time interval after SAH

Time after SAH	Neurological complication	Systemic complication
0–3 days	Direct effects of SAH Brain edema Acute hydrocephalus Rebleed Diabetes insipidus	Hypertension Cardiac arrhythmia Respiratory arrest Respiratory irregularity Pulmonary edema Decreased platelet count
4–14 days	Angiographic vasospasm Symptomatic vasospasm (Cerebral ischemia or infarction) Rebleed	Temperature elevation Hyponatremia Blood leukocytosis
> 15 days	Normal pressure hydrocephalus Seizure	Gastrointestinal complications Water imbalance
Whenever		Thromboembolism

Revised from Youmans[9].

Table 11.2. Causes of death and disability in patients with SAH

Cause	Death (%)	Disability (%)	Total (%)
Direct effect of bleed	7.0	3.6	10.6
Vasospasm	7.2	6.3	13.5
Rebleed	6.7	0.8	7.5
Hydrocephalus	0.3	1.4	1.7
Cerebral hemorrhage	1.0	1.0	2.0
Operative complications	1.7	2.3	4.0
Medical complications	0.7	0.1	0.7
Others	1.3	1.1	2.4
Total	26.0	16.3	42.3

Revised from Kassell et al.[8]. Percentage of 3251 hospitalized patients.

Vasospasm is one of the neurological complications which remain to be solved. International cooperative study revealed that vasospasm remains the leading cause of mortality and morbidity in SAH (Table 11.2)[8]. Angiographic vasospasm, (Figure 11.1) defined as focal or diffuse narrowing of the major cerebral arteries, requires several days before it becomes evident. The onset of vasospasm occurs at 4 to 10 days after the onset of SAH and persists for 2 to 3 weeks. Approximately 60% of patients with SAH exhibit such angiographically evident vasospasm. Nearly one half of patients who showed angiographic vasospasms produce permanent or temporary delayed ischemic neurological deficits (DIND) that is also referred to as "symptomatic vasospasm"[1,9]. There is a correlation between the site of major subarachnoid clot and the occurrence and severity of vasospasm. Therefore the occurrence of vasospasm can be predicted by the grading system of an amount of subarachnoid clot as seen by the initial CT scan images according to Fisher et al.[10] (Figure 11.2).

Subarachnoid hemorrhage 169

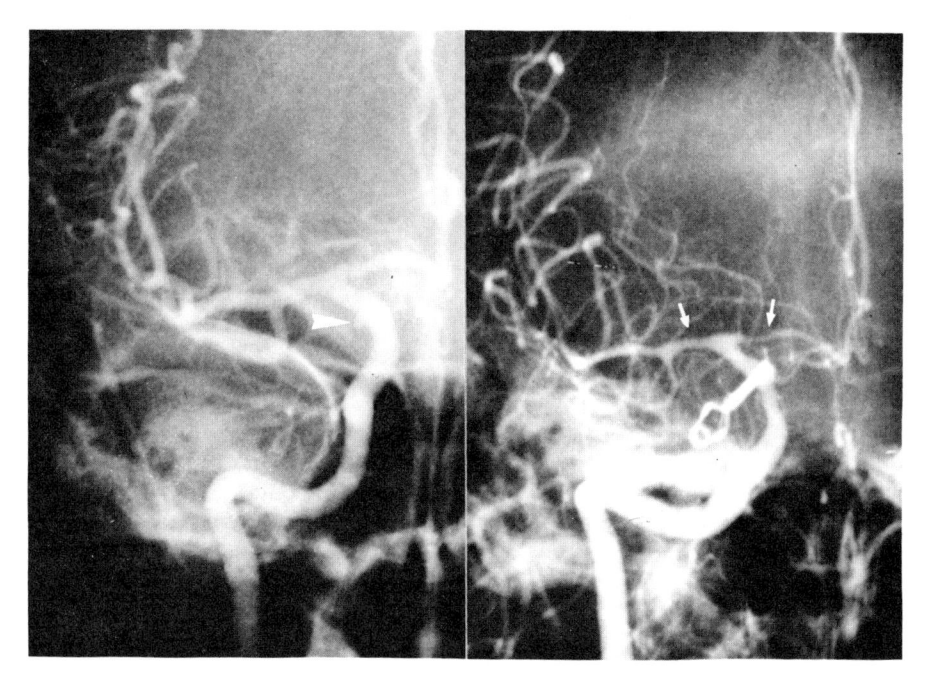

Figure 11.1. Angiographic vasospasm in a patient who showed symptomatic vasospasm. Right internal carotid angiogram obtained one day after the onset of SAH (left) shows an aneurysm in the posterior wall of internal carotid artery (arrow head). No vasospasm was noted. The angiogram obtained on 17 days after the onset of SAH (right) shows severe diffuse narrowing in the first segment of anterior and middle cerebral arteries (arrows). Aneurysm was successfully clipped at day 1 of SAH.

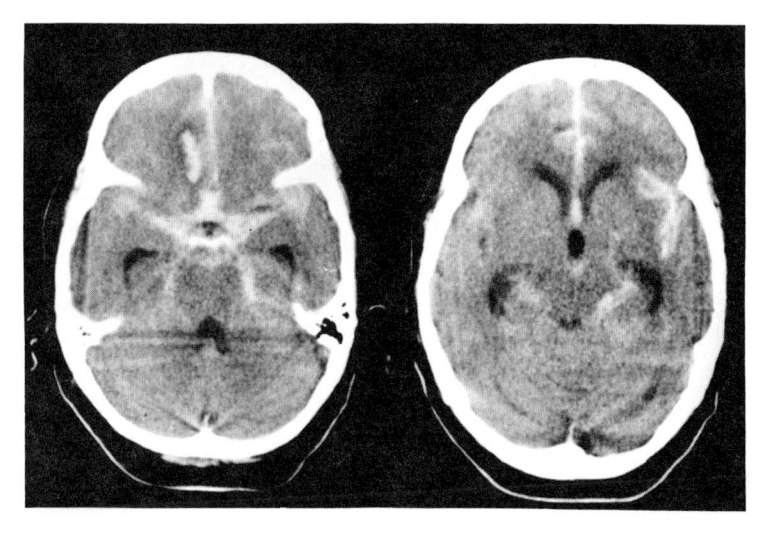

Figure 11.2. CT scan images in a patient with SAH. Note that the amount of subarachnoid clot can be detected on the initial CT scan images.

PATHOGENESIS OF VASOSPASM

Cerebral vasospasm in SAH has several distinctive features: arterial narrowing appears later than 4 days after the onset of SAH, is diffuse in location, is prolonged in duration (lasting 2 weeks or more), and is not relieved by the multitude of vasodilating drugs in human patients[11]. The etiology of arterial narrowing (angiographic vasospasm) has been extensively studied. There is little doubt that the blood in the subarachnoid space is related to the development of vasospasm[1,10,12]. Various blood cells and many spasmogenic substances that are created by the biochemical processes involved in clotting and subsequent lysis of blood have been implicated as the cause of vasospasm. These include epinephrine, norepinephrine, serotonin, oxyhemoglobin, free radicals, and platelet activating factor, and many others[1,11-14]. Numerous attempts at preventing vasospasm have been made using many drugs, including prostaglandins, calcium antagonists, free radical scavengers, and others[15]. Despite these extensive studies, the cause of arterial narrowing remains unclear. Therefore the pathogenesis of cerebral vasospasm is thought to be multifactorial. The possible factors involved may include contraction of cerebral artery smooth muscle cells induced by a putative spasmogen, impairment of vasodilatation, proliferative vasculopathy, and other inflammatory reactions[9].

Recent observations have revealed certain morphological changes in spastic arteries. Spastic arteries are difficult to obtain from humans for study and recent studies vary in their conclusions[16,17]. However, experimental studies consistently reveal endothelial vacuolation, disrupted tight junctions, and fragmentation of the internal elastic lamina on transmission electron microscopy[18,19] (Figure 11.3). Thickening of the intimal layer, smooth muscle cell vacuolation, myonecrosis are also noted frequently[19]. Permeability changes in major cerebral arteries and blood-brain barrier disruptions have also been reported[20-22]. All of these findings suggest that cerebral vasospasm represent not only prolonged functional contraction of the vessels but also coexisting vasculopathy.

The concept of endothelium-dependent vasodilatation was introduced by Furchgott[23] who suggested that the endothelium plays an important role in regulating vascular tone. On the basis of the fact that morphological changes were seen in the endothelium of spastic arteries, studies of the vasodilatory function of the endothelium have been undertaken. Kassell and his group reported that the vasodilatory response to ATP was suppressed in basilar arteries in rabbits sacrificed 2 days after SAH[24]. They postulated that the impairment of endothelium-dependent vasodilatation was due to the inhibition of spontaneously released endothelium-derived relaxing factor (EDRF) by hemoglobin[25,26]. They also found that the spastic basilar artery had an enhanced contractile response to serotonin. Kim et al. performed a series of experiments which proved that in spastic arteries there is no endothelium-dependent relaxation, however, the release of EDRF was maintained in basilar arteries of dogs 8 days after they received two intracisternal blood injections[27,28]. They hypothesized that reduced production of cyclic guanosine monophosphate (cGMP) in smooth muscle cells impairs the responsiveness of smooth muscle cells to EDRF[29]. Edwards et al.[30] showed that cGMP levels are reduced by intraluminal application of hemoglobin *in vitro* to a preparation of a pig cerebral artery. However, they also had some controversial results, that cGMP levels in isolated spastic cerebral arteries in pigs were not reduced

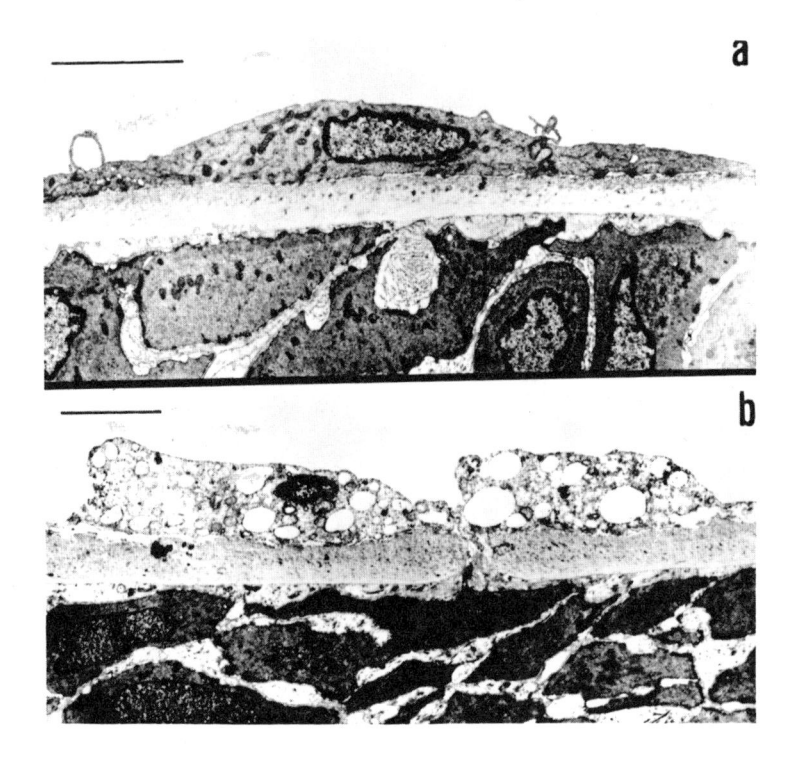

Figure 11.3. Ultrastructural changes of the endothelium of the basilar artery in the rabbit SAH model. a) endothelium in normal rabbit basilar artery. b) endothelium of basilar artery in rabbits 2 days after receiving intracisternal injection of autologous blood. Marked vacuolation, disruption of tight junctions, and fragmentation of the internal elastic lamina are observed.

after *in vivo* exposure to hemoglobin or to whole blood for 2 days. Hatake et al.[31], studied the vasodilatory responses to various drugs by human basilar arteries obtained from SAH patients who died within 1 day of SAH onset. They revealed that endothelium-dependent relaxation responses to thrombin, bradykinin, and calcium ionophore A23187 were impaired, however, the endothelium-independent response to sodium nitroprusside did not differ from the control. Their findings suggested, in contrast to Kim's, that cGMP in the wall of human cerebral arteries is not altered after SAH. Thus their study suggested that decrease in the production of EDRF may reflect the loss of endothelium-dependent relaxation. On the other hand, several reports indicated that the protein kinase C-dependent smooth muscle contraction participated the occurrence of vasospasm[32,33]. They postulated that the sustained contraction of the cerebral arteries may be caused by protein kinase C-dependent smooth muscle contraction other than phosphorylation of 20-kDa myosin light chain in SAH.

Though no definite conclusions have been drawn from these diverse results, considering these data together with our knowledge of endothelin makes it plausible that functional disturbances of endothelium have a significant role in the pathogenesis of arterial narrowing.

ENDOTHELIN AND CEREBRAL VASOSPASM

Since endothelin was first isolated from endothelial cells[34], its potent and long-lasting vasoconstrictor activity implicated it as the candidate substance which causes the cerebral arterial narrowing seen following SAH. Cerebral arteries in various species, including humans, showed dose-dependent vasoconstriction in response to endothelin that occurs only at low concentrations *in vitro*[35-37]. In an *in vivo* study, intracisternal injection of endothelin produced dose-dependent vasoconstriction in dog basilar artery, which lasted for at least 3 days[38]. Mima et al.[39] also found that intracisternal injection of endothelin induced severe prolonged basilar artery constriction in cats and dogs, however, if the endothelin was given in vertebral arteries, no arterial constriction was observed. The findings suggested that vasoconstriction by endothelin was elicited only when endothelin was applied to the outside of vessels. The phenomenon was explained by the presence of the blood-brain barrier (BBB) which is impermeable to endothelin[40]. A recent study, however, revealed that dog coronary artery was constricted by topical application of endothelin, but not by intracoronary administration of endothelin[41]. This study showed that the phenomenon is seen not only in cerebral arteries but also in other arteries. They suggested that intraluminal administration of endothelin stimulates EDRF induction to antagonize vasoconstriction by endothelin. Furthermore, Yamaura et al.[42] found that the level of immunoreactive endothelin-1 is increased significantly in the basilar artery wall of mongrel dogs sacrificed 2 days after the initial intracisternal injection of autologous blood, but was not increased in arteries obtained 7 days after SAH. In addition, they applied topically AwETN40, mouse monoclonal antibody to endothelin-1, to exposed vasospastic basilar arteries. The experiments revealed that application of endothelin antibody relaxed these arteries significantly at 2 days after SAH, though, not much relaxation was seen at 7 days after SAH. Moreover, phosphramidon, an inhibitor of the specific converting enzyme of big endothelin-1, and endothelin ET_A receptor antagonists FR139317 were proven to prevent the occurrence of cerebral vasospasm *in vivo* model[43,44]. Clozel et al. reported that an endothelin ET_A receptor antagonist BQ123 and a novel orally active endothelin receptor antagonist Ro 46-2005 both prevented cerebral vasoconstriction after experimental SAH in rat. However, it is necessary to confirm the late onset of angiographic cerebral vasospasm, they only proved that the drugs had inhibitory effects on the reduction of cerebral blood flow during the first 2 hours following the induction of intrathecal blood in rats[45,46]. Most of the described experiments suggested that endothelin-1 serves some role in the origin of cerebral vasospasm, particulary during the early phase of arterial narrowing.

Endothelin has fascinated many researchers because it may serve a significant role in the physiology of human health and the pathogenesis of many diseases. Several methods of measuring human endothelin and related compounds have been introduced[47-49]. Endothelin-1 and related compounds have been detected in the plasma, cerebrospinal fluid (CSF), and urine of healthy human subjects, suggesting that endothelin is a circulating hormone which regulates vascular tone in man. Our group reported endothelin-1 levels in patients with SAH and recently reported more precisely levels in plasma and CSF of endothelin-1 in patients with SAH[50,51]. Thus, several groups have published endothelin levels in patients with SAH, although the results are controver-

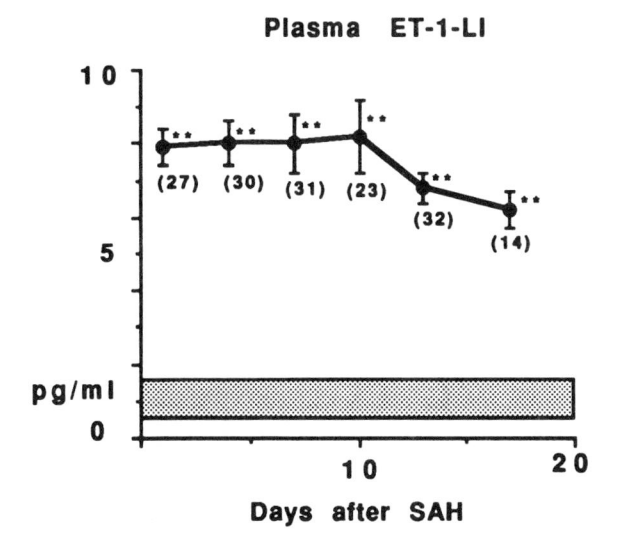

Figure 11.4. Plasma endothelin-1-LI levels in patients with SAH. Plasma endothelin-1 levels were elevated significantly during the whole study period. The shadowed area is normal value (1.1 +/− 0.5 pg/ml). **: p < 0.01 compared to the normal value. Number of patients studied in each period are shown in parenthesis.

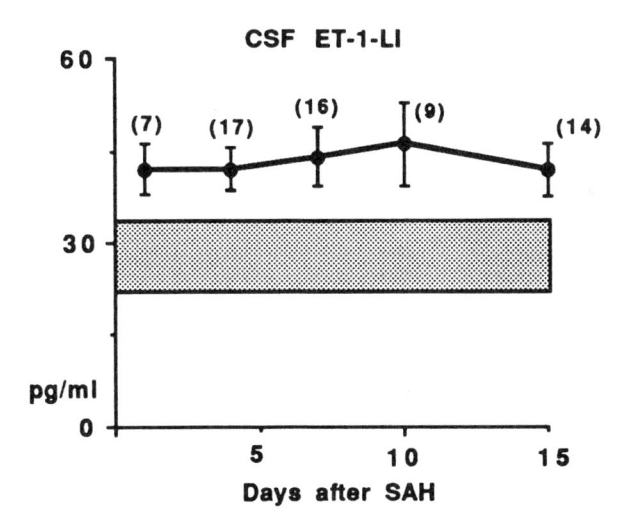

Figure 11.5. CSF endothelin-1-LI levels in 17 patients. CSF endothelin-1 levels were not elevated at any time during the study period. The normal range is 28 +/− 5 pg/ml.

sial. Serial measurement of CSF endothelin-1 levels revealed the highest values to occur several days after SAH coincide with the occurrence of symptomatic vasospasm[52,53]. Others, however, have reported that the CSF endothelin-1 level does not increase at all in SAH[54,55]. Reports of plasma endothelin-1 levels were mostly negative, though

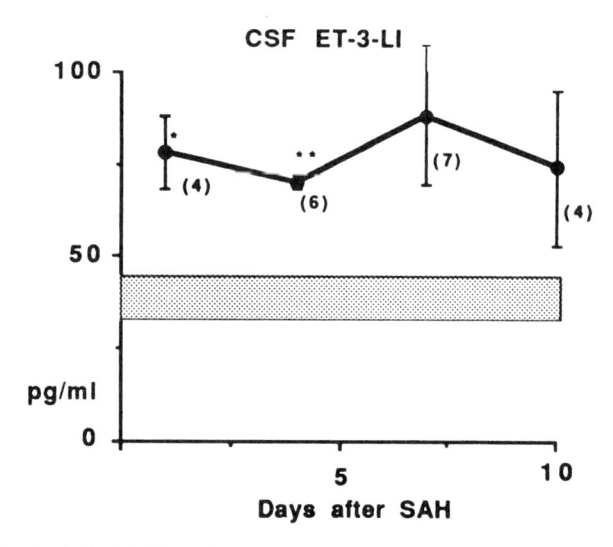

Figure 11.6. CSF endothelin-3-LI levels in 7 patients with SAH are elevated significantly during the first week of the disease, *: $p < 0.05$, **: $p < 0.01$.

Table 11.3

Substances measured	Method	No. of cases
Plasma endothelin-1-LI	RIA[47,58]	36
CSF endothelin-1-LI	RIA[49,57]	17
CSF endothelin-3-LI	RIA[49]	7

LI: like immunoreactivity, RIA: radioimmunoassay, CSF: cerebrospinal fluid.

Fujimori et al.[54] found significantly higher levels of plasma endothelin-1 in patients with vasospasm than in those without vasospasm during the second week of SAH. Humann et al. reported that there was no elevation of big endothelin in plasma and CSF in patients with SAH[56]. However, CSF endothelin-3 levels in patients with SAH were consistently reported to be elevated[53,55].

Our recent data obtained from 36 patients with SAH (Table 11.3) are shown in figure 11.4–8. We used radioimmunoassay (RIA) to measure plasma and CSF endothelin-1[47,57], and endothelin-3 levels[49]. Among 36 patients, 12 sustained delayed ischemic neurological deficits (DIND) due to vasospasm (symptomatic vasospasm).

Plasma endothelin-1-L1 levels were elevated significantly from the onset of SAH for two weeks (Figure 11.4), while, CSF endothelin-1-L1 levels were not elevated during the observation period (Figure 11.5). These results suggest that SAH induces the synthesis of endothelin-1. Endothelin-1 may be secreted from the endothelium in local cerebral vessels into blood stream. Since endothelin-1 does not cross the BBB, CSF endothelin-1 levels remain unchanged. However, this early elevation of plasma endothelin-1 may not cause arterial narrowing. This is because plasma endothelin levels do not reach the

Plasma ET-1-LI

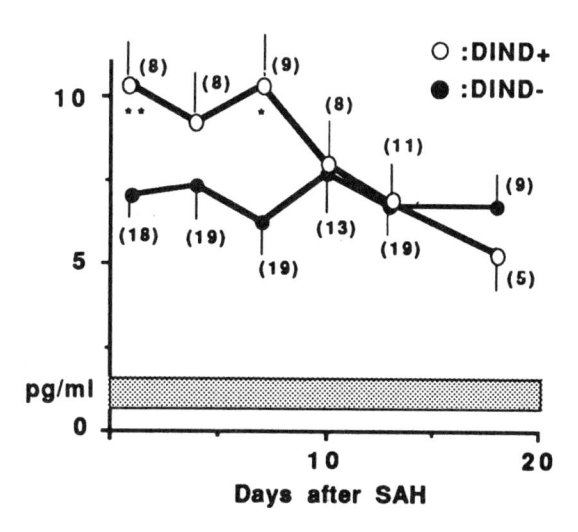

Figure 11.7. Plasma endothelin-1-LI levels in patients with and without DIND. In the former, higher endothelin-1 levels are seen during the first week of disease. *: p < 0.05, **: p < 0.01.

concentrations that produce vasoconstriction. This may explain why endothelin does not produce significant cerebral arterial constriction when applied from the luminal side. Finally, the time courses of vasospasm and elevation of plasma endothelin levels do not coincide.

In contrast to CSF endothelin-1, CSF endothelin-3 levels seem to be elevated during the first week of SAH (Figure 11.6). An elevation of endothelin-3 levels in the CSF can be interpreted as SAH stimulating endothelin-3 synthesis in the neural tissues, or anterior pituitary cells[49,59]. However, the role of endothelin-3 in the pathophysiology of vasospasm remains unclear.

Correlation between the endothelin-1 level and the occurrence of DIND (symptomatic vasospasm) was assessed, and the following results were obtained. The plasma endothelin-1 levels in patients with DIND were significantly higher than in those without DIND during the first week of their disease (Figure 11.7). Thereafter the plasma levels of endothelin-1 were decreased. The occurrence of DIND correlated well with the amount of subarachnoid clot (Figure 11.2)[10], and it was proven that plasma levels of endothelin-1 are higher in patients with thick subarachnoid clot than in patients with thin subarachnoid clot[51]. According to these facts, early elevation of plasma endothelin-1 in patients with DIND may only reflect the amount of subarachnoid clot. On the other hand, changes in CSF endothelin-1 levels explain more plausibly the occurrence of DIND. During the first few days CSF endothelin-1 levels were within normal range in both patient groups, though, CSF endothelin-1 levels in patients with DIND gradually increased during the second week (Figure 11.8). However, CSF endothelin-1 levels in patients without DIND remain within normal range throughout the observation period. There are two manners in which elevation of

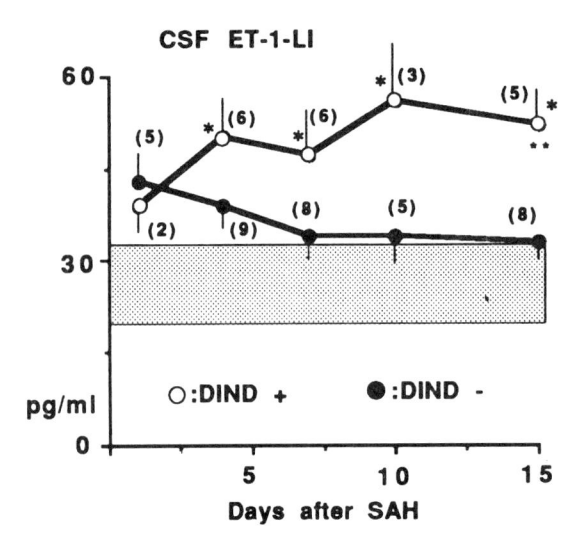

Figure 11.8. CSF endothelin-1-LI levels in patients with and without DIND. In the early periods, both were within normal range. Then, for two weeks after SAH, CSF endothelin-1 increased gradually in patients with DIND **: p < 0.01, compared between the two groups. *: p < 0.01, compared to the normal value.

CSF endothelin-1 may be delayed. First of all, endothelin-1 expression may be induced in brain tissue or in smooth muscle cells by unknown stimulants that occur several days after the onset of SAH. The other possibility is that the permeability of the BBB has increased to endothelin-1, which is continuously secreted from vascular endothelial cells, as the result of endothelial injury. After integrating the facts obtained so far, the latter explanation seems more plausible. However, the concentration of CSF endothelin-1 in patients with DIND did not reach the vasoconstrictive level. Endothelin can act through autocrine action to constrict cerebral vessels locally, although, the mechanism may not be so simple. Other factors may participate to enhance vasoconstriction by endothelin.

CURRENT CONCEPT OF THE OCCURRENCE OF VASOSPASM

Many biological reactions occur after the initiation of SAH. There have been discovered a number of substances thought to participate in the progression of the disease. Table 11.4. comprises a list of the main substances which may serve an important role in vasospasm and have an effect on endothelium or endothelin.

We can conclude that red blood cells in the subarachnoid space are essential for causing cerebral vasospasm following aneurysmal SAH and that endothelial injury which serves a key role in causing vasospasm, does certainly occur but requires several days to become complete. On the basis of these idea, we hypothesize the following concept (Figure 11.9).

Oxyhemoglobin has been postulated to be the most potent trigger of vasospasm[65]. Oxyhemoglobin releases superoxide anions when it is autoxidized to methemoglobin.

Table 11.4 Interactions of the substances with endothelium

Substance	Origin	Interaction with endothelium
Thrombin	Subarachnoid clost	Stimulate ET induction
Hemoglobin	Subarachnoid clot	Inhibit EDRF induction
Oxyhemoglobin	Hemoglobin	Inhibit EDRF induction
		Stimulate ET induction
Superoxide anion	Oxyhemoglobin	Endothelial injury
	Inflammatory cells	Inactive EDRF
		Induce peroxinitrite
Cytokines	Leukocyte	Stimulate ET induction
Endothelin-1	Endothelium	Stimulate EDRF induction
Endothelin-3	Neural tissue?	?
Nitric oxide	Endothelium	Cellular injury
		Inhibit ET induction

ET: endothelin, EDRF: endothelium-derived relaxing factor[60-64].

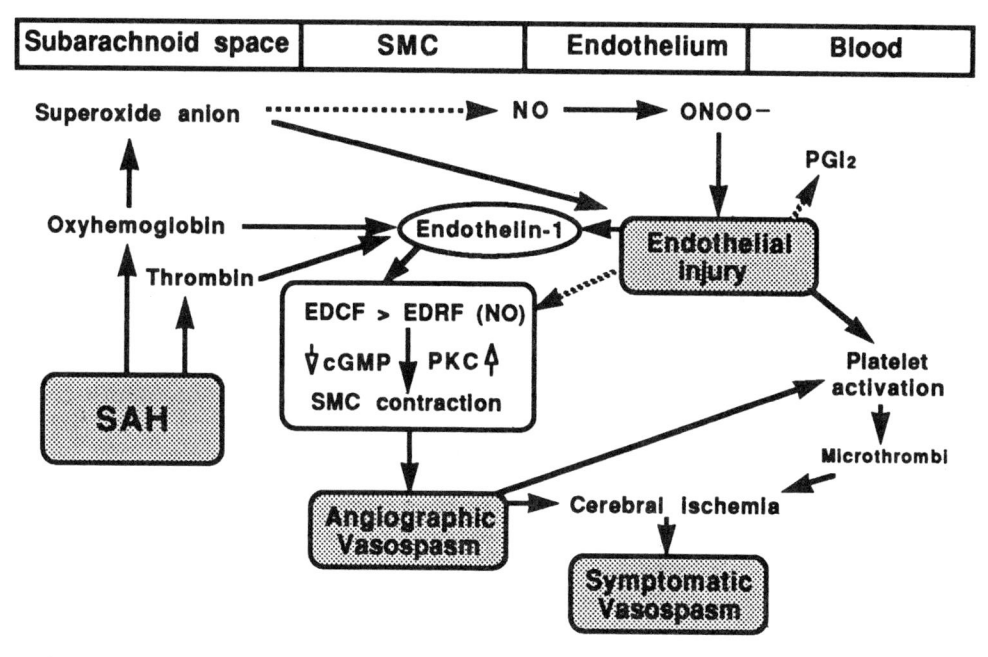

Figure 11.9. Schematic representation of the biological reactions relating angiographic vasospasm (arterial narrowinng), and symptomatic vasospasm (delayed ischemic neuroligical deficit; DIND). Arrows with solid line; promoting effect, with dotted line; inhibitory effect.

A superoxide anion generates more active free radicals that may then initiate the chain reaction of lipid peroxidation in the arterial wall[66,67] it also interacts with nitric oxide to induce peroxynitrite which may induce endothelial injury[60,68]. These reactions caused an inactivation of EDRF[69,70]. Simultaneously endothelin induction is stimulated by an excess amount of thrombin, shear stress, and tissue hypoxia due to endothelial injury[34,71-73]. As a results of these reactions cause an imbalance between EDRF and endothelium-derived contracting factor (EDCF, endothelin). After endothelial injury, endothelin can reach the smooth muscle cells in the arterial wall through the pathologically permeable BBB and inhibition of EDFR enhances endothelin-mediated contraction[74]. Then, cerebral arteries contracted, namely angiographic vasospasm occur. The parallel progression of endothelial injury and arterial narrowing activates platelet aggregation[75], and decreases prostacyclin (PGI2) production in the arterial wall[76]. Inactivation of nitric oxide and PGI2 in the endothelium may enhance platelet adhesion in the arterial wall[77], resulting in cerebral microthrombi formation. Subsequently, focal ischemic neurological deficits, namely symptomatic vasospasm, develop. In severe cases, the neurological deficit become permanent as proliferative angiopathy may have developed. However, in cases with good recovery, the subarachnoid clot resolves over the time and the endothelial injury is repaired. Then the spastic artery recovers its normal function as the vasoconstriction remits.

THE ROLE OF ENDOTHELIN IN SAH

As reviewed in Table 11.1, various systemic complications other than vasospasm are seen following SAH. It is understandable that intracranial disasters cause significant reactions throughout the body. However, the means by which these systemic reactions occur are not clearly understood. Recently many new bioactive substances have been identified, including endothelin, cytokines, and natriuretic peptides. Our data which show that plasma endothelin levels are elevated in patients with SAH suggests that endothelin works not only to regulate vascular tone, but also acts as a paracrine hormone to mediate intracranial signals to the heart, kidney, endocrine organs, and other vital organs. We have summarized in Table 11.5 the possible role of endothelin in systemic complications of SAH. As we learn the vascular regulatory function of endothelium, we understand further the pathophysiology of this disastrous disease. However, the goal stands a little further.

Table 11.5 The possible role of endothelin in systemic complications of SAH

Complications	Role of Endothelin
Circulation	Enhances release of catecholamine[78]
Hypertension	Potentiates the action of norepinephrine and
Arrhythmia	serotonin[79]
Hyponatremia	Stimulates release of atrial natriuretic peptide[80]
Water imbalance	Stimulates vasopressin secretion[81]
Pulmonary edema	Augments pulmonary hypertension[82]

References

1. Kassell, N. F., Sasaki, T., Colohan, A. R. T, Nazar, G. (1985) Cerebral vasospasm following aneurysmal subarachnoid hemorrhage. *Stroke*, **16**, 562–572.
2. Kiyohara, Y., Kazuo, U., Hasuo, Y., Wada, J., Kawano, H., Kato, I., Shinkawa, A., Ohmura, T., Iwamoto, H., Omae, T., Fujishima M. (1989) Incidence and prognosis of subarachnoid hemorrhage in a Japanese rural community. *Stroke*, **20**, 1150–1155.
3. Whisnant, J., Sacco, S., O'Fallon, M., Fode, N., Sundt, T. M. Jr. (1993) Referral bias in aneurysmal subarachnoid hemorrhage. *J Neurosurg*, **78**, 726–732.
4. Estanol, B., Marin, O. (1975) Cardial arrhythmias and sudden death in subarachnoid hemorrhage. *Stroke*, **6**, 382–386.
5. Oppenheimer, S., Cechetto, D., Hachinski V. (1990) Cerebrogenic cardiac arrhythmias. *Arch Neurol*, **47**, 513–519.
6. Garcia-Uria, J., Hoff, J., Miranda, S., Nishimura, M. (1981) Experimental neurogenic pulmonary edema. Part 2: The role of cardiopulmonary pressure change. *J Neurosurg*, **54**, 632–636.
7. Nelson, B., Seif, S., Gutai, J., Robinson, A. (1984) Hyponatremia with natriuresis following subarachnoid hemorrhage in a monkey model. *J Neurosurg*, **60**, 233–237.
8. Kassell, N. F., Torner, J. C., Haley, E. C., Jane, J. A., Adams, H. P., Kongable, G. L. (1990) The international co-operative study on the timing of aneurysm surgery. Part I, Overall management results. *J Neurosurg*, **73**, 18–36.
9. Youmans, J. (1990) Neurological Surgery (Third edition). ed. J. Youmans. Vol. 3. Philadelphia, WB. Saunders Company.
10. Fisher, C. M., Kistler, J. P., Davis, J. M. (1980) Relation of cerebral vasospasm to subarachnoid hemorrhage visualized by computed tomographic scanning. *Neurosurgery*, **6**, 1–9.
11. Wilkins, R. H. (1988) Cerebral vasospasm. *Comptemp Neurosurg*, **10**, 1–6.
12. Duff, T. A., Louie, J., Feilbach, J. A., Scott, G. (1988) Erythrocytes are essential for development of cerebral vasculopathy resulting fron subarachnoid hemorrfhage in cats. *Stroke*, **19**, 68–72.
13. Asano, T., Tanishima, T., Sasaki, T., Sano, K. (1980) Possible participation of free radical reactions initiated by clot lysis in the pathogenesis of vasospasm after subarachnoid hemorrhage. In: *Cerebral Arterial Spasm*, R. H. Wilkins, Editor, pp. 190–201. Baltimore, Williams & Wilkins Co.
14. Hirashima, Y., Endo, S., Otsuji, T., Karasawa, K., Nojima, S., Takaku, A. (1993) Platelet-activating factor and cerebral vasospasm following subarachnoid hemorrhage. *J Neurosurg*, **78**, 592–597.
15. Wilkins, R. H. (1986) Attempts at prevention or treatment of intracranial arterial spasm, and update. *Neurosurgery*, **18**, 808–825.
16. Eldevik, O., Kristiansen, K., Torvik, A. (1981) Subarachnoid hemorrhage and cerebrovascular spasm. Morphological study of intracranial arteries based on animal experiments and human autopsies. *J Neurosurg*, **55**, 869–876.
17. Smith, R. R, Clower, B. R, Peeler, D. F, Yoshioka J. (1983) The angiography of subarachnoid hemorrhage, angiographic and morophologic correlates. *Stroke*, **14**, 240–245.
18. Findlay, J. M., Weir, B. K. A., Kanamaru, K., Espinosa F. (1989) Arterial wall changes in cerebral vasospasm. *Neurosurgery*, **25**, 736–746.
19. Tanabe, Y., Sakata, K., Yamada, H., Ito, T., Takada, M. (1978) Cerebral vasospasm and ultrastructual changes in cerebral arterial wall. *J Neurosurg*, **49**, 229–238.
20. Germano, A., d'Avella, D., Cicciarello, R., Hayes, R., Tomasello, F. (1992) Blood-brain barrier permeability changes after experimental subarachnoid hemorrhage. *Neurosurgery*, **30**, 882–886.
21. Ohta, T., Satoh, G., Kuroiwa, T. (1992) The premeability changes of major cerebral arteries in experimental vasospasm. *Neurosurgery*, **30**, 331–336.
22. Sasaki, T., Kassell, N. F., Zuccarello, M., Nakagomi, T., Fujiwara, S., Colohan, A. R. T., Lehman, R. M. (1986) Barrier disruption in the major cerebral arteries in the acute stage after experimental subarachnoid hemorrhage. *Neurosurgery*, **19**, 177–184.
23. Furchgott, R. F., Zawadzki, J. V. (1980) The obilgatory role of endothelial cells in the relaxation of arterial smooth muscle by acetylcholine. *Nature*, **288**, 373–376.
24. Nakagomi, T., Kassell, N. F, Sasaki, T. Fujiwara, S. Lehman, R. M. Johshita, H. *et al.* (1987) Effects of subarachnoid hemorrhage on endothelium-dependent vasodilation. *J Neurosurg*, **66**, 915–923.
25. Fujiwara, S., Kassell, N., Sasaki, T., Nakagomi, T., Lehman, R. M. (1986) Selective hemoglobin inhibition of endothelium-dependent vasodilation of rabbit basilar artery. *J Neurosurg*, **64**, 445–452.
26. Hongo, K., Kassell, N. F., Nakagomi, T., Sasako, T., Tsukahara, T., Ogawa, H., Vollmer, D., Lehman, R. M. (1988) Subarachonoid hemorrhage inhibition of endothelium-derived relaxing factor in rabbit basilar artery. *J Neurosurg*, **69**, 247–253.
27. Kim, P., Sundt, T. M. Jr, Vanhoutte, P. M. (1988) Alterations in endothelium-dependent responsiveness of the canine basilar artery after subarachnoid hemorrhage. *J Neurosurg*, **69**, 239–246.

28. Kim, P., Lorenz, R. R., Sundt, T. M. J., Vanhoutte, P. M. (1989) Release of endothelium-derived relaxing factor after subarachnoid hemorrhage. *J Neurosurg*, 70, 108–114.
29. Kim, P., Schini, V., Sundt, T. M. Jr, Vanhoutte, P. M. (1992) Reduced production of cyclic GMP explains the loss of endothelium-dependent relaxations in the canine basilar artery after subarachnoid hemorrhage. *Circ Res*, 70, 248–256.
30. Edwards, D. H., Byrne, J. V., Griffith, T. M. (1992) The effect of chronic subarachnoid hemorrhage on basal endothelium-derived relaxing factor activity in intrathecal cerebral arteries. *J Neurosurg*, 76, 830–837.
31. Hatake, K., Wakabayashi, I., Kakishita, E., Hishida, S. (1992) Impairment of endothelium-dependent relaxation in human basilar artery after subarachnoid hemorrhage. *Stroke*, 23, 1111–1117.
32. Matui, T., Takuwa, Y., Johshita, H., Yamashita, K., Asano, T. (1991) Possible role of protein kinase C-dependent smooth muscle contraction in the pathogenesis of chronic cerebral vasospasm. *J Cereb Blood Flow Metab*, 11, 143–149.
33. Takuwa, Y., Matui, T., Abe, Y., Nagafuji, T., Yamashita, K., Asano, T. (1993) Alterations in protein kinase C activity and membrane lipid metabolism in cerebral vasospasm after subarachnoid hemorrhage. *J Cereb Blood Flow Metab*, 13, 409–415.
34. Yanagisawa, M., Kurihara H., Kimura, S., Tomobe, Y., Kobayashi, M., Mitsui, Y., et al. (1988) A novel potent vasoconstrictor peptide produced by vascular endothelial cells. *Nature*, 332, 411–415.
35. De Aguilera, E. M., Iruruzun, A., Vila, J. M., Aldasoro, M., Galeote, M. S., Lluch, S. (1990) Role of endothelium and calcium channels in endothelin-induced contraction of human cerebral arteries. *Br J Pharmacol*, 99, 439–440.
36. Papadopoulos, S., Gilbert, L., Webb, R., D'Amato, C. (1990) Characterization of contractile responses to endothelin in human cerebral arteries: implications for cerebral vasospasm. *Neurosurgery*, 26, 810–815.
37. Saito, A., Shiba, R., Kimura, S., Yanagisawa, M. Goto, K. Masaki, T. (1989) Vasoconstrictor response of large cerebral arteries of cats to endothelin, and endothelium-derived vasoactive peptide. *Eur J Pharmacol*, 162, 353–358.
38. Asano, T., Ikegaki, I., Suzuki, Y., Satoh, S., Shibuya, M. (1989) Endothelin and the production of cerebral vasospasm in dogs. *Biochem Biophys Res Commun*, 159, 1345–1351.
39. Mima, T., Yanagisawa, M., Shigeno, T., Saito, A., Goto, K., Takakura, K., Masaki, T. (1989) Endothelin acts in feline and canine cerebral arteries from the adventitial side. *Stroke*, 20, 1553–1556.
40. Koseki, C., Imai, M., Hirata, Y., Yanagisawa, M., Masaki, T. (1989) Autoradiographic distribution in rat tissues of binding sites for endothelin: a neuropeptide? *Am J Physiol*, 256, R858–R866.
41. Lamping, K. G., Clothier, J. L., Eastham, C. L., Marcus, M. L. (1992) Coronary microvascular response to endothelin is dependent on vessel diameter and route of administration. *Am J Physiol*, 263, H703–H709.
42. Yamaura, I., Tani, E., Maeda, Y., Minami, N., Shindo, H. (1992) Endothelin-1 of canine basilar artery in vasospasm. *J Neurosurg*, 76, 99–105.
43. Matsumura, Y., Ikegawa, R., Suzuki, Y., Takaoka, M., Uchida, T., Kido, H., et al. (1991) Phos- phoramidon prevents cerebral vasospasm following subarachonoid hemorrhage in dogs: The relationship to endothelin-1 levels in the cerebrospinal fluid. *Life Science*, 49, 841–848.
44. Nirei, H., Hamada, K., Shoubo, N., Sogabe, K., Notsu, Y., Ono, T. (1993) An endothelin ETA receptor antagonist, FR139317, ameliorates cerebral vasospasm in dogs. *Life Science*, 52, 1869–1874.
45. Clozel, M., Breu, V., Burri, K., Casal, J., Fischli, W., Gray, G., et al. (1993) Pathophysiological role of endothelin revealed by the first orally active endothelin receptor antagonist. *Nature*, 365, 759–761.
46. Clozel, M., Watanabe, H. (1993) BQ 123, a peptidic endothelin ETA receptor antagonist, prevents the early cerebral vasospasam following subarachnoid hemorrhage after intracisternal but not intravenous injection. *Life Science*, 52, 825–834.
47. Ando, K., Hirata, Y., Shichiri, M., Emori, T., Marumo, F. (1989) Presence of immunoreactive endothelin in human plasma. *FEBS Lett*, 245, 164–166.
48. Suzuki, N., Matsumoto, H., Kitada, C., Masaki, T., Fujino, M. (1989) A sensitive sandwich-enzyme immunoassay for human endothelin. *J Immunol Meth*, 118, 245–250.
49. Togashi, K., Hirata, Y., Ando, K., Matsunaga, T., Kawakami, M., Marumo, F. (1990) Abundance of endothelin-3 in human cerebrospinal fluid. *Biomed Res*, 11, 243–246.
50. Masaoka, H., Suzuki, R., Hirata, Y., Emori, T., Marumo, F., Hirakawa, K. (1989) Raised plasma endothelin in aneurysmal subarachnoid hemorrhage. *Lancet*, 334, 1402.
51. Suzuki, R., Masaoka, H., Hirata, Y., Marumo, F., Isotani, E., Hirakawa, K. (1992) The role of endothelin-1 in the origin of cerebral vasospasm in patients with aneurysmal subarachnoid hemorrhage. *J Neurosurgl*, 77, 96–100.
52. Suzuki, H., Sato, S., Suzuki, Y. Takekoshi, K. Ishihara, N., Shimoda, S. (1990) Increased endothelin concentration in CSF from patients with subarachnoid hemorrhage. *Acta Neurol Scand*, 81, 553–554.
53. Ehrenreich, H., Lange, M., Near, K., Anneser, F., Schoeller, L., Schmid, R., et al. (1992) Longterm

monitoring of immunoreactive endothelin-1 and endothelin-3 in ventricular cerebrospinal fluid, plasma, and 24-h urine of patients with subarachnoid hemorrhage. *Res Exp Med (Berl)*, **192**, 257–268.
54. Fujimori, A., Yanagisawa, M., Saito, A., Goto, K. Masaki, T., Mima, T. (1990) Endothelin in plasma and cerebrospinal fluid of patients with subarachnoid hemorrhage. *Lancet*, **336**, 633.
55. Kraus, G. E., Bucholz, R. D., Yoon, K., Knuepfer, M. M., Smith, K. R. (1991) Cerebrospinal fluid endothelin-1 and endothelin-3 levels in normal and neurosurgical patients, a clinical study and literature review. *Surg Neurol*, **35**, 20–29.
56. Hamann, G., Isenberg, E., Strittmatter, M., Schimrigk, K. (1993) Abscence of elevation of big endothelin in subarachnoid hemorrhage. *Stroke*, **24**, 383–386.
57. Hirata, Y., Matsunaga, T., Ando, K., Furukawa, H. Tsukagoshi, H., Marumo, F. (1990) Presence of endothelin-like immunoactivity in human cerebrospinal fluid. *Biochem Biophys Res Commun*, **166**, 1274–1278.
58. Ando, K., Hirata, Y., Takei, Y., Kawakami, M., Marumo, F. (1991) Endothelin-1-Like immunoreactivity in human urine. *Nephron*, **57**, 36–39.
59. Matsumoto, H., Suzuki, N., Onda, H., Fujino, M. (1989) Abundance of endothelin-3 in rat intestine, pituitary gland and brain. *Biochem Biophys Res Commun*, **164**, 74–80.
60. Beckman, J. S. Beckman, T. W., Chen, J., Marshell, P. S., Freeman, B. S. (1990) Apparent hydroxyl radical production by peroxynitrite: implications for endothelial injury from nitric oxide and superoxide. *Proc Natl Acad Sci USA*, **87**, 1620–1624.
61. Mathiesen, T., Andersson, B., Loftenius, A., Holst, H. (1993) Increased interleukin-6 levels in cerebrospinal fluid following subarachnoid hemorrhage. *J Neurosurg*, **78**, 562–567.
62. Ohlstein, E. H., Storer, B. L. (1992) Oxyhemoglobin stimulation of endothelin production in cultured endothelial cells. *J Neurosurg*, **77**, 274–278.
63. Peterson, J. W., Kwun, B.-D., Hackett, J. D., Zervas, N. T. (1990) The role of inflammation in experimental cerebral vasospasm. *J Neurosurg*, **72**, 767–774.
64. Yoshizumi, M., Kurihara, H., Morita, T., Yamashita, T. Oh-hashi, Y., Sugiyama, T. et al. (1990) Interleukin 1 increases the production of endothelin-1 by cultured endothelial cells. *Biochem Biophys Res Commun*, **166**, 324–329.
65. Macdonald, R. L., Weir, B. K. A. (1991) A review of hemoglobin and the pathogenesis of cerebral vasospasm. *Stroke*, **22**, 971–982.
66. Sasaki, T., Asano, T., Sano, K. (1980) Cerebral vasospasm and free radical reactions. *Neurol Med Chir (Tokyo)*, **20**, 145–153.
67. Shishido, T., Suzuki, R., Qian, L., Hirakawa, K. (1994) The role of superoxide anions in the pathogenesis of cerebral vasospasm. *Stroke*, **25**, 864–868.
68. Rubanyi, G. M., Vanhoutte, P. M. (1986). Oxygen-derived free radicals, endothelium, and respon- siveness of vascular smooth muscle. *Am J Physiol*, **250**, H815–H821.
69. Gryglewski, R. J., Palmer, R. M. J., Moncada, S. (1986) Superoxide anion is involved in the breakdown of endothelium-derived vascular relaxing factor. *Nature*, **320**, 454–456.
70. Rubanyi, G. M., Vanhoutte, P. M. (1986) Superoxide anions and hyperoxia inactivate endothelium-derived relaxing factor. *Am J Physiol*, **250**, H822–H827.
71. Yoshizumi, M., Kurihara, H., Sugiyama, T., Takaku, F., Yanagisawa, M., Masaki, T., Yazaki, Y. (1989) Hemodynamic shear stimulates endothelin production by cultured endothelial cells. *Biochem Biophys Res Commun*, **161**, 1859–864.
72. Kourembana, S., Marsden, P. A., McQuillan, L. P., Faller, D. V. (1991) Hypoxia induces endothelin gene expression and secretion in cultured human endothelium, *J Clin Invest*, **88**, 1054–1057.
73. Lerman, A., Bernett, J. C. Jr (1992) Intact and altered endothelium in regulation of vasomotion. *Circulation*, **86** (Suppl III), 12–19.
74. Lerman, A., Sandok, E., Hildebrand, F. J., Burnett, J. C. Jr. (1992) Inhibition of endothelium derived relaxing factor enhances endothelin-mediated vasoconstriction. *Circulation*, **85**, 1894–1898.
75. Ohkuma, H., Suzuki, S., Kimura, M., Sobata, E. (1991) Role of platelet function in symptomatic cerebral vasospasm following aneurysmal subarachnoid hemorrhage. *Stroke*, **22**, 854–859.
76. Sasaki, T., Murota, S., Wakai, S., Asano, T. Sano, K. (1981) Evaluation of prostaglandin biosynthetic activity in canine basilar artery following subarachnoid injection of blood. *J Neurosurg*, **55**, 771–778.
77. Radomski, M. W., Palmer, R. M. J., Moncada, S. (1987) Endogenous nitric oxide inhibits human platelet adhesion to vascular endothelium. *Lancet*, **2**, 1057–1058.
78. Takeuchi, A., Kimura, T., Satoh, S. (1992) Enhancement by endothelin-1 of the release of catecholamines from the canine adrenal gland in response to splanchnic nerve stimulation. *Clin Exp Pharmacol Physiol*, **19**, 663–666.
79. Yang, Z. H., Richard, V., von Segesser, L., Bauer, E., Stulz, P., Turina, M., Luscher, T. F. (1990) Threshold concentration of endothelin-1 potentiate contractions to norepinephrine and serotomin in human arteries. A new mechanism of vasospasm. *Circulation*, **82**, 188–195.

80. Kohno, M., Muruakawa, K., Horio, T., Kurihara, N., Yokokawa, K., Yasunari, K., *et al.* (1990) Endothelin stimulates release of arterial natriuretic factor in anesthetized rats. *Metabolism*, **391**, 557–559.
81. Shichiri, M., Hirata, Y., Kanno, K. (1989) Effect of endothelin-1 on release of arginin-vasopressin from perfused rat hypothalamus. *Biochem Biophys Res. Commun*, **163**: 1332–1337.
82. Luscher, T. F. (1992) Endothelin: systemic arterial and pulmonary effects of a new peptide with potent biologic properties. *Am Rev Respir Dis*, **146**, S56–S60.

12 Neurological and Psychiatric Aspects of Endothelin Research

Toshihiro Yoshizawa and *Ichiro Kanazawa

Department of Neurology, Institute of Clinical Medicine, University of Tsukuba, Tsukuba City, 305, Japan

*Department of Neurology, Institute of Brain Research, Faculty of Medicine, University of Tokyo, Tokyo, 113, Japan

INTRODUCTION

Endothelin-1 (ET-1) is a 21-amino acid vasoconstrictor peptide, originally isolated from vascular endothelium[1]. Biological activity of ET-1 is not confined to vascular constriction. Recent studies indicated that ET-1 has a wide spectrum of pharmacological effects including the effects on the central nervous system (CNS)[2]. Screening of genomic DNA library disclosed the presence of other isoforms of endothelin, i.e., endothelin-2 (ET-2) and endothelin-3 (ET-3)[3]. Northern blot analysis showed the different patterns of tissue expression of these endothelin isopeptides[4]. In addition, different classes of endothelin receptors were recently identified and were present in various tissues including the CNS, which corresponded with the former studies of endothelin binding[5]. All of these data suggest the essential role of endothelin in the CNS as well as in other tissues.

In this chapter, I briefly summarize the basic aspect of endothelin research in the CNS and review the studies directed to elucidating the relationships between endothelin and the CNS diseases.

ENDOTHELIN IN THE CENTRAL NERVOUS SYSTEM

Pharmacological effects of endothelin on the spinal cord neurons

Although ET-1 was first isolated from vascular endothelium and was characterized as a vasoconstrictor peptide, we thought that ET-1 would have any function in the CNS since a variety of neuropeptides have physiological roles both in the CNS and the peripheral tissues. Therefore, in 1988, we started to investigate the direct action of ET-1 on the spinal neurons with an *in vitro* spinal cord preparation of the newborn rat[6]. As a result, we found that bath-applied ET-1 produced a ventral root depolarization. The ET-1-induced ventral root depolarization was dose-dependent and was depressed by the dihydropyridine sensitive Ca^{2+} channel blocker, nicardipine or the substance P antagonist, spantide. ET-2 and ET-3 produced similar ventral root depolarization. These results suggested that ET-1 may act directly on the spinal neurons and cause substance P release probably through the activation of dihydropyridine-sensitive Ca^{2+} channels[7].

Presence of endothelin in the spinal cord

Because ET-1 was proved to have a direct action on the spinal cord neurons, we tried to isolate endothelin isopeptides from the porcine spinal cord with high performance liquid chromatography (HPLC) and radioimmunoassay (RIA) with antisera raised against endothelin-related peptides. Both ET-1 and ET-3 were detected based on their chromatographic retention times and characteristics of immunoreactivities to the antisera. The concentrations of immunoreactive ET-1 and immunoreactive ET-3 were estimated to be 0.120 pmol/g tissue and 0.009 pmol/g tissue, respectively. From the peak of immunoreactive ET-1, we isolated a single peptide by successive HPLC and RIA, which was identified as ET-1 itself by a gas phase sequencer.

Next, we investigated the porcine spinal cord immunohistochemically to elucidate the localization of ET-1. We found ET-1-like immunoreactivity in motoneurons, dorsal horn neurons and dot- and fiber-like structures in the dorsal horn as well as in the endothelium of spinal cord vessels[7,8]. Giaid et al. also examined the human spinal cord by in situ hybridization and found the presence of ET-1 mRNA in motoneurons, dorsal horn neurons and in the neurons of dorsal root ganglia[9], which confirmed our data in the porcine spinal cord. The presence of ET-1 mRNA and ET-1-like immunoreactivity in the spinal neurons indicated the actual production of ET-1 in neurons.

Presence of endothelin in the brain

We also isolated both ET-1 and ET-3 from porcine brain by HPLC and RIA[10]. The concentrations of immunoreactive ET-1 and immunoreactive ET-3 were 0.140 pmol/g tissue and 0.005 pmol/g tissue. We could not detect any ET-2-like immunoreactivity in the homogenate of porcine brains.

A general immunohistochemical survey for endothelin in rat and porcine CNS revealed that endothelin-like immunoreactivity was most prominent in the paraventricular and supraoptic nuclear neurons and their terminals in the posterior pituitary. Chemical identification of endothelin in porcine hypothalamus by HPLC and RIA indicated the presence of ET-1. Moreover, in situ hybridization demonstrated ET-1 mRNA in porcine paraventricular nuclear neurons. In the rat, endothelin-like immunoreactivity in posterior pituitary was depleted by water deprivation, suggesting a release of endothelin under physiological conditions[11]. These data indicated that ET-1 is produced by porcine hypothalamic neurons and is released from their terminals and suggested that ET-1 may involve the neurosecretory functions.

We also found weak endothelin-like immunoreactivities in neurons of porcine hippocampus and Purkinje cells in cerebellum[12]. Giaid et al. also demonstrated the wide distribution of endothelin mRNA and peptide immunoreactivity in neurons of the human brain[13]. They found that many neurons were labelled by *in situ* hybridization with cRNA probes specific to ET-1, ET-2 or ET-3. Especially, the labelled neurons were distributed in lamina III-IV of cerebral cortex, hypothalamic nuclei, caudate nucleus, amygdala, hippocampus, basal nucleus of Meynert, substantia nigra, raphe nuclei and Purkinje cell layer of the cerebellum. Immunoreactive neurons to endothelin were reported to the fewer than neurons labelled by *in situ* hybridization. However, the distribution of the neurons with ET-like immunoreactivity was similar to that of endothelin mRNA. A similar result was reported by Lee *et al.* in which the expression of ET-1 mRNA in the human brain was examined[14].

The prominent expression of endothelin in the hypothalamus may suggest a role of endothelin in the neurosecretory function or the central vasoregulatory control. On the other hand, the widespread distribution of endothelin may imply the fundamental role in regulating the neuronal functions. Several reports also described the production of endothelin and its mRNA by cultured astroglial cells[15,16]. These data suggest that the physiological roles of endothelin may not only be related to the neuronal functions, but also to the astroglial functions.

Presence of endothelin in cerebrospinal fluid

A number of neuropeptides exist in cerebrospinal fluid (CSF) and change their content under various states of neurological diseases. Previous studies indicated the production of endothelin in the CNS and suggested a role of endothelin as a novel neuropeptide. Therefore, it is reasonable to imagine that endothelin exists in CSF. The presence of immunoreactive ET-1 and ET-3 in CSF has been shown by several reports[17-23]. The mean concentration of ET-1 in CSF in control subjects varied with the assay system. Our data showed that the mean ET-1 concentration in CSF in control subjects was 0.194 pg/ml which was lower than that in plasma[23].

Endothelin receptors in the central nervous system

Several autoradiographic studies with [^{125}I]ET-1 disclosed the widespread distribution of the binding sites for ET-1 in the CNS[24-27]. Especially, high densities were found in hippocampus, cerebellum, brain stem, choroid plexus and subfornical organ. Subcellular fractionation of whole rat brain showed the enrichment of ET-1 binding sites in the synaptosomal fraction[28]. Because these reported binding sites for ET-1 were not similar to the distribution of vasculature, the specific receptors for endothelin in the CNS seems to be related to the neuronal functions.

The binding sites for endothelin were also found in the endothelial cells from brain microvessels[29] and glial cells[16,30-34]. Physiological roles of endothelin in glial cell functions have not been unclear. However, a few data suggested the trophic effects of endothelin on glial cells[15,33,34].

Recently, cDNAs encoding two classes of endothelin receptor (ET_A and ET_B) were cloned[35,36]. Both of these classes of receptors were reported to be expressed in the brain. The functions of these receptors in the brain should be elucidated in future.

Other pharmacological effects and possible physiological role of endothelin in the central nervous system

Several lines of the pharmacological effects of endothelin in the CNS have been reported, which suggested the physiological roles of endothelin in the CNS. These studies are mainly classified as follows: (1) central cardiovascular control (2) neurosecretory effects. These subjects will be reviewed in other chapters of this book. Therefore, we do not deal with these subjects in this chapter.

POSSIBLE RELATIONSHIP BETWEEN ENDOTHELIN AND NEUROPSYCHIATRIC DISEASES

Cerebrospinal fluid endothelin-1 in Alzheimer's disease and senile dementia of Alzheimer type

Alzheimer's disease (AD) and senile dementia of Alzheimer type (SDAT) are neurodegenerative disorders characterized by progressive dementia which occur in middle and late life. Neuropathological and neurochemical analysis disclosed the degeneration of cerebral cortical neurons and several neurotransmitter systems including neuropeptides which may be involved in the pathogenesis of dementia. Alterations in neurotransmitter markers or neuropeptides in CSF were also reported, which may reflect the degenerations of specific neuronal systems in CNS. However, there is no information for an alteration in the CSF ET-1 level or the CNS ET-1 system in AD and SDAT. Therefore, we determined CSF ET-1 concentrations in patients with AD and SDAT compared with those of disease control[23].

Eleven patients with Alzheimer type dementia (ATD) and seven patients of disease control without dementia admitted were included in this study. All patients diagnosed as ATD met NINCDS/ADRDA diagnostic criteria for probable Alzheimer's disease[37]. ATD patients were divided into the following two groups according to the age of onset: (1) Alzheimer's disease (AD) group; 5 patients (5 women) whose onsets were before the age of 65 years. Mean age of patients ± standard deviation (SD) was 64 ± 8.2. (2) senile dementia of Alzheimer type (SDAT) group; 6 patients (1 man and 5 women) whose onsets were after the age of 65 years. Mean age ± SD was 77.5 ± 4.7. Disease control (DC) group included 7 non-demented patients whose mean age ± SD was 58.9 ± 9.5. The mean age in AD group was not significantly different from that in DC group. However, the mean age in SDAT group was higher than that in DC and AD group ($p < 0.05$, unpaired t test).

CSF samples were obtained by lumbar puncture around noon. Blood samples were obtained from 4 AD patients and 6 SDAT patients before lumbar puncture. Each sample was collected in a polypropylene tube containing 300 KIU/ml of aprotinin and 2 mg/dl of EDTA. After centrifugation at 1000 × g for 10 minutes, supernatant of CSF or plasma was stored at $-80°C$ until assayed.

CSF and plasma ET-1 concentrations were determined with sandwich-enzyme immunoassay (sandwich-EIA) for human ET-1[38]. A value of ET-1 in each group was given as mean ± SD. Statistical analysis was performed using a 2-tailed unpaired Student's t test. Correlation coefficient was calculated by the data analysis software of Stat View II.

The CSF ET-1 concentrations in DC, AD and SDAT were 0.194 ± 0.026 pg/ml (range, 0.15 to 0.22 pg/ml), 0.142 ± 0.030 pg/ml (range, 0.09 to 0.17 pg/ml) and 0.198 ± 0.087 pg/ml (range, 0.12 to 0.31 pg/ml), respectively. The CSF ET-1 level was significantly lower in AD group than in DC group ($p < 0.05$). However, the CSF ET-1 level in SDAT group was not significantly different from that in DC or AD group.

Concerning the correlation coefficients between the CSF ET-1 levels and various factors (age, duration from onset, systolic blood pressure, CSF protein level, plasma ET-1 level), none of these factors had significant correlations with CSF ET-1 levels in AD or SDAT group ($p < 0.05$). On the other hand, in DC group, only the age of patient was negatively correlated with the CSF ET-1 level ($p < 0.05$) (correlation coefficient: -0.928).

Because the age distribution in AD group is not significantly different from that in DC group, it is possible to suppose that the lower level of CSF ET-1 level was not correlated with the plasma ET-1 level in AD or SDAT, it is unlikely that CSF ET-1 is derived from plasma ET-1. There is rather a possibility that CSF ET-1 could be derived from the CNS neurons and could reflect the condition of the CNS ET-1 system. In AD, extensive degeneration of cortical and hypothalamic neurons which was reported to express ET-1 mRNA was recognized. The lower level of CSF ET-1 in AD group may reflect the degeneration of these neurons.

In contrast to AD group, the CSF ET-1 level in SDAT group was not significantly different from that in DC group. Since we could not collect data from disease control patients whose ages were matched with that of SDAT patients, the present data in DC group was not always adequate to the statistical analysis in DC and SDAT groups. In consideration of each level of CSF ET-1 in SDAT group, 4 out of 6 indicated the lower levels than that in DC group. However, 2 out of 6 in SDAT group showed higher levels in CSF ET-1. These two patients were bed-ridden for more than two years. From these relevant informations, other factors might influence the CSF ET-1 levels in these patients.

Plasma endothelin-1 levels during upright tilt in patients with multiple system atrophy presenting orthostatic hypotension

Shichiri et al. reported that the plasma ET-1 concentration increased with upright posture and decreased with volume expansion in healthy volunteers[39]. There results raised the possibility that ET-1 is a circulating hormone involved in the control of arterial blood pressure.

Kaufmann et al. examined the plasma levels of ET-1 during upright tilt in healthy subjects and in the patients with multiple system atrophy who showed the impairment of baroreceptor reflex[40]. They found that the arterial blood pressure did not change and the plasma ET-1 significantly increased during upright tilt in normal subjects. In patients with multiple system atrophy, although the arterial blood pressure fell considerably during tilt, plasma ET-1 remained unchanged. From these results, they considered that the increase in plasma ET-1 induced by upright tilt is mediated by baroreceptor reflex. The failure in increase of ET-1 during upright posture in patients with multiple system atrophy is probably due to the impairment of baroreceptor reflex. The source of increased ET-1 may be the release from posterior pituitary because the patients with diabetes inspidus did not show the increase in ET-1 during upright tilt.

The contribution of the lack of increase in plasma ET-1 during upright tilt to orthostatic hypotension in patients with multiple system atrophy was not clear at present. Since baroreceptor-mediated vasopressin release in normal subjects is important for the postural control of arterial blood pressure, baroreceptor-mediated ET-1 release may also be important for the maintenance of arterial blood pressure during postural change.

Plasma and cerebrospinal endothelin in cerebral vasospasm following subarachnoid hemorrhage

Subarachnoid hemorrhage (SAH) often induces the severe cerebral vasospasm which affects the prognosis of patients suffered from SAH. Although the pathophysiology of cerebral vasospasm following SAH has not been fully elucidated, endothelin isopeptides which produce potent and long-term vasoconstriction are supposed to be important causal factors of vasospasm after SAH. Mima et al. reported that intracisternally administered ET-1 produced the long-lasting basilar artery contraction in cats and dogs. On the other hand, infusion of ET-1 into the vertebral artery had no effect on basilar artery caliber[41]. De novo synthesis of ET-1 in endothelial cells may be induced by SAH and may produce the vasospasm.

In fact, Suzuki et al. reported the raised concentration of CSF ET-1 in patients with SAH[20]. The highest concentration was observed within 4 to 6 days after the attack of SAH. Kraus et al. reported the increase in CSF ET-3 concentration in patients with SAH[22]. These data partly support the hypothesis in which endothelin isopeptides produce delayed vasospasm after the attack of SAH.

However, Fujimori et al. did not observe the significant correlation between CSF ET-1 and vasospasm after SAH[18]. Hamann et al. reported that there were no elevations of big ET-1 in plasma and CSF obtained from patients with acute SAH[42]. They did not observe the significant differences of big ET-1 between patients with and without vasospasm.

From the above results, we cannot conclude that CSF ET-1 increases after SAH and directly contributes to the production of delayed vasospasm. The vasospasm after SAH is probably seen as a multifactorial development. Since a recent study showed that an intracisternally administered ET_A receptor antagonist prevents the early cerebral vasospasm following experimental SAH in rats, ET-1 may be one of the causal factor of delayed vasospasm after SAH[43].

Acute ischemic stroke and endothelin

Ziv et al. measured the plasma levels of ET-1 and ET-3 in patients with acute ischemic stroke (cerebral infarction) within the first 72 hours after the onset and found a marked elevation in plasma ET-1 levels in the patients compared with those in the control subjects[44]. According to their report, plasma ET-1 levels in the patients with more severe neurological impairment tended to be higher than the levels in the patients with milder impairment. However, plasma ET-3 levels were below the detection threshold of the assay in all subjects. They discussed the possibility that the ischemic insult may induce the production and release of ET-1 from injured endothelial cells of the involved cerebral microvessels. In fact, the increasing density of ET-1 immunoreactivity in the ischemic area was recognized by Giuffrida et al. in Mongolian gerbils after the occlusion of the common carotid artery of one side[45]. The denser ET-1 immunoreactivity in the area of neuronal degeneration compared with that in the surrounding area was also recognized twelve hours after the reopening of common carotid artery. These data possibly suggest that the ischemia-induced ET-1 production in the ischemic area may cause the elevation of plasma ET-1 levels and the constriction of collateral vessels which may contribute to the worsening of neurological deficits. The drugs which modify the ischemia-induced ET-1 production or the ET-1 induced vasoconstriction would be beneficial in breaking the vicious circle.

Cerebrospinal fluid endothelin-1 in depressive patients

Hoffman et al. reported that the depressive patients had significantly lower CSF concentrations of ET-1 compared with healthy volunteers[17]. According to their report, the mean concentration of CSF ET-1 in control subjects was 8.0 pg/ml. This value was higher than that reported by other groups[21,23]. Therefore, we cannot simply compare this result with the data obtained by other groups. However, the lower concentration of CSF ET-1 could reflect the disease status in depression.

Glioma and endothelin

Kurihara et al. first demonstrated a single class of high-affinity binding sites for [^{125}I]ET-1 in surgical specimens of human astrocytoma and glioblastoma[46]. Although low numbers of [^{125}I]ET-1 binding sites were detected in the gray matter of normal human cortex, relatively high numbers of [^{125}I]ET-1 binding sites were present in the tissue sections derived from glioma. Several studies demonstrated that ET-1 induced intracellular calcium rise and inositol 1,4,5-triphosphate formation in cultured glioma cells[30]. In conjunction with the data showing the production of ET-1 and its mRNA in cultured glial cells[15,16], ET-1 may act on glial cells autologously and may promote the glial growth which may be related to the increase of the human glioma.

FUTURE ASPECTS OF ENDOTHELIN RESEARCH IN NEURO-PSYCHIATRIC DISORDERS

In this chapter, we summarize the possible relationship between endothelin and the human CNS disease. Previous studies suggest a role of endothelin as a neuropeptide which may be functioning in the specific neuronal system such as in the posterior pituitary system. Recent reports suggest that endothelin may have more broad and fundamental functions in cells other than neurons, for example, vascular endothelium of cerebral vessels and glial cells. In future, antagonists for endothelin receptors may be useful tools for elucidating the pathophysiology of the human CNS disease and may become a novel class of therapeutic drugs.

References

1. Yanagisawa, M., Kurihara, H., Kimura, S., Tomobe, Y., Kobayashi, M., Mitsui, Y., et al. (1988) Endothelin: a novel potent vasoconstrictor peptide produced by vascular endothelial cells. *Nature*, **332**, 411–415.
2. Masaki, T., Yanagisawa, M. and Goto, K. (1992) Physiology and Pharmacology of endothelins. *Med. Res. Rev.*, **12**, 391–421.
3. Inoue, A., Yanagisawa, M., Kimura, S., Kasuya, Y., Miyauchi, T., Goto, K., et al. (1989) The human endothelin family: Three structurally and pharmacologically distinct isopeptides predicted by three separate genes. *Proc. Natl. Acad. Sci. USA*, **86**, 2863–2867.
4. Goto, K., Sakurao, T. and Kasuya, Y. (1992) Molecular pharmacology of endothelin in the cardiovascular system. *Nippon Yakurigaku Zasshi*, **100**, 205–218.
5. Sakurai, T., Yanagisawa, M. and Masaki, T. (1992) Molecular characterization of endothelin receptors. *Trends. Pharmacol. Sci.*, **13**, 103–108.
6. Yoshizawa, T., Kimura, S., Kanazawa, I., Yanagisawa, M. and Masaki, T. (1989) Endothelin-1 depolarizes a ventral root potential in the newborn rat spinal cord. *J. Cardiovasc. Pharmacol.*, **13 (Suppl 5)**, S216–S217.
7. Yoshizawa, T., Kimura, S., Kanazawa, I., Uchiyama, Y., Yanagisawa, M. and Masaki, T. (1989) Endothelin localizes in the dorsal horn and acts on the spinal neurones: possible involvement of dihydropyridine-sensitive calcium channels and substance P release. *Neurosci. Lett.*, **102**, 179–184.
8. Shinmi, O., Kimura, S., Yoshizawa, T., Sawamura, T., Uchiyama, Y., Sugita, Y., et al. (1989) Presence of endothelin-1 in porcine spinal cord: isolation and sequence determination. *Biochem. Biophys. Res. Commun.*, **162**, 340–346.
9. Giaid, A., Gibson, S. J., Ibrahim, N. B. N., Legon, S., Bloom, S. R., Yanagisawa, M., et al. (1989) Endothelin-1, and endothelium-derived peptide, is expressed in neurons of the human spinal cord and dorsal root ganglia. *Proc. Natl. Acad. Sci. USA*, **86**, 7634–7638.
10. Shinni, O., Kimura, S., Sawamura, T., Sugita, Y., Yoshizawa, T., Uchiyama, Y., et al. (1989) Endothelin-3 is a novel neuropeptide: isolation and sequence determination of endothelin-1 and endothelin-3 in porcine brain. *Biochem. Biophys. Res. Commun.*, **164**, 587–593.
11. Yoshizawa, T., Shinmi, O., Giaid, A., Yanagisawa, M., Gibson, S. J., Kimura, S., et al. (1990) Endothelin: a novel peptide in the posterior pituitary system. *Science*, **247**, 462–464.
12. Kanazawa, I., Yoshizawa, T. and Masaki, T. (1991) Localization of endothelin in the posterior pituitary system. In *New Trends in Autonomic Nervous System Research*, edited by M. Yoshikawa, pp. 423–425. Amsterdam: Elsevier Science Publishers B.V.
13. Giaid, A., Gibson, S. J., Herrero, M. T., Gentleman, S., Legon, S., Yanagisawa, M., et al. (1991) Topographical localization of endothelin mRNA and peptide immunoreactivity in neurones of the human brain. *Histochemistry*, **95**, 303–314.
14. Lee, M.-E., de la Monte, S. M., Ng, S.-H., Bloch, K. D. and Quertermous, T. (1990) Expression of the potent vasoconstrictor endothelin in the human central nervous system. *J. Clin. Invest.*, **86**, 141–147.
15. MacCumber, M. W., Ross, C. A. and Snyder, S. H. (1990) Endothelin in brain: receptors, mitogenesis and biosynthesis in glial cells. *Proc. Natl. Acad. Sci. USA*, **87**, 2359–2363.
16. Ehrenreich, H., Kehrl, J. H., Anderson, R. W., Rieckmann, P., Vitkovic, L., Coligan, J. E., et al. (1991) A vasoactive peptide, endothelin-3, is produced by and specifically binds to primary astrocytes. *Brain Res.*, **538**, 54–58.
17. Hoffman, A., Keiser, H. R., Grossman, E., Goldstein, D. S., Gold, P. W. and Kling, M. (1989) Endothelin concentrations in cerebrospinal fluid in depressive patients. *Lancet*, **2**, 1519.
18. Fujimori, A., Yanagisawa, M., Saito, A. Goto, K., Masaki, T., Mima, T., et al. (1990) Endothelin in plasma and cerebrospinal fluid of patients with subarachnoid haemorrhage. *Lancet*, **336**, 633.
19. Hirata, Y., Matsunaga, T., Audo, K., Furukawa, T., Tsukagoshi, H. and Marumo, F. (1990) Presence of endothelin-1-like immunoreactivity in human cerebrospinal fluid. *Biochem. Biophys. Res. Commun.*, **166**, 1274–1278.
20. Suzuki, H., Sato, S., Suzuki, Y., Takekoshi, K., Ishihira, N. and Shimoda, S. (1990) Increased endothelin concentration in CSF from patients with subarachnoid hemorrhage. *Acta Neurol. Scand.*, **81**, 553–554.
21. Yamaji, T., Johshita, H., Ishibashi, M., Takaku, F., Ohno, H., Suzuki, N., Matsumoto, H. and Fujino, M. (1990). Endothelin family in human plasma and cerebrospinal fluid. *J. Clin. Endoclinol. Metab.*, **71**, 1611–1615.
22. Kraus, G. E., Bucholz, R. D., Yoon, K. W., Knuepfer, M. M. and Smith, . R. Jr. (1991) Cerebrospinal fluid endothelin-1 and endothelin-3 levels in normal and neurosurgical patients: a clinical study and literature review. *Surgical Neurology*, **35**, 20–29.
23. Yoshizawa, T., Iwamoto, H., Mizusawa, H., Suzuki, H., Matsumoto, H. and Kanazawa, I. (1992)

Cerebrospinal fluid endothelin-1 in Alzheimer's disease and senile dementia of Alzheimer type. *Neuropeptides*, **22**, 85–88.
24. Koseki, C., Imai, M., Hirata, Y., Yanagisawa, M. and Masaki, T. (1989) Autoradiographic distribution in rat tissues of binding sites for endothelin: a neuropeptide? *Am. J Physiol.* 256, R858–866.
25. Jones, C. R., Hiley, C. R., Pelton, J. T. and Mohr, M. (1989) Autoradiographic visualization of the binding sites for [^{125}I]endothelin in rat and human brain. *Neurosci. Lett.*, **97**, 276–279.
26. Kohzuki, M., Chai, S. Y., Paxinos, G., Karavas, A., Casley, D. J., Johnston, C. I., et al. (1991) Localization and characterization of endothelin receptor binding sites in the rat brain visualized by *in vitro* autoradiography. *Neuroscience*, **42**, 245–260.
27. Niwa, M., Kawaguchi, T., Fujimoto, M., Kataoka, Y. and Taniyama, K. (1991) Receptors of endothelin in the central nervous system. *J. Cardiovasc. Pharmacol.*, **17 (Suppl. 7)**, S173–S179.
28. Bolger, G. T., Berry, R. and Jaramillo, J. (1992) Regional and subcellular distribution of [^{125}I]endothelin binding sites in rat brain. *Brain. Res. Bull.*, **28**, 789–797.
29. Vigne, P., Ladoux, A. and Frelin, C. (1991) Endothelin activates Na + /H + exchange in brain capillary endothelial cells via a high affinity endothelin-3 receptor that is not coupled to phospholipase. *J. Biol. Chem.*, **266**, 5925–5928.
30. Marsault, R., Vigue, P., Breittmayer, J. P. and Frelin, C. (1990) Astrocytes are target cells for endothelins and sarafotoxin. *J. Neurochem.*, **54**, 2142–2144.
31. Hosli, E. and Hosli, L. (1991) Autoradiographic evidence for endothelin receptors on astrocytes in cultures of rat cerebellum, brainstem and spinal cord. *Neurosci. Lett.*, **129**, 55–58.
32. Hosli, L., Hosli, E., Lefkovitgs, M. and Wagner, S. Electrophysiological evidence for existence of receptors for endothelin and vasopressin on cultured astrocytes of rat spinal cord and brainstem. *Neurosci. Lett.*, **131**, 193–195.
33. Hama, H., Sakurai, T., Kasuya, Y., Fujiki, M., Masaki, T. and Goto, K. (1993) Action of endothelin-1 on rat astrocytes through the ET$_B$ receptor. *Biochem. Biophys. Res. Commun.*, **186**, 355–362.
34. Levin, E. R., Frank, H.J. and Pedram, A. (1992) Endothelin receptors on cultured fetal rat diencephalic glia. *J. Neurochem.*, **58**, 659–666.
35. Arai, H., Hori, S., Aramori, I., Ohkubo, H. and Nakanishi, S. (1990) Cloning and expression of a cDNA encoding an endothelin receptor. *Nature*, **348**, 730–732.
36. Sakurai, T., Yangisawa, M., Takuwa, Y., Miyazaki, H., Kimura, S., Goto, K. et al. (1990) Cloning of a cDNA encoding a non-isopeptide-selective subtype of the endothelin receptor. *Nature*, **348**, 732–735.
37. Mckhann, G., Drachman, D., Flostein, M., Katzman, R., Price, D. and Stadlan, M. (1984) Clinical diagnosis of Alzheimer's disease: report of the NINCDS-ADRDA work group under the auspices of department of health and human services task force on Alzheimer's disease. *Neurology*, **34**, 939–944.
38. Suzuki, N., Matsumoto, H., Kitada, C., Masaki, T. and Fujino, M. (1989) A sensitive sandwich-enzyme immunoassay for human endothelin. *J. Immunol. Methods*, **118**, 245–250.
39. Shichiri, M., Hirata, Y., Ando, K., Kanno, K., Emori, T., Ohta, K., et al. (1990) Postural change and volume expansion affect plasma endothelin levels. *JAMA*, **263**, 661.
40. Kaufmann, H., Oribe, E. and Oliver, J. A. (1991) Plasma endothelin during upright tilt: relevance for orthostatic hypotension? *Lancet*, **338**, 1542–1545.
41. Mima, T., Yanagisawa, M., Shigeno, T., Saito, A., Goto, K., Takakura, K., et al. (1989) Endothelin acts in feline and canine cerebral arteries from the adventitial side. *Stroke*, **20**, 1553–1556.
42. Hamann, G., Isenberg, E., Strittmatter, M. and Schimrigk, K. (1993) Absence of elevation of big endothelin in subarachnoid hemorrhage. *Stroke*, **24**, 383–386.
43. Clozel, M. and Watanabe, H. (1992) BQ-123, a peptidic endothelin ET$_A$ receptor antagonist, prevents the early cerebral vasospasm following subarachnoid hemorrhage after intracisternal but not intravenous injection. *Life Sci.*, **52**, 825–834.
44. Ziv, I., Fleminger, G., Djaldetti, R., Aciron, A., Melamed, E. and Sokolovsky, M. (1992) Increased plasma endothelin-1 in acute ischemic stroke. *Stroke*, **23**, 1014–1016.
45. Giuffrida, R., Bellomo, M., Polizzi, G. and Malatino, L. S. (1992) Ischemia-induced change in the immunoreactivity for endothelin and other vasoactive peptides in the brain of the Mongolian gerbil. *J. Cardiovasc. Pharmacol.*, **Suppl. 12**, S41–S44.
46. Kurihara, M., Ochi, A., Kawaguchi, T., Niwa, M., Kataoka, Y. and Mori, K. (1990) Localization and characterization of endothelin receptors in human gliomas: a growth factor? *Neurosurgery*, **27**, 275–281.

13 Endothelin Mechanisms in the Heart: Role in Pathophysiology

Anil Gulati

Department of Pharmaceutics and Pharmacodynamics (m/c 865), The University of Illinois at Chicago, 833 South Wood Street, Chicago, IL 60612, USA

INTRODUCTION

Endothelin (ET) is widely distributed throughout many tissues. The synthesis of ET is regulated by ET genes and analysis of these genes has revealed that three distinct ET genes exist and encode different mature ET sequences (ET-1, ET-2 and ET-3). There are no species differences among isoforms of human, porcine, rat, bovine or dog[1]. Messenger ribonucleic acid (mRNA) encoding preproET has been shown to be present in the endothelial cells of blood vessels in various mammalian tissues including the heart[2]. Several factors like epinephrine, thrombin and angiotensin II can enhance the production of preproET. PreproET is cleaved by an endopeptidase to form proET (big ET) and finally an ET converting enzyme cleaves proET to form mature ET.

ET exerts its biological actions by acting on specific receptors on the cell membranes. ET binding sites have been identified in the heart[3], lung, kidney, adrenal gland and central nervous system (CNS)[4,5]. The intracellular mechanism of action of ET is linked to increases in inositol triphosphate and diacylglycerol, which is accompanied with the increases in intracellular calcium and activation of protein kinase C.

The major biological action of ET described is vasoconstriction. However, in addition, ET has several important cardiovascular, renal and endocrine functions[5,6]. ET has modulatory actions on the renin-angiotensin-aldosterone system and has antinatriuretic effects[7]. ET has been reported to stimulate the secretion of atrial natriuretic peptide from cultured rat atrial myocytes[8]. Plasma ET-1 level increases in various pathological conditions associated with cardiovascular system[9]. Increases in circulating ET have been documented in states of severe cardiovascular stress, including cardiogenic and septic shock[10,11], acute myocardial infarction[12,13] and pulmonary hypertension[14] implicating it in several disease conditions associated with cardiovascular system. Although the clinical significance of elevated levels of ET in these diseases is not clear, however, studies do indicate that ET has biological actions at pathophysiological concentration[6] implicating a possible role of ET mechanisms in the pathogenesis of cardiovascular disorders.

The functional importance of ET increases because of its mitogenic potential, which could contribute to structural changes within the cardiovascular system. ET-1 has been shown to be a smooth muscle mitogen and its synthesis can be increased by damage to the endothelium. Thus, it may play a role in genesis of atherosclerosis and in forms of hypertension in which smooth muscle proliferation has been implicated[15]. ET has also been reported to stimulate the proliferation of fibroblasts, glomerular mesangial and human carcinoma cells with the expression of proto- oncogenes (c-myc, c-fos) in these cells[16].

ET AND MYOCARDIAL CELL HYPERTROPHY

ET has been demonstrated to induce hypertrophy with concomitant increases in the transcripts of muscle-specific genes and a proto-onco-gene, c-fos, as well as augmenting DNA and protein synthesis in cultured neonatal rat cardiomyocytes[17]. ET-1 (10^{-9} to 10^{-7} M) induced dose dependent increases in the gene expression of myosin light chain 2, α-actin, and troponin I. ET-1 also dose-dependently stimulated accumulation of total inositol phosphates in cardiomyocytes. The surface area of cardiomyocytes was significantly increased without any cell proliferation[17]. In another study, the effect of ET-1 on myocardial cell hypertrophy was studied using neonatal rat myocardial cell model. The hypertrophic response was assessed using several parameters. It was found that ET-1 (0.1 to 10 nM concentrations) showed a dose-dependent increase in the number of cells displaying hypertrophy with organized sarcomeric structures. ET-1 (1 nM) resulted in the rapid and transient expression of an immediate early gene expression of an immediate early gene program. Thus, ET-1 activated the immediate early gene expression and sarcomere assembly. Besides, ET-1 also activated the transcription of cardiac genes[18]. Rat cardiac myocytes culture showed an increase in the rate of protein synthesis, morphological size, contraction rate and Ca^{2+} uptake when ET-1 was added[19]. The effect of ET-1 on cardiac myosin heavy chain gene expression was examined in cultured neonatal rat myocardial cells. ET-1 was found to stimulate both α- and β-myosin heavy chain gene expression. Myocardial cells treated with ET-1 (1 to 100 nM) increased the transcription rate of α- and β-myosin heavy chain genes in a dose-dependent manner[20]. ET-1 was also found to increase the cell surface area, ^{3}H-leucine incorporation and gene expression. The increase in ^{3}H-leucine incorporation by ET-1 could be attenuated by BQ-123[21]. Most of the studies were performed on the cultured neonatal rat ventricular myocytes. Sugden et al.[22] studied the effects of ET-1 on protein synthesis and phosphoinositide hydrolysis in ventricular myocytes obtained from adult rat hearts. ET-1 (10^{-11} to 10^{-7} M) produced a dose-dependent increase in phosphoinositide hydrolysis and the rate of protein synthesis. The above studies clearly indicate that ET can lead to hypertrophy of myocardial cells obtained from neonatal or adult animals. The induction of cardiac hypertrophy by ET-1 appears to be mediated through the enhanced Ca^{2+} entry through the sarcolemmal T-type Ca^{2+} channel, possibly through a pathway involving activation of protein kinase C[23].

Recently, both ET_A and ET_B types of receptors have been shown to be present in cardiac fibroblasts with ET_B predominating[24]. It was also found that ET-1 and ET-3 increased the synthesis of type I and III collagens and ET-1 but not ET-3 reduced collagenase activity. The effect of ET on collagen synthesis in cardiac fibroblasts may be mediated through both ET_A and ET_B types of receptors, whereas their effect on collagenase seems to be mediated through ET_A receptors[25].

EFFECT OF ET ON THE HEART

Positive chronotropic effect of ET

ET-1 has been shown to possess positive chronotropic effect[26,27]. The positive chronotropic effect of ET-1 was not affected by the L-type Ca^{2+} channel antagonist, nicardipine. Reid et al.[27] have reported that ET-1 decreases the chronotropic responses to stimulation of intramural sympathetic nerves by approximately 60% in rat and 10–15% in guinea pig atria, but does not affect the stimulation induced release of norepinephrine. The reduction of stimulation induced chronotropic responses by ET-1 appeared to be dependent on the increase in basal rate and the ability of ET-1 to facilitate the norepinephrine uptake.

Ventricular arrhythmias are generally attributed to severe ischemia, the fact that specific ET receptors have also been identified in cardiac myocytes[28,29] and in the cardiac conducting system[30] raises the possibility that ET might possess electrophysiological properties. ET-1 infused into the left circumflex coronary artery or left anterior descending coronary artery produced a dose dependent decrease in blood flow and ECG changes typical of myocardial ischemia. ET-1 when administered to left anterior descending artery produced fatal arrhythmias even in lower doses and several animals died. In contrast, when ET-1 was administered to left circumflex artery no deaths occurred even though the decrease in flow was comparable[31]. The direct effect of ET-1 on the isolated dog right bundle branch, false tendon, ventricular muscle and atrial muscle preparation was studied. ET-1 prolonged the duration of action potentials in all the tissues except atrial muscle, the spontaneous firing of the right bundle branch was suppressed by ET-1 and the prolongation of action potential duration was far more marked in the right bundle branch than in other tissues and it was followed by the development of early after depolarization[32]. The development of early after depolarization might be responsible for the direct actions of ET on the myocardial cells to cause arrhythmias.

Positive inotropic effect of ET

In the heart ET acts as a positive inotropic agent[33,34]. ET exerts a prominent stimulatory action on the isolated heart preparations from rats[35], guinea pigs[33], humans[36], rabbits[37] and ferrets[38]. However, ET-1 could not elicit any effect on the dog ventricular myocardium[39]. The positive inotropic effect of ET was not affected by adrenergic, muscarinic, histaminergic and serotonergic antagonists[33,35,40]. This indicates that the release of endogenous catecholamines, acetylcholine, histamine or serotonin is not involved in the positive inotropic effect of ET.

ET-1 produced a pronounced positive inotropic effect on the rabbit papillary muscle, intermediate one in the guinea pig and rat and none in dog. The rank order of ET-1 induced positive inotropic effects in these species was found to be consistent with that of the density of ET-1 receptors determined by radioreceptor assay[39]. The isoforms of ET (ET-1, ET-2 and ET-3) were found to be equieffective and equipotent in eliciting a positive inotropic response in rabbit[39] suggesting that the subtype of ET receptors responsible for the inotropic effect may be different from those in vascular smooth muscle cells, where ET-1 produces contraction with a much higher potency than ET-3[41].

The characteristics of ET induced positive inotropic effect on mammalian ventricular myocardium were found to be very similar to those of myocardial α-adrenoceptor stimulation[39,42]. ET has been found to influence adrenergic responses[5,43].

The subcellular mechanism of ET induced positive inotropic effect appears to involve phosphoinositide hydrolysis[39,40,44]. ET-1 catalyzed phosphoinositide hydrolysis in a concentration and time dependent manner in rabbit ventricular myocardium. A striking similarity was noted between the characteristic of ET-1 and myocardial α_1-adrenoceptor mediated acceleration of phosphoinositide hydrolysis and regulation of myocardial contractility[45]. Thapsigargin, an inotropic agent, was found to completely antagonize the positive inotropic effect and Ca^{2+} mobilizing action of 100 nM of ET-1. Thapsigargin had no effect on the basal or ET-1 stimulated production of inositol phosphates[46]. Recently, it has been found that there are two components in the positive inotropic effect of ET-1 in guinea pig atria. ET-1 at concentrations of 10 nM and higher produced an initial increasing phase (early component) and a second greater positive inotropic phase (late component). The two components may be mediated by different mechanisms. Stimulation of phosphoinositide hydrolysis and subsequent activation of protein kinase C seems to play a key role in the late component. However, the early component appears to be independent of the protein kinase C activation but may be due to prolongation of the duration of action potential[47]. The potent positive inotropic effect of ET-1 on the mammalian heart has also been demonstrated to be mediated through the apparent sensitization of cardiac myofilaments to intracellular calcium[48] which is in part due to stimulation of the sarcolemmal Na^+-H^+ exchanger by a protein kinase C mediated pathway[44].

When ET is administered into perfused rat heart preparations, it causes a negative inotropic effect because of its vasoconstrictor effect[49]. In dogs, ET produced a potent vasoconstriction of the resistance coronary vessels producing a redistribution of transmural blood flow and a decrease in myocardial contractility secondary to ischemia[50]. Intracoronary injection of ET-1 in swine at a dose producing an extensive coronary vasoconstriction produced no change in regional or global myocardial contractile function[51]. These authors concluded that in spite of strong *in vitro* evidence of positive inotropic effect due to ET-1 the effect is probably not relevant *in vivo*. However, it could be species related as *in vitro* studies do not show any positive inotropic effect in dog ventricle despite the presence of ET-1 binding sites.

ET AND PULMONARY HYPERTENSION

Pulmonary hypertension is a progressive condition, characterized by an increase in pulmonary vascular resistance. The increase in resistance is so marked that it ultimately leads to right heart failure. Although factors initiating pulmonary hypertension vary in different patients, the common factor is the proliferation of smooth muscle cells in the vascular media and intima[52]. The thickening of vascular wall reduces the caliber of blood vessels and increases the vascular resistance. The increase in pulmonary vascular resistance may also be due to elevated levels of potent vasoconstrictor substances. The most potent vasoconstrictor is ET-1[2] which is also a mitogen for smooth muscle and other cells[15,53,54]. Normal lung removes ET from the circulation[55], however, in pulmonary hypertension studies have shown that there is an increased production and release of ET-1 into the pulmonary circulation[56]. ET concentrations were found to be similar in plasma samples obtained from pulmonary artery and left superior pulmonary vein indicating that there is not net pulmonary clearance of ET in patients undergoing coronary artery bypass grafting[57]. Yoshibayashi et al.[58] found plasma ET-1 levels were elevated in patients with pulmonary hypertension, the elevation was due to the increased production of ET-1 in pulmonary circulation. Venous plasma ET concentrations in patients with primary pulmonary hypertension were significantly greater than those with Eisenmenger syndrome (pulmonary hypertension secondary to congenial heart defect), although they had lower mean pulmonary arterial pressure[59]. Plasma ET-1 levels and pulmonary arterial pressures were synchronously elevated in patients with valvular heart disease according to the severity of pulmonary hypertension, and both of them decreased soon after surgical correction of the diseased valve in the heart[60]. A close correlation between plasma ET-1 level and mean pulmonary artery wedge pressure and total pulmonary vascular resistance was observed in patients of myocardial infarction with cardiac and pulmonary circulatory distress[61]. On the other hand, no evidence of increase in circulating plasma ET and 24 hour urinary ET was found in children with pulmonary hypertension[62].

It has been demonstrated that a marked increase in intrapulmonary ET-1 production occurs in fawn hooded rats with idiopathic pulmonary hypertension[63]. The pharmacological profile of ET-1 suggests that it could act not only to increase pulmonary vascular tone[64], but also to stimulate proliferation of vascular smooth muscle cells[15,54,65], both these phenomenon are closely associated with pulmonary hypertension. On the contrary, it is also possible that ET-1 could be acting as an endogenous vasodilator to counteract the pulmonary hypertension. Chang et al.[60] concluded that ET-1 was a reactive mediator the release of which was stimulated by altered pulmonary venous drainage. Low doses have been shown to produce dilation of the preconstricted pulmonary blood vessels[66,67,68]. The increased production of ET during pulmonary hypertension could be due to endothelial injury because of the shear stress induced by pulmonary hypertension. Although the role of ET-1 in the pathogenesis of pulmonary hypertension is speculative but there is evidence which implicates ET in the pathophysiology of pulmonary hypertension.

Pulmonary hypertension was found to be associated with the increased expression of ET-1 in vascular endothelial cells providing further evidence that local production of ET-1 may be contributing to the vascular abnormalities associated with pulmonary hypertension[69]. Giaid et al.[70] found that ET-1 like immunoreactivity and ET-1mRNA were present in pulmonary vascular endothelial cells, particularly in specimens from patients with pulmonary hypertension. In patients they found a significant co-relation between ET-1 like immunoreactivity and histological parameters of disease activity.

Postobstructive pulmonary vasculopathy was produced by chronic ligation of one pulmonary artery of dogs. Plasma ET-1 levels distal to the ligation were not different from those of the control pulmonary artery. ET-1 like immunoreactivity was more intense in the pulmonary arteries and new bronchial vessels of ligated lungs[71] indicating that ET-1 may be playing a role in the bronchial neovascularization during pulmonary vasculopathy. Pulmonary ET-1 concentrations were significantly higher in patients with pulmonary hypertension irrespective of its cause and there was a positive correlation between ET-1 concentration and pulmonary vascular resistance[72]. These findings do suggest a role for cell specific expression of ET-1 in the pathogenesis of pulmonary hypertension and that excessive local production of ET-1 in the lungs might be contributing to the vascular abnormalities associated with pulmonary hypertension.

ET IN CONGENITAL HEART DEFECTS

Patients with congenial heart defects may have altered pulmonary blood flow due to left to right shunts, that can lead to be development of pulmonary hypertension. Studies have been performed to determine ET levels in children with congenital heart disease. Plasma ET levels were measured in blood samples obtained from various sites during cardiac catheterization in patients with congenital heart defects with an without pulmonary hypertension. It was found that plasma ET-1 levels were elevated in patients with congenital heart defects with pulmonary hypertension in comparison to those without pulmonary hypertension[58]. Cacoub et al.[59] found that venous plasma ET-1 levels were significantly elevated in patients with primary pulmonary hypertension and pulmonary hypertension secondary to congenital heart defect (Eisenmenger syndrome). Patients with Eisenmenger syndrome had pulmonary arterial pressure of 71 ± 5 mmHg and those with primary pulmonary hypertension had 57 ± 5 mmHg of pulmonary artery pressure, but ET-1 levels were significantly greater in primary pulmonary hypertension than in patients of Eisenmenger syndrome. Another study also indicates that plasma ET concentrations are not related to increased pulmonary artery pressure but are related to increased pulmonary blood flow in children with congenital heart defects[73]. In contrast, there is a report showing no evidence of any change in plasma or urinary ET levels in children with congenital heart disease[74]. The same group reports that cardiopulmonary by pass in patients with pulmonary hypertension and congenital heart disease is associated with an immediate postoperative increase in circulating ET and that patients who had a high pulmonary blood flow before the operation were particularly vulnerable to more injurious effect on lung[75].

ET AND CONGESTIVE HEART FAILURE

Congestive heart failure (CHF) is a clinical syndrome characterized by reduced peripheral perfusion, increased peripheral vascular resistance, impaired cardiac performance and decreased cardiac output[76]. CHF is usually accompanied with an increased vascular tone due to activation of sympathetic nervous system and by increased plasma concentrations of neurohumoral factors such as angiotensin II, norepinephrine and arginine vasopressin leading to hypoperfusion[77,78] and decrease in cardiac output. ET, a potent vasoconstrictor peptide[2] when infused intravenously in rats[2] and in dogs[79,80] produced intense and sustained vasoconstriction and increased peripheral vascular resistance. Studies have reported increased plasma ET levels during CHF in animals[81] and humans[82,83] supporting a possible role of ET in the neurohumoral adaptations to CHF. However, another study reported no increase in circulating ET in humans with severe but stable CHF[10].

The role of ET in the pathophysiology of congestive heart failure is now supported by several studies indicating an elevation of plasma levels in human and in experimental situations[81,84-86]. In anesthetized dogs CHF produced by rapid ventricular pacing, the circulating ET levels were found to be increased compared with normal controls. It was found that a plasma ET level of more than 14 pg/ml was a sensitive and specific indicator of significant CHF. The right atrial pressure and pulmonary capillary wedge pressure correlated independently with circulating ET levels[84]. In another study, CHF was produced in dogs by thoracic inferior vena caval constriction, a model of low cardiac output CHF. Plasma ET levels were found to be significantly increased in dogs with CHF. Exogenous infusion of ET (5 ng/kg/min) produced a systemic and renal vasoconstrictor response in dogs with CHF. Atrial natriuretic factor prevented the systemic vascular and arterial pressure responses of ET but the potent renal vasoconstricting action of ET was not affected[87]. In rats with high output heart failure plasma ET levels were found to be significantly elevated and there was a down regulation (decreased density) of renal glomerular ET receptors[88].

Studies conducted in human subjects also showed that ET levels in plasma were significantly elevated in patients with CHF. Increased circulating plasma ET was found to be particularly relevant to the range of pulmonary vasoconstriction encountered in CHF[89,90]. Plasma ET levels were determined in patients with severe CHF and in age- and sex- matched healthy volunteers. ET levels were 6.4 ± 0.3 pmol/l in healthy volunteers but in patients with CHF ET levels (12.4 ± 0.6 pmol/l) were significantly elevated. Plasma ET levels did not increase with exercise. There was no correlation between plasma ET and plasma atrial natriuretic factor, serum urea or serum creatinine in patients with CHF. There was a significant renal extraction of ET in patients with CHF[91]. In another study, plasma ET was estimated in 71 healthy control subjects and 56 patients with CHF. The mean plasma ET levels in healthy subjects was 7.1 ± 0.1 pg/ml but in patients with CHF ET levels were (12.6 ± 0.6 pg/ml) significantly elevated[92]. Further analysis showed that 24 patients had mild CHF and plasma ET levels were 11.1 ± 0.7 pg/ml and 32 patients had severe CHF and plasma ET levels were found to be 13.8 ± 0.9 pg/ml. There was significant negative correlation between plasma concentration of ET and left ventricular ejection fraction[92]. Plasma ET-1 levels were rapidly increased in normal human subjects within 5 min of postural change indicating a role of ET-1 in neurohumoral compensation for hemodynamic stress. Patients with CHF had markedly higher levels of circulating ET-1 and there was no further increase on postural change[86]. Plasma ET-1 levels were also found to be increased in patients with end stage heart failure compared with age matched controls. ET-1 levels increased further following heart transplantation the increase was sustained for 3-12 months after heart transplantation[93]. Big ET-1 was also found to be significantly elevated in patients with CHF, this increase was not related to increase in blood pressure but correlated with right atrial pressure, pulmonary capillary wedge pressure, left ventricular ejection fraction, effort capacity and severity of CHF[94].

Infusion of 1 to 2.5 ng/kg/min of ET resulted in circulating ET levels of 3 to 10 pmol/l and produced significant systemic and renal hemodynamics effects in humans and animals[6,95,96]. Low dose infusion of ET (2.5 ng/kg/min) resulted in a two fold increase in plasma ET concentration and significant increases in systemic and renal vascular resistance and decreases in cardiac output[97]. Thus, a two fold increase in plasma ET levels in patients with CHF will be able to produce significant hemodynamic effects and therefore might be playing a role in the pathophysiology of CHF.

If ET contributes towards tissue hypoperfusion in CHF then some evidence of alterations in ET receptors in the cardiovascular system should be present. CHF was produced in rabbits by combined aortic valvular insufficiency and stenosis. Plasma ET levels were found to be elevated in CHF and ET concentrations in the left ventricle and kidney were decreased and in the right ventricle were increased. ET receptor affinity was unchanged in the ventricles but density was decreased in the left and right ventricles and kidney during CHF[98]. In another study CHF was produced in rats by myocardial ischemia. ET receptor density was significantly decreased in the mesenteric arteries but were not affected in the heart of rats with CHF. The pressor response to bolus injection of ET-1 was significantly less in rats with CHF[99]. These results indicate that elevated ET levels during CHF could be responsible for the down regulation of ET receptors in the blood vessels leading to decreased vascular ET- receptor function.

The mechanism responsible for increased circulating levels of ET in CHF may be due to (1) diminished clearance of ET due to a decreased blood flow to the lung and kidneys which are important for the metabolism of ET[100], (2) stimulation of ET release by an elevation in the circulating levels of angiotensin II and arginine vasopressin, which are known to stimulate production of ET[101] and (3) stimulation of ET release by hypoxia due to pulmonary congestion[102,103].

The vasoconstricting effects of ET may be beneficial in early heart failure by augmenting preload through venoconstriction and sodium retention and by increasing systemic vascular resistance to maintain perfusion pressure. Long term effects of ET may be influenced by the action of ET as a growth factor, which may contribute to the remodelling of the cardiovascular system; these effects may exceed the limit leading to continuing deterioration in cardiac function[104]. ET has also been shown to produce a profound loss of plasma volume, independent of renal excretion, by increasing transudation of fluid into the extrapulmonary interstitial space presumably by increasing hydrostatic pressure[105]. The loss of plasma volume will lead to a decrease in circulating volume which will decrease the preload. The ultimate effect of ET on preload is based on the additive effects of two opposing actions[106,107] and is dependent on the dose or concentration of ET.

ET AND CARDIAC TRANSPLANTATION

Cardiac transplantation is usually performed at the end stage of CHF. Cardiac transplantation results in the improvement of cardiac functions and partly restores the neurohumoral activation. Studies have been performed to determine whether the increased levels of ET during CHF remains elevated or not following cardiac transplantation. Lerman et al.[93] found that ET concentrations are increased in patients with CHF and increase further after heart transplantation. The plasma ET concentrations increased within 1 day and remained elevated 3 to 12 months following heart transplantation. In another study ET-1 levels were found to be significantly increased after successful orthotopic cardiac transplantation[108]. Since the introduction of cyclosporine the survival rate (1 year) after heart transplantation has increased to more than 80%[109]. However, cyclosporine causes renal vasoconstriction leading to renal insufficiency[110] and hypertension[111]. Cyclosporine also damages endothelial cells causing cell lysis and detachment[112].

It could be possible that the increase in plasma ET concentration following heart transplantation is due to the effects of cyclosporine. Some studies have demonstrated that cyclosporine increases plasma and urinary ET[113-115]. The increase in plasma ET-1 concentration after heart transplantation did not correlate with hemodynamic variables, serum creatinine or cyclosporine levels[108]. Edwards et al.[116] also found that chronic cyclosporine therapy is not associated with sustained activation of circulating ET and that post transplantation hypertension and renal insufficiency do not correlate with circulation ET levels. Further studies are needed to determine the factors responsible for the increase in ET levels following cardiac transplantation.

ET MECHANISMS IN CORONARY ARTERY ASSOCIATED DISORDERS

ET-1 when applied topically on the epicardium of beating canine heart, induced a dose-dependent elevation of the ST segment of electrocardiogram and severe constriction of the coronary microvessels[117]. Using an intravital fluorescence videomicroscope system it was found that ET-1 produced a dose-dependent narrowing of coronary microvessels of isolated beating hearts of rats[118]. Intravenous administration of ET-1 to anesthetized dogs produced significant elevation in ST segment in lead II, III and aVf of electrocardiogram, these changes could be blocked by cromakalin, a potassium activator[119]. Intracoronary administration of ET-1 (5 µg) induced ST segment elevation of the electrocardiogram due to coronary artery contraction and arrhythmias involving atrio-ventricular block, ventricular premature contraction and ventricular fibrillations. These effects could be attenuated by antianginal drugs like KRN2391, nicorandil and diltiazem[120]. ET has been demonstrated to be a potent vasoconstrictor of coronary arteries from man[121-123]. Bolus injections of ET evoked a biphasic response, an initial dilation and then constriction of large and small coronary arteries of conscious dogs, while infusion of ET produced only vasoconstriction[124]. Intracoronary administration of ET produced a marked vasoconstriction of coronary blood vessels and a more pronounced reduction of blood flow in the subepicardium compared with the subendocardium[125]. The reduction of coronary blood flow by intracoronary bolus administration of ET was similar but longer lasting that Bay K8644 or U 46619 and was only partially antagonized by nitrendipine[126]. Both ET_A and ET_B types of receptors have been found to mediate coronary vasoconstriction. The large conduit arteries in dogs produce vasoconstriction through ET_A receptors while

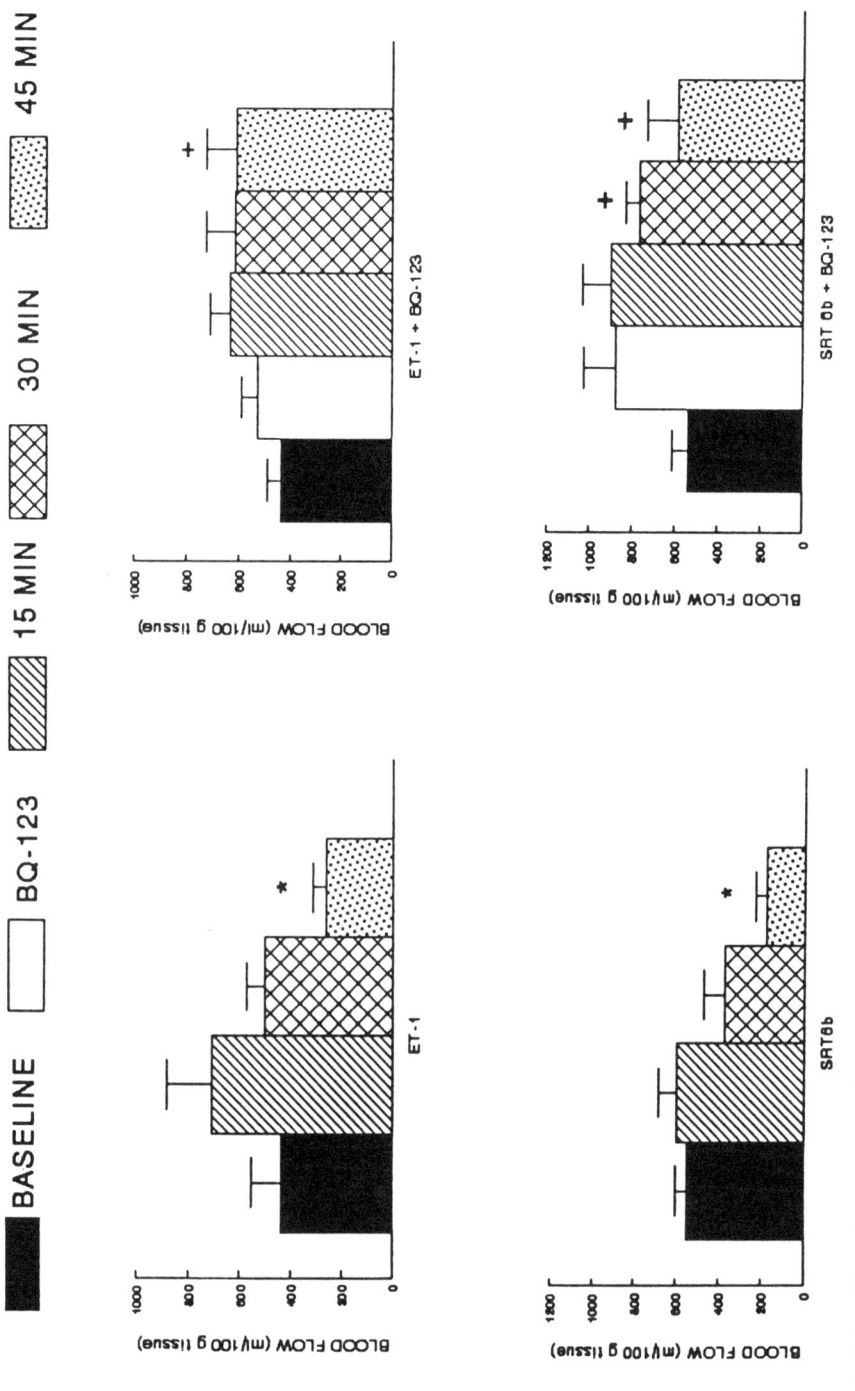

Figure 13.1. Effect of intravenous infusion of ET-1 (250 ng/kg/min) and sarafotoxin 6b (SRT 6b) (250 ng/kg/min) on blood flow to the heart at 15, 30 and 45 min of control (left panel) and BQ-123 treated (right panel) rats. BQ-123 (5 mg/kg/h) infusion was started 15 min prio to ET-1 or SRT 6b administration and continued till the end of experiment. ET-1 and SRT 6b produced a significant (*) decrease in coronary blood flow which was significant (+) attenuated by BQ-123.

the smaller coronary vessels involve both ET_A and ET_B[127]. Pernow and Modin[128] found that the contraction of pig coronary arteries is mediated through ET_A and Teerlink et al.[129] have shown that ET_B receptors are also involved in the vasoconstriction of canine coronary blood vessels. Studies conducted in our laboratory indicate that the decrease in blood flow produced by infusion of ET-1 (250 ng/kg/min) or sarafotoxin 6b (250 ng/kg/min) can be attenuated by BQ-123, a specific ET_A antagonist (Fig. 13.1). Since ET-1 acts mainly on ET_A type of receptors while sarafotoxin 6b acts mainly on ET_B type of receptors, it appears that several types of ET receptors are involved in the regulation of coronary blood vessels.

ET and coronary angioplasty

Percutaneous transluminal coronary angioplasty (PTCA) is frequently associated with vasoconstriction involving large vessels as well as microcirculation. Circulating ET in the coronary sinus and the femoral artery was measured in patients who underwent PTCA. ET levels in the coronary sinus were significantly elevated after PTCA, this increase was present but not significant in femoral artery samples. ET levels in the coronary sinus were not related to the plasma thromboglobulin, plasma thrombin-antithrombin complex, mean blood pressure or heart rate[130]. Ameli et al.[131] found that there was no change in plasma ET levels after angiography alone, but there was a significant increase after PTCA. The increase was associated with an increase in its counter-regulatory hormone, atrial natriuretic factor[132-134] and a decrease in epinephrine and norepinephrine levels. Circulating ET levels did not correlate with the percent coronary stenosis before or after PTCA or the presence or absence of angiographically visible thrombus. These results indicate that the increase in plasma ET in the coronary sinus or femoral artery is not through thrombin but could be due to direct endothelial injury by PTCA. PTCA of the left anteriodescending coronary artery was performed and plasma ET-1 levels were determined in 24 patients. The ratio of the diameter of the inflated balloon and the diameter of the dilated artery correlated with plasma ET concentrations after PTCA[135], providing further evidence that the release of ET appears to be due to direct endothelial injury by PTCA. It will be critical that dilatation of the coronary artery during PTCA should correspond with diameter of the artery and over dilatation should be avoided. Another evidence is provided by a study where the cardiac venus ET concentration was found to be increased after PTCA[136]. However there are some studies showing that no change in ET concentration was observed following PTCA[137,138].

ET and myocardial infarction (MI)

The role ET in the pathophysiology of MI is not clear, several reports provide evidence in favor or against the involvement of ET mechanisms in MI. Although Miyauchi et al.[12] found a marked increase in venous plasma levels of ET-1 in patients with acute MI but found no change in plasma ET-1 levels in the coronary sinus or aorta of coronary artery ligated dogs[139]. Patients with stable or unstable angina did not show any change in the systemic or coronary venous blood ET levels[140]. Plasma ET-1 levels in patients with stable coronary disease were not different from those of normal subjects. However, plasma ET-1 levels rose sharply after MI, reaching a peak at 6 hours after the onset of chest pain and returning rapidly towards normal range by 24 hours. Patients with complicated infarction also showed a rapid rise and the plasma ET-1 levels remained elevated till 72 hours after infarction. There was no correlation between peak increases in creatine kinase and ET-1[141]. Plasma ET levels are increased in the acute phase of MI but are not altered in stable or unstable angina[142]. Salminen et al.[13] also found that ET levels increased immediately after MI with peak reaching between 1 to 4 hours and then declining.

In patients with acute MI the plasma ET levels were elevated in the acute phase and were highest on the day of onset. The plasma ET level showed a positive correlation with the wall motion abnormality index, thrombin-antithrombin III complex and beta thromboglobulin[143]. ET levels were significantly elevated in patients of acute MI at the time of admission as compared to healthy controls. Plasma ET levels remained elevated for at least 2 days after acute MI. The highest concentration of ET was at 1 hour after admission. All patients received thrombolytic therapy. Reperfusion of the infarct-related artery markedly influenced ET concentrations. In patients without early perfusion plasma ET concentrations were significantly higher during the first hours after acute MI than those with early perfusion. In patients who did not have early perfusion the peak ET concentrations correlated with the angiographic left ventricular ejection fraction, maximum creatinine kinase MB mass concentrations and creatinine kinase activities[144,145]. It appears that plasma ET levels are increased in acute phase of MI and the cardiac dysfunction, an activated coagulation system and platelet hyperactivity may be associated with the increase in plasma ET. Naruse et al.[146] determined plasma levels of two endothelium derived substances, ET and thrombomodulin in control and acute MI. ET but not thrombomodulin levels were found to be elevated in acute MI, indicating that increases in plasma ET is not due to simple injury of the endothelium.

In an experimental study on dogs the plasma ET concentrations from central vein were increased by 2.2 fold at 60 min after release of the ligated left anterior descending coronary artery. However, occlusion by itself did not cause any increase in the plasma ET concentration[147]. Plasma ET levels in samples obtained from venous blood were found to be increased during reperfusion following a brief coronary artery ligation in pigs, however, ET levels in samples obtained from aortic arch were decreased[148]. It was found that no net removal or production of ET occurred in the pulmonary circulation, however, there was a marked increase in plasma ET concentration from the left atrium to the aortic arch control conditions. This increase shifted to a marked reduction during early reperfusion following brief ischemia[149]. It might be possible that endocardial endothelial cells, like other endothelial cells, are able to synthesize and release ET[150]. A role for ET in evolving MI is strongly indicated by studies of coronary ligation in the rat, where the myocardial ET content increases after MI and the extent of ventricular damage is reduced by the use of ET antibodies[151]. ET binding sites showed significant regional differences within the myocardium and a specific down regulation of ET binding sites occurred in the left atrium following myocardial infarction in rats[152]. Coronary occlusion causes not only myocardial ischemia, but also endothelial dysfunction[153], and after release of the occlusion increased coronary flow and shear stress. These factors could affect ET concentration as observed in several studies, since hypoxia[102] and shear stress[154] have been shown to induce ET production from cultured endothelial cells.

In order to elucidate the pathogenic contribution of ET-1 to coronary spasm, spasm was provoked by administration of acetylcholine in the coronary artery of patients with a tentative diagnosis of vasospastic angina. Patients without ischemic heart disease showed no change in plasma ET-1 levels in samples obtained from coronary sinus and aortic root following acetylcholine (100 µg) induced coronary artery spasm. However, patients having myocardial lactate production during acetylcholine induced spasm showed a significant increase in ET-1 levels in the coronary sinus but not in aortic root[155]. In another study, the plasma ET-1 levels in venous and coronary sinus blood of the spasm provoked (by acetylcholine or ergonovine) patients were 1.71 fold and 2.16 fold higher, respectively, than those of non-provoked cases. No change in ET-1 levels was observed in patients in whom spasm could not be provoked[156].

Although studies clearly indicate that ET levels are elevated in early phase of myocardial infarction, the exact role of ET in the pathogenesis of myocardial infarction remains unclear. ET is an extremely potent vasoconstrictor of coronary and systemic blood vessels and could initiate or aggravate acute myocardial ischemia. It could be argued that increase in the circulating concentrations of ET in humans are not sufficient enough to induce vasoconstriction. However, the primary role of ET may be as an autacoid, acting locally on the smooth muscles of the coronary blood vessels with the circulating peptide resulting from spillover into the vascular lumen. ET-1 concentration was found to significantly increase in plasma obtained from left atrium to aortic arch in pigs[149]. This favors the view that endocardial endothelial cells are able to synthesize and release ET and this ET could influence myocardial function if released abluminally or indirectly if released into the cavity and then entering the coronary circulation. The elevation of ET levels in early myocardial infarction could be due to stress reaction to myocardial infarction. Elevated ET levels have been associated with surgeries[157] increase in catecholamines[2], thrombin or thrombus products[2,158]. Some reports do not favor the view that ET-1 production is related to coronary thrombus formation but is related to thrombolysis[159]. In contrast, early reflow and reversion of myocardial ischemia using thrombolytic therapy was found to be associated with a reduced ET release in patients with acute myocardial infarction[144]. The production of ET will also be influenced by the severity of lesion and the degree of endothelial cell perturbation[160].

The elevation of ET in early myocardial infarction is not likely to be due to the release of stored ET from endothelial cells since endothelial cells lack secretory granules and little ET has been identified intracellulary[161]. The de novo synthesis of ET is also not possible since in culture cell media it takes several hours to detect stimulated levels of ET[102,162]. It has been shown that the ratio of big ET to ET in plasma is in the range of 2 to 2.5[163,164]. Enzymes from leukocytes have been shown to facilitate the conversion of big ET to ET[165-167]. If leucocytic enzymes promote the conversion of big ET to ET then elevated levels of ET could be rapidly possible because increased activities of these enzymes are likely to occur during ischemia and reperfusion. Ischemic/reperfusion injury to the heart is known to cause migration of neutrophils and may contribute to impaired coronary vasodilator reserve[168]. Neutrophils have been shown to convert big ET to ET[169] and this could be responsible for the early increase in plasma ET levels observed in acute MI which might be playing a role in the pathophysiology of MI. Phosphoramidon, an ET converting enzyme inhibitor, when given intravenously to rats subjected to coronary occlusion and reperfusion was found to significantly reduce the size of infarct 24 hours post ischemia[170].

ET IN OTHER CARDIAC DISORDERS

Plasma ET concentrations were determined in the pulmonary artery, left atrium, ascending aorta and femoral vein before and after balloon dilatation of the mitral valve in patients with mitral stenosis. Plasma ET concentrations were higher in patients with mitral stenosis than healthy volunteers and the increase was found to be proportional to left atrial pressure. After balloon dilatation of the mitral valve an abrupt increase in plasma ET in femoral vein and pulmonary artery was observed but ET levels did not change in left atrial or aortic blood samples[171].

In open chest operations involving various surgical procedures the elevation of plasma ET-1 level occurred and it appear that increased thrombin formation by surgical tissue damage[172] might be partly contributing to an increase in the production of ET-1 in these patients[173].

Konthe et al.[174] found that ET levels are higher in older patients when compared to younger ones with similar biometric data. No correlation existed between plasma ET and catecholamine levels and hemodynamics during and after aortocoronary bypass grafting in younger or older patients.

SUMMARY

The physiological effects of ET are complicated. ET can act directly or in concert with other regulatory agents. Studies conducted in animal models and in patients clearly indicate that ET is increased in heart failure and after heart transplantation. Whether this increase is responsible for the significant regional or systemic vasoconstriction and represents an adaptive or deleterious response in heart failure remains to be investigated. The role of ET in the pathophysiology of pulmonary hypertension and in acute MI is becoming more evident. The mitogenic potential of ET along with its ability to produce significant cardiovascular effects could contribute to structural changes within the cardiovascular system. Various strategies including the development of ET converting enzyme inhibitors, decreasing the stimuli to ET secretion and development of specific ET receptor antagonists are likely to emerge in near future for the treatment of cardiovascular disorders.

Acknowledgements

The author is grateful to Baxter Healthcare Corporation, Miles Incorporated and National Institutes of Health for providing research funds to our laboratory and to Shruti Gulati for helping in preparation of bibliography.

References

1. Masaki, T. (1993) Overview: Reduced sensitivity of vascular response to endothelin. *Circulation*, **87 (Suppl V)**, V33–V35.
2. Yanagisawa, M., Kurihara, H., Kimura, S., Tomobe, Y., Kobayashi, M., Mitsui, Y., Yazaki, Y., Goto, K. & Masaki, T. (1988) A novel potent vasoconstrictor peptide produced by vascular endothelial cells. *Nature*, **332**, 411–415.
3. Wharton, J., Rutherford, R. A., Gordon, L., Moscoso, G., Schiemberg, I., Gaer, J. A., Taylor, K. M. & Polak, J. M. (1991) Localization of endothelin binding sites and endothelin-like immunoreactivity in human fetal heart. *J Cardiovasc Pharmacol*, **17 (Suppl. 7)**, S378–S384.
4. MacCumber, M. W., Ross, C. A., Glaser, B. M. & Snyder, S. H. (1989) Endothelin: visualization of mRNAs by *in situ* hybridization provides evidence for local action. *Proc Natl Acad Sci USA*, **86**, 7285–7289.
5. Gulati, A. & Srimal, R. C. (1992) Endothelin mechanisms in the central nervous system: A target for drug development. *Drug Develop Res*, **26**, 361–387.
6. Lerman, A., Hildebrand, F. L., Jr., Aarhus, L. L. & Burnett, J. C., Jr. (1991) Endothelin has biological actions at pathophysiological concentrations. *Circulation*, **83**, 1808–1814.
7. Lerman, A., Hildebrand, F. L., Jr., Margulies, K. B., O'Murchu, B., Perrella, M. A., Heublein, D. M., Schwab, T. R. & Burnett, J. C., Jr (1990) Endothelin: a new cardiovascular regulatory peptide. *Mayo Clin Proc*, **65**, 1441–1455.
8. Fukuda, Y., Hirata, Y., Yoshimi, H., Kojima, T., Kobayashi, Y., Yanagisawa, M. & Masaki, T. (1988) Endothelin is a potent secretagogue for atrial natriuretic peptide in cultured rat atrial myocytes. *Biochem Biophys Res Commun*, **155**, 167–172.
9. Battistini, B., D'Orleans Juste, P. & Sirois, P. (1993) Endothelins: circulating plasma levels and presence in other biologic fluids. *Lab Invest*, **68**, 600–628.
10. Cernacek, P. & Stewart, D. J. (1989) Immunoreactive endothelin in human plasma: marked elevations in patients in cardiogenic shock. *Biochem Biophys Res Commun*, **161**, 562–567.
11. Pernow, J., Hemsën, A., Hallén, A. & Lundberg, J. M. (1990) Release of endothelin-like immunoreactivity in relation to neuropeptide Y and catecholamines during endotoxin shock and asphyxia in the pig. *Acta Physiol Scand*, **140**, 311–322.
12. Miyauchi, T., Yanagisawa, M., Tomizawa, T., Sugishita, Y., Suzuki, N., Fujino, M., Ajisaka, R., Goto, K. & Masaki, T. (1989) Increased plasma concentrations of endothelin-1 and big endothelin-1 in acute myocardial infarction. *Lancet*, **2**, 53–54.
13. Salminen, K., Tikkanen, I., Saijonmaa, O., Nieminen, M., Fyhrquist, F. & Frick, M. H. (1989) Modulation of coronary tone in acute myocardial infarction by endothelin. *Lancet*, **2**, 747.
14. Barnard, J. W., Barman, S. A., Adkins, W. K., Longenecker, G. L. & Taylor, A. E. (1991) Sustained effects of endothelin-1 on rabbit, dog, and rat pulmonary circulations. *Am J Physiol*, **261**, H479–H486.
15. Komuro, I., Kurihara, H., Sugiyama, T., Yoshizumi, M., Takaku, F. & Yazaki, Y. (1988) Endothelin stimulates c-fos and c-myc expression and proliferation of vascular smooth muscle cells. *FEBS Lett*, **238**, 249–252.
16. Shichiri, M., Hirata, Y., Nakajima, T. et al. (1991) Endothelin-1 is an autocrine/paracrine growth factor for human cancer cell lines. *J Clin Invest*, **87**, 1867–1895.
17. Ito, H., Hirata, Y., Hiroe, M., Tsujino, M., Adachi, S., Takamoto, T., Nitta, M., Taniguchi, K. & Marumo, F. (1991) Endothelin-1 induces hypertrophy with enhanced expression of muscle-specific genes in cultured neonatal rats cardiomyocytes. *Circ Res*, **69**, 209–215.
18. Shubeita, H. E., McDonough, P. M., Harris, A. N., Knowlton, K. U., Glembotski, C. C., Brown, J. H. & Chien, K. R. (1990) Endothelin induction of inositol phospholipid hydrolysis, sarcomere assembly, and cardiac gene expression in ventricular myocytes. A paracrine mechanism for myocardial cell hypertrophy. *J Biol Chem*, **265**, 20555–20562.
19. Suzuki, T., Hoshi, H., Sasaki, H. & Mitsui, Y. (1991) Endothelin-1 stimulates hypertrophy and contractility of neonatal rat cardiac myocytes in a serum-free medium. II. *J Cardiovasc Pharmacol*, **17 (Suppl 7)**, S182–S186.
20. Wang, D. L., Chen, J. J., Shin, N. L., Kao, Y. C., Hsu, K. H., Huang, W. Y. & Liew, C. C. (1992) Endothelin stimulates cardiac alpha- and beta- myosin heavy chain gene expression. *Biochem Biophys Res Commun*, **183**, 1260–1265.
21. Ito, H., Hiroe, M., Hirata, Y., Adachi, S., Tujino, M. & Marumo, F. (1992) Endothelin-1 as an autocrine factor in hypertrophy of cardiomyocytes. *Jpn Circ J*, **56 (Suppl 5)**, 1314–1318.
22. Sugden, P. H., Fuller, S. J., Mynett, J. R., Hatchett, R. J., Bogoyevitch, M. A. & Sugden, M. C. (1993) Stimulation of adult rat ventricular myocyte protein synthesis and phosphoinositide hydrolysis by the endothelins. *Biochem Biophys Acta*, **1175**, 327–332.
23. Furukawa, T., Ito, H., Nitta, J., Tsujino, M., Adachi, S., Hiroe, M., Marumo, F., Sawanobori, T.

& Hiraoka, M. (1992) Endothelin-1 enhances calcium entry through T-type calcium channels in cultured neonatal rat ventricular myocytes. *Circ Res*, **71**, 1242–1253.
24. Katwa, L. C., Guarda, E. & Weber, K. T. (1993) Endothelin receptors in cultured adult rat cardiac fibroblasts. *Cardiovasc Res*, **27**, 2125–2129.
25. Guarda, E., Katwa, L. C., Myers, P. R., Tyagi, S. C. & Weber, K. T. (1993) Role of endothelins on collagen turnover in cardiac fibroblasts. *Cardiovasc Res*, **27**, 2130–2134.
26. Ishikawa, T., Yanagisawa, M., Kimura, S., Goto, K. & Masaki, T. (1988) Positive chronotropic effects of endothelin, a novel endothelium-derived vasoconstrictor peptide. *Pflugers Arch*, **413**, 108–110.
27. Reid, J. J., Wong Dusting, H. K. & Rand, M. J. (1989) The effect of endothelin on noradrenergic transmission in rat and guinea-pig atria. *Eur J Pharmacol*, **168**, 93–96.
28. Galron, R., Kloog, Y., Bdolah, A. & Sokolovsky, M. (1989) Functional endothelin/sarafotoxin receptors in rat heart myocytes: structure-activity relationships and receptor subtypes. *Biochem Biophys Res Commun*, **163**, 936–943.
29. Hirata, Y., Fukuda, Y., Yoshimi, H., Emori, T., Shichiri, M. & Marumo, F. (1989) Specific receptor for endothelin in cultured rat cardiocytes. *Biochem Biophys Res Commun*, **160**, 1438–1444.
30. Yamasaki, H., Niwa, M., Yamashita, K., Kataoka, Y., Shigematsu, K., Hashiba, K. & Ozaki, M. (1989) Specific ^{125}I-endothelin-1 binding sites in the atrioventricular node of the porcine heart. *Eur J Pharmacol*, **168**, 247–250.
31. Salvati, P., Chierchia, S., Dho, L., Ferrario, R. G., Parenti, P., Vicedomini, G. & Patrono, C. (1991) Proarrhythmic activity of intracoronary endothelin in dogs: relation to the site of administration and to changes in regional flow. *J Cardiovasc Pharmacol*, **17**, 1007–1014.
32. Yorikane, R., Koike, H. & Miyake, S. (1991) Electrophysiological effects of endothelin-1 on canine myocardial cells. *J Cardiovasc Pharmacol*, **17 (Suppl 7)**, S159–S162.
33. Ishikawa, T., Yanagisawa, M. Kimura, S., Goto, K. & Masaki, T. (1988) Positive inotropic action of novel vasoconstrictor peptide endothelin on guinea-pig atria. *Am J Physiol*, **255**, H970–H973.
34. Shomisch, M. C., Reynolds, E., Stewart, R. & Bond, M. (1989) Endothelin is a positive inotropic agent in human and rat heart *in vitro*. *Biochem Biophys Res Commun*, **159**, 14–18.
35. Hu, J. R., Von Harsdorf, R. & Lang, R. E. (1988) Endothelin has potent inotropic effects in rat atria. *Eur J Pharmacol*, **158**, 275–278.
36. Moravec, C. S., Reynolds, E. E., Stewart, R. W. & Bond, M. (1989) Endothelin is a positive inotropic agent in human and rat heart *in vitro*. *Biochem Biophys Res Commun*, **159**, 14–18.
37. Watanabe, T., Kusumoto, K., Kitayoshi, T. & Shimamoto, N. (1989) Positive inotropic and vasoconstrictive effects of endothelin-1 in *in vivo* and *in vitro* experiments: characteristics and the role of L-type calcium channels. *J Cardiovasc Pharmacol*, **13 (Suppl 5)**, S108–11 discussion s123.
38. Shah, A. M., Lewis, M. J. & Henderson, A. H. (1989) Inotropic effects of endothelin in ferret ventricular myocardium. *Eur J Pharmacol*, **163**, 365–367.
39. Takanashi, M. & Endoh, M. (1991) Characterization of positive inotropic effect of endothelin on mammalian ventricular myocardium. *Am J Physiol*, **261**, H611–H619.
40. Vigne, P., Lazdunski, M. & Frelin, C. (1989) The inotropic effect of endothelin-1 on rat atria involves hydrolysis of phosphatidylinositol. *FEBS Lett*, **249**, 143–146.
41. Le Monnier de Gouville, A. C., Lippton, H., Cohen, G., Cavero, I. & Hyman, A. (1990) Vasodilator activity of endothelin-1 and endothelin-3: rapid development of cross-tachyphylaxis and dependence on the rate of endothelin administration. *J Pharmacol Exp Ther*, **254**, 1024–1028.
42. Endoh, M. & Takanashi, M. (1991) Inotropic effects of endothelin on mammalian ventricular contractility. *Basic Res Cardiol*, **86 (Suppl 1)**, 173–178.
43. Gulati, A. & Srimal, R. C. (1993) Endothelin antagonizes the hypotension and potentiates the hypertension induced by clonidine. *Eur J Pharmacol*, **230**, 293–300.
44. Kramer, B. K., Smith, T. W. & Kelly, R. A. (1991) Endothelin and increased contractility in adult rat ventricular myocytes. Role of intracellular alkalosis induced by activation of the protein kinase C-dependent Na(+)-H+ exchanger. *Circ Res*, **68**, 269–279.
45. Takanashi, M. & Endoh, M. (1992) Concentration- and time-dependence of phosphoinositide hydrolysis induced by endothelin-1 in relation to the positive inotropic effect in the rabbit ventricular myocardium. *J Pharmacol Exp Ther*, **262**, 1189–1194.
46. Vigne, P., Breittmayer, J. P. & Frelin, C. (1992) Thapsigargin, a new inotropic agent, antagonizes action of endothelin-1 in rat atrial cells. *Am J Physiol*, **263**, H1689–H1694.
47. Hattori, Y., Nakaya, H., Nishihira, J. & Kanno, M. (1993) A dual-component positive inotropic effect of endothelin-1 in guinea pig left atria: a role of protein kinase C. *J Pharmacol Exp Ther*, **266**, 1202–1212.
48. Kelly, R. A., Eid, H., Kramer, B. K., O'Neill, M., Liang, B. T., Reers, M. & Smith T. W. (1990) Endothelin enhances the contractile responsiveness of adult rat ventricular myocytes to calcium by a pertussis toxin-sensitive pathway. *J Clin Invest*, **86**, 1164–1171.

49. Baydoun, A. R., Peers, S. H., Cirino, G. & Woodward, B. (1989) Effects of endothelin-1 on the rat isolated heart. *J Cardiovasc Pharmacol*, **13 (Suppl 5)**, S193–S196.
50. Domenech, R. J., Macho, P., Gonzalez, R. & Huidobro-Toro, J. P. (1991) Effect of endothelin on total and regional coronary resistance and on myocardial contractility. *Eur J Pharmacol*, **192**, 409–416.
51. Ricou, F. J., Murata, K., Oh, B. H., Kambayashi, M. & Peterson, K. L. (1992) Evaluation of inotropic effect of endothelin-1 *in vivo*. *J Cardiovasc Pharmacol*, **20**, 671–677.
52. Wagenvoort, C. A. (1981) Grading of pulmonary vascular lesions – a reappraisal. *Histopathology*, **5**, 595–598.
53. Dubin, D., Pratt, R. E., Kooke, J. P. & Dzau, V. J. (1989) Endothelin, a potent vasoconstrictor, is a vascular smooth muscle mitogen. *J Vasc Biol Med*, **1**, 150–154.
54. Hirata, Y., Takagi, Y., Fukuda, Y. & Marumo, F. (1989) Endothelin is a potent mitogen for rat vascular smooth muscle cells. *Atherosclerosis*, **78**, 225–228.
55. de Nucci, G., Thomas, R., D'Orleans Juste, P., Antunes, E., Walder, C., Warner, T. D. & Vane, J. R. (1988) Pressor effects of circulating endothelin are limited by its removal in the pulmonary circulation and by the release of prostacyclin and endothelium-derived relaxing factor. *Proc Natl Acad Sci USA*, **85**, 9797–9800.
56. Stewart, D. J., Levy, R. D., Cernacek, P. & Langleben, D. (1991) Increased plasma endothelin-1 in pulmonary hypertension: marker or mediator of disease? *Ann Intern Med*, **114**, 464–469.
57. Ray, S. G., McMurray, J. J., Morton, J. J. & Dargie, H. J. (1992) Circulating endothelin is not extracted by the pulmonary circulation in man. *Chest*, **102**, 1143–1144.
58. Yoshibayashi, M., Nishioka, K., Nakao, K., Saito, Y., Matsumura, M., Temma, S., Shirakami, G., Imura, H. & Mikawa, H. (1991) Plasma endothelin concentrations in patients with pulmonary hypertension associated with congenital heart defects. Evidence for increased production of endothelin in pulmonary circulation. *Circulation*, **84**, 2280–2285.
59. Cacoub, P., Dorent, R., Maistre, G., Nataf, P., Carayon, A., Piette, C., Godeau, P., Cabrol, C. & Gandjbakhch, I. (1993) Endothelin-1 in primary pulmonary hypertension and the Eisenmenger syndrome. *Am J Cardiol*, **71**, 448–450.
60. Chang, H., Wu, G. J., Wang, S. M. & Hung, C. R. (1993) Plasma endothelin levels and surgically correctable pulmonary hypertension. *Ann Thorac Surg*, **55**, 450–458.
61. Tomoda, H. (1993) Plasma endothelin-1 in acute myocardial infarction with heart failure. *Am Heart J*, **125**, 667–672.
62. Adatia, I. & Haworth, S. G. (1991) Endothelin in pulmonary hypertensive congenital disease. *Am Rev Respir Dis*, **143**, A403.
63. Stelzner, T. J., O'Brien, R. F., Yanagisawa, M., Sakurai, T., Sato, K., Webb, S., Zamora, M., McMurtry, I. F. & Fisher, J. H. (1992) Increased lung endothelin-1 production in rats with idiopathic pulmonary hypertension. *Am J Physiol*, **262**, L614–L620.
64. Horgan, M. J., Pinheiro, J. M. & Malik, A. B. (1991) Mechanism of endothelin-1-induced pulmonary vasoconstriction. *Circ Res*, **69**, 157–164.
65. Bobik, A., Grooms, A., Millar, J. A., Mitchell, A. & Grinpukel, S. (1990) Growth factor activity of endothelin on vascular smooth muscle. *Am J Physiol*, **258**, C408–C415.
66. Hasunuma, K., Rodman, D. M., O'Brien, R. F. & McMurtry, I. F. (1990) Endothelin 1 causes pulmonary vasodilation in rats. *Am J Physiol*, **259**, H48–H54.
67. Lippton, H. L., Hauth, T. A., Summer, W. R. & Hyman, A. L. (1989) Endothelin produces pulmonary vasoconstriction and systemic vasodilation. *J Appl Physiol*, **66**, 1008–1012.
68. Deleuze, P. H., Adnot, S., Shiiya, N., Roudot Thoraval, F., Eddahibi, S., Braquet, P., Chabrier, P. E. & Loisance, D. Y. (1992) Endothelin dilates bovine pulmonary circulation and reverses hypoxic pulmonary vasoconstriction. *J Cardiovasc Pharmacol*, **19**, 354–360.
69. Giaid, A., Yanagisawa, M., Langleben, D., Michel, R. P., Levy, R., Shennib, H., Kimura, S., Masaki, T., Duguid, W. P. & Stewart, D. J. (1993) Expression of endothelin-1 in the lungs of patients with pulmonary hypertension. *N Engl J Med*, **328**, 1732–1739.
70. Giaid, A., Michel, R. P., Stewart, D. J., Sheppard, M., Corrin, B. & Hamid, Q. (1993) Expression of endothelin-1 in lungs of patients with cryptogenic fibrosing alveolities. *Lancet*, **341**, 1550–1554.
71. Giaid, A., Stewart, D. J. & Michel, R. P. (1993) Endothelin-1-like immunoreactivity in postobstructive pulmonary vasculopathy. *J Vasc Res*, **30**, 333–338.
72. Cacoub, P., Dorent, R., Nataf, P. & Carayon, A. (1993) Endothelin-1 in pulmonary hypertension. *N Engl J Med*, **329**, 1967–1968.
73. Vincent, J. A., Ross, R. D., Kassab, J., Hsu, J. M. & Pinsky, W. W. (1993) Relation of elevated plasma endothelin in congenital heart disease to increased pulmonary blood flow. *Am J Cardiol*, **71**, 1204–1207.
74. Adatia, I. & Haworth, S. G. (1993) Circulating endothelin in children with congenital heart disease. *Br Heart J*, **69**, 233–236.
75. Komai, H., Adatia, I. T., Elliott, M. J., de Leval, M. R. & Haworth, S. G. (1993) Increased plasma levels

of endothelin-1 after cardiopulmonary bypass in patients with pulmonary hypertension and congenital heart disease. *J Thorac Cardiovasc Surg*, **106**, 473–478.
76. Zelis, R. & Flaim, S. F. (1982) Alterations in vasomotor tone in congestive heart failure. *Prog Cardiovasc Dis*, **24**, 437–459.
77. Francis, G. S., Goldsmith, S. R., Levine, T. B., Olivari, M. T. & Cohn, J. N. (1984) The neurohumoral axis in congestive heart failure. *Ann Intern Med*, **101**, 370–377.
78. Greager, M. A., Faxon, D. P., Cutler, S. S., Kohlmann, O., Ryan, T. J. & Garvas, H. (1986) Contribution of vasopressin to vasoconstriction in patients with congestive heart failure: Comparison with the renin-angiotensin system. *J Am Coll Cardiol*, **7**, 758–765.
79. Miller, W. L., Redfield, M. M. & Burnett, J. C. J. (1989) Integrated cardiac, renal, and endocrine actions of endothelin. *J Clin Invest*, **83**, 317–320.
80. Goetz, K. L., Wang, B. C., Madwed, J. B., Zhu, J. L. & Leadley, R. J. J. (1988) Cardiovascular, renal, and endocrine responses to intravenous endothelin in conscious dogs. *Am J Physiol*, **255**, R1064–R1068.
81. Cavero, P. G., Miller, W. L., Heublein, D. M., Margulies, K. B. & Burnett, J. C. J. (1990) Endothelin in experimental congestive heart failure in the anesthetized dog. *Am J Physiol*, **259**, F312–F317.
82. Robertson, R., Susawa, T., Sugiura, M., Haile, V. & Ingami, T. (1990) Circulating endothelin levels: modulation by heart failure in man. *Clin Res*, **38**, 414A.
83. Nakamura, M., Arakawa, N., Yoshida, H., Funakoshi, T., Chiba, M., Abe, Y., Makita, S., Aoki, H. & Hiramori, K. (1993) Increased plasma endothelin concentrations in patients with acute heart failure after myocardial infarction. *Jpn Circ J*, **57**, 371–378.
84. Margulies, K. B., Hildebrand, F. L., Jr., Lerman, A., Perrella, M. A. & Burnett, J. C., Jr. (1990) Increased endothelin in experimental heart failure. *Circulation*, **82**, 2226–2230.
85. Hiroe, M., Hirata, Y., Fujita, N., Umezawa, S., Ito, H., Tsujino, M., Koike, A., Nogami, A., Takamoto, T. & Marumo, F. (1991) Plasma endothelin-1 levels in idiopathic dilated cardiomyopathy. *Am J Cardiol*, **68**, 1114–1115.
86. Stewart, D. J., Cernacek, P., Costello, K. B. & Rouleau, J. L. (1992) Elevated endothelin-1 in heart failure and loss of normal response to postural change. *Circulation*, **85**, 510–517.
87. Underwood, R. D., Aarhus, L. L., Heublein, D. M. & Burnett, J. C. J. (1992) Endothelin in thoracic inferior vena caval constriction model of heart failure. *Am J Physiol*, **263**, H951–H955.
88. Gauquelin, G., Thibault, G. & Garcia, R. (1991) Renal glomerula endothelin receptors in rats with high-output heart failure. *Regul Pept*, **35**, 73–79.
89. Cody, R. J., Haas, G. J., Binkley, P. F., Capers, Q. & Kelley, R. (1992) Plasma endothelin correlates with the extent of pulmonary hypertension in patients with chronic congestive heart failure. *Circulation*, **85**, 504–509.
90. Cody, R. J. (1992) The potential role of endothelin as a vasoconstrictor substance in congestive heart failure. *Eur Heart J*, **13**, 1573–1578.
91. McMurray, J. J., Ray, S. G., Abdullah, I., Dargie, H. J. & Morton, J. J. (1992) Plasma endothelin in chronic heart failure. *Circulation*, **85**, 1374–1379.
92. Rodeheffer, R. J., Lerman, A., Heublein, D. M. & Burnett, J. C. J. (1992) Increased plasma concentrations of endothelin in congestive heart failure in humans. *Mayo Clin Proc*, **67**, 719–724.
93. Lerman, A., Kubo, S. H., Tschumperlin, L. K. & Burnett, J. C. J. (1992) Plasma endothelin concentrations in humans with end-stage heart failure and after heart transplantation. *J Am Coll Cardiol*, **20**, 849–853.
94. Pacher, R., Bergler, Klein, J., Globits, S., Teufelsbauer, H., Schuller, M., Krauter, A., Ogris, E., Rodler, S., Wutte, M. & Hartter, E. (1993) Plasma big endothelin-1 concentrations in congestive heart failure patients with or without systemic hypertension. *Am J Cardiol*, **71**, 1293–1299.
95. Tsuchiya, K., Naruse, M., Sanaka, T., Naruse, K., Kato, Y., Zeng, Z. P., Nitta, K., Shizume, K., Demura, H. & Sugino, N. (1990) Effects of endothelin on renal hemodynamics and excretory functions in anesthetized dogs. *Life Sci*, **46**, 59–65.
96. Vierhapper, H., Wagner, O., Nowotny, P. & Waldhausl, W. (1990) Effect of endothelin-1 in man. *Circulation*, **18**, 1415–1418.
97. Lerman, A., Hildebrand, F. L., Aarhus, L. L. & Burnett, J. C. (1990) Endothelin is a vasoconstrictor at physiologic concentration. *Am J Hypertens*, **3 (Suppl A)**, 97A.
98. Loffler, B. M., Roux, S., Kalina, B., Clozel, M. & Clozel, J. P. (1993) Influence of congestive heart failure on endothelin levels and receptors in rabbits. *J Mol Cell Cardiol*, **25**, 407–416.
99. Fu, L. X., Sun, X. Y., Hedner, T., Feng, Q. P., Liang, Q. M., Hoebeke, J. & Hjalmarson, A. (1993) Decreased density of mesenteric arteries but not of myocardial endothelin receptors and function in rats which chronic ischemic heart failure. *J Cardiovasc Pharmacol*, **22**, 177–182.
100. Masaki, T., Kimura, S., Yanagisawa, M. & Goto, K. (1991) Molecular and cellular mechanism of endothelin regulation. Implications for vascular function. *Circulation*, **84**, 1457–1468.
101. Emori, T., Hirata, Y., Ohta, K., Shichiri, M. & Marumo, F. (1989) Secretory mechanism of immunoreactive endothelin in cultured bovine endothelial cells. *Biochem Biophys Res Commun*, **160**, 93–100.

102. Hieda, H. S. & Gomez Sanchez, C. E. (1990) Hypoxia increases endothelin release in bovine endothelial cells in culture, but epinephrine, norepinephrine, serotonin, histamine and angiotensin II do not. *Life Sci*, **47**, 247–251.
103. Shirakami, G., Nakao, K., Saito, Y., Magaribuchi, T., Jougasaki, M., Mukoyama, M., Arai, H., Hosoda, K., Suga, S., Ogawa, Y. et al. (1991) Acute pulmonary alveolar hypoxia increases lung and plasma endothelin-1 levels in conscious rats. *Life Sci*, **48**, 969–976.
104. Weber, K. T., Anversa, P., Armstrong, P. W., Brilla, C. G., Burnett, J. C., Jr., Cruickshank, J. M., Devereux, R. B., Giles, T. D., Korsgaard, N., Leier, C. V. et al. (1992) Remodeling and reparation of the cardiovascular system. *J Am Coll Cardiol*, **20**, 3–16.
105. Zimmerman, R. S., Martinez, A. J., Maymind, M. & Barbee, R. W. (1992) Effect of endothelin on plasma volume and albumin escape. *Circ Res*, **70**, 1027–1034.
106. Zimmerman, R. S., Maymind, M. & Barbee, R. W. (1992) The role of endothelin in hemorrhagic shock. *Am J Hypertens*, **5**, 102A.
107. Zimmerman, R. S. (1992) A potential role for endothelin in congestive heart failure. *Mayo Clin Proc*, **67**, 801–803.
108. Haas, G. J., Wooding-Scott, M., Binkley, P. F., Myerowitz, P. D., Kelley, R. & Cody, R. J. (1993) Effects of successful cardiac transplantation on plasma endothelin. *Am J Cardiol*, **71**, 237–240.
109. Heck, C. F., Shumway, S. J. & Kaye, M. P. (1989) The Registry of the International Society for Heart Transplantation: sixth official report 1989. *J Heart Transplant*, **8**, 271–276.
110. Myers, B. D., Ross, J., Newton, L., Luetscher, J. & Perlroth, M. (1984) Cyclosporine-associated chronic nephropathy. *N Engl J Med*, **311**, 699–705.
111. Olivari, M. T., Antolick, A. & Ring, W. S. (1989) Arterial hypertension in heart transplant recipients treated with triple-drug immunosuppressive therapy. *J Heart Transplant*, **8**, 34–39.
112. Zoja, C., Furci, L., Ghilardi, F., Zilio, P., Benigni, A. & Remuzzi, G. (1986) Cyclosporine induced endothelial cell injury. *Lab Invest*, **55**, 455–462.
113. Lau, D. E. W., Wong, H. L. & Hwang, W. S. (1989) Cyclosporine toxicity on cultured rat microvascular endothelial cells. *Kidney Int*, **35**, 604–613.
114. Benigni, A., Perico, N., Ladny, J. R., Imberti, O., Bellizzi, L. & Remuzzi, G. (1991) Increased urinary excretion of endothelin-1 and its precursor, big-endothelin-1, in rats chronically treated with cyclosporine. *Transplantation*, **52**, 175–177.
115. Kon, V., Sugiura, M., Inagami, T., Harvie, B. R., Ichikawa, I & Hoover, R. L. (1990) Role of endothelin in cyclosporine-induced glomerular dysfunction. *Kidney Int*, **37**, 1487–1491.
116. Edwards, B. S., Hunt, S. A., Fowler, M. B., Valantine, H. A., Anderson, L. M. & Lerman, A. (1991) Effect of cyclosporine on plasma endothelin levels in humans after cardiac transplantation. *Ann J Cardiol*, **67**, 782–784.
117. Hori, S., Kyotani, S., Inoue, S., Fukuda, K., Ohnishi, Y., Kusuhara, M., Aikawa, N., Yamaguchi, K., Nakamura, Y. & Handa, S. (1991) Subepicardial microischemia formation induced by epicardial application of endothelin-1. *J Cardiovasc Pharmacol*, **17 (Suppl 7)**, S300–S301.
118. Homma, S., Miyauchi, T., Goto, K., Sugishita, Y., Sato, M. & Ohshima, N. (1991) Effects of endothelin-1 on coronary microcirculation in isolated beating hearts of rats. *J Cardiovasc Pharmacol*, **17 (Suppl 7)**, S276–S278.
119. Tsunetoshi, T., Otsuka, A., Mikami, H., Katahira, K., Moriguchi, A. & Ogihara, T. (1991) Effect of cromakalim (BRL 34915) on hemodynamic and electrocardiographic changes induced by endothelin in dogs. *Basic Res Cardiol*, **86**, 49–55.
120. Harada, K., Miwa, A., Kaneta, S., Izawa, T., Fukushima, H. & Ogawa, N. (1993) Effects of KRN2391, nicorandil and diltiazem on the changes in the electrocardiogram caused by endothelin-1 in anaesthetized rats. *Br J Pharmacol*, **109**, 679–684.
121. Cocks, T. M., Broughton, A., Dib, M., Sudhir, K. & Angus, J. A. (1989) Endothelin is blood vessel selective: studies on a variety of human and dog vessels *in vitro* and on regional blood flow in the conscious rabbit. *Clin Exp Pharmacol Physiol*, **16**, 243–246.
122. Franco Cereceda, A. (1989) Endothelin- and neuropeptide Y-induced vasoconstriction of human epicardial coronary arteries *in vitro*. *Br J Pharmacol*, **97**, 968–972.
123. Chester, A. H., O'Neil, G. S., Allen, S. P., Luu, T. N., Tadjkarimi, S. & Yacoub, M. H. (1992) Effect of endothelin on normal and diseased human coronary arteries. *Eur J Clin Invest*, **22**, 210–213.
124. Wang, J., Zeballos, G. A., Kaley, G. & Hintze, T. H. (1991) Dilation and constriction of large coronary arteries in conscious dogs by endothelin. *Am J Physiol*, **261**, H1379–H1386.
125. Clozel, J. P. & Clozel, M. (1989) Effects of endothelin on the coronary vascular bed in open-chest dogs. *Circ Res*, **65**, 1193–1200.
126. Hom, G. J., Touhey, B. & Rubanyi, G. M. (1992) Effects of intracoronary administration of endothelin in anesthetized dogs: comparison with Bay k 8644 and U 46619. *J Cardiovasc Pharmacol*, **19**, 194–200.

127. Haynes, W. G., Davenport, A. P. & Webb, D. J. (1993) Endothelin: progress in pharmacology and physiology. *Trends Pharmacol Sci*, **14**, 225–228.
128. Pernow, J. & Modin, A. (1993) Endothelial regulation of coronary vescular tone *in vitro* – contribution of endothelin receptor subtypes and nitric oxide. *Eur J Pharmacol*, **243**, 281–286.
129. Teerlink, J. R., Breu, V., Sprecher, U., Clozel, M. & Clozel, J. (1994) Potent vasoconstriction mediated by endothelin ET_B receptors in canine coronary arteries. *Circ Res*, **74**, 105–114.
130. Tahara, A., Kohno, M., Yanagi, S., Itagane, H., Toda, I., Akioka, K., Teragaki, M., Yasuda, M., Takeuchi, K. & Takeda, T. (1991) Circulating immunoreactive endothelin in patients undergoing percutaneous transluminal coronary angioplasty. *Metabolism*, **40**, 1235–1237.
131. Ameli, S., Kaul, S., Castro, L., Arora, C., Mirea, A. & Shah, P. K. (1993) Effect of percutaneous transluminal coronary angioplasty on circulating endothelin levels. *Am J Cardiol*, **72**, 1352–1356.
132. Zimmerman, R. S., Martinez, A. J., MacPhee, A. A. & Barbee, R. W. (1990) Atrial natriuretic factor blocks the pressor action of endothelin. *J Cardiovasc Pharmacol*, **16**, 865–870.
133. Saijonmaa, O., Ristimaki, A. & Fyhrquist, F. (1990) Atrial natriuretic peptide, nitroglycerine, and nitroprusside reduce basal and stimulated endothelin production from cultured endothelial cells. *Biochem Biophys Res Commun*, **173**, 514–520.
134. Opgenorth, T. J. & Novosad, E. I. (1990) Atrial natriuretic factor and endothelin interactions in control of vascular tone. *Eur J Pharmacol*, **191**, 351–357.
135. Chmielk, Z., Pszona, B., Dabrowski, M., Witkowski, A. & Ruzyö, W. (1993) Percutaneous coronary angioplasty and levels of endothelin-1 in blood. *Kardiol Pol*, **39**, 252–6; discussion 256–7.
136. Kaul, S., Ameli, S., Arora, C., Castro, L., Mirea, A. & Shah, P. K. (1991) Does PTCA increase circulating endothelin level in man? *Circulation*, **84**, II–726.
137. Ryan, T. J., Vekshtein, V. I., Yeung, A. C., Bittl, J. A., Selwyn, A. P. & Ganz, P. (1991) The role of endothelin-1 in coronary vasoconstriction following balloon angioplasty. *Eur Heart J*, **12**, 160.
138. Spielberg, C., Schwenn, K., Hensen, J. & Linderer, T. (1991) Endothelin levels in the coronary sinus during PTCA of the left descending coronary artery. *Circulation*, **84**, II–726.
139. Miyauchi, T., Doi, T., Suzuki, N., Kakihana, M., Yamaguchi, I., Sugishita, Y., Mitsui, T., Hori, M., Masaki, T. & Goto, K. (1992) Plasma endothelin-1 concentrations in the coronary sinus in dogs with artificially induced myocardial infarction. *Peptides*, **13**, 1013–1015.
140. Stewart, J. T., Nisbet, J. A., & Davies, M. J. (1991) Plasma endothelin in coronary venous blood from patients with either stable or unstable angina. *Br Heart J*, **66**, 7–9.
141. Stewart, D. J., Kubac, G., Costello, K. B. & Cernacek, P. (1991) Increased plasma endothelin-1 in the early hours of acute myocardial infarction. *J Am Coll Cardiol*, **18**, 38–43.
142. Ray, S. G., McMurray, J. J., Morton, J. J. & Dargie, H. J. (1992) Circulating endothelin in acute ischaemic syndromes. *Br Heart J*, **67**, 383–386.
143. Yasuda, M., Kohno, M., Tahara, A., Itagane, H., Toda, I., Akioka, K., Teragaki, M., Oku, H., Takeuchi, K. & Takeda, T. (1990) Circulating immunoreactive endothelin in ischemic heart disease. *Am Heart J*, **119**, 801–806.
144. Lechleitner, P., Genser, N., Mair, J., Maier, J., Artner Dworzak, E., Dienstl, F. & Puschendorf, B. (1993) Plasma immunoreactive endothelin in the acute and subacute phases of myocardial infarction in patients undergoing fibrinolysis. *Clin Chem*, **39**, 955–959.
145. Lechleitner, P., Genser, N., Mair, J., Maier, J., Artner Dworzak, E., Dienstl, F. & Puschendorf, B. (1992) Endothelin-1 in patients with complicated and uncomplicated myocardial infarction. *Clin Investig*, **70**, 1070–1072.
146. Naruse, M., Kawana, M., Hifumi, S., Naruse, K., Yoshihara, I., Oka, T., Monzen, C., Kurimoto, F., Ohsumi, K. *et al.* (1991) Plasma immunoreactive endothelin, but not thrombomodulin, is increased in patients with essential hypertension and ischemic heart disease. *J Cardiovasc Pharmacol*, **17 (Suppl 7)**, S471–S474.
147. Tsuji, S., Sawamura, A., Watanabe, H., Takihara, K., Park, S. E. & Azuma, J. (1991) Plasma endothelin levels during myocardial ischemia and reperfusion. *Life Sci*, **48**, 1745–1749.
148. Tonnessen, T., Naess, P. A., Kirkeboen, K. A., Offstad, J., Ilebekk, A. & Christensen, G. (1993) Release of endothelin from the porcine heart after short term coronary artery occlusion. *Cardiovasc Res*, **27**, 1482–1485.
149. Tonnessen, T., Naess, P. A., Kirkeboen, K. A., Ilebekk, A. & Christensen, G. (1993) Alterations in plasma endothelin during passage through the left heart chambers before and after brief myocardial ischemia. *Cardiovasc Res*, **27**, 2160–2163.
150. Kramer, B. K., Nishida, M., Kelly, R. A. & Smith, T. W. (1992) Endothelins. Myocardial actions of a new class of cytokines. *Circulation*, **85**, 350–356.
151. Watanabe, T., Suzuki, N., Shimamoto, N., Fujino, M. & Imada, A. (1990) Endothelin in myocardial infarction. *Nature*, **344**, 114.
152. Nambi, P., Pullen, M., Egan, J. W. & Smith, E. F. (1991) Identification of cardiac endothelin binding

sites in rats: downregulation of left atrial endothelin binding sites in response to myocardial infarction. *Pharmacology*, **43**, 84–89.
153. Dauber, I. M., Vanbenthuysen, K. M., McMurtry, I. F. et al. (1990) Functional coronary microvascular injury evident as increased permeability due to brief ischemia and reperfusion. *Circ Res*, **66**, 986–998.
154. Yosizumi, M., Kurihara, H., Sugiyama, T., Takaku, F., Yanagisawa, M., Masaki, T. & Yazaki, Y. (1989) Hemodynamic shear stress stimulates endothelin production by cultured endothelial cells. *Biochem Biophys Res Commun*, **161**, 859–864.
155. Matsuyama, K., Yasue, H., Okumura, K., Saito, Y., Nakao, K., Shirakami, G. & Imura, H. (1991) Increased plasma level of endothelin-1-like immunoreactivity during coronary spasm in patients with coronary spastic angina. *Am J Cardiol*, **68**, 991–995.
156. Toyo-oka, T., Aizawa, T., Suzuki, N., Hirata, Y., Miyauchi, T., Shin, W. S., Yanagisawa, M., Masaki, T. & Sugimoto, T. (1991) Increased plasma level of endothelin-1 and coronary spasm induction in patients with vasospastic angina pectoris. *Circulation*, **83**, 476–483.
157. Pittet, J. F., Morel, D. R., Hemsen, A., Gunning, K., Lacroix, J. S., Suter, P. M. & Lundberg, J. M. (1991) Elevated plasma endothelin-1 concentrations are associated with the severity of illness in patients with sepsis. *Ann Surg*, **213**, 261–264.
158. Kurihara, H., Yoshizumi, M., Sugiyama, T., Takaku, F., Yanagisawa, M., Masaki, T., Hamaoki, M., Kato, H. & Yazaki, Y. (1989) Transforming growth factor-beta stimulates the expression of endothelin mRNA by vascular endothelial cells. *Biochem Biophys Res Commun*, **159**, 1435–1440.
159. Tomoda, H. (1993) Coronary thrombolysis and endothelin-1 release. *Angiology*, **44**, 441–446.
160. Vane, J. R., Anggard, E. E. & Botting, R. M. (1990) Mechanisms of disease: regulatory functions of the vascular endothelium. *N Engl J Med*, **323**, 27–36.
161. Hexum, T. D., Hoeger, C., Rivier, J. E., Baird, A. & Brown, M. R. (1990) Characterization of endothelin secretion by vascular endothelial cells. *Biochem Biophys Res Commun*, **167**, 294–300.
162. Kourembanas, S., Marsden, P. A., McQuillan, L. P. & Faller, D. V. (1991) Hypoxia induces endothelin gene expression and secretion in cultured human endothelium. *J Clin Invest*, **88**, 1054–1057.
163. Suzuki, T., Toyo-oka, T., Shin, W. S. & Sugimoto, T. (1991) Cell growth-dependent expression of endothelin-1 provocable Ca2+ channels in cloned vascular smooth muscle cells. *J Cardiovasc Pharmacol*, **17 (Suppl 7)**, S187–S189.
164. Watanabe, T., Suzuki, N., Shimamoto, N., Fujino, M. & Imada, A. (1991) Contribution of endogenous endothelin to the extension of myocardial infarct size in rats. *Circ Res*, **69**, 370–377.
165. Kaw, S., Hecker, M. & Vane, J. R. (1992) The two-step conversion of big endothelin-1 to endothelin 1 and degradation of endothelin 1 by subcellular fractions from human polymorphonuclear leukocytes. *Proc Natl Acad Sci USA*, **89**, 6886–6890.
166. Sessa, W. C., Kaw, S., Zembowicz, A., Anggard, E., Hecker, M. & Vane, J. R. (1991) Human polymorphonuclear leukocytes generate and degrade endothelin-1 by two distinct neutral proteases. *J Cardiovasc Pharmacol*, **17 (Suppl 7)**, S34–S38.
167. Wypij, D. M., Nichols, J. S., Novak, P. J., Stacy, D. L., Berman, J. & Wiseman, J. S. (1992) Role of mast cell chymase in the extracellular processing of big-endothelin-1 to endothelin-1 in the perfused rat lung. *Biochem Pharmacol*, **43**, 845–853.
168. Kloner, R. A., Giacomelli, F., Alker, K. J., Hale, S. L., Matthews, R. & Bellows, S. (1991) Influx of neutrophils into the walls of large epicardial coronary arteries in response to ischemia/reperfusion. *Circulation*, **84**, 1758–1772.
169. Uprichard, A., Chi, L. & Lucchesi, B. (1993) Functional consequence of big endothelin conversion: Demonstration with isolated neutrophils but not in a postinfarction model. *Pharmacology*, **47**, 277–285.
170. Grover, G. J., Sleph, P. G., Fox, M. & Trippodo, N. C. (1992) Role of endothelin-1 and big endothelin-1 in modulating coronary vascular tone, contractile function and severity of ischemia in rat hearts. *J Pharmacol Exp Ther*, **263**, 1074–1082.
171. Kinoshita, O., Yoshimi, H., Nagata, S., Ishikura, F., Kimura, K., Yamabe, T., Takagaki, K., Miyatake, K. & Omae, T. (1993) Rapid increase in plasma endothelin concentrations during percutaneous ballon dilatation of the mitral valve in patients with mitral stenosis. *Br Heart J*, **69**, 322–326.
172. Kambayashi, J., Sakon, M., Yokota, M., Shiba, E., Kawasaki, T. & Mori, T. (1990) Activation of coagulation and fibrinolysis during surgery, analyzed by molecular markers. *Thromb Res*, **60**, 157–167.
173. Onizuka, M., Miyauchi, T., Mitsui, K., Suzuki, N., Ueno, H., Goto, K., Masaki, T. & Hori, M. (1993) Plasma levels of endothelin-1 and thrombin-antithrombin III complex in patients undergoing open chest operations. *J Thorac Cardiovasc Surg*, **105**, 559–560.
174. Knothe, C. H., Boldt, J., Zickmann, B., Ballesteros, M., Dapper, F. & Hempelmann, G. (1992) Endothelin plasma levels in old and young patients during open heart surgery: Correlations to cardiopulmonary and endocrinology parameters. *J Cardiovasc Pharmacol*, **20**, 664–670.

14 Role of Endothelin in Regional Vascular System

Avadhesh C. Sharma and Anil Gulati

Department of Pharmaceutics and Pharmacodynamics (M/C 865), The University of Illinois at Chicago, 833 South Wood Street, Chicago, Illinois 60612-7231, USA

INTRODUCTION

Vasomotor tone regulates the overall cardiovascular system, and provides differential flow to regional vascular beds at times of normal stress (e.g. exercise) and physiological stress (e.g. congestive heart failure). Vascular tone permits abrupt and large shifts to vascular volume particularly during hemorrhage. Recently, extensive data has been generated which indicate that the vascular tone is regulated locally at the site of blood vessels. The control of vascular tone can be endothelium-dependent or endothelium-independent. Endothelium dependent regulation can involve a number of vasoactive substances acting simultaneously, in an independent or interdependent fashion[1,2]. Some substances are responsible for vasoconstrictor action (e.g. endothelin), while others are responsible for dilation of the blood vessels [e.g. prostaglandins (PGI_2) and endothelium derived relaxing factor (EDRF or nitric oxide (NO))]. This chapter will focus on the function of endothelin as a regulator of regional blood circulation.

The discovery of endothelin (ET), a 21-amino acid peptide, by Yanagisawa et al.[3] has helped in improving our knowledge about local regulation of vascular tone by blood vessels. ETs, a family of three structurally related peptides (ET-1, ET-2 and ET-3), have been demonstrated to be of potential significance in the regulation of circulation under physiological and pathological conditions. ETs are produced by cultured endothelial cells at a slow basal rate. Due to high vasoconstrictor potency and long lasting action, the continuous release of small amounts of ET from endothelial cells towards the underlying smooth muscle cells may contribute to the maintenance of vascular tone and blood pressure[4]. Under physiological conditions the basal tone maintained by ET was balanced by the release of EDRF[1] and other vasoactive agents.

ETs have been reported to possess both vasodilator and constrictor action. In particular ETs are found to be one of the most potent activators of vascular smooth muscle cells. ETs do not contribute to acute endothelium-dependent changes in the tension as they are not stored in endothelial cells. However, it has been found that removal of endothelium augments the ET-1-induced vasoconstriction, which suggests the release of a relaxing factor by ET-1 itself. In the isolated perfused mesenteric artery of rat[5] and perfused aorta of the rabbit, ET-1 and ET-3 release EDRF and ET-1 was found to be more potent than ET-3[6]. ETs act on two types of receptors, ET_A receptors, which have high affinity for ET-1 as compared to ET-3[7] and ET_B receptors, which have equal affinity for ET-1 and ET-3[8]. ET_A receptors have been demonstrated to be present on the smooth muscles[7], whereas, ET_B receptors were found on the endothelial cells[8]. Recently ET_B receptors have also been shown to be present on the vascular smooth muscles[9].

ET biosynthesis and release can be modulated by a number of vasoactive substances which contribute to homeostasis. In endothelial cells, NO inhibits the synthesis of ET[10]. The extent of ET-induced effects appear to be maintained by NO because during simultaneous stimulation of NO and ET, NO inhibits the production of ET[11]. Thrombin which causes endothelium-dependent relaxation has been found to have potent interaction with NO[12] and stimulates the biosynthesis and release of ETs[13]. Several vasoactive agents have been demonstrated to modulate thrombin-induced increase in ET biosynthesis. N^G-mono-metyl-L-arginine (L-NMMA), a NO inhibitor, has been demonstrated to stimulate the thrombin-induced production of ET from the porcine aorta. Superoxide dismutase, an oxygen free radical scavenger has been found to inhibit thrombin-induced ET production[14]. Besides, angiotensin II has also been found to activate the production of ETs[15]. Angiotensin II-induced ET gene expression in porcine aortic cell cultures and also from endothelial cells obtained from spontaneously hypertensive rats[3,16]. Angiotensis II has also shown to stimulate, though much weaker than other agents, the production of ETs and augments the vascular reactivity to ET-1[17]. Moreover, other agents like low density lipoproteins, inhibit the production of ETs in and cGMP independent mechanism indicating that NO interfers with ET biosynthesis. ETs have also been found to stimulate the production of eicosanoids, particularly, prostacyclin and thromboxane A_2 in isolated perfused kidney and spleen[18]. However, cyclooxygenase inhibitor, indomethacin, potentiates the ET-1 induced pressor responses suggesting a role for the prostanoids in the *in vivo* effects of ETs[19]. These potent interactions of ETs with both cGMP dependent and independent vasoactive agents in isolated organs as well as in endothelial cell cultures indicate the importance of ETs in the regulation of vascular tone, and suggest that ETs may play a key role in the maintenance of blood pressure and regional circulation *in vivo*.

ET MECHANISMS: ROLE IN SYSTEMIC HEMODYNAMICS

Intravenous injection of ET-1 causes an initial decrease in blood pressure followed by a prolonged pressor response[20] both in anesthetized, chemically denervated and in conscious rats[21-23]. ET administered intravenously, is eliminated promptly from the circulation with a half life of about 7 min. It disappears rapidly by means of first pass effect of the lungs and kidneys[24]. The hemodynamic responses of ET last for long duration, demonstrating a high affinity binding of ET to the receptors on the vascular smooth muscle cells, which finally internalize in the cells[25]. ET produces a dose-dependent increase in systemic vascular resistance and mean arterial blood pressure in several species including squirrel monkeys, dog, goats and rats[26-29]. The blood pressure responses to ET-1, administered intravenously in rats, were biphasic with an initial, transient decrease in blood pressure followed by a well sustained pressor response. These responses were dose-dependent and the pressor effect of ET-1 was due to an increase in the total peripheral resistance with no change in heart rate or cardiac output[30]. The hemodynamic effects of ET-1 and ET-3 assessed in conscious, Long Evans and Brattleboro (i.e. vasopressin-deficient) rats suggested that ET-3 produces pressor response in the systemic hemodynamics and causes initial hypotension and hindquarters vasodilation similar to that seen with ET-1. However, the subsequent pressor effects were demonstrated to be less marked with ET-3 in both strains of rat[31]. The systemic vasodilator responses to both (ET-1 and ET-3) peptides were reported to be independent of activation of muscarinic, β_2-adrenergic, cyclooxygenase products and platelet-activating factor, but involve contributions from EDRF or prostacyclin released by the endothelium[32], due to a stimulus provided by ET itself. Although ET-1 and ET-3 were initially reported as vasoconstrictor peptides, studies are available suggesting that ET-1 and ET-3 act differently in the systemic vascular beds. ET has been shown to produce a unique and potent systemic vasodilator activity in rabbits[33]. In another study, it was observed that lower dose of ET-1 (25 pmol/kg/min) produced an increase in mean arterial pressure which was completely blocked by higher dose of Cyclo(D-Asp-L-Pro-D-Val-L-Leu-D-Trp) (BQ-123) (0.25 mg/kg/min)[34]. These studies suggested the involvement of ET_A receptors in the maintenance of blood pressure in normal and anesthetized rats.

ET MECHANISMS: ROLE IN REGIONAL CIRCULATION

It is well known that ET receptors have wide spread distribution and are recognized as ET_A and ET_B receptors. ET receptors are found to be present both in the periphery and in the central nervous system[35-36]. However, it is still debatable, whether ETs produce similar vascular effects in the vascular beds of various organ systems. Vasoconstriction induced by ETs has been assessed in several isolated blood vessels including strips of rat aorta, cat basilar artery, rabbit and dog mesenteric arteries, and human mesentric and pulmonary arteries. The ET receptor specificity and selectivity of ET receptors subtypes in various blood vessels in distinct studies has been shown in Tables 14.1, 14.2 and 14.3.

Brain

ETs are known to be synthesized in the cerebral vessels[37]. ET-1 and ET-3 have been identified in neurones[38,39] and glia[40,41]. Binding sites for ETs are also found in the CNS neurones, glia and cerebrovascular smooth muscles[41-43]. It has been suggested that conversion of bigET-1 to ET-1 in the brain is essential for the expression of hemodynamic actions, and that a metalloprotease enzyme capable of converting bigET-1 to ET-1 is present in the rat brain[44].

Studies using *in vivo*, *in situ* and *in vivo* techniques have demonstrated that ET-1 is a potent vasoconstrictor of cerebral blood vessels and is capable of reducing the

Table 14.1 Response of ET agonists, antagonists and receptor specificity demonstrated in *in vitro* preparations in a variety of animal models. (+) = constriction, (−) = relaxation, (N) = not used, (---) = not specified, (B) = antagonizd, (NB) = not antagonized, P = partially antagonized

Vascular preparation/Species	ET agonists	Response	Antagonists	Receptor	References
Cerebral arteries					
(dog)	ET-1, ET-2, ET-3	+	N	---	Saito et al.[52]
(cat)	ET	+	N	---	Kauser et al.[53]
(goat)	RT-1	+	N	---	Dieguez et al.[28]
(human)	ET	+	N	---	Papadopoulos et al.[54]
Coronary artery					
(dog, hypoxic)	ET-1, ET-3, SRT6c	+	BO-123(NB)	non ET_A	Douglas et al.[55]
(human)	ET-1, ET-2, ET-3	+	N	---	Hemsen et al.[46]
(porcine)	ET-1, SRT6b	+	BQ-123(P)	ET_A/ET_B	Ihara et al.[57]
(goat)	ET-1	+	N	---	Dieguez et al.[28]
Pulmonary artery					
(rat)	ET-1	+	N	---	Itoh et al.[58]
(dog, hypoxic)	ET-1, ET-3, SRT6c	+	BQ-123(B)	ET_A	Douglas et al.[55]
(porcine)	SRT6b	−	N	ET_B	Saeki et al.[59]
(sheep)	ET	+	N	---	Toga et al.[60]
(guinea pig)	ET-1, ET-2	+	FR139317(B)	ET_A	Cardell et al.[61]
Pulmonary vein					
(sheep)	ET	+	N	---	Toga et al.[60]
Carotid artery					
(rat)	ET-1	−	BQ-123(NB)	non ET_A	Douglas et al.[62]
Aorta					
(rat, SHR)	ET-1	+	N	---	Cargnelli et al.[63]
(rat)	SRT6b		N	ET_B	Watanabe et al.[64]
(rat)	ET-1,	−	IRL1038(B)	ET_A	Karaki et al.[65,66]
(rabbit)	AgII	+	BQ-123(B)	---	Webb et al.[67]
(guinea pig)	ET-1	+	BQ-123(B)	ET_A	Hay et al.[70]
Saphenous vein					
(rabbit)	ET-1, SRT6b	+	N	non ET_A	Moreland et al.[68]
(human)	ET-1, SRT6b	+	BQ-123(NB)	non ET_A	Bax et al.[69]
Jugular vein					
(rabbit)	ET-1, ET-3, [Ala^{1,3,11,15}]ET-1	+	BQ-123(NB)	ET_A/ET_B	Sumner et al.[9]
Mesenteric arteries (SHR)	ET-1	+	N	---	Dohi et al.[71]
Cutaneous and ear arteries					
(rabbit)	ET-1	+	N	---	Monge et al.[72]

cerebral blood flow[41-49]. The vasoconstrictor effects implicate ET-1 as an important mediator of cerebral vasospasm and/or post-ischemic hypoperfusion[50]. ET-1 induced a potent cerebral vasoconstriction *in vivo* probably by acting directly on vascular musculature. This vasoconstriction was found to be attenuated during hypercapnia and hypertension but was potentiated during hypotension[28,51]. ET-1 (25 μl; 10^{-7}–10^{-4} M), when applied to adventitial surface of middle cerebral artery produced a severe dose-dependent reduction in the cerebral blood flow[48]. Application of ET-1 over the middle cerebral artery caused dose-dependent ischemic brain damage suggesting the role of ET in the pathogenesis of cerebral ischemia[49]. In another study carried out in

Table 14.2 Response of ET agonists, antagonists and receptor specificity demonstrated in a variety of *in vivo* animal models. (+) = constriction, (−) = relaxation, (N) = not used, (- - -) = not specified, (NB) = not antagonized

In vivo models/Species	ET agonists	Response	Antagonists	Receptor	References
Cerebral vasculature					
(dog)	ET-1	+	N	- - -	Willette et al.[50]
(cat, dog)	ET	+	N	- - -	Mima et al.[73]
(goat)	ET-1	+	N	- - -	Salom et al.[74]
Basilar artery					
(dog)	ET-1	+	N	- - -	Yamaura et al.[75]
Coronary vascular bed					
(dog, hypoxic)	ET-1,ET-3	+	N	- - -	Clozel and Clozel[27]
Pulmonary circulation					
(human)	ET-1	+	N	non ET$_A$	Wagner et al.[76]
Mesenteric bed					
(rat)	ET-1	+	BQ-123(NB)	- - -	Douglas et al.[55]
Hepatic microcirculation					
(rats)	ET-1, ET-3	+	BQ-123(NB)	non ET$_A$	Kurihara et al.[77,78]
Splanchnic					
(monkeys)	ET-1	+	N	- - -	Clozel and Clozel[26]
(human)	ET-1	+	N		Wagner et al.[76]
Renal Vasculature					
(rat)	ET-1	+	N	- - -	Lippton et al.[79]

Table 14.3 Response of ET agonists, antagonists and receptor specificity demonstrated using ligand binding, mRNA determination and related techniques in a variety of animal models. (N) = not used, (- - -) = not specified

Region (binding/mRNA studies)	Agonists	Antagonists	Receptors	References
Brain capillary endothelial calls (rats)	ET-1	BQ-123	ET$_A$	Vigne et al.[80]
Vascular smooth muscle cells	ET-1	BQ-123	ET$_A$	Eguchi et al.[81]
(rats)	ET-1	FR139317	ET$_A$	Sogabe et al.[82]
Aorta (rabbit)	ET-1	FR139317	ET$_A$	Sogabe et al.[82]
Basilar smooth muscle cells	ET-1, ET-2 & ET-3	N	- - -	Takenaka et al.[83]
Kidney arcuate artery	ET-1	N	ET$_A$	Tereda et al.[35]
Kidney (human)	ET-1 BQ3020	BQ-123	Predominantly ET$_B$	Karet et al.[84]
Saphenous Vein (rabbit)	ET-1, ET-3 & SRT6c	- - -	70% ET$_A$ and 30% ET$_B$	Webb et al.[85]

goats, injection of ET-1 directly into the cerebral circulation decreased cerebral blood flow and increased cerebrovascular resistance in a dose-dependent manner[51]. Infusion of calcium channel blocker, nicardipine, attenuated the ET-1-induced reductions in cerebral blood flow. These observations suggested that ET-1 reduces cerebral blood flow due to constriction of cerebral arteries by a direct action on smooth muscle. The cerebral vasoconstriction appears to be modulated by the endothelium and depends partially on the activation of Ca^{2+} influx through the dihydropyridine-sensitive channels[74]. ET_A receptor antagonists BQ-485 and FR-139317, have been found to reverse the narrowing of basilar artery in experimental vasospasm model in animals[86,87]. Clozel and Watanabe[88] suggested that BQ-123 does not cross blood brain barrier because it prevented the early cerebral vasospasm during subarachnoid hemorrhage following intracisternal but not when administered intravenously to rats. The ability ETs to markedly reduce cerebral blood flow, may cause severe brain damage implicating this peptide in the cerebrovascular sequelae and neuronal injury associated with subarachnoid hemorrhage, ischemic stroke and related cerebrovascular disorders.

Heart

ET-1 (1 nM) when infused intravenously into anaesthetized open-chest rabbits decreased the myocardial contractile force[89]. ET-1 increased coronary blood flow due to either an increase in cardiac output, redistribution of cardiac output or both[29,30]. In isolated rat heart, ET-1 causes marked and long-lasting constriction of coronary blood vessels. The effect is not influenced by sympathetic or Ca^{2+}-channel blockade, is enhanced by inhibiting prostaglandin synthesis, and is reduced by angiotensin converting enzyme inhibition[90]. Other studies have demonstrated that ET-1 produces coronary vasoconstriction *in vivo* and *in vitro* by acting directly on vascular musculature in goats[28]. Clozel and Clozel[27] observed the coronary vasoconstrictor effect of ET-1, with a selective effect on the subepicardium and suggested that at least part of the increase in the coronary vascular resistance is due to constriction of the large coronary arteries in dogs. The existence of both ET_A and ET_B receptors have been found to mediate coronary vasoconstriction. It is observed that constriction of large conduit arteries in dogs is regulated through ET_A receptors and constriction of coronary vascular bed involves ET_A and ET_B receptors in dogs and rat[91]. Pernow and Modin[92] studied the functional effects of ET-1, ET-3 and ET_B agonist, [Ala^{1,3,11,15}]ET-1 on the porcine coronary arteries, and indicated that ET-1 induced contraction was reversed by BQ-123 suggesting that the contractile response is mediated through ET_A receptors. It has been shown that ET_B receptor mediated responses are modulated by NO suggesting both ET_A and ET_B receptors mediate coronary contractions[92]. In human coronary arteries and ventricular and atrial muscles using autoradiographic technique, it was found that ET_A and ET_B receptor binding sites are present in these tissues. However, these investigators demonstrated that sarafotoxin-6b, a structurally related peptide, binds to a non ET_A and non ET_B binding site with a high affinity for BQ-123 and ET_B agonist[69].

Gastrointestinal tract

ET analogues produced sustained and potent vasoconstriction of gastric vasculature[93]. ET-1 (0.01–1 nmol/kg/min) administration to rabbits produced severe vasoconstriction of the gastrointestinal tract (stomach and colon), which may contribute to the induction of the gastric damage[29]. Sirois *et al.*[94] suggested that the effect of ET-1 on vascular permeability, in specific vascular beds including stomach, duodenum is partly mediated and/or modulated by the secondary release of TXA_2, whereas its action on arterial blood pressure appears to be independent of prostanoid release in conscious rats[94]. Infusion of ET-1 reduced blood flow in the isolated perfused rat stomach[95]. ET-1 (0.1 and 1 nmol/kg) increased dose-dependently vascular permeability in the stomach and duodenum (up to 240%) as measured by the extravazation of Evans blue dye[96]. The highest dose of ET-3 induces hemorrhagic gastric mucosal lesions, periods of hyper- and hypo-tension and mortality in the rat. Medium and low doses of ET-3 caused vascular injury, and dose-dependently potentiated the vascular and hemorrhagic mucosal lesions caused by dilute HCl and ethanol[97]. ET-3 causes endothelial damage in the capillaries and venules of rat stomach and predisposes it to mucosal damage even after exposure to dilute ethanol or HCl. ET is more potent than leukotrienes and histamine in this effect and thus may play an important role in the mechanism of acute gastric mucosal injury and protection where the vascular network appears to be a major target[97]. Gastric mucous cell cultures have been reported to secrete ET-1[98]. In another study, Masuda et al.[99] suggested that ethanol may stimulate the release of ET from gastric vasculature and may cause gastric ischemia due to vasoconstriction resulting in acute gastric mucosal injury.

Liver

ET is a potent agonist in the liver eliciting both a sustained vasoconstriction of the hepatic vasculature and a significant increase in hepatic glucose output[100]. ET-1 increased blood flow to the liver due to either an increase in cardiac output or redistribution of cardiac output or both[30]. ET-1 (0.01–0.1 nmol/kg; i.v.) in rabbits showed a severe decrease in the hepatic arterial blood flow using the microsphere technique[89]. Using Laser doppler blood flow meter, Kurihara et al.[78] demonstrated that in rats ET-3-produced a greater decrease in the hepatic blood flow than ET-1. ET-3-induced decrease in hepatic blood flow was found to be inhibited by indomethacin and thromboxane synthetase inhibitor, OKY-046. These investigators suggested that ET-1 caused decrease in the hepatic blood flow due to the direct effect on hepatic blood vessels, while ET-3 produced its effect through TXA_2 receptors demonstrating an interaction between prostaglandins and ETs[78].

Renal circulation

The renal blood vessels have been observed to be about 10 times more sensitive to ET-1-induced vasoconstriction than other regions. ET-1 stimulates mesangial cell contraction via pharmaco-mechanical coupling and activates phospholipase A_2 to produce PGE_2, $PGF_{2\alpha}$, and TXB_2[101]. ET-1 also amplified β adrenergic-stimulated cAMP accumulation in a PGE_2-dependent mechanism[101]. ET-1 affects the renovascular permeability mediated and/or modulated by the secondary release of TXA_2, whereas its action on arterial blood pressure appears to be independent of prostanoid release in conscious rats[94,96]. Besides, ET inhibits the release of norepinephrine during a slight increase in renal nerve activity, while it does not affect α-adrenoceptor mediated vasoconstriction in the dog kidney[102]. Pollock and Opgenorth[34] reported that ET-1 induced renal vasoconstrictor effect was not affected by BQ-123. However in our study, we observed that ET-1 produced significant decrease in blood flow to the kidneys and increase in the regional vascular resistance of renal blood vessels, which could be partly blocked by BQ-123 (Fig. 14.2). These observations lead to the conclusion the ET-1-induced renovascular constriction may not be solely related to ET_A receptors. A study is available suggesting that ET affects renal blood flow, preferentially at the cortex[103]. Administration of ET (600 ng/kg/h) in the renal artery reduced ipsilateral renal excretion of water, sodium and potassium, and decreased the glomerular filtration rate and effective renal plasma flow in chronic hypoxic SHR rats, indicating that ET may play a role in the regulation of renal function[104]. Cirino et al.[105] reported that ET-1 caused transient vasodilator followed by a prolonged vasoconstrictor response in the renal blood vessels of rats. The pressor response was not mediated by a secondary release of either leukotriene D_4 or thromboxane A_2. This response, however, could be inhibited in a dose-dependent fashion by a selective ET_A antagonist, BQ-153 (cyclo-D-sulphalanine-L-Pro-D-Val-L-Leu-D-Trp). Following blockade by BQ-153 the vasodilator response and the residual pressor response were unaffected, suggesting that either one or both of these effects were mediated either through and ET_B or as yet undefined ET receptor[105].

BigET-1 may affect renal vascular resistance by a direct effect and following phosphoramidon-sensitive conversion to ET-2. The vasoconstrictor effect of bigET-1 might be expressed during the conversion of bigET to mature ET. Metalloproteases are also involved in degradation of ET and this could be another mechanism responsible for the potentiation of in vivo effects of ET-1 by phosphoramidon[106]. Infusion of ET-specific antibodies into SHR rats decreased mean arterial pressure by approximately 10% and increased renal vascular resistance by approximately 35%. Glomerular filtration rate and renal plasma flow both increased by approximately 50% over control suggesting that ET plays an important role in the modulation of systemic blood pressure and renal function in genetic hypertension[107]. ET-1 has a short half-life with very high regional plasma clearance, which limits detection of its overflow into the systemic circulation. However, the release of ET-1 reaching vasoconstrictor levels seems to occur during circulatory changes in the newborn and in septic shock[108]. Pretreatment with N^G-nitro-L-arginine (L-NNA) abolished the ET-3 induced renal vasodilation. Renal blood flow decreased immediately after the start of ET-3 infusion into animals treated with L-NNA. ET-3 acts as a diuretic and renal vasodilator peptide, the vascular effects of which may be mediated through the production of endothelial NO in the kidney[109]. Endogenous ET may contribute to the adaptive modulation of sodium excretion by a renal tubular action, and of renin release in association with a change in sodium balance[110]. The renal vasoconstrictor action, but not the tubular action of ET is functionally coupled with the activation of dihydropyridine-sensitive calcium channels[111]. Infusion of ET-1 (120 pmol/h) to conscious, Long Evans and Brattleboro rats caused progressive hypertension and vasoconstriction of renal vascular bed[31]. In a study on human subjects, when ET-1 was infused intravenously in a dose of 4 pmol/kg/min for 20 min, the mean arterial blood pressure increased, while splanchnic and renal blood flows were reduced, which returned to basal values after about 1 hr in the splanchnic and about 3 hrs in the kidneys[112]. ET-1-induced vasoconstriction in the kidney was attenuated by nifedipine (100 µg/kg) in rats[113,114]. ET-1 causes a dose-dependent vasoconstriction in several vascular beds with a more pronounced effect on the renal circulation[113]. Infusion of the higher dose of ET-2 or sarafotoxin 6b produced an increase in mean blood pressure along with constriction in the renal, mesenteric, and hindquarter vascular beds. It was found that sarafotoxin 6b is more potent than ET-2 for vasodilator response *in vivo*; despite this, sarafotoxin 6b also exerts a more marked vasoconstrictor effect than ET-2[115]. Bolus intravenous injections of ET-1 produce elevation in the plasma renin, aldosterone, adrenocorticotropic hormone, cortisol, catecholamine and arginine vasopressin in a dose-dependent manner[116]. In another study, it has been suggested that unlike other human tissues, kidney contains predominantly ET_B receptors[84] (Table 14.3). Above studies provide sufficient evidence for the potent renal vasoconstrictor action of ET. Besides, ET is also an important regulator of renal functions and may be involved in the pathophysiology of renovascular disorders.

ET RECEPTORS IN THE REGULATION OF SYSTEMIC HEMODYNAMICS AND REGIONAL CIRCULATION

ET-1 is believed to be mainly involved in the regulation of regional blood flow as vasoconstrictors of peripheral vessels. It can also modulate and balance the vasodilator action of nitric oxide and prostacyclin since all of them are produced by the endothelial cells[117]. BQ-123 antagonizes ET-1 induced contraction of porcine isolated coronary artery strips and has greater affinity for ET_A receptros in porcine aortic smooth muscle than for ET_B receptors[57]. However, plasma concentration of ET-1 is too low to maintain vascular tone[118] and ET_A antagonist, BQ-123, when injected intravenously to rats did not affect the basal blood pressure[57], reinforcing that circulating ET-1 is not a major factor in the maintenance of vascular tone. Several factors have been suggested to stimulate the production of ET-1 in endothelial cells which is released on the basal side of the endothelium and acts upon the underlying smooth muscles to produce vasoconstriction[119,120]. ET-1 might therefore be participating in the maintenance of blood flow of peripheral small resistance vessels in a paracrine manner[32].

We investigated the effect of BQ-123, a specific ET_A receptor antagonist, on the regional circulatory and systemic hemodynamic changes induced by ET-1 (250 ng/kg/min i.v.) in male Sprague-Dawley rats, using a radioactive microsphere technique[121–123]. ET-1 (250 ng/kg/min) produced a significant increase in blood pressure and decrease in cardiac output and stroke volume. Total peripheral resistance was also found to increase significantly. Pretreatment with BQ-123 did not affect the increase in blood pressure, but blocked the decrease in cardiac output, stroke volume and increase in total peripheral resistance induced by ET-1 (Figure 14.1).

Coronary blood flow was found to increase (28 ± 8%) after 15 minute of administration of ET-1 followed by decrease (−45 ± 11%) at 45 min. The hepatic blood flow increased (32 ± 7%) at 15 min followed by decrease (−50 ± 11%) at 45 min. A significant decrease in blood flow to the kidneys, GIT, skin and musculoskeletal system was observed following ET-1 infusion. Cerebral blood flow was not affected except at 45 min of infusion when a decrease in blood flow (−36 ± 6%) was observed. An increase in the vascular resistance was observed in the coronary vascular bed, kidneys, GIT and musculo-skeletal system. However, no change in the vascular resistance was observed in the cerebral and hepatic blood vessels. (Figure 14.2).

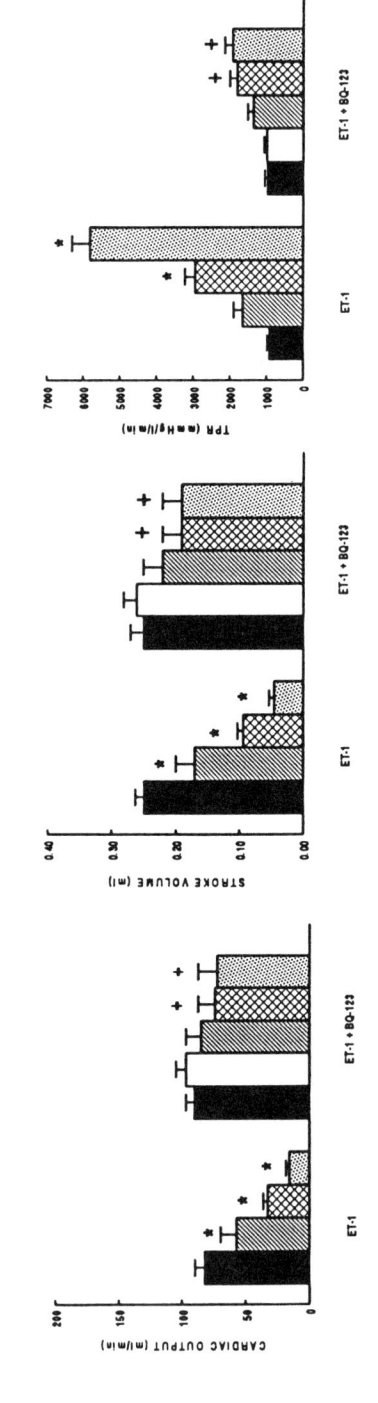

Figure 14.1. Effect of intravenous infusion of ET-1 (250 ng/kg/min) on systemic hemodynamics at 15, 30 and 45 min of control and BQ-123 treated rats. BQ-123 (5 mg/kg/h) infusion was started 15 min prior to ET-1 administration and continued till the end of experiment. *Indicates significantly different compared to baseline and + indicates significantly different compared to control.

Regional vascular system 225

Figure 14.2. Effect of intravenous infusion of ET-1 (250 ng/kg/min) on percent change in regional blood flow and vascular resistance at 15, 30 and 45 min of control and BQ-123 treated rats. BQ-123 (5 mg/kg/h) infusion was started 15 min prior to ET-1 administration and continued till the end of experiment. *Indicates significantly different compared to baseline and + indicates significantly different compared to control.

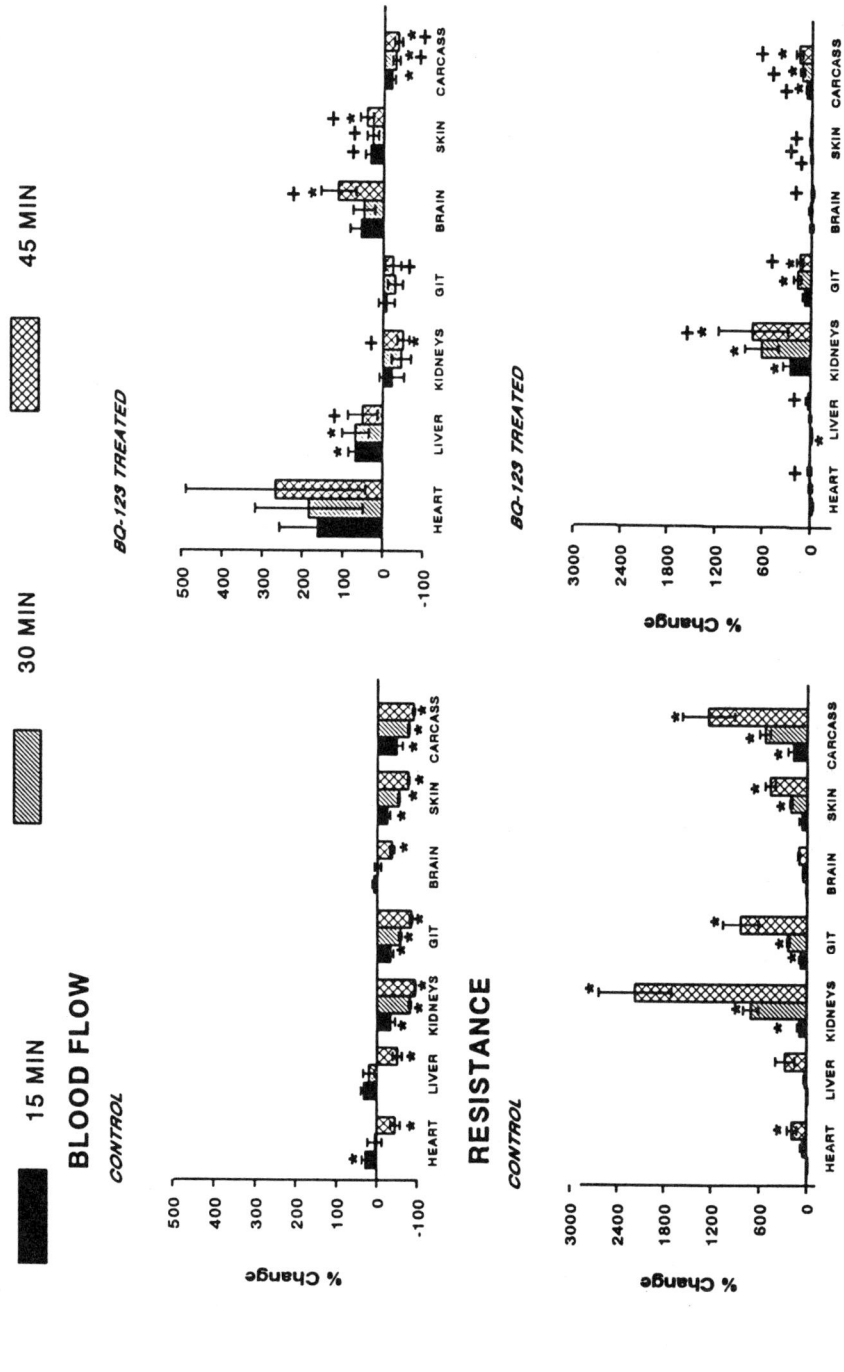

BQ-123 pretreatment blocked the decrease in blood flow induced by ET-1 to the kidneys, liver, GIT, brain, skin and musculo-skeletal system. ET-1 induced decrease in blood flow to the musculo-skeletal system was partially affected by BQ-123 pretreatment (Figure 14.2). ET-1 increased vascular resistance in the heart, kidneys, GIT, skin and musculo-skeletal system. BQ-123 pretreatment significantly attenuated the increase in vascular resistance induced by ET-1 in the heart, liver, kidneys, GIT, brain, skin and musculo-skeletal system. However, in some vascular beds the attenuation was more marked than in others (Figure 2). These observations are consistent with earlier studies suggesting that ET-1 produces markedly different effects on blood circulation in different regions[31,116,124-127].

The regional vascular effects of ET-1 encompassed widespread vasoconstriction (especially to the kidneys, GIT, liver, skin and musculo-skeletal system). ET-1 induced vasoconstriction to several regions has also been demonstrated by Hof et al.[29]. However, it has been suggested that ET-1 can cause either vasodilatation or vasoconstriction depending on the region[20,116]. It appears that higher concentrations of ET-1 lead to vasoconstriction due to a direct action on ET_A receptors located at the vascular smooth muscles. It is also possible that ETs can stimulate the release of vasodilators like prostacyclin and EDRF/NO[19]. EDRF/NO has also been reported to inhibit the release/synthesis of ET-1[10]. The influence of other vasoactive factors (like thrombin, arg-vasopressin, angiotensin II, oxyhemoglobin), which stimulate the production of ET-1[128] could also attribute to the differences in the responses of ET-1 in various vascular beds.

CONCLUSIONS AND FUTURE PROSPECTS

The potent and widespread vascular reactivity observed with ET has made it an important peptide which may be involved in the pathophysiology of several central and cardiovascular disorders. It is well established that ET causes regional blood flow alterations by acting on the smooth muscles of large and small blood vessels. However, *in vivo* studies related to regional circulatory effects of ET indicate that different vascular beds show variable responses to ET. Since, ET is one of the vasoactive agents released from endothelium, the role of ET in maintenance of vascular tone and its interaction with other vasoactive agens (e.g. EDRF/NO and thromboxanes and prostaglandins) has been emphasized in recent years. It appears that different vascular beds have different types of ET receptors. However, not enough studies have been performed to demonstrate the types of ET receptors in various vascular beds. Since several selective ET_A or ET_B receptor antagonists are now available, it is likely that the regional specificity of ET_A, ET_B or other types of ET receptors mediated vascular effects may be useful for the development of new therapeutic agents for the cardiovascular disorders.

Acknowledgements

The authors are grateful to Baxter Healthcare Corporation, Miles Incorporated and National Institutes of Health for providing research funds to our laboratory.

References

1. Vanhoutte, P. M., Auch-Schweik, W., Boulanger, C. M. (1989) Does endothelin-1 mediate endothelium dependent contractions during anoxia? *Journal of Cardiovascular Pharmacology*, (Suppl 5), **13**, S124–S128.
2. Vanhoutte, P. M. (1993) Other endothelium-derived vasoactive factors. *Circulation*, (Suppl V), **87**, V-9–V-17.
3. Yanagisawa, M., Kurihara, H., Kimura, S., Tomobe, Y., Kobayashi, M., Mitsui, Y. et al. (1988) A novel potent vasoconstrictor peptide produced by vascular endothelial cells. *Nature*, **332**, 411–415.
4. Rubanyi, G. M. (1992) Potential physiological and pathological significance of endothelins. *Drugs of Future*, **17**, 915–936.
5. Kitazumi, K., Shiba, T., Nishiki, K., Furukawa, Y., Takasaki, C., Tasaka, K. (1990) Vasodilator effects of sarafotoxins and endothelin-1 in spontaneously hypertensive rats and rat isolated perfused mesentery. *Biochemical Pharmacology*, **40**, 1843–1847.
6. Warner, T. F., Mitchell, J. A., de Nucci, G., Vane, J. R. (1989) Endothelin-1 and endothelin-3 release EDRF from isolated perfused arterial vessels of the rat and rabbit. *Journal of Cardiovascular Pharmacology (Suppl. 5)*, **13**, 85–88.
7. Arai, H., Hori, S., Aramori, I., Ohkubo, H., Nakanishi, S. (1990) Cloning and expression of a cDNA encoding an endothelin receptor. *Nature*, **348**, 730–732.
8. Sakurai, T., Yanagisawa, M., Takuwa, Y., Kimura, S., Goto, K., Masaki, T. (1990) Cloning of cDNA encoding a non-isopeptide-selective subtype of the endothelin receptor. *Nature*, **348**, 732–735.
9. Sumner, M. J., Cannon, T. R., Mundin, J. W., White, D. G., Watts, I. S. (1992) Endothelin ET_A and ET_B receptors mediate vascular smooth muscle contraction. *British Journal of Pharmacology*, **107**, 858–860.
10. Boulanger, C. M., Luscher, T. F. (1990) Release of endothelin from the porcine aorta: inhibition by endothelium-derived nitric oxide. *Journal of Clinical Investigation*, **252**, 587–590.
11. Luscher, T. F., Boulanger, C. M., Yang, Z., Noll, G., Dohi, Y. (1993) Interactions between endothelium-derived relaxing and contracting factors in health and cardiovascular disease. *Circulation (Suppl. 5)*, V-36–V-45.
12. Luscher, T. F., Diederich, D., Siebenmann, R., Lehmann, K., Stulz, P., von Segesser, L. et al. (1988) Differences between endothelium-dependent relaxation in arterial and in venous coronary bypass grafts, *New England Journal of Medicine*, **319**, 462–467.
13. Schini, V. B., Hendrickson, H., Heublein, D., Burnett, J. Jr., Vanhoutte, P. (1989) Thrombin enhances the release of endothelin-1 from cultured porcine aortic endothelial cells. *European Journal of Pharmacology*, **165**, 333–334.
14. Gryglewski, R. J., Palmer, R. M. J., Moncada, S. (1986) Superoxide anion is involved in the breakdown of endothelium-derived relaxing factor. *Nature*, **320**, 454–456.
15. Kohno, M., Yasunari, K., Yokokawa, K., Murakawa, K. I., Horio, T., Takeda, T. (1991) Inhibition by atrial and brain natriuretic peptides of endothelin-1 secretion after stimulation with angiotensin II and thrombin of cultured human endothelial cells. *Journal of Clinical Investigation*, **87**, 1999–2004.
16. Dohi, Y., Hahn, A. W. A., Boulanger, C. M., Buhler, F. R. Luscher, T. F. (1992) Endothelin stimulated by angiotensin-II augments contractility of spontaneously hypertensive rat resistance arteries. *Hypertension*, **19**, 131–137.
17. Sawamura, T., Lasuya, Y., Matshushita, Y., Suzuki, N., Shinmi, O., Kishi, N. et al. (1991) Phosphoramidon inhibits the intracellular conversion of big endothelin-1 to endothelin-1 in cultured endothelial cells. *Biochemical and Biophysical Research Communications*, **1741**, 779–784.
18. Rae, G. A., Trybulec, M., de Nucci, G., Vane, J. R. (1989) Endothelin-1 releases eicosanoids from rabbit isolated kidneys and spleen. *Journal of Cardiovascular Pharmacology*, (Suppl 5), **13**, 89–92.
19. deNucci, G., Thomas, R., D'orlians-Juste, P. E., Walder, C., Warner, T. D., Vane, J. R. (1988) Pressor effects of circulating endothelin are limited by its removal in the pulmonary circulation and by the release of prostacyclin and endothelium-derived relaxing factor. *Proceedings of National Academy of Science USA*, **85**, 9797–9800.
20. Inoue, A., Yanagisawa, M., Kimura, S., Kasuya, Y., Miyauchi, T., Goto, K. et al., (1989) The human endothelin family, three structurally and pharmacologically distinct isopeptides predicted by three separate genes. *Proceeding of National Academy of Science USA*, **86**, 2863–2867.
21. Miyauchi, T., Ishikawa, T., Tomobe, Y., Yanagisawa, M., Kimura, S., Sigishita, Y. et al. (1989) Characteristic pressor response to endothelin in spontaneously hypertensive and Wistar-Kyoto rats. *Hypertension*, **14**, 427–434.
22. Rohmeiss, P., Photiadis, J., Rohmeiss, S., Unger, T. (1990) Hemodynamic actions of intravenous endothelin in rats, comparison with sodium nitroprusside and methoxamine. *American Journal of Physiology*, **258**, H337–H346.

23. King, A. J., Pfeffer, J. M., Pfeffer, M. A., Brenner, B. M. (1990) Systemic hemodynamic effects of endothelin in rats. *American Journal of Physiology*, **258**, H788–H792.
24. Shiba, R., Yanagisawa, T., Miyauchi, Y., Ishii, S., Kimura, Y., Uciyama, T. *et al.* (1989) Elimination of intravenously injected endothelin-1 from the circulation of the rat. *Journal of Cardiovascular Pharmocology (Suppl 5)*, **13**, S88–S93.
25. Hirata, Y., Yishimi, H., Emori, T, Shichiri, M., Marumo, F. (1988) Binding and receptor down regulation of a novel vasoconstrictor endothelin in cultured rat vascular smooth muscle cells. *FEBS Letters*, **239**, 13–17.
26. Clozel, M., Clozel, J. P. (1989) Effects of endothelin on regional blood flows in squirrel monkeys. *Journal of Pharmacology and Experimental Therapeutics*, **250**, 1125–1131.
27. Clozel, J. P., Clozel, M. (1989) Effects of endothelin on the coronary vascular bed in open-chest dogs. *Circulation Research*, **65**, 1193–200.
28. Dieguez, G., Garcia, J. L., Fernandez, N., Garcia-Villalon A. L., Monge, L., Gomez, B. (1992) Cerebrovascular and coronary effects of endothelin-1 in the goat. *American Journal of Physiology*, **263**, R834–R839.
29. Hof, R. P., Hof, A., Takiguchi, Y. (1990) Attenuation of endothelin-induced regional vasoconstriction by isradipine, a nonspecific antivasoconstrictor effect. *Journal of Cardiovascular Pharmacology*, **15 (Suppl 1)**, S48–S54.
30. MacLean, M. R., Randall, M. D., Hiley, C. R. (1989) Effects of moderate hypoxia, hypercapnia and acidosis on haemodynamic changes induced by endothelin-1 in the pithed rat. *British Journal of Pharmacology*, **98**, 1055–1065.
31. Gardiner, S. M., Compton, A. M., Bennett, T. (1990) Regional haemodynamic effects of endothelin-1 and endothelin-3 in conscious Long Evans and Brattleboro rats. *British Journal of Pharmacology*, **99**, 107–112.
32. Masaki, T. (1993) Endothelins, homeostatic and compensatory actions in the circulatory and endocrine systems. *Endocrine Reviews*, **14**, 256–267.
33. Lippton, H. L., Ohlstein, E. H., Summer, W. R., Hyman, A. L. (1991) Analysis of responses to endothelins in the rabbit pulmonary and systemic vascular beds. *Journal of Applied Physiology*, **70**, 331–341.
34. Pollock, D. M., Opgenorth, T. J. (1993) Evidence for endothelin-induced renal vasoconstriction independent of ET_A receptor activation. *American Journal of Physiology*, **264**, R222–R226.
35. Terada, Y., Tomita, K., Murumo, F. (1992) Endothelin, EDRF, CGRP. *Nippon-Rinsho*, **50**, 2901–2908.
36. Gulati, A., Srimal, R. C. (1992) Endothelin mechanisms in the central nervous system: A target for drug development. *Drug Development and Research*, **26**, 361–387.
37. Yoshimoto, S., Ishikzaki, Y., Kurihara, H., Sasaki, T., Yoshizumi, M., Yanagisawa, M., *et al.* (1990) Cerebral microvessel endothelium is producing endothelin. *Brain Research*, **508**, 283–285.
38. Giaid, A., Gibson, S. J., Ibrahim, N., Legon, S., Bloom, S., Yanagisawa, M. *et al.* (1989) Endothelin-1 and endothelium-derived peptide is expressed in neurons of the human spinal cord and dorsal root ganglia. *Proceedings of National Academy of Science U.S.A.*, **86**, 7634–7638.
39. Lee, M.-E., de la Monte, S. M., Ng, S. C., Bloch, K. D., Quertermous, T. (1990) Expression of the potent vasoconstrictor endothelin in the human central nervous system. *Journal of Clinical Investigation*, **86**, 141–147.
40. MacCumber, M. W., Ross, C. A., Snyder, S. H. (1990) Endothelin in brain: Receptors, mitogenesis, and biosynthesis in glial cells. *Proceedings of National Academy of Science U.S.A.*, **87**, 2359–2363.
41. Ehrenreich, H., Kehrl, J. H., Anderson, R. W., Rieckmann, P., Vitkovic, L., Coligan, J. E. *et al.* (1991) A vasoactive peptide, endothelin-3, is produced by and specifically binds to primary astrocytes. *Brain Research*, **538**, 54–58.
42. Davenport, A. P., Morton, A. J. (1991) Binding sites for $[I^{125}]$ET-1, ET-2, ET-3 and vasoactive intestinal contractor are present in adult rat brain and neuron-enriched primary cultures of embryonic brain cells. *Brain Research*, **554**, 278–285.
43. Hoyer, D., Waeber, C., Palacios, J. M. (1989) $[I^{125}]$-endothelin-1 binding sites: autoradiographic studies in the brain and periphery of various species including humans. *Journal of Cardiovascular Pharmacology*, **13 (Suppl 5)**, S162–S165.
44. Hashim, M. A. Tadepalli, A. S. (1991) Functional evidence for the presence of a phosphoramidon-sensitive enzyme in rat brain that converts big endothelin-1 to endothelin-1. *Life Science*, **49**, L207–L211.
45. Asano, T., Ikegaki, I., Suzuki, Y., Satoh, S. Shibuya, M. (1989) Endothelin and the production of cerebral vasospasm in dogs. *Biochemical and Biophysical Research Communications*, **159**, 1345–1351.
46. Robinson, M. J., McCulloch, J. (1990) Contractile responses to endothelin in feline cortical vessels *in situ*. *Journal of Cerebral Blood Flow and Metabolism*, **10**, 285–289.
47. Willette, R. N., Sauermelch, C. (1990) Abluminal effects of endothelin in cerebral microvascular assessed by laser-doppler flowmetery. *American Journal of Physiology*, **259**, H1688–H1693.

48. Macrae, I. M., Robinson, M. J., Graham, D. J., Reid, J. L., McCulloch, J. (1993) Endothelin-1-induced reduction in cerebral blood flow, dose dependency, time course, and neuropathological consequences. *Journal of Cerebral Blood Flow and Metabolism*, **13**, 276–284.
49. Macrae, I. M., Robinson, M. J., McAuley, M., Reid, J. L., McCulloch, J. (1993) Effects of intracisternal endothelin-1 injection on blood flow to the lower brain stem. *European Journal of Pharmocology*, **203**, 85–91.
50. Willette, R. N., Sauermelch, C., Ezekiel, M., Feuerstein, G., Ohlstein, E. H. (1990) Effect of endothelin on cortical microvascular perfusion in rats. *Stroke*, **21**, 451–458.
51. Garcia, J. L., Gomez, B., Monge, L., Garcia-Villalon, A. L., Dieguez, G. (1991) Endothelin action on cerebral circulation in unanesthetized goats. *American Journal of Physiology*, **261**, R581–R587.
52. Saito, A; Shiba, R; Yanagisawa, M; et al. (1991) Endothelins: vasoconstrictor effects and localization in canine cerebral arteries. *British Journal of Pharmocology* 103, 1129–1135.
53. Kauser, K., Rubanyi, G. M, Harder, D. R. (1990) Endothelin-dependent modulation of endothelin-induced vasoconstriction and membrane depolarization in cat cerebral arteries. *Journal of Pharmacology and Experimental Therapeutics*, **252**, 93–97.
54. Papadopoulos, S. M., Gilbert, L. L, Webb, R. C., D'Amato, C. J. (1990) Characterization of contractile responses to endothelin in human cerebral arteries: implications for cerebral vasospasm. *Neurosurgery*, **26**, 810–815.
55. Douglas S. A., Vickery Clark, L. M., Ohlstein, E. H. (1993) Endothelin-1 does not mediate hypoxic vasoconstriction in canine isolated blood vessels: effect of BQ-123. *British Journal of Pharmacology*, **108**, 418–21.
56. Hemsen, A., Franco-Cereceda, A., Metran, R., Rudehill, A., Lundberg, J. M. (1990) Occurrence, specific binding sites and functional effects of endothelin in human cardiopulmonary tissue. *European Journal of Pharmocology*, **191**, 319–328.
57. Ihara, M., Noguchi, K., Saeki, T., Eukuroda, T., Tsuchida, S., Kimura, S. et al. (1992) Biological profiles of highly potent novel endothelin antagonists selective for the ET_A receptor. *Life Science*, **50**, 247–255.
58. Itoh, H., Haraoka, N., Higuchi., H., Ito, M., Konishi, T., Nakano, T. (1992) Contractile actions of endothelin-1 in isolated helical strips from rat pulmonary artery: potentiation of serotonin-induced contraction. *Journal of Cardiovascular Pharmacology*, **20**, 1–6.
59. Saeki, T. Ihara, M. Fukuroda, T. Yamagiwa, M. Yano, M. (1991) [Ala^{1,3,11,15}]endothelin-1 analogs with ET_B agonistic activity. *Biochemical Biophysical Research Communication*, **179**, 286-92.
60. Toga, H., Ibe, B. O., Raj, J. U. (1992) In vitro responses of ovine intrapulmonary arteries and veins to endothelin-1. *American Journal of Physiology*, **263**, L15–L21.
61. Cardell, L. O., Uddman, R., Edvinsson, L. (1993) A novel ET_A-receptor antagonsit, FR 139317, inhibits endothelin-induced contractions of guinea-pig pulmonary arteries, but not trachea. *British Journal of Pharmacology*, **108**, 448–452.
62. Douglas, S. A., Elliott, J. D., Ohlstein, E. H. (1992) Regional vasodilation to endothelin-1 is mediated by a non-ET_A receptor subtype in the anaesthetized rat: effect of BQ-123 on systemic haemodynamic responses. *European Journal of Pharmacology*, **221**, 315–324.
63. Cargnelli, G., Rossi, G., Bova, S., Pessina, A. C. (1990) In vitro vascular reactivity to endothelin: a comparison between young and old normotensive and hypertensive rats. *Clinical and Experimental Hypertension [A]*, **12**, 1437–51.
64. Watanabe, K., Hoshi N., Suzuki, T. (1993) Epithelioid angiosarcoma of the intestinal tract with endothelin-1-like immunoreactivity. *Virchows Archives A Pathological Anatomy and Histopathology*, **423**, 309–314.
65. Karaki, H. Sudjarwo S. A., Hori, M., Takai, M., Urade, Y., Okada, T. (1993) Induction of endothelium-dependent relaxation in the rat aorta by IRL 1620, a novel and selective agonist at the endothelium ET_B receptor. *British Journal of Pharmacology*, **109**, 486–490.
66. Karaki, H., Sudjarwo, S. A., Hori, M., Sakata, K., Urade, Y., Takai, M. et al. (1993) ET_B receptor antagonist, IRL 1038, selectively inhibits the endothelin-induced endothelin-dependent vascular relaxation. *European Journal of Pharmacology*, **231**, 371–374.
67. Webb ML, Dickinson KE, Delaney CL, et al. (1992) The endothelin receptor antagonist, BQ-123, inhibits angiotensin II-induced contractions in rabbit aorta. *Biochemical Biophysical Communications*, **185**, 887–892.
68. Moreland S, McMullen DM, Delaney CL, Lee VG, Hunt JT. (1992) Venous smooth muscle contains vasoconstrictor ET_B-like receptors. *Biochemical Biophysical Research Communications*, **184**, 100–106.
69. Bax, W. A. Bruinvels, A. T., Vansuylen, R. J., Saxena, P. R. Hoyer, D. (1993) Endothelin receptor in the human coronary artery, ventricle and atrium – a quantitative autoradiographic analysis. *Naunyn-Schmiedbergs Archives of Pharmacology*, **348**, 403–410.
70. Hay, D. W. (1992) Pharmacological evidence for distinct endothelin receptors in guinea-pig bronchus and aorta. *British Journal of Pharmacology*, **106**, 759–761.

71. Dohi, Y., Criscione, L., Luscher, T. F. (1991) Renovascular hypertension impairs formation of endothelium-derived relaxing factors and sensitivity to endothelin-1 in resistance arteries. *British Journal of Pharmacology*, **104**, 349–354.
72. Monge, L., Garcia Villalon, A. L., Montoya, J. J., Garcia, J. L., Gomez, B., Dieguez, G. (1991) Response of rabbit ear artery to endothelin-1 during cooling. *British Journal of Pharmacology*, **104**, 609–612.
73. Mima, T., Yanagisawa, M., Shigeno, T., et al. (1989) Endothelin acts in feline and canine cerebral arteries from the adventitial side. *Stroke*, **20**, 1553–1556.
74. Salom, J. B., Torregrosa, G., Miranda, F. J., Alabadi, J. A., Alvarez, C., Alborch, E. (1991) Effects of endothelin-1 on the cerebrovascular bed of the goat. *European Journal of Pharmacology*, **192**, 39–45.
75. Yamaura, I., Tani, E., Maeda, Y., Minami, N., Shindo, H. (1992) Endothelin-1 of canine basilar artery in vasospasm. *Journal of Neurosurgery*, **76**, 99–105.
76. Wagner, O. F., Vierhapper, H., Gasic, S., Nowotny, P., Waldhausl, W. (1992) Regional effects and clearance of endothelin-1 across pulmonary and splanchnic circulation. *European Journal of Clinical Investigations*, **22**, 277–282.
77. Kurihara, T., Akimoto, M., Ishiguro, H., Niimi, A., Maeda, A., Sagemoto, M. et al. (1992) Relationship between endothelin and thromoboxane-A$_2$ in rat liver microcirculation. *Life Science*, **51**, L281–L285.
78. Kurihara, T., Akimoto, M., Kurokawa, K., Ishiguro, H., Niimi, A., Maeda, A. et al. (1992) ET-3 sensitive reduction of tissue bold flow in rat liver. *Life Science*, **51**, L101–L106.
79. Lippton, H., Goff, J., Hyman, A. (1988) Effects of endothelin in the systemic and renal vascular beds in vivo. *European Journal of Pharmacology*, **155**, 197–199.
80. Vigne, P., Breittmayour, J. P., Freilin, C. (1993) Competitive and non-competitive interactions of BQ-123 with ET$_A$ receptors. *European Journal of Pharmacology*, **245**, 229–232.
81. Eguchi, S., Hirata, Y., Ihara, M., Yano, M., Marumo, F. (1992) A novel ET$_A$ antagonist (BQ-123) inhibits endothelin-1-induced phosphoinositide breakdown and DNA synthesis in rat vascular smooth muscle cells. *FEBS Letters*, **3021**, 243–246.
82. Sogabe, K., Nirei, H., Shoubo, M. et al. (1993) Pharmacological profile of FR 139317, a novel, potent endothelin ET$_A$ receptor antagonist. *Journal of Pharmacology and Experimental Therapeutics*, **264**, 1040–1046.
83. Takenaka, K., Kishino, J., Arita, H. et al. (1993) Biological activity of the endothelin family in cultured basilar arterial smooth muscle cells. *Neurol Research*, **15**, 29–32.
84. Karet, F. E, Kuc, R. E, Davenport, A. P. (1993) Novel ligands BQ-123 and BQ-3020 characterize endothelin receptor subtypes ET$_A$ and ET$_B$ in human kidney. *Kidney International*, **44**, 36–42.
85. Webb, M. L., Liu, E. C., Monshizadegan, H. et al. (1993) Expression of endothelin receptor subtypes in rabbit saphenous vein. *Molecular Pharmacology*, **44**, 959–66.
86. Itoh, S., Sasaki, T., Ide, Ishikawa, K., Nishikibe, M., Yano, M. (1993) A novel endothelin ET$_A$ receptor antagonist, BQ-485, and its preventive effect on experimental cerebral vasospasm in dogs. *Biochemical and Biophysical Research Communications*, **195**, 969–975.
87. Nieri, H., Hamada, K., Shoubo, M., Sogabe, K., Notsu, Y., Ono, T. (1993) An endothelin ET$_A$ receptor antagonist FR 139317, ameliorates cerebral vasospasm in dogs. *Life Sciences*, **52**, 1869–1874.
88. Clozel, J. P., Watanabe, H. (1993) BQ-123, a peptidic endothelin ET$_A$ receptor antagonist, prevents the early cerebral vasospasm following subarrachnoid hemorrhage after intracisternal but not intravenous injection. *Life Science*, **52**, 822–834.
89. Hof, R. P., Hof, A. Takiguchi, Y. (1989) Massive regional differences in the vascular effects of endothelin. *Journal of Hypertension*, (**Suppl 7**), S274–S275.
90. Neubauer, S., Ertl, G., Haas, U., Pulzer, F., Kochsiek, K. (1990) Effects of endothelin-1 in isolated perfused rat heart. *Journal of Cardiovascular Pharmacology*, **16**, 1–8.
91. Haynes, W. G., Davenport, A. P. Webb, D. J. (1993) Endothelin: progress in pharmacology and physiology. *Trends in Pharmacological Sciences*, **14**, 225–228.
92. Pernow, J., Modin, A. (1993) Endothelial regulation of coronary vascular tone in vitro – contribution of endothelin receptor subtypes and nitric oxide. *European Journal of Pharmacology*, **243**, 281–286.
93. Wood, J. G., Yan, Z. Y., Cheung, L. Y. (1992) Relative potency of endothelin analogues on changes in gastric vascular resistance. *American Journal of Physiology*, **262**, G977–G982.
94. Sirois, M. G., Filep, J. G., Rousseau, A., Fournier, A., Plante, G. E., Sirois, P. (1992) Endothelin-1 enhances vascular permeability in conscious rats, role of thromboxane A$_2$. *European Journal of Pharmacology*, **214**, 119–125.
95. Peskar, B. M., Nowak, P., Lambrecht, N. (1992) Effect of prostaglandins and capsaicin on gastric vascular flow and mucosal injury in endothelin-1-treated rats. *Agents Actions (Suppl.)*, **37**, 85–91.
96. Filep, J. G., Sirois, M. G., Rousseau, A., Fournier, A., Sirois, P. (1991) Effects of endothelin-1 on vascular permeability in the conscious rat, interactions with platelet-activating factor. *British Journal of Pharmacology*, **104**, 797–804.
97. Morales, R. E., Johnson, B. R., Szabo, S. (1992) Endothelin induces vascular and mucosal lesions,

enhances the injury by HCl/ethanol, and the antibody exerts gastroprotection. *FASEB Journal*, **6**, 2354–60.
98. Ota, S., Hirata, Y., Sugimoto, T., Kohmoto, O., Hata, Y., Yoshiura, K. et al. (1991) Endothelin-1 secretion from cultured rabbit gastric epithelial cells. *Journal of Cardiovascular Pharmacology*, **17, (Suppl. 7)**, S406–S407.
99. Masuda, E., Kawano, S., Nagano, K., Tsuji, S., Ishigami, Y., Hayashi, N. et al., (1991) Effect of ethanol on endothelin-1 release from gastric vasculature. *Japnese Journal of Gastroenterology*, **26 (Suppl 3)**, 81–82.
100. Gandhi, C. R., Stephenson, K., Olson, M. S. (1990) Endothelin, a potent peptide agonist in the liver. *Journal of Biological Chemistry*, **265**, 17432–17435.
101. Simonson, M. S., Dunn, M. J. (1990) Endothelin-1 stimulates contraction of rat glomerular mesangial cells and potentiates beta-adrenergic-mediated cyclic adenosine monophosphate accumulation. *Journal of Clinical Investigation*, **85**, 790–797.
102. Takagi, H., Hisa, H., Satoh, S. (1991) Effects of endothelin on adrenergic neurotransmission in the dog kidney. *European Journal of Pharmacology*, **203**, 291–294.
103. Tsuchiya, K., Naruse, M., Sanaka, T., Naruse, K., Nitta, K., Demura, H., Sugino, N. (1989) Effects of endothelin on renal regional blood flow in dogs. *European Journal of Pharmacology*, **166**, 541–543.
104. Chen, C. F., Chien, C. T., Wu, M. S. (1992) Direct renal effects of endothelin in chronic hypoxic spontaneously hypertensive rats. *Clinical and Experimental Pharmacology and Physiology*, **19**, 809–813.
105. Cirino, M., Motz, C., Maw, J., Ford-Hutchinson, A. W., Yano, M. (1992) BQ-153, a novel endothelin (ET) antagonist, attenuates the renal vascular effects of endothelin-1. *Journal of Pharmacy and Pharmacology*, **44**, 782–785.
106. Salvati, P., Dho, L., Calabresi, M., Rosa, B., Patrono, C. (1992) Evidence for a direct vasoconstrictor effect of big endothelin-1 in the rat kidney. *European Journal of Pharmacology*, **221**, 267–273.
107. Ohno, A., Naruse, M., Kato, S., Hosaka, M., Naruse, K., Demura, H. et al. (1992) Endothelin-specific antibodies decrease blood pressure and increase glomerular filtration rate and renal plasma flow in spontaneously hypertensive rats. *Journal of Hypertension*, **10**, 781–5.
108. Lundberg, J. M., Ahlborg, G., Hemsen, A., Nisell, H., Lunell, N. O., Pernow, J., Rudehill, A., Weitzberg, E. (1991) Evidence for release of endothelin-1 in pigs and humans. *Journal of Cardiovascular Pharmacology*, **17 (Suppl 7)**, S350–S353.
109. Yamashita, Y., Yukimura, T., Miura, K., Okumura, M., Yamamoto, K. (1991) Effects of endothelin-3 on renal functions. *Journal of Pharmacology and Experimental Therapeutics*, **259**, 1256–1260.
110. Yamada, K., Yoshida, S. (1991) Role of endogenous endothelin in renal function during altered sodium balance. *Journal of Cardiovascular Pharmacology*, **17 (Suppl. 7)**, S290–S292.
111. Yukimura, T., Miura, K., Yamashita, Y., Shimmen, T., Okumura, M., Yamanaka, S. et al. (1991) Effects of the calcium channel antagonist nicardipine on renal action of endothelin in dogs. *Contribution to Nephrology*, **90**, 105–110.
112. Weitzberg, E., Ahlborg, G., Lundberg, J. M. (1991) Long-lasting vasoconstriction and efficient regional extraction of endothelin-1 in human splanchnic and renal tissues. *Biochemical and Biophysical Research Communications*, **1801**, 1298–1303.
113. Pernow, J., Franco-Cereceda, A., Matran, R., Lundberg, J. M. (1989) Effect of endothelin-1 on regional vascular resistances in the pig. *Journal of Cardiovascular Pharmacology*, **13 (Suppl 5)**, S205–S206.
114. Madeddu, P., Yang, X. P., Anani, V., Troffa, C., Pazzo, A. A., Soro, A. et al. (1990) Efficacy of nifedipine to prevent systemic and renal vasoconstrictor effects of endothelin. *American Journal of Physiology*, **259**, F304–F311.
115. Gardiner, S. M., Compton, A. M., Bennett, T. (1990) Regional hemodynamic effects of endothelin-2 and sarafotoxin-S6b in conscious rats. *American Journal of Physiology*, **258**, R912–R917.
116. Nakamoto, H., Suzuki, H., Murakami, M., Kageyama, Y., Ohishi, A., Fukuda, K. et al. (1989) Effects of endothelin on systemic and renal haemodynamics and neuroendocrine hormones in conscious dogs. *Clinical Sciences*, **77**, 567–72.
117. Vane, J. R., Botting, R. M. (1991) Endothelium-derived vasoactive factors and the control of circulation. *Seminars Perinatology*, **15**, 4–10.
118. Fukuda, Y., Hirata, Y., Yoshimi, H., Kijima, T., Kibayashi, Y., Yanagisawa, M. et al. (1988) Endothelin is a potent secretagogue for atrial natriuretic peptide in cultured rat atrial myocytes. *Biochemical and Biophysical Research Communications*, **16**, 167–172.
119. Yoshimoto, S., Ishikzaki, Y., Sasaki, T., Murota, S. (1991) Effects of carbon dioxide and oxygen on endothelin production by cultured porcine cerebral endothelial cells. *Stroke*, **22**, 378–383.
120. Wagner, O. F., Christ, G., Wijta, J., Vierhapper, H., Parzer, S., Nowotny, J. et al. (1992) Polar secretion of endothelin-1 by cultured endothelial cells. *Journal of Biological Chemistry*, **267**, 16066–16068.
121. Saxena, P. R., Schamhardt, H. C., Forsyth, R. P., Loeve, J. (1980) Computer programs for the radioactive microsphere technique. *Computer Programs in Biomedicine*, **12**, 63–84.

122. Gulati, A., Agarwal, S. K., Shukla, R. Srimal, R. C., Dhawan, B. N. (1985) The mechanism of opening of the blood-brain barrier by hypertonic saline. *Neuropharmacology*, **24**, 909–913.
123. Sharma, A. C., Gulati, A. (1994) Effects of diaspirin cross-linked hemoglobin and norepinephrine in systemic hemodynamics and regional circulation in rats. *Journal of Laboratory and Clinical Medicine*, **123**, 299–308.
124. Wright, C. E., Fozard, J. R. (1990) Differences in regional vascular sensitivity to endothelin-1 between spontaneously hypertensive and normotensive Wistar-Kyoto rats. *British Journal of Pharmacology*, **100**, 107–113.
125. LeMonnier de Gouville, A. C., Mondot, S., Lippton, H., Hyman, A., Cavero, I. (1989) Hemodynamic and pharmacological evaluation of the vasodilator and vasoconstrictor effects of endothelin-1 in rats. *Journal of Pharmacology and Experimental Therapeutics*, **252**, 300–311.
126. Minkes, R. K., Kadowitz, P. J. (1989) Influence of endothelin on systemic arterial pressure and regional blood flow in the cat. *European Journal of Pharmacology*, **163**, 163–166.
127. Minkes, R. K., Coy, D. H., Murphy, W. A., McNamara, D. B., Kadowitz, P. J. (1989) Effects of porcine and rat endothelin and an analog on blood pressure in the anesthetized cat. *European Journal of Pharmacology*, **164**, 571–575.
128. Miller, R. C., Pelton, J. T., Huggins, J. P. (1993) Endothelins – from receptors to medicine. *Trends in Pharmacological Sciences*, **141**, 54–60.

15 Role of Endothelin in Renal Disorders

Ananda P. Sen and Anil Gulati

Department of Pharmaceutics and Pharmacodynamics (m/c 865), The University of Illinois at Chicago, 833 South Wood Street, Chicago, IL 60612, USA

INTRODUCTION

Endothelin (ET) peptides (21 amino-acids) are amongst the most potent peptides[1] which display a profound and important role on the renal functions. ET family consists of three isoforms, ET-1, ET-2, and ET-3[2]. A recent autoradiographic study has revealed the presence of all the three ET-1, ET-2, and ET-3 isoforms in the kidneys of human, baboon, monkey, tree shrew, pig, and rat[3]. However, ET-1 is the major isoform responsible for most of the pathophysiology associated with altered ET production in the kidneys. ET-1 is secreted at several sites in the kidneys like endothelial cells[4], mesangial cells[5], glomerular epithelial cells[6] and tubular epithelial cells[7-10]. In the kidneys ET-1 acts in a paracrine and autocrine signaling mode on target cells[11], and is also a mitogen for glomerular mesangial cells[12,13]. The kidneys contribute to the clearance of ET-1 and contain ET-degrading enzymes[14-16]. ET peptides regulate renal functions through multiple mechanisms, like controlling renal blood flow (RBF), glomerular filtration rate (GFR), and by regulating sodium and water excretion. ET also appears to contribute to renal dysfunction during certain pathophysiological states like acute and chronic renal failure, hypertension, cyclosporine-induced renal toxicity, diabetes, pre-eclampsia, radio-contrast nephropathy, septic shock, ureteric obstruction, neonatal injury, and glomerulonephritis.

ENDOTHELIN RECEPTORS IN THE KIDNEY

ET acts by binding irreversibly to specific cell-surface receptors[17,18]. Two major ET-receptor subtypes, ET_A and ET_B, have been isolated and cloned. ET_A receptors were initially cloned in the bovine lung[19] and rat A10 cells[20] and later in human placenta[21]. ET_B receptors have been initially studied in the rat lung[22] and also in human intestine and liver[23-25]. The ET_A receptor recognizes the ETs in the order ET-1 > ET-2 ≫ ET-3[19-21], while the ET_B recognizes all the three isoforms with the same affinity[22-25].

A third subtype of ET receptor, ET_C, has been speculated in the rat renal papilla, with a high affinity for the ET-3 isoform[26]. The human kidneys have predominantly ET_B receptor subtype in the cortex and medulla[27]. In rat kidneys, the glomerulus has both ET_A and ET_B receptor subtypes[28], while the inner medullary collecting ducts have ET_B receptor subtype[29], and the renal medullary interstitial cells possess the ET_A receptor subtype[30]. ET_B receptor subtypes have also been found on the rat cortical collecting ducts and outer medullary collecting ducts[30]. Both ET_A and ET_B receptors have been observed in the rat kidney cortex in an equal ratio[31]. In rats mRNA expression for ET_A receptors have been observed in renal vascular smooth muscles and glomerular arterioles, while mRNA for ET_B receptors have been observed in endothelial cells of glomeruli, vasa recta bundles, and Henle's loop[32].

ENDOTHELIN AND RENAL CIRCULATION

Renal vascular tone is regulated by the sympathetic output, and by vasoactive compounds like angiotensin II, prostaglandins, arginine vasopressin, atrial natriuretic peptide, and ET. ET is the most potent vasoconstrictor amongst these[33,34]. Amongst the vascular beds the renal vasculature is most sensitive to ET[35]. ET exerts control over renal functions, both under physiological and pathophysiological conditions. ET regulates the long-term control of RBF, GFR, and sodium and water balance. Systemic infusion of ET-1 led to a reduction in RBF, and increase in renal vascular resistance *in vitro* in isolated perfused rabbit[36] and rat kidneys[37-40], and also *in vivo* in rats[41-46], dogs[42,47-49] and rabbits[50,51]. This is often preceded by a transient renal vasodilation. The reduction of RBF flow is due to the constriction of the afferent and efferent renal arterioles, a calcium-dependent reduction in the glomerular capillary surface area available for ultrafiltration[36,37,42,46], increases in cytosolic free calcium[17,18,52], and proliferation of mesangial cells[41]. These changes were accompanied by a sustained reduction in sodium excretion, an increased plasma renin activity, and an increase in renal vascular resistance[53,54]. Infusion of lower dose (10 ng/kg/min) of ET-1 in rats produced an increase in mean arterial pressure, natriuresis and diuresis[44,55-58]. The enhanced natriuresis and diuresis are due to reduction of proximal tubular sodium reabsorption, and are probably mediated through a renal arterial pressure related phenomena (pressure natriuresis and diuresis)[59], enhanced release of atrial natriuretic peptide[55], and inhibition of the renal response to antidiuretic hormone[60]. In contrast, a bolus dose of big ET-1 to conscious rats did not change RBF or renal vascular resistance, thus indicating a different mechanisms of action[61]. However, big ET-1 showed vasoconstrictor effects in the isolated rat kidneys[62]. A bolus dose of ET-1 administered intravenously to rats showed a biphasic systemic pressor response, characterized by an initial rapid and transient vasodilation followed by a sustained rise in arterial blood pressure[44]. While the renal vascular bed is highly sensitive to the vasoconstrictor activity of exogenously administered ET-1, data on the effects of endogenously synthesized ET-1 in normal humans is lacking. When ET-1 is infused directly into the renal artery of rats[55,58,63,64] or dogs[33,64], both renal plasma flow and GFR declined. The role of endogenous renal ET-1 in producing alteration in renal hemodynamics has been shown during thyroid dysfunctions[65].

Whether ET increases or decreases glomerular capillary hydraulic pressure is not clear and contradictory findings have been reported. Using *in vivo*[66,67] and *in vitro*[37,68] models of rat hydronephrotic kidneys, a calcium-dependent[37,68] high sensitivity of renal afferent arterioles than efferent arterioles to the constricing of ET-1 was observed, with a reduction of GFR[37]. Higher sensitivity of the afferent renal arterioles to ET-1 than the efferent arterioles has been observed *in vitro* in rats[69]. Increased mean arterial pressure and decreased GFR and RBF in response to ET-1 infusion has been observed *in vivo* in rabbit kidneys, probably by preferential constriction of afferent renal arterioles[51]. Opposite results have also been reported in rabbit[36] and in rat[41,44] renal arterioles, where the efferent arterioles show a higher sensitivity than afferent arterioles to ET-1 induced constriction. These studies provide evidence that arteriolar vasoconstriction plays a predominant role in the regulation of glomerular function following ET-1 challenge.

It is still unclear as to which receptors are involved in ET-1 induced vasoconstriction in the kidneys. Studies conducted *in vivo* on rats show that the vasoconstriction is mediated through ET_B receptors[70,71], though ET_A receptors are involved in the maintenance of renal arterial pressure and vascular resistance[71]. Studies conducted *in vitro* show that the vasoconstriction is mediated through ET_A receptors in the rabbit kidneys[72] and both ET_A and ET_B receptors in the rat kidneys[73].

ENDOTHELIN AND GLOMERULAR FUNCTIONS

Single nephron glomerular filtration rate (SNGFR) is the product of net filtration pressure across the glomerular capillary and the ultrafiltration coefficient. ET-1 regulates SNGFR by affecting both these variables. Systemic administration of ET-1 produced a decrease in GFR in rats[41,42,48,74] and dogs[42,48]. Similar results have been observed by the intra-renal infusion of ET-1 into rats[55,63,64] and dogs[33,64] *in vivo*, and also *in vitro* in perfused rat kidneys[38–40]. Sub-pressor doses of ET-1 caused a proportionately greater increase in efferent than afferent arteriolar contraction without any alteration in the SNGFR[44]. Higher doses of ET-1 caused an increase in afferent and efferent resistance thereby reducing GFR[44,55]. Several micropuncture studies have reported that ET-1 reduces the glomerular ultrafiltration coefficient thereby contributing to the fall in GFR[44,55].

ENDOTHELIN AND MESANGIAL CELL FUNCTIONS

Mesangial cells are specialized microvascular pericytes located in the central region of the glomerular tuft between capillary loops. They regulate GFR, process macromolecules trapped within the mesangium, and control the viscoelastic properties of the glomerulus[75]. The regulation of glomerular mesangial cell activity is amongst the most important renal functions of ET. ET has both contractile and mitogenic properties in mesangial cells[12,13,18,55,76–79]. ET is also a growth factor for mesangial cells in culture[12,18].

Though mesangial cells express both ET_A and ET_B receptors[80], the receptor subtype responsible for the actions of ET is still not certain[12,18,78]. The mitogenic property of ET illustrates that these peptides can also induce long term changes in cell phenotype that require differential regulation of gene expression[52].

ET-1 induces several genes in quiescent mesangial cells which include *fos* and *jun* family genes[81], collagenase[81], platelet-derived growth factor A and B chains[79], and prostaglandin endoperoxide synthase[82]. ET causes contraction of mesangial cells cultured on collagen gels and it is hypothesized that this phenomena mimics a wound healing response, and that ET-induced mitogenesis in the mesangium might contribute to the glomerular response to injury[83]. ET-1 evokes release of arachidonic acid and production of PGE_2 from mesangial cells[12], which might attenuate ET-1 induced contraction[76,77]. Thus, release of ET from the glomerular endothelial cells might be an important paracrine determinant for the prostaglandin biosynthetic capacity of mesangial cells.

ENDOTHELIN AND SODIUM EXCHANGE

Kidneys regulate the extracellular fluid volume (ECFV) and thus mean arterial pressure. ECFV is dependent upon the availability of exchangeable sodium ions, and so alterations in renal sodium excretion by ET regulate ECFV and thereby the mean arterial pressure. ET appears to have a pleiotropic effect on renal sodium handling and the precise role of ET-1 on sodium exchange is not clear. Systemic infusion of ET-1 decreased sodium excretion[84,85], by a reduction of filtered sodium load, increased secretion of aldosterone, sodium reabsorption, and a reduction of peritubular capillary Starling gradient in favor of sodium reabsorption. Intra-renal infusion of ET-1 produced no change in sodium excretion but decreased natriuresis at higher doses[33,63]. Other studies show a natriuretic effect despite a fall in RBF and GFR in intact[44,58,86], and isolated perfused[38-40] kidneys. It is speculated that in hypertensive patients with normal renal function, renal ET increases sodium excretion by suppressing sodium reabsorption in the ducts[87]. A bolus injection of big ET-1 has a natriuretic effect, which shows that intra-renal processing of big ET-1 to ET-1 takes place at local effector sites[61]. The natriuretic effects of ET-1 are probably mediated through an inhibition of renin secretion by a direct effect of ET-1 on juxtaglomerular cells[88], increased atrial natriuretic peptide secretion[89], and inhibition of prostaglandin-mediated Na^+K^+-ATPase activity in medullary collecting ducts[90]. It could be possible that ET-1 acting in an intra-renal, paracrine, or autocrine mode would be natriuretic, and while acting in an endocrine mode, ET-1 would be anti-natriuretic. The available studies favors an intra-renal role of ET in the kidneys, and it is speculated that the physiological role of ET in the renal sodium exchange would be natriuresis, but which is possibly influenced by other intra-renal and extra-renal mechanisms.

ENDOTHELIN AND WATER EXCHANGE

The water balance and plasma osmolality by the kidneys are maintained by changes in pituitary arginine vasopressin (AVP) release, which in turn controls the permeability of collecting ducts to water. ET-1 enhances diuresis despite a decrease in RBF and GFR, by inhibiting water reabsorption[41,91]. ET-1 inhibits AVP-mediated cAMP accumulation in the cortical collecting duct, outer medullary collecting duct, and inner medullary collecting duct of isolated nephrons, thus raising the possibility that ET regulates water exchange independent of its effects on sodium reabsorption or renal hemodynamics[92]. Direct evidence for inhibition of AVP-stimulated water permeability comes from studies in microperfused inner medullary collecting duct segments where ET-1 reversibly inhibited the increase in osmotic water permeability by AVP, whereas ET-1 has no effect on water permeability *per se*[93]. It may be speculated that ET acts *in vitro* to enhance water excretion by inhibiting the actions of AVP. This might partly explain the ability of ET-1 to induce diuresis despite a decrease in RBF and GFR.

ENDOTHELIN AND KIDNEY DISORDERS

In recent years extensive research on ET has focussed on its potential role in renal diseases. ET affects three major aspects of renal physiology: vascular and mesangial tone, mitogenesis of mesangial and probably other cells, and sodium and water balance. The actions of ET in the kidney appear to be mainly mediated by paracrine and autocrine mechanisms. Thus, endothelial cell derived ET would regulate adjacent vascular smooth muscle tone, while glomerular endothelial, epithelial, and mesangial cell ET would effect glomerular cell proliferation, and tubular cell-derived ET would modulate sodium and water transport. Alterations in regional ET production and actions could have diverse, and even opposite effects on kidney function. It is important that the actions of ET should be studied in the context of its local production and effects.

The circulating levels of ET are elevated in several pathophysiological states to a level at which renal effects are manifested[94]. In several pathophysiological states involving the kidney elevated urinary levels of ET-1 have been observed, though the plasma ET-1 levels are quite low in comparison to target cells. Pathogenically high plasma ET-1 level has been observed only in patients with malignant hypertension[95]. However, it is still unclear whether these alterations in urinary ET-1 levels are of pathophysiological significance. Numerous studies indicate that ET-1 may be an important mediator of renal dysfunction. We have reviewed the role of ET-1 in the pathophysiology of several renal disorders.

Acute renal failure

Hypoxemic vasomotor nephropathy

Acute renal failure may be defined as acute decrease in GFR. Based on sites of primary disorder i.e., circulation, renal parenchyma, or urinary outflow, the causes of acute renal failure may be prerenal, intrinsic, or postrenal failure, respectively. Prerenal failure or hypoxemic vasomotor nephropathy, accounts for more than one-third of the cases of pediatric acute renal failure[96]. ET probably plays a role in hypoxic vasomotor nephropathy. ET-antibody, administered intravenously to neonatal rabbits, prevented the increase in afferent and efferent arteriolar resistance and the decrease in single-nephron GFR 48 hours after a 25 minute clamping of the renal artery, a procedure which mimicked hypoxemia[55]. Also, ET-1 antiserum, when infused in animals followed by hypoxemic stress, the symptoms of hypoxemia are attenuated[96].

Aortic cross-clamping

Aortic cross-clamping is a clinically relevant animal model of altered systemic and renal functions. This model is similar to the surgical procedure used during perpheral arterial revascularization and reconstruction, and is associated with profound systemic and renal vasoconstriction, acute renal failure, and an increase in circulating ET levels[97-100]. Elevated plasma level of ET-1 have been observed in patients with acute renal failure[60]. Acute renal failure with elevated ET-1 levels have been reported in animal models using dogs[97] and rats[98,101]. The acute renal failure were attenuated by the ET_A antagonist BQ-123[97,98]. Renal ET-1 but not ET-2 and ET-3 mRNA has been found to be elevated following renal ischemia[102]. These findings support a functional role for increased endogenous ET-1 acting through the ET_A receptors in the regulation of renal vascular tone associated with acute renal failure.

Chronic renal failure

Elevated plasma and urinary ET-1 levels have been observed in patients with chronic renal failure, specially those on dialysis and chronic ambulatory peritoneal dialysis[103-107]. Amongst the possible explanations for this are impaired metabolism and excretion of ET-1 due to renal insufficiency, and increased release of ET-1 from the vascular endothelial cells probably mediated by uremic toxins. Urinary ET-1 excretion may serve as a potential marker for chronic renal failure though a pathophysiological role of this peptide in chronic renal failure remains to be established.

Cyclosporine-mediated renal toxocity

Cyclosporine is widely used as an immunosuppressant after organ transplantation, though it is a nephrotoxic agent. It decreases GFR, RBF, and produces a chronic, progressive deterioration in renal function. ET is an important mediator of acute cyclosporine-induced nephrotoxicity, though in chronic cyclosporine-induced nephrotoxicity other non-ET mechanisms are likely to be involved[108]. Acute cyclosporine stimulates ET-1 release from cultured endothelial, epithelial, and mesangial cells[109-111]. Anti-ET serum, when infused into rat renal artery ameliorated the acute cyclosporine-induced decrease in SNGFR as well as increase in renal arteriolar resistance[55,112]. ET antibody showed protective effect against acute cyclosporine-induced deteriorations in SNGFR in a model of ischemic renal failure[55,112]. ET antibody also ameliorated renal vasoconstriction induced by cyclosporine in the rat kidneys[55,112]. Similarly, ET antibody ameliorated the reduction in GFR and RBF following cyclosporine administration to the isolated perfused rat kidneys[39]. Acute cyclosporine toxicity is probably related to ET-1 interaction with the ET_A receptor since cyclosporine-induced hemodynamic changes were attenuated by the ET_A receptor antagonist BQ-123[113] and PED-3512-PI[114] in rats. In studies conducted on isolated rat renal arterioles, BQ-123 inhibited the cyclosporine-induced vasoconstriction[69]. Exposure to cyclosporine caused an increase in myosin light chain phosphorylation, a biochemical marker of contraction in mesangial cells, but it was ameliorated when pretreated with BQ-123[115]. These studies suggest that ET_A receptors are likely to be involved in acute cyclosporine-induced nephrotoxicity.

Renal dysfunction during pre-eclampsia

Pre-eclampsia or gestational proteinuric hypertension, is a syndrome occurring in 5% of first pregnancies and 1% of multigravid women and is amongst the most common cause of maternal and fetal morbidity and mortality. The major clinical symptoms include hypertension and impaired renal function with decreased uric acid secretion and glomerular endothelial cell injury, but the cause of pre-eclampsia is still not known. Elevated levels of circulating ET have been observed in pre-eclamptic women which correlated closely with serum uric acid levels and measures of renal dysfunction[116]. It is possible that ET may be involved in the systemic vasoconstriction, reduction in renal and placental blood flow, and elevated plasma uric acid levels associated with pre-eclampsia.

Glomerulonephritis

ET is involved in the cellular proliferation observed in several forms of kidney diseases. A number of inflammatory mediators can stimulate ET-1 production[5,117-119]. Renal ET-1 mRNA expression and urinary ET-1 excretion are increased in several experimental[120] and human glomerulonephritis[94,106]. NZB/W F1 mice serve as animal models for human systemic lupus erythematosus, characterized by mesangial cell proliferation and mononuclear cell infiltration of the kidneys. In these mice the renal concentrations of ET-1 increase with age[120]. ET-1 may activate monocytes[121], which, along with macrophages and leukocytes, are capable of secreting ET-1[122,123]. Thus, by exerting direct effects on glomerular cells, as well as recruiting inflammatory cell infiltration and activation, ET-1 may induce glomerular cell proliferation. Further studies with chronic administration of ET antibody or ET antagonists are needed to determine the precise role of ET in glomerulonephritis.

Hypertensive nephropathy

Hypertension frequently coexists with glomerulonephritis and is the major factor leading to renal dysfunctions. Though the renal vasculature is able to cope with altered systemic blood pressure by an autoregulatory mechanism regulating intraglomerular pressure and arteriolar resistance, they are unable to do so in diseased kidneys. This condition leads to renal hyperhemodynamics. Several studies have attempted to link increased plasma ET-1 levels to the development and maintenance of hypertension. Plasma ET-1 levels in hypertensive patients directly correlate with the degree of reduction in GFR[124]. Studies on experimental animal models of hypertension have shown either no response[125,126] or increased sensitivity[127] to the vasoconstrictor effect of ET-1. ET-1 evokes a greater increase in intracellular calcium concentration in isolated mesangial and vascular smooth muscle cells[128]. Infusion of ET antibody increases GFR and RBF in spontaneously hypertensive rats[129]. In a rat model of experimental nephritis (mesangial proliferation) induced by antithymocyte serum, the renal hemodynamic alterations were marked with exogenous ET-1 as compared to control rats[130].

Renal-tubule-derived ET-1 may play a role in the development and maintenance of hypertension. Inner medullary ET-1 and ET-1 mRNA production is reduced in hypertensive rats[128,131] and humans[132]. ET-1 may inhibit sodium and water reabsorption by the collecting ducts in an autocrine manner[133], and any reduction in ET-1 production by the inner medullary collecting ducts might lead to enhanced sodium and water retention. It is not clear whether altered ET-1 production by the inner medullary collecting ducts contributes to enhanced sodium and water retention in hypertension.

It is speculated that hypertension itself causes endothelial cell damage and increases endothelial cell ET-1 release. The increased ET-1 levels combined with hypertension induced enhanced vascular sensitivity to ET-1, causes further vasoconstriction, thereby exacerbating existing hypertension. Alterations in renal medullary hemodynamics may exacerbate hypertension by enhancing the reabsorption of sodium and water by the collecting ducts. A reduction of medullary flow would increase medullary tonicity which may, in turn, reduce ET-1 production by the inner medullary collecting ducts, and decrease autocrine inhibition of sodium and water transport in the inner medullary collecting ducts by ET-1. The net result would be retention of salt and water, thereby contributing to the pathogenesis and maintenance of hypertension.

Progressive renal disease

Most human renal diseases progress to end-stage renal insufficiency which is often independent from the initial insult. This is particularly true for diseases which manifest with increased glomerular permeability to macromolecules. The kidneys' adaptive response to surgical ablation is often used as a condition mimicking human progressive renal diseases. In rats with surgically ablated renal mass, a progressively increasing urinary ET-1 release and ET-1 gene expression were observed with an excessive urinary excretion of the corresponding protein and parallel signs of renal injury like proteinuria and glomerulosclerosis[134,135]. In patients with chronic renal failure the urinary excretion of ET-1 has been found to be enhanced[106] and elevated levels of ET-1 and ET-3 have been found in the plasma of patients undergoing hemodialysis[136]. The ET_A receptor antagonist FR 139317 reduced the abnormal permeability to proteins, limited glomerular injury and prevented renal function deterioration in rats with surgically ablated kidney[135]. Thus, ET_A receptors are mainly involved in mediating the deleterious effect of ET in the kidneys. Glomerular endothelial and mesangial cells express ET_B receptors[32] and so the potential role of ET_B receptors in pathophysiology of renal diseases cannot yet be excluded. This finding can have major clinical implications as ET-1 antagonists could eventually prove useful as renoprotective agents in progressive renal diseases.

Radiocontrast nephropathy

Experimental radiocontrast nephropathy has been produced in rats by application of radiocontrast agents along with other multiple insults, which reduce medullary oxygen supply and predispose hypoxic medullary injury[137]. Contributing to these may be the ability of radiocontrast agents to release ET-1 from renal vascular endothelial cells. High plasma ET-1 levels have been found in rats subjected to multiple insults like uninephrectomy and salt depletion, followed by the administration of radiocontrast agents like sodium iothalamate, ioxaglate and ioversol[137]. ET has been speculated in the pathophysiology of radiocontrast-induced nephropathy in humans[138]. The radiocontrast agents have been shown to stimulate the release ET-1 in cell culture studies[137]. Humans[138] and animals[139] with other cardio-renal risk factors are likely to be more susceptible to radiocontrast-induced nephropathy with enhanced renal ET-1 levels. It is hypothesized that ET-1 might be a marker for cellular toxicity, and a by-product rather than the the cause of nephrotoxicity.

Septic shock

Septic shock or endotoxemia is a life-threatening condition, during which an increase in cardiac output is insufficient to compensate for a decrease in peripheral vascular tone, resulting in hypotension, maldistribution of blood flow, regional ischemia, and is associated with severe renal vasoconstriction and acute renal failure[140,141]. The vasodilation has been related to the release or increased production (by injured and activated endothelium and macrophages) of endothelium-derived relaxing factors. Highly increased production and release of ET-1 has been observed during septic shock in humans[141], animals[142-144], and also in culture studies[143]. Endotoxin directly stimulates ET-1 release from endothelial cells[143], which were ameliorated by ET antibody[55]. Tumor necrosis factor, which is markedly increased in sepsis, directly stimulates ET-1 release from endothelial and mesangial cells[5,119]. The increased levels of ET-1 during septic shock might have been caused by, amongst others, intravascular coagulation, thrombin formation and activated leukocytes[145], also by increased shear stress during high blood flows, hypoxia, and activation of the sympathetic nervous system[141]. A correlation has been observed between ET-1 and leukocyte counts in patients with septic shock[141].

Diabetic nephropathy

Increased levels of plasma immunoreactive ET has been observed in patients of diabetes mellitus[146], probably due to endothelial cell damage due to the occurrence of angiopathy in these patients. However, no correlation has been found between the plasma immunoreactive ET-1 levels and blood glucose levels, blood pressure, urinary microalbumin, retinopathy, or duration of diabetes mellitus[147]. On the contrary, high glucose levels decrease ET-1 production by cultured bovine endothelial cells[148]. Decreased ET-like immunoreactivity has been observed in a rat model of streptozotocin-induced diabetes mellitus, but increased in dexamethasone-induced diabetes mellitus[147]. Increased sensitivity to ET-1 has been found in the isolated kidneys of streptozotocin-diabetic rats[149]. Insulin directly stimulated ET-1 gene expression by endothelial cells[150]. It is not clear whether ET plays any significant role in the pathogenesis of diabetic complications.

Ureteric obstruction

Reduced GFR and RBF have been observed following unilateral release of bilateral ureteral obstruction in rats. These were partially prevented by the infusion of an anti-ET antibody[151]. Enhanced urinary ET-1 exertion has been found in pigs after unilateral ureteral obstruction[152]. These studies suggest a possible role of ET in the hemodynamic changes associated with urinary tract obstruction.

Neonatal injury

The ontogenesis of urinary ET-1 like immunoreactivity has been studied in mature and premature one week old neonates and also in sick neonates with renal dysfunction secondary to neonatal asphyxia. ET-1 like immunoreactivity was observed to the same extent in the mature and premature neonates but it was elevated in the sick neonates[153]. Earlier studies in normal humans have shown that saline infusion did not affect urinary ET-1 excretion rate[106]. Also, studies in rats have shown that exogenously administered ET-1 is not excreted by the kidney and an enhanced urinary ET-1 excretion represents increased renal production[154]. The enhanced ET-1 excretion observed in the sick neonates may be a reflection of the renal damage and ET-1 may be a non-specific marker of renal injury in the neonates.

CONCLUSIONS

The biological actions of ET in the kidneys include severe vasoconstriction, mesangial cell contraction, glomerular cell proliferation, and enhanced sodium and water retention. Alteration in the concentration of ET in several renal disorders has been demonstrated. However, it appears that ET does not contribute to the pathophysiology of renal disorders but ET levels are altered as a result of the renal diseases and may be contributing to further renal complications. Specific inhibitors of ET synthesis and ET receptor antagonist need to be developed which would help in elucidating the involvement of mechanisms of ET in renal pathophysiology.

Acknowledgements

The authors are grateful to Baxter Healthcare Corporation, Miles Incorporated and National Institutes of Health for providing research funds to our laboratory.

References

1. Yanagisawa, M., Kurihara, H., Kimura, S., Tomobe, Y., Kobayashi, M., Mitsui, Y., Yazaki, Y., Goto, K & Masaki, T. (1988) A novel potent vasoconstrictor peptide produced by vascular endothelial cells. *Nature*, **332**, 411–415.

2. Inoue, A., Yanagisawa, M., Takuwa, Y., Mitsui, Y., Kobayashi, M. & Masaki, T. (1989) The human preproendothelin-1 gene. Complete nucleotide sequence and regulation of expression. *J Biol Chem*, **264**, 14954–14959.
3. Fuchs, E., Grone, H. J., Simon, M. & Laue, A. (1992) Distribution of 125I-endothelin-1,-2,-3 binding sites in mammalian kidneys. *Comp Biochem Physiol A*, **101**, 775–778.
4. Shiba, R., Sakurai, T., Yamada, G., Morimoto, H., Saito, A., Masaki, T. & Goto, K. (1992) Cloning and expression of rat preproendothelin-3 cDNA. *Biochem Biophys Res Commun*, **186**, 588–594.
5. Kohan, D. E. (1992) Production of endothelin-1 by rat mesangial cells: regulation by tumor necrosis factor. *J Lab Clin Med*, **119**, 477–484.
6. Kasinath, B. S., Fried, T. A., Davalath, S. & Marsden, P. A. (1992) Glomerular epithelial cells synthesize endothelin peptides. *Am J Pathol*, **141**, 279–283.
7. Kohan, D. E. & Fiedorek, F. T. J. (1991) Endothelin synthesis by rat inner medullary collecting duct cells. *J Am Soc Nephrol*, **2**, 150–155.
8. Kohan, D. E. (1991) Endothelin synthesis by rabbit renal tubule cells. *Am J Physiol*, **261**, F221–F226.
9. Ujiie, K., Terada, Y., Nonoguchi, H., Shinohara, M., Tomita, K. & Marumo, F. (1992) Messenger RNA expression and synthesis of endothelin-1 along rat nephron segments. *J Clin Invest*, **90**, 1043–1048.
10. Uchida, S., Takemoto, F., Ogata, E. & Kurokawa, K. (1992) Detection of endothelin-1 mRNA by RT-PCR in isolated rat renal tubules. *Biochem Biophys Res Commun*, **188**, 108–113.
11. Tejada, I. S. D., Mueller, J. D., Morenas, A. D. L., Machado, M., Moreland, R. B., Krane, R. J., Wolfe, H. J. & Traish, A. M. (1992) Endothelin in the urinary bladder: I. Synthesis of endothelin-1 by epithelia, smooth muscle and fibroblasts suggests autocrine and paracrine cellular regulation. *The Journal of Urology*, **148**, 1290–1298.
12. Simonson, M. S. & Dunn, M. J. (1990) Endothelin-1 stimulates contraction of rat glomerular mesangial cells and potentiates beta-adrenergic-mediated cyclic adenosine monophosphate accumulation. *J Clin Invest*, **85**, 790–797.
13. Lopez-Farre, A., Gomez-Garre, D., Bernabeu, F., Montanes, I., Millas, I. & Lopez-Novoa, J. M. (1991) Renal effects and mesangial cell contraction induced by endothelin are mediated by PAF. *Kidney Int*, **39**, 624–630.
14. Abassi, Z. A., Klein, H., Golomb, E. & Keiser, H. R. (1993) Regulation of the urinary excretion of endothelin in the rat. *Am J Hypertens*, **6**, 453–457.
15. Deng, Y. & Jeng, A. Y. (1992) Soluble endothelin degradation enzyme activities in various rat tissues. *Biochem Cell Biol*, **70**, 1385–1389.
16. Deng, Y., Martin, L. L., DelGrande, D. & Jeng, A. Y. (1992) A soluble protease identified from rat kidney degrades endothelin-1 but not proendothelin-1. *J Biochem (Tokyo)*, **112**, 168–172.
17. Simonson, M. S., Kester, M., Baldi, E., Osanai, T., Thomas, C. P., Mene, P. & Dunn, M. J. (1992) Endothelins: renal and cardiovascular actions. *Adv Nephrol Necker Hosp*, **21**, 177–194.
18. Simonson, M. S. & Dunn, M. J. (1992) The molecular mechanisms of cardiovascular and renal regulation by endothelin peptides. *J Lab Clin Med*, **119**, 622–639.
19. Arai, H., Hori, S., Aramori, I., Ohkubo, H. & Nakanishi, S. (1990) Cloning and expression of a cDNA encoding an endothelin receptor. *Nature*, **348**, 730–732.
20. Lin, H. Y., Kaji, E. H., Winkel, G. H., Ives, H. E. & Lodish, H. F. (1991) Cloning and functional expression of a vascular smooth muscle endothelin-1 receptor. *Proc Natl Acad Sci USA*, **88**, 3185–3189.
21. Hosoda, K., Nakao, K., Tamura, N., Arai, H., Ogawa, Y., Suga, S., Nakanishi, S. & Imura, H. (1992) Organization, structure, chromosomal assignment, and expression of the gene encoding the human endothelin-A receptor. *J Biol Chem*, **267**, 18797–18804.
22. Sakurai, T., Yanagisawa, M., Takuwa, Y., Miyazaki, H., Kimura, S., Goto, K. & Masaki, T. (1990) Cloning of a cDNA encoding a non-isopeptide-selective subtype of the endothelin receptor. *Nature*, **348**, 732–735.
23. Sakamoto, A., Yanagisawa, M., Sakurai, T., Takuwa, Y., Yanagisawa, H. & Masaki, T. (1991) Cloning and functional expression of human cDNA for the ET_B endothelin receptor. *Biochem Biophys Res Commun*, **178**, 656–663.
24. Nakamuta, M., Takayanagi, R., Sakai, Y., Sakamoto, S., Hagiwara, H., Mizuno, T., Saito, Y., Hirose, S., Yamamoto, M. & Nawata, H. (1991) Cloning and sequence analysis of a cDNA encoding human non-selective type of endothelin receptor. *Biochem Biophys Res Commun*, **177**, 34–39.
25. Ogawa, Y., Nakao, K., Arai, H., Nakagawa, O., Hosoda, K., Suga, S., Nakanishi, S. & Imura, H. (1991) Molecular cloning of a non-isopeptide-selective human endothelin receptor. *Biochem Biophys Res Commun*, **178**, 248–255.
26. Woodcock, E. A. & Land, S. (1991) Endothelin receptors in rat renal papilla with a high affinity for endothelin-3. *Eur J Pharmacol*, **208**, 255–260.
27. Karet, F. E., Kuc, R. E. & Davenport, A. P. (1993) Novel ligands BQ123 and BQ3020 characterize endothelin receptor subtypes ET_A and ET_B in human kidney. *Kidney Int*, **44**, 36–42.

28. Terada, Y., Tomita, K., Nonoguchi, H. & Marumo, F. (1992) Different localization of two types of endothelin receptor mRNA in microdissected rat nephron segments using reverse transcription and polymerase chain reaction assay. *J Clin Invest*, **90**, 107–112.
29. Cassals, M., Wikes, B. M., Hart, D., Vander Molen, M., Barnett, R. L. & Nord, E. P. (1990) Mechanism of endothelin action in inner medullary collecting duct cells. *J Am Soc Nephrol*, **1**, 467A
30. Wilkes, B. M., Ruston, A. S., Mento, P., Girardi, E., Hart, D., Vander Molen, M., Barnett, R. & Nord, E. P. (1991) Characterization of endothelin-1 receptor and signal transduction mechanisms in rat medullary interstitial cells. *Am J Physiol*, **260**, F579–F589.
31. Nambi, P., Wu, H. L., Pullen, M., Aiyar, N., Bryan, H., & Elliott, J. (1992) Identification of endothelin receptor subtypes in rat kidney cortex using subtype-selective ligands. *Mol Pharmacol*, **42**, 336–339.
32. Hori, S., Komatsu, Y., Shigemoto, R., Mizuno, N. & Nakanishi, S. (1992) Distinct tissue distribution and cellular localization of two messenger ribonucleic acids encoding different subtypes of rat endothelin receptors. *Endocrinology*, **130**, 1885–1895.
33. Stacy, D. L., Scott, J. W. & Granger, J. P. (1990) Control of renal function during intrarenal infusion of endothelin. *Am J Physiol*, **258**, F1232–F1236.
34. Yanagisawa, M. & Masaki, T. (1989) Endothelin, a novel endothelium-derived peptide. Pharmacological activities, regulation and possible roles in cardiovascular control. *Biochem Pharmacol*, **38**, 1877–1883.
35. Lerman, A., Hildebrand, F. L., Jr., Margulies, K. B., O'Murchu, B., Perella, M. A., Heublein, D. M., Schwab, T. R. & Burnett, J. C., Jr. (1990) Endothelin: a new cardiovascular regulatory peptide. *Mayo Clin Proc*, **65**, 1441–1455.
36. Edwards, R. M., Trizna, W. & Ohlstein, E. H. (1990) Renal microvascular effects of endothelin. *Am J Physiol*, **259**, F217–F221.
37. Loutzenhiser, R., Epstein, M., Hayashi, K. & Horton, C. (1990) Direct visualization of effects of endothelin on the renal microvasculature. *Am J Physiol*, **258**, F61–F68.
38. Nitta, K., Naruse, M., Sanaka, T., Tsuchiya, K., Naruse, K., Zeng, Z. P., Demura, H. & Sugino, N. (1989) Natriuretic and diuretic effects of endothelin in isolated perfused rat kidney. *Endocrinol Jpn*, **36**, 887–890.
39. Perico, N., Dadan, J. & Remuzzi, G. (1990) Endothelin mediates the renal vasoconstriction induced by cyclosporine in the rat. *J Am Soc Nephrol*, **1**, 76–83.
40. Perico, N., Dadan, J., Gabanelli, M. & Remuzzi, G. (1990) Cyclooxygenase products and atrial natriuretic peptide modulate renal response to endothelin. *J Pharmacol Exp Ther*, **252**, 1213–1220.
41. Badr, K. F., Murray, J. J., Breyer, M. D., Takahashi, K., Inagami, T. Harris, R. C. (1989) Mesangial cells, glomerular and renal vascular responses to endothelin in the rat kidney. *J Clin Invest*, **83**, 336–342.
42. Cao, L. Q. & Banks, R. O. (1990) Cardiorenal actions of endothelin, Part II: Effects of cyclooxygenase inhibitors. *Life Sci*, **46**, 585–590.
43. King, A. J. & Brenner, B. M. (1991) Endothelium-derived vasoactive factors and the renal vasculature. *Am J Physiol*, **260**, R653–R662.
44. King, A. J., Brenner, B. M. & Anderson, S. (1989) Endothelin: a potent renal and systemic vasoconstrictor peptide. *Am J Physiol*, **256**, F1051–F1058.
45. Yamada, K. & Yoshida, S. (1991) Role of endogenous endothelin in renal function during altered sodium balance. *J Cardiovasc Pharmacol*, **17 (Suppl 7)**, S290–S292.
46. Madeddu, P., Yang, X. P., Anania, V., Troffa, C., Pazzola, A., Soro, A., Manunta, P., Tonolo, G., Varoni, M. V. & et al. (1990) Efficacy of nifedipine to prevent systemic and renal vasoconstrictor effects of endothelin. *Am J Physiol*, **259**, F304–F311.
47. Miura, K., Yukimura, T., Yamashita, Y., Shimmen, T., Okumura, M., Yamanaka, S., Imanishi, M. & Yamamoto, K. (1991) Renal and femoral vascular responses to endothelin-1 in dogs: role of prostaglandins. *J Pharmacol Exp Ther*, **256**, 11–17.
48. Chou, S. Y., Dahhan, A. & Porush, J. G. (1990) Renal actions of endothelin: interaction with prostacyclin. *Am J Physiol*, **259**, F645–F652.
49. Tsuchiya, K., Naruse, M., Sanaka, T., Naruse, K., Zeng, Z. P., Nitta, K., Demura, H., Shizume, K. & Sugino, N. (1990) Renal and hemodynamic effects of endothelin in anesthetized dogs. *Am J Hypertens*, **3**, 792–795.
50. Denton, K. M. & Anderson, W. P. (1990) Vascular actions of endothelin in the rabbit kidney. *Clin Exp Pharmacol Physiol*, **17**, 861–872.
51. Rogerson, M. E., Cairns, H. S., Fairbanks, L. D., Westwich, J. & Neild, G. H. (1993) Endothelin-1 in the rabbit: interactions with cyclo-oxygenase and NO-synthase products. *Br J Pharmacol*, **108**, 838–843.
52. Simonson, M. S. & Dunn, M. J. (1990) Cellular signaling by peptides of the endothelin gene family. *FASEB J*, **4**, 2989–3000.
53. Suzuki, N., Miyauchi, T., Tomobe, Y., Matsumoto, H., Goto, K., Masaki, T. & Fujino, M. (1990) Plasma concentrations of endothelin-1 in spontaneously hypertensive rats and DOCA-salt hypertensive rats. *Biochem Biophys Res Commun*, **167**, 941–947.

54. Miura, K., Yukimura, T., Yamashita, Y., Shichino, K., Shimmen, T., Saito, M., Okumura, M., Imanishi, M., Yamanaka, S. & Yamamoto, K. (1990) Effects of endothelin on renal hemodynamics and renal function in anesthetized dogs. *Am J Hypertens*, **3**, 632–634.
55. Kon, V. & Badr, K. F. (1991) Biological actions and pathophysiologic significance of endothelin in the kidney. *Kidney Int*, **40**, 1–12.
56. Harris, P. J., Zhuo, J., Mendelsohn, F. A. & Skinner, S. L. (1991) Haemodynamic and renal tubular effects of low doses of endothelin in anaesthetized rats. *J Physiol (Lond)*, **433**, 25–39.
57. Takabatake, T., Ise, T., Ohta, K. & Kobayashi, K. (1992) Effects of endothelin on renal hemodynamics and tubuloglomerular feedback. *Am J Physiol*, **263**, F103–F108.
58. Perico, N., Cornejo, R. P., Benigni, A., Malanchini, B., Ladny, J. R. & Remuzzi, G. (1991) Endothelin induces diuresis and natriuresis in the rat by acting on proximal tubular cells through a mechanism mediated by lipoxygenase products. *J Am Soc Nephrol*, **2**, 57–69.
59. Uzuner, K. & Banks, R. O. (1993) Endothelin-induced natriuresis and diuresis and pressure-dependent events in the rat. *Am J Physiol*, **265**, R90–R96.
60. Tomita, K., Nonoguchi, H. & Marumo, F. (1990) Effects of endothelin on peptide-dependent cyclic adenosine monophosphate accumulation along the nephron segments of the rat. *J Clin Invest*, **85**, 2014–2018.
61. Hoffman, A., Grossman, E. & Keiser, H. R. (1990) Opposite effects of endothelin-1 and Big-endothelin-(1-39) on renal function in rats. *Eur J Pharmacol*, **182**, 603–606.
62. Salvati, P., Dho, L., Calabresi, M., Rosa, B. & Patrono, C. (1992) Evidence for a direct vasoconstrictor effect of big endothelin-1 in the rat kidney. *Eur J Pharmacol*, **221**, 267–273.
63. Katoh, T., Chang, H., Uchida, S., Okuda, T. & Kurokawa, K. (1990) Direct effects of endothelin in the rat kidney. *Am J Physiol*, **258**, F397–F402.
64. Banks, R. O. (1990) Effects of endothelin on renal function in dogs and rats. *Am J Physiol*, **258**, F775–F780.
65. Singh, G., Sharma, A. C., Thompson, E. B. & Gulati, A. (1994) Renal endothelin mechanism in altered thyroid states. *Life Sci*, **54**, 1901–1908.
66. Gulbins, E., Hoffend, J., Zou, A. P., Dietrich, M. S., Schlottmann, K., Cavarape, A. & Steinhausen, M. (1993) Endothelin and endothelium-derived relaxing factor control of basal renovascular tone in hydronephrotic rat kidneys. *J Physiol (Lond)*, **469**, 571–582.
67. Bloom, I. T., Bentley, F. R., Wilson, M. A. & Garrison, R. N. (1993) In vivo effects of endothelin on the renal microcirculation. *J Surg Res*, **54**, 274–280.
68. Takenaka, T., Forster, H. & Epstein, M. (1993) Protein kinase C and calcium channel activation as determinants of renal vasoconstriction by angiotensin II and endothelin. *Circ Res*, **73**, 743–750.
69. Lanese, D. M. & Conger, J. D. (1993) Effects of endothelin receptor antagonist on cyclosporine-induced vasoconstriction in isolated rat renal arterioles. *J Clin Invest*, **91**, 2144–2149.
70. Cristol, J. P., Warner, T. D., Thiemermann, C. & Vane, J. R. (1993) Mediation via different receptors of the vasoconstrictor effects of endothelins and sarafotoxins in the systemic circulation and renal vasculature of the anaesthetized rat. *Br J Pharmacol*, **108**, 776–779.
71. Pollock, D. M. & Opgenorth, T. J. (1993) Evidence for endothelin-induced renal vasoconstriction independent of ET_A receptor activation. *Am J Physiol*, **264**, R222–R226.
72. Telemaque, S., Gratton, J. P., Claing, A. & D'Orleans-Juste, P. (1993) Endothelin-1 induces vasoconstriction and prostacyclin release via the activation of endothelin ET_A receptors in the perfused rabbit kidney. *Eur J Pharmacol*, **237**, 275–281.
73. Warner, T. D., Allcock, G. H., Corder, R. & Vane, J. R. (1993) Use of the endothelin antagonists BQ123 and PD 142893 to reveal three endothelin receptors mediating smooth muscle contraction and the release of EDRF. *Br J Pharmacol*, **110**, 777–782.
74. Madeddu, P., Pala, F., Troffa, C., Pinna Parpagliam P., Pazzola, A., Soro, A., Manunta, P., Tonolo, G., Melis, M. G. & Demontis, M. P. (1990) Protectice effect of a calcium antagonist against renal vasoconstriction induced by endothelin in the normotensive rat. *Boll Soc Ital Biol Sper*, **66**, 671–678.
75. Mene, P., Simonson, M. S. & Dunn, M. J. (1989) Physiology of the mesangial cell. *Physiol Rev*, **69**, 1347–1424.
76. Dunlop, M. E. & Larkins, R. G. (1990) Insulin-dependent contractility of glomerular mesangial cells in response to angiotensin II, platelet-activating factor and endothelin is attenuated by prostaglandin E2. *Biochem J*, **272**, 561–568.
77. Dunlop, M. E. & Larkins, R. G. (1990) Insulin-dependent contractility of glomerular mesangial cells in response to angiotensin. *Biochem J*, **272**, 561–568.
78. Simonson, M. S., Wann, S., Mene, P., Dubyak, G. R., Kester, M., Nakazato, Y. & Sedor, J. R. (1989) Endothelin stimulates phospholipse C, Na^+/H^+ exchange, c-fos expression, and mitogenesis in rat mesangial cell. *J Clin Invest*, **83**, 708–712.

79. Jaffer, F. E., Knauss, T. C., Poptic, E. & Abboud, H. E. (1990) Endothelin stimulates PDGF secretion in cultured human mesangial cell. *Kidney Int*, **38**, 1193–1198.
80. Baldi, E. & Dunn, M. J. (1991) Endothelin binding and receptor down regulation in rat glomerular mesangial cells. *J Pharmacol Exp Ther*, **256**, 581–586.
81. Simonson, M. S., Jones, J. M. & Dunn, M. J. (1992) Differential regulation of *fos* and *jun* gene expression and AP-1 cis-element activity by endothelin isopeptides. Possible implications for mitogenic signaling by endothelin. *J Biol Chem*, **267**, 8643–8649.
82. Simonson, M. S., Wolfe, J. A., Konieczkowski, M., Sedor, J. R. & Dunn, M. J. (1991) Regulation of prostaglandin endoperoxide synthase gene expression in cultured rat mesangial cells: induction by serum via a protein kinase-C-dependent mechanism. *Mol Pharmacol*, **5**, 441–451.
83. Shibouta, Y., Suzuki, N., Shino, A., Matsumoto, H., Terashita, Z., Kondo, K. & Nishikawa, K. (1990) Pathophysiological role of endothelin in acute renal failure. *Life Sci*, **46**, 1611–1618.
84. Hirata, Y., Matsuoka, H., Kimura, K., Fukui, K., Hayakawa, H., Suzuki, E., Sugimoto, T., Yanagisawa, M. & Masaki, T. (1989) Renal vasoconstriction by the endothelial cell-derived peptide endothelin in spontaneously hypertensive rats. *Circ Res*, **65**, 1370–1379.
85. Miller, W. L., Redfield, M. M. & Burnett, J. C. J. (1989) Integrated cardiac, renal, and endocrine actions of endothelin. *J Clin Invest*, **83**, 317–320.
86. Garcia, R., Lachance, D. & Thibault, G. (1990) Positive inotropic action, natriuresis and atrial natriuretic factor release induced by endothelin in the conscious rat. *J Hypertens*, **8**, 725–731.
87. Saito, I., Mizuno, K., Niimura, S. & Fukuchi, S. (1993) Urinary endothelin and sodium excretion in essential hypertension. *Nephron*, **65**, 152–153.
88. Moe, O., Tejedor, A., Campbell, W. B. Alpern, R. J. & Henrich, W. L. (1991) Effects of endothelin on *in vitro* renin secretion. *Am J Physiol*, **260**, E521–E525.
89. Sei, C. A. & Glembotski, C. C. (1990) Calcium dependence of phenylephrine-, endothelin-, and potassium chloride-stimulated atrial natriuretic factor secretion from long term primary neonatal rat atrial cardiocytes. *J Biol Chem*, **265**, 7166–7172.
90. Zeidel, M. L., Brady, H. R., Kone, B. C., Gullans, S. R. & Brenner, B. M. (1989) Endothelin, a peptide inhibitor of Na^+-K^+-ATPase in intact renal tubular epithelial cells. *Am J Physiol*, **257**, C1101–C1107.
91. Schnermann, J., Lorenz, J. N., Briggs, J. P. & Keiser, J. A. (1992) Induction of water diuresis by endothelin in rats. *Am J Physiol*, **263**, F516–F526.
92. Goetz, K., Wang, B. C., Leadley, R., Jr., Zhu, J. L., Madwed, J. & Bie, P. (1989) Endothelin and sarafotoxin produce dissimilar effects on renal blood flow, but both block the antidiuretic effects of vasopressin. *Proc Soc Exp Biol Med*, **191**, 425–427.
93. Oishi, R., Nonoguchi, H., Tomita, K. & Marumo, F. (1991) Endothelin-1 inhibits AVP-stimulated osmotic water permeability in rat inner medullary collecting duct. *Am J Physiol*, **261**, F951–F956.
94. Lerman, A., Hildebrand, F. L., Jr., Aarhus, L. L. & Burnett, J. C., Jr. (1991) Endothelin has biological actions at pathophysiological concentrations. *Circulation*, **83**, 1808–1814.
95. Yokokawa, K., Tahara, H., Kohno, M., Murakawa, K., Yasunari, K., Hamada, T., Otani, S., Yanagisawa, M. & Takeda, T. (1991) Endothelin-secreting tumor. *J Cardiovasc Pharmacol*, **17 (Suppl 7)**, S398–S401.
96. Guignard, J. P., Semama, D., Joh, E. & Huet, F. (1993) Acute renal failure. *Crit Care Med*, **21**, S349–S351.
97. Stingo, A. J., Clavell, A. L., Aarhus, L. L. & Burnett, J. C., Jr. (1993) Biological role for the endothelin-A receptor in aortic cross-clamping. *Hypertension*, **22**, 62–66.
98. Mino, N., Kobayashi, M., Nakajima, A., Amano, H., Shimamoto, K., Ishikawa, K., Watanabe, K., Nishikibe, M., Yano, M. & Ikemoto, F. (1992) Protective effect of a selective endothelin receptor antagonist, BQ-123, in ischemic acute renal failure in rats. *Eur J Pharmacol*, **221**, 77–83.
99. Sandok, E. K., Lerman, A., Stingo, A. J., Perrella, M. A., Gloviczki, P. & Burnett, J. C., Jr. (1992) Endothelin in a model of acute ischemic renal dysfunction: modulating action of atrial natriuretic factor. *J Am Soc Nephrol*, **3**, 196–202.
100. Nambi, P., Pullen, M., Jugus, M. & Gellai, M. (1993) Rat kidney endothelin receptors in ischemia-induced acute renal failure. *J Pharmacol Exp Ther*, **264**, 345–348.
101. Lopez-Farre, A., Gomez-Garre, D., Bernabeu, F. & Lopez-Novoa, J. M. (1991) A role for endothelin in the maintenance of post-ischemic renal failure in the rat. *J Physiol (Lond)*, **444**, 513–522.
102. Firth, J. D. & Ratcliffe, P. J. (1992) Organ distribution of the three rat endothelin messenger RNAs and the effects of ischemia on renal gene expression. *J Clin Invest*, **90**, 1023–1031.
103. Deray, G., Carayon, A., Maistre, G., Benhmida, M., Masson, F., Barthelemy, C., Petitclerc, T. & Jacobs, C. (1992) Endothelin in chronic renal failure. *Nephrol Dial Transplant*, **7**, 300–305.
104. Saito, Y., Kazuwa, N., Shirakami, G., Mukoyama, M., Arai, H., Hosoda, K., Suga, S., Ogawa, Y.

& Imura, H. (1991) Endothelin in patients with chronic renal failure. *J Cardiovasc Pharmacol*, **17 Suppl 7**, S437–S439.
105. Stockenhuber, F., Gottsauner-Wolf, M., Marosi, L., Liebisch, B., Kurz, R. W. & Balcke, P. (1992) Plasma levels of endothelin in chronic renal failure and after renal transplantation: impact on hypertension and cyclosporine A-associated nephrotoxicity. *Clin Sci (Colch)*, **82**, 255–258.
106. Ohta, K., Hirata, Y., Shichiri, M., Kanno, K., Emori, T., Tomita, K. & Marumo, F. (1991) Urinary excretion of endothelin-1 in normal subjects and patients with renal disease. *Kidney Int*, **39**, 307–311.
107. Naruse, K., Naruse, M., Watanabe, Y., Yoshihara, I., Ohsumi, K., Horiuchi, J., Monzen, C., Kato, Y., Nakamura, N. & Sugino, N. (1991) Molecular form of immunoreactive endothelin in plasma and urine of normal subjects and patients with various disease states. *J Cardiovasc Pharmacol*, **17 (Suppl 7)**, S506–S508.
108. Fisch, J., Gulmi, F. A., Chou, S. Y., Mooppan, U. M., Kester, R. R. & Kim, H. (1993) The renal hemodynamic response to endothelin in chronic cyclosporine-treated dogs. *J Urol*, **149**, 878–883.
109. Bunchman, T. E. & Brookshire, C. A. (1991) Cyclosporine-induced synthesis of endothelin by cultured human endothelial cells. *J Clin Invest*, **88**, 310–314.
110. Moutabarrik, A., Ishibashi, M., Fukunaga, M., Kameoka, H., Takano, Y., Kokado, Y., Takahara, S., Jiang, H., Sonoda, T. & Okuyama, A. (1991) FK 506 mechanism of nephrotoxicity: stimulatory effect on endothelin secretion by cultured kidney cells and tubular cell toxicity *in vitro*. *Transplant Proc*, **23**, 3133–3136.
111. Nakahama, H., Fukuaga, M., Kakihara, M., Horio, M., Fujiwara, Y., Fukuhara, Y., Ueda, N., Orita, Y. & Kamada, T. (1991) Comparative effects of cyclosporine A and FK-506 on endothelin secretion by a cultured renal cell line, LLC-PK1. *J Cardiovasc Pharmacol*, **17 (Suppl 7)**, S172–S173.
112. Kon, V. & Awazu, M. (1992) Endothelin and cyclosporine nephrotoxicity. *Ren Fail*, **14**, 345–350.
113. Fogo, A., Hellings, S. E., Inagami, T. & Kon, V. (1992) Endothelin receptor antagonism is protective *in vivo* acute cyclosporine toxicity. *Kidney Int*, **42**, 770–774.
114. Bloom, I. T., Bentley, F. R. & Garrison, R. N. (1993) Acute cyclosporine-induced renal vasoconstriction is mediated by endothelin-1. *Surgery*, **114**, 480–7; discussion 487–8.
115. Takeda, M., Breyer, M. D., Noland, T. D., Homma, T., Hoover, R. L., Inagami, T. & Kon, V. (1992) Endothelin-1 receptor antagonist: effects on endothelin- and cyclosporine-treated mesangial cells. *Kidney Int*, **41**, 1713–1719.
116. Clark, B. A., Halvorson, L., Sachs, B. & Epstein, F. H. (1992) Plasma endothelin levels in preeclampsia: elevation and correlation with uric acid levels and renal impairment. *Am J Obstet Gynecol*, **166**, 962–968.
117. Lamas, S., Michel, T., Collins, T., Brenner, B. M. & Marsden, P. A. (1992) Effects of interferon-gamma on nitric oxide synthase activity and endothelin-1 production by vascular endothelial cells. *J Clin Invest*, **90**, 879–887.
118. Sakamoto, H., Sasaki, S., Nakamura, Y., Fushimi, K. & Marumo, F. (1992) Regulation of endothelin-1 production in cultured rat mesangial cells. *Kidney Int*, **41**, 350–355.
119. Marsden, P. A. & Brenner, B. M. (1992) Transcriptional regulation of the endothelin-1 gene by TNF-alpha. *Am J Physiol*, **262**, C854–C861.
120. Nakamura, T., Ebihara, I., Fukui, M., Osada, S., Tomino, Y., Masaki, T., Goto, K., Furuichi, Y. & Koide, H. (1993) Renal expression of mRNAs for endothelin-1, endothelin-3 and endothelin receptors in NZB/WF1 mice. *Renal Physiol Biochem*, **16**, 233–243.
121. Achmad, T. H. & Rao, G. S. (1992) Chemotaxis of human blood monocytes toward endothelin-1 and the influence of calcium channel blockers. *Biochem Biophys Res Commun*, **189**, 994–1000.
122. Martin Nizard, F., Houssaini, H. S., Lestavel Delattre, S., Duriez, P. & Fruchart, J. C. (1991) Modified low density lipoproteins activate human macrophages to secrete immunoreactive endothelin. *FEBS Lett*, **293**, 127–130.
123. Sessa, W. C., Kaw, S., Zembowicz, A., Anggard, E., Hecker, M. & Vane, J. R. (1991) Human polymorphonuclear leukocytes generate and degrade endothelin-1 by two distinct neutral proteases. *J Cardiovasc Pharmacol*, **17 (Suppl 7)**, S34–S38.
124. Kohno, M., Yasunari, K., Murakawa, K., Yokokawa, K., Horio, T., Fukui, T. & Takeda, T. (1990) Plasma immunoreactive endothelin in essential hypertension. *Am J Med*, **88**, 614–618.
125. Dohi, Y., Criscione, L. & Luscher, T. F. (1991) Renovascular hypertension impairs formation of endothelium-derived relaxing factors and sensitivity to endothelin-1 in resistance arteries. *Br J Pharmacol*, **104**, 349–354.
126. Bolger, G. T., Liard, F., Jodoin, A & Jaramillo, J. (1991) Vascular reactivity, tissue levels, and binding sites for endothelin: a comparison in the spontaneously hypertensive and Wistar-Kyoto rats. *Can J Physiol Pharmacol*, **69**, 406–413.
127. Yokokawa, K., Kohno, M., Murakawa, K., Yasunari, K., Inoue, T. & Takeda, T. (1990) Effects of

endothelin on blood pressure and renal hemodynamics in DOCA-salt hypertensive rats under conscious and unrestrained condition. *Clin Exp Hypertens [A]*, **12**, 1049–1062.
128. Goligorsky, M. S., Iijima, K., Morgan, M., Yanagisawa, M., Masaki, T., Nasjletti, A., Kaskel, F., Frazer, M. & Badr, K. F. (1991) Role of endothelin in the development of Dahl hypertension. *J Cardiovasc Pharmacol*, **17 (Suppl 7)**, S484–S491.
129. Ohno, A., Naruse, M., Kato, S., Hosaka, M., Naruse, K., Demura, H. & Sugino, N. (1992) Endothelin-specific antibodies decrease blood pressure and increase glomerular filtration rate and renal plasma flow in spontaneously hypertensive rats. *J Hypertens*, **10**, 781–785.
130. Kanai, H., Okuda, S., Kiyama, S., Tomooka, S., Hirakata, H. & Fujishima, M. (1993) Effects of endothelin and angiotension II on renal hemodynamics in experimental mesangial proliferative nephritis. *Nephron*, **64**, 609–614.
131. Hughes, A. K., Cline, R. C. & Kohan, D. E. (1992) Alterations in renal endothelin-1 production in the spontaneously hypertensive rat. *Hypertension*, **20**, 666–673.
132. Hoffman, A., Grossman, E., Ohman, K. P., Marks, E. & Keiser, H. R. (1990) The initial vasodilation and the later vasoconstriction of endothelin-1 are selective to specific vascular beds. *Am J Hypertens*, **3**, 789–791.
133. Kohan, D. E. & Padilla, E. (1992) Endothelin-1 is an autocrine factor in rat inner medullary collecting ducts. *Am J Physiol*, **263**, F607–F612.
134. Orisio, S., Benigni, A., Bruzzi, I., Corna, D., Perico, N., Zoja, C., Benatti, L. Remuzzi, G. (1993) Renal endothelin gene expression is increased in remnant kidney and correlates with disease progression. *Kidney Int*, **43**, 354–358.
135. Benigni, A., Zoja, C., Corna, D., Orisio, S., Longaretti, L., Bertani, T. & Remuzzi, G. (1993) A specific endothelin subtype A receptor antagonist protects against injury in renal disease progression. *Kidney Int*, **44**, 440–444.
136. Suzuki, N., Matsumoto, H., Miyauchi, T. Goto, K., Masaki, T., Tsuda, M. & Fujinom M. (1990) Endothelin-3 concentrations in human plasma: the increased concentrations in patients undergoing haemodialysis. *Biochem Biophys Res Commun*, **169**, 809–815.
137. Heyman, S. N., Clark, B. A., Cantley, L., Spokes, K., Rosen, S., Brezis, M. & Epstein, F. H. (1993) Effects of ioversol versus iothalamate on endothelin release and radiocontrast nephropathy. *Invest Radiol*, **28**, 313–318.
138. Nord, E. P. (1993) Renal actions of endothelin. *Kidney Int*, **44**, 451–463.
139. Margulies, K. B., Hildebrand, F. L., Heublein, D. M. & Burnett, J. C. J. (1991) Radiocontrast increases plasma and urinary endothelin. *J Am Soc Nephrol*, **2**, 1041–1045.
140. Badr, K. F. (1992) Sepsis-associated renal vasoconstriction: potential targets for future therapy. *Am J Kidney Dis*, **20**, 207–213.
141. Voerman, H. J., Stehouwer, C. D., van Kamp, G. J., Strack van Schijndel, R. J., Groeneveld, A. B. & Thijs, L. G. (1992) Plasma endothelin levels are increased during septic shock. *Crit Care Med*, **20**, 1097–1101.
142. Takahashi, K., Silva, A., Cohen, J., Lam, H. C., Ghatei, M. A. & Bloom, S. R. (1990) Endothelin immunoreactivity in mice with gram-negative bacteraemia: relationship to tumour necrosis factor-alpha. *Clin Sci (Colch)*, **79**, 619–623.
143. Sugiura, M., Inagami, T. & Kon, V. (1989) Endotoxin stimulates endothelin-release *in vivo* and *in vitro* as determined by radioimmunoassay. *Biochem Biophys Res Commun*, **161**, 1220–1227.
144. Pernow, J., Hemsen, A., Hallen, A. & Lundberg, J. M. (1990) Release of endothelin-like immunoreactivity in relation to neuropeptide Y and catecholamines during endotoxin shock and asphyxia in the pig. *Acta Physiol Scand*, **140**, 311–322.
145. Ehrenreich, H., Anderson, R. W., Fox, C. H., Rieckmann, P., Hoffman, G. S., Travis, W. D., Coligan, J. E., Kehrl, J. H. & Fauci, A. S. (1990) Endothelins, peptides with potent vasoactive properties, are produced by human macrophages. *J Exp Med*, **172**, 1741–1748.
146. Takahashi, K., Ghatei, M. A., Lam, H. C., O'Halloran, D. J. & Bloom, S. R. (1990) Elevated plasma endothelin in patients with diabetes mellitus. *Diabetologia*, **33**, 306–310.
147. Takahashi, H., Nishimura, M., Nakanishi, T., Habuchi, Y., Tanaka, H., Ikegaki, I. & Yoshimura, M. (1991) Effects of intracerebroventricular and intravenous injections of endothelin-1 on blood pressure and sympathetic activity in urethane-anesthetized rats. *J Cardiovasc Pharmacol*, **17 (Suppl 7)**, S287–S289.
148. Molinatti, P. A., Porta, M., Takahashi, K., Kanse, S. M., Brooks, R. A., Bloom, S. R. & Kohner, E. M. (1990) Reduced synthesis of endothelin-1 by retinal capillary endothelial cells cultured in high glucose. *Med Sci Sec Spring Meet Brit Diab Assoc*, , A32.
149. Tammesild, P. J., Hodgson, W. C. & King, R. G. (1992) Increased sensitivity to endothelin-1 in isolated Kreb's-perfused kidneys of streptozotocin-diabetic rats. *Clin Exp Pharmacol Physiol*, **19**, 261–265.
150. Oliver, F. J., de la Rubia, G., Feener, E. P., Lee, M. E., Loeken, M. R., Shiba, T., Quertermous, T. & King,

G. L. (1991) Stimulation of endothelin-1 gene expression by insulin in endothelial cells. *J Biol Chem*, **266**, 23251–23256.
151. Reyes, A. A. & Klahr, S. (1992) Renal function after release of ureteral obstruction: role of endothelin and the renal artery endothelium. *Kidney Int*, **42**, 632–638.
152. Kelleher, J. P., Shah, V., Godley, M. L., Wakefield, A. J., Gordon, I., Ransley, P. G., Snell, M. E. & Risdon, R. A. (1992) Urinary endothelin (ET-1) in complete ureteric obstruction in the miniature pig. *Urol Res*, **20**, 63–65.
153. Kojima, T., Isozaki-Fukuda, Y., Sasai, M., Hirata, Y., Matsuzaki, S. & Kobayashi, Y. (1993) Urinary endothelin-1-like immunoreactivity excretion in the newborn period. *Am J Perinatol*, **10**, 220–223.
154. Benigni, A., Perico, N. & Gaspari, F. (1990) Increased renal endothelin (ET) production in rats with renal mass reduction (RMR). *J Am Soc Nephrol*, **1**, 411.

16 Role of Endothelin in Pulmonary Diseases

Douglas W. P. Hay[1] and Roy G. Goldie[2]

[1]*Department of Inflammation & Respiratory Pharmacology, SmithKline Beecham Pharmaceuticals, 709 Swedeland Road, King of Prussia, PA 19406, USA*

[2]*Department of Pharmacology, University of Western Australia, Perth, Nedlands 6009, Western Australia, Australia*

INTRODUCTION

In 1988 Yanagisawa and co-workers described the isolation, purification, cloning and expression, and initial pharmacological characterization of a potent vasoconstrictor 21-amino acid peptide, designated endothelin (ET), which was released from porcine aortic endothelial cells[1]. It was demonstrated subsequently that this novel substance was member of a mammalian family of vasoconstrictor peptides, designated ET-1, ET-2 and ET-3, which are encoded by three distinct ET-related genes and which bear a close structural and functional homology to a group of snake venom toxins, the sarafotoxins; ET-1 is the original porcine/human ET, ET-2 differs by two amino acid substitutions from ET-1, and ET-3 differs by six amino acids[2-4].

Since the discovery of ET-1 there has been an enormous amount of research conducted (over 3000 publications) on the putative physiological and pathophysiological actions of the ETs. Not surprisingly, in light of its recognized potent vasoconstrictor properties and the fact that it was originally isolated from endothelial cells, the focus of initial interest was on its activity and potential pathophysiological relevance in the cardiovascular system. However, it quickly became apparent that the ETs possess a broad spectrum of biological activities and exert diverse effects in a variety of tissues and systems. One such area is in the pulmonary system, in which there is growing interest and research on the effects of the ETs. Accordingly, in this chapter a comprehensive review of our understanding of the influence of the ETs in various cells in the pulmonary system will be given, with particular attention being paid to their potential pathophysiological relevance in respiratory tract disorders.

DISTRIBUTION, SYNTHESIS, RELEASE, METABOLISM, UPTAKE AND CLEARANCE

Distribution

The lung is one of the sites in the body in which the ET levels are among the highest noted[5-7]. For example, in rat lung the level of immunoreactive (ir)-ET was calculated to be 42.0 ± 3.7 pg/mg[7], and in the pig, 1.5 ± 0.07 pmol/g, which was the highest amount detected in the several tissues examined[8]. Interestingly, ET-1 mRNA was detected in human lung homogenates[9]. The cellular origins of ET released in the bronchial wall have still to be clarified, although it appears that they include the endothelium, epithelium and some inflammatory cells. ET-like immunoreactivity is present in the majority of epithelial cells in the conducting airways of rat and mouse[10]. There is intense staining in mucous, serous and Clara cells, but little or no immunoreactivity in basal cells and most ciliated cells. In rabbit trachea ET-1 immunoreactivity was detected in cells scattered throughout the epithelium, and was also detected in cultured tracheal epithelial cells[11]. Furthermore, consistent with the location of ET at these sites is the presence in rat fetal lung of large amounts of ET mRNA, localized in respiratory epithelial cells of bronchioles and also blood vessels[12]. Interestingly, in this study Northern blot analysis detected two forms of ET mRNA (2.5-kilobase and 3.7-kilobase forms) in rat tissues, both of which were present in lung.

Immunocytochemical techniques have also demonstrated ir-ET in human airway epithelial and endocrine cells. Furthermore, mRNA for the three ET isoforms have been detected in these cells. Immunoreactivity was observed predominantly in pulmonary endocrine cells and was less evident in the airway epithelium (in about 50% of human adults)[13]. The amounts of immunoreactivity and mRNA present in vascular endothelial cells was highest in the developing lung, started to decrease before birth and was minimal in adults. It was proposed that ET may play a role in growth regulation.

In addition to the above locations, the expression and release of ET-1 from human macrophages – an inflammatory cell commonly found in the lung – has been demonstrated[14]. In the same study the expression but not the release of ET-3 was noted. Furthermore, ir-ET-1, but not ir-ET-3, is present in mouse primary bone marrow mast cells in large quantities (600–800 pg/10^8 cells), although there was little basal release of ET-1[15]. This contrasts with endothelial cells which have little storage capacity for ET-1 but secrete basally significant quantities of the peptide.

Synthesis

In the first publication on ET-1 it was proposed that the mature peptide was synthesized *via* an unusual proteolytic process involving a two-step pathway (Figure 16.1). The initial stage involved the formation of a 39-amino acid residue intermediate, designated "big endothelin", from a 203-residue preproendothelin *via* the activity of an endopeptidase(s) specific for the paired dibasic amino acid residues[1]; note, the human form of preproendothelin consists of 212-amino acid residues[16]. Big endothelin then undergoes a previously unknown type of cleavage between Trp[73] and Val[74], *via* the activity of a putative endopeptidase with chymotrypsin-like activity, which was designated as "endothelin-converting enzyme" or "ECE". ET-1, Big ET-1 and the carboxyterminal of Big ET-1 (big ET[22-39]) have been detected on the supernatant of cultured endothelial cells[17,18] and in human plasma[19]. The vasoconstrictor potency of big ET-1 in isolated blood vessels is appreciably less (>100-fold) than ET-1[20,21], suggesting that the formation of ET-1 is critical for the realization of the potent biological activity of the ET system. The presence of mRNA

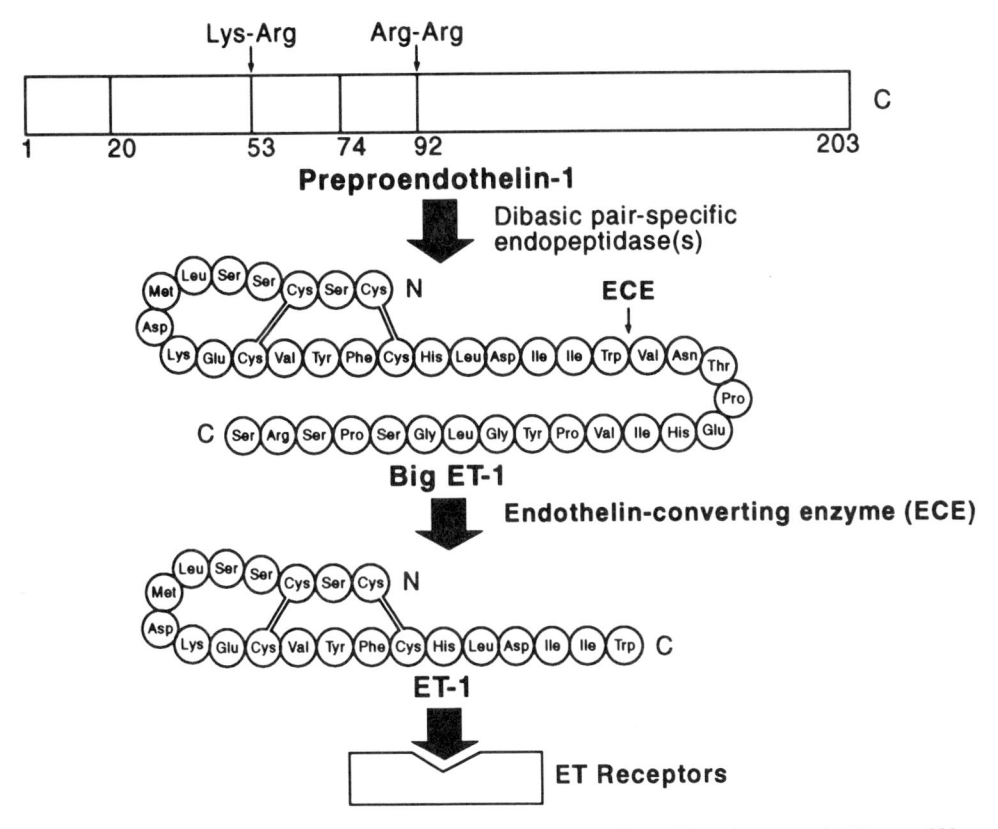

Figure 16.1. Biosynthetic pathway for endothelin-1. Adapted from Yanagisawa et al., *Nature*, **332**, 411–415 (1988).

encoding preproendothelin ET in endothelial cells provided evidence that ET is generated by *de novo* synthesis and is not stored preformed in this tissue, with the regulation of synthesis predominantly at the mRNA transcription level. This is supported by the apparent lack of secretory granules in the endothelial cells[22] and the minimal quantities of ET-1 and big ET-1 that are detected intracellularly[23,24].

Controversy persists as to the identity, location and characteristics of the putative ECE. Evidence has been presented suggesting the existence of at least three ECE-like enzymatic activities, two of which are cytosolic and the other membrane-associated, with a membrane-bound, neutral metalloprotease, which is sensitive to phosphoramidon, the most attractive candidate is the physiologically relevant ECE[4,24]. A phosphoramidon-sensitive (IC$_{50}$ = 0.5 µM) neutral protease which was able to convert big ET-1 to ET-1 was identified in rat lung, with a relative abundance in the membrane versus the cytosol of 4:1[25]. Furthermore, recently, the partial solubilization and purification of ECE from porcine lung was reported[26] and successful purification to homogeneity of ECE from rat lung microsomes was demonstrated[27]. In the latter study, the purified enzyme had a molecular weight of 130 kD and specifically catalyzed the conversion of big ET-1 to ET-1 *via* a mechanism which was inhibited by phosphoramidon and metal chelators. It was concluded that ECE is a neutral metalloprotease[27].

In the airways there is further evidence *in vivo* and using perfused lungs that the ECE responsible for the conversion of big ET-1 to ET-1 is sensitive to phosphoramidon. For example, big ET-1 was converted to ET-1 in rabbit perfused lung *via* a mechanism which was blocked by phosphoramidon[28]. Similar findings were observed in guinea-pigs in which it was noted that proteolytic conversion of big ET-1, *via* a phosphoramidon-sensitive pathway, was essential for bronchoconstrictor and pressor responses following intravenous administration[29]. In addition, phosphoramidon abolished the increase in ET-1 release induced by ischemia-hypoxia in isolated guinea-pig lungs[30].

In addition, the presence of an aspartic protease with ECE activity in rat lung was reported[31]. Studies using gel filtration chromatography indicated that there is a novel enzyme present in the soluble fraction of porcine lung which degraded big ET-1 by cleavage at the bond between Val^{22} and Asn^{23}. The enzyme was a serine protease sensitive to diisopropylfluorophosphate and was designated ET-Val-generating endopeptidase[32]. It was also suggested that lung mast cell-derived chymase can produce that was termed "physiologically relevant" extracellular processing of big ET-1 to ET-1 in the perfused rat lung[33].

Once the nature of physiologically important ECE, or ECEs, has been clarified this enzyme may provide a reasonable molecular target to design novel drugs to control the release and activities of the ETs in diseases.

Release

ET-1 is released basally from cultured porcine, canine[34] and human bronchial[35] and guinea-pig[36,37] and rabbit tracheal epithelial cells[38]. In addition, ET-3 was detected in supernatants from canine and porcine cultured tracheal epithelial cells[34]. ET-1 is also released from murine cultured bone marrow-derived mast cells following long-term incubation with IgE (10-fold increase after 20 hr) *via* a mechanism that is not directly linked to degranulation[15]. The release of ET is increased by endotoxin, thrombin, and various cytokines[36-38]. In the comprehensive analysis of the effects of several cytokines, it was noted that they possessed a spectrum of activities. Thus, IL-8, TNF-α and TGF-β transiently stimulated the synthesis of ET-1, whereas EGF, PDGF and GM/CSF promoted the proliferation of the epithelial cells. Furthermore, IL-1 increased the synthesis of big-ET-1, while IL-2, IL-6 and IGF-1 induced the synthesis of big ET-1 and mitogenesis[37]. The regulatory role of the cytokines on ET-1 synthesis and release may be important in inflammation and tissue repair associated with many pulmonary disorders, processes in which the cytokines are thought to play a key role. The ET amounts released into the culture medium appear to be appreciably less than those required to elicit a bronchoconstrictor response: for example, ET release from human bronchial epithelial cells over 72 hours is 1.12 ± 0.19 pmol/ml/10^6 cells, whereas the EC$_{50}$ for producing contraction of human bronchus is in the nM range (*vide infra*). However, *in vivo* local concentrations of the ETs will be much higher and perhaps sufficient to elicit bronchospasm. In addition, some effects of the ETs, for example stimulation of mitogenesis[39], occur in lower concentrations than required to cause contraction of airway smooth muscle.

Metabolism

Our laboratory originally demonstrated that the epithelium inhibited contractile responses induced by ET-1 in guinea-pig trachea *via* a mechanism which was sensitive to phosphoramidon, an inhibitor of neutral endopeptidase (NEP; EC 3.4.24.11)[40]. It was speculated that this phenomenon was attributed to ET-1 being metabolized by epithelium-derived NEP. The ETs were subsequently shown to be good substrates for NEP[41,42]. Other researchers have provided further functional data in support of a modulatory role of epithelium-derived NEP on ET-1-induced contraction in guinea-pig trachea[43,44]. For example, recombinant human NEP decreased ET-1-induced contraction[43]. These observations have been extended to *in vivo* studies in which it has been demonstrated that phosphoramidon potentiates ET-1-induced bronchoconstriction in guinea-pigs[45]. In human bronchus, evidence was provided to indicate that NEP is involved in the local metabolism of ET-3 but not ET-1. Thus, phosphoramidon potentiated responses elicited by the former but not the latter agonist; similar findings were observed in rabbit bronchus[46]. However, the status of the integrity of the airway epithelium in these experiments was not indicated, and this may have markedly influenced the results obtained. Indeed, another study demonstrated that phosphoramidon did potentiate ET-1-induced contraction in human bronchus[47]. Interestingly, these and other data suggest strongly that two phosphoramidon-sensitive enzymes have opposing effects in the control of ET-1 levels in airways: thus, as indicated above, the putative ECE responsible for the formation of ET-1 from big ET-1 is a neutral metalloprotease sensitive to phosphoramidon, whereas NEP appears to be involved in the breakdown of ET-1.

Although, it appears that NEP is the major enzyme involved in ET-1 degradation in the airways, other pathways may exist. For example, ET-1 was metabolized by activated, but not non-stimulated, human polymorphonuclear neutrophils (PMNs)[48]. Soybean trypsin inhibitor essentially abolished the degradation of ET-1, whereas phosphoramidon was without effect, suggesting that cathepsin G, rather than NEP, is involved in ET-1 metabolism by these cells. The levels of cathepsin G in these cells have been estimated to be about 300- to 3600-fold higher than those of NEP.

Uptake and clearance

Intravenously administered ET-1 was reported to be rapidly eliminated from the circulation in rats, with accumulation predominantly in the lungs and in the kidneys[49-51]. It was calculated that 82% of [^{126}I]-ET-1 was taken up by the lungs[51]. Evidence was provided in guinea-pig and rat isolated perfused lungs for substantial removal of ET-1 by the pulmonary circulation (>50% in a single passage)[52]. Furthermore, in rabbits significant uptake of ET-1 was demonstrated by the pulmonary but not the coronary circulation[53]. In contrast, in pig it was concluded that during infusion of ET-1 there was no clearance in the lungs[8]. Similarly, following analysis of ET concentrations at several points in the circulation is was concluded that ET was not extracted by the pulmonary system in humans[55]. Thus, it appears that marked species differences exist in the contribution of the pulmonary circulation to the uptake and clearance of ET.

Receptor localization

Numerous studies employing binding and autoradiographic techniques have revealed significant quantities of a single class of high-affinity ET-1 binding sites in the respiratory tract of several species including humans[55-60]. In human bronchial tissues, labeling of [^{125}I]-ET-1 was localized largely to airway and vascular smooth muscle, with little or no binding on cartilage, connective tissues, the submucosal layer, including glandular cells, and epithelium[55,57] (Figure 16.2); similar observations were obtained in tracheal sections from mouse, rat guinea-pig[57]. In contrast, recent studies in sheep trachea have revealed high densities of specific binding sites for ET-1 in cells associated with submucosal glands and in the submucosa immediately below the epithelium (lamina propria) (Figure 16.3). In addition, in human, and also rat and guinea-pig airways, it was noted that there was significant binding associated with alveolar septae and with parasympathetic ganglia, and also with paravascular nerves and nerves in the connective tissues[55,57,61,62]. A single, specific high affinity binding site for [^{125}I]-ET-1 was detected on cultured human bronchial smooth muscle cells, with an apparent binding affinity, K_d, of 0.11 nM, and a maximum binding capacity, B_{max} = 22.1 fmol/10^6 cells[35]. Evidence has been presented in support of at least two binding sites for the ETs in guinea-pig airway[60]. In that study some diffuse binding in the tracheal epithelium was noted although the density of binding was 16% of that demonstrated in the smooth muscle and only 6% of that in the submucosal region[60]. Similarly, significant labeling of [^{125}I]-ET in rat airway epithelium was noted[49]. However, it is generally the case that the levels of specific ET-1 binding to epithelium are low compared to airway smooth muscle in most species studied so far. Following, *in vivo* labeling studies in rats the highest density of labeling was observed in the lung and kidney[49]. Furthermore, in a comparison of [^{125}I]-ET binding to various tissue membrane fractions, the highest density of binding was demonstrated in trachea followed by lung parenchyma and *vas deferens*[63].

Receptor subtypes

In light of the quantitative and qualitative differences apparent in the pharmacological profile of the ET isoforms, it was proposed that the many biological activities of the ETs may be mediated *via* multiple ET receptors which possess different tissue distributions[3,4]. In addition to functional results, biochemical and molecular biological data in a variety of cells and tissues, including lung, provided unequivocal evidence for the existence of distinct ET receptor subtypes. The lung has been widely used in studies investigating ET receptor characterization and subtyping, in large part due to its high densities of ET receptors. Cross-linking affinity labeling studies in rat lung membranes provided evidence for two ET receptors, a 44 kD type which had higher affinity for ET-1 and ET-2 than ET-3 and another with a molecular weight of 32 kD which had a higher affinity for ET-3[64]. Ligand binding and affinity labelling studies in porcine lung and other tissues have also suggested the presence of two distinct ET receptor subtypes, an ET-1-specific receptor and a receptor that was common to the ET/sarafotoxin family[65]. Furthermore, using several systems, including rat and bovine lung, the cloning and expression of cDNA for a selective and also for

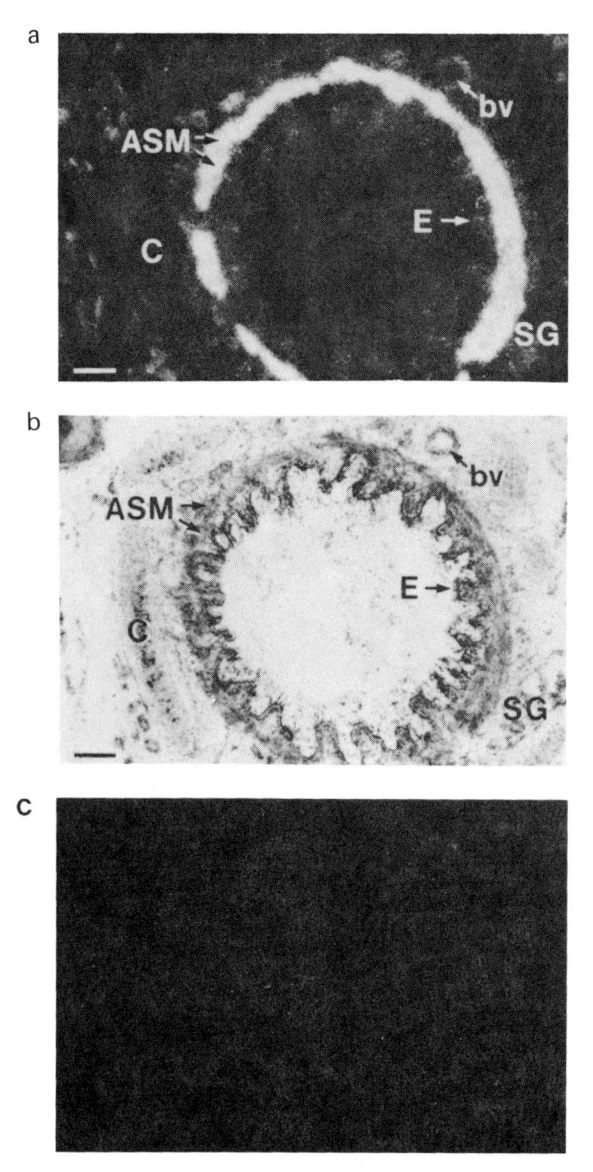

Figure 16.2. (a) Dark-field photomicrograph of a 10 μm frozen section of human isolated bronchus showing the distribution and localization of autoradiographic grains derived from [^{125}I]-endothelin-1 binding ([^{125}I]-ET-1; 0.5 nM, 60 min incubation). (b) Bright-field photomicrograph of the above section. ASM = airway smooth muscle, E = epithelium, SG = submucosal gland, bv = blood vessel, C = cartilage. (c) Dark-field photomicrograph showing the distribution of non-specific autoradiographic grains in a neighboring section incubated with [^{125}I]-ET-1 (0.5 nM) in the combined presence of the ET$_A$ receptor antagonist BQ-123 (1 μM) and the ET$_B$ receptor agonist, sarafotoxin S6c (100 nM). Bar = 200 μm.

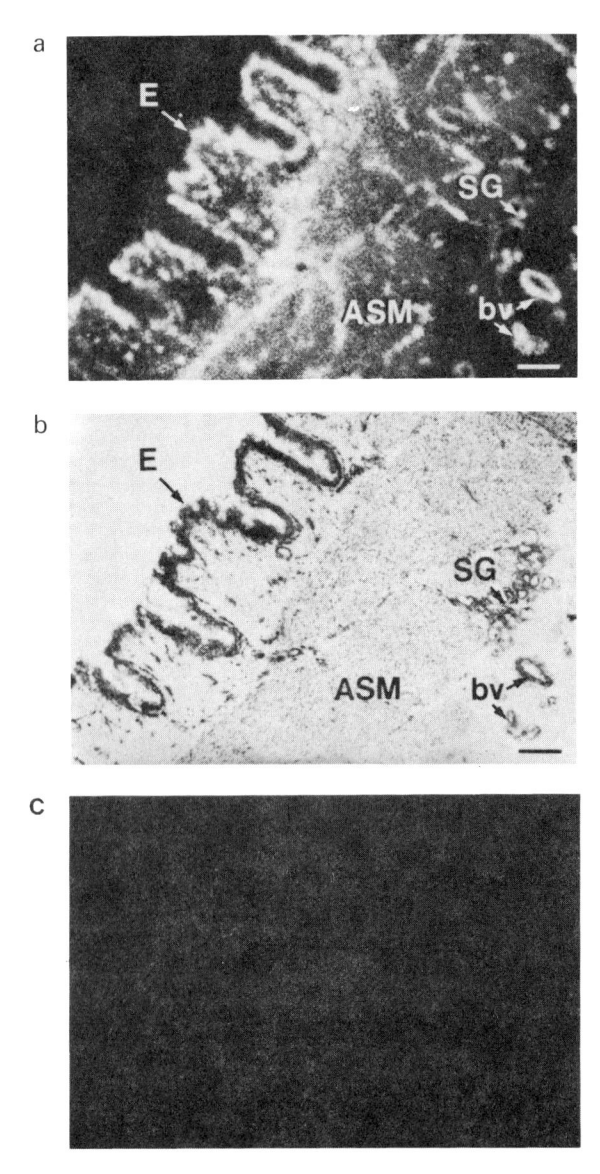

Figure 16.3. (a) Dark-field photomicrograph of a 10 μm frozen section of ovine isolated trachea showing the distribution and localization of autoradiographic grains derived from [^{125}I]-endothelin-1 binding ([^{125}I]-ET-1; 0.5 nM, 60 min incubation). (b) Bright-field photomicrograph of the above section. ASM = airway smooth muscle, E = epithelium, SG = submucosal gland, bv = blood vessel, C = cartilage. (c) Dark-field photomicrograph showing the distribution of non-specific autoradiographic grains in a neighboring section incubated with [^{125}I]-ET-1 (0.5 nM) in the combined presence of the ET$_A$ receptor antagonist BQ-123 (1 μM) and the ET$_B$ receptor agonist, sarafotoxin S6c (100 nM). Bar = 200 μm.

a non-selective ET receptor, designated ET_A and ET_B, respectively, has been achieved[4,66-69]. The ET_A receptor has a higher affinity for ET-1 or ET-2 compared with ET-3, whereas the ET_B receptor has equal affinity for the various ET isoforms. Both receptors belong to the superfamily of G-protein-linked, seven transmembrane domain receptors[4,69]. Evidence has also been provided in rat cultured anterior pituitary cells and rat PC12 pheochromocytoma cells, for an ET receptor subtype, designated ET_C[4], which is selective for ET-3[70,71]. This receptor has recently been cloned from *Xenopus laevis* dermal melanophores[72]. The solubilization of ET_A and ET_B receptors from rat lung[73] and the purification of the ET_B receptor (52 kD) from bovine lung[74,75] have been reported. *In vivo* functional evidence has now been provided for the existence of ET_A-like and ET_C-like receptors in the cat pulmonary vascular beds[76].

Using immunohistochemical and immunoprecipitation techniques with an ET_B-specific antiserum, it was calculated that about 70% of the ET receptors in bovine lung were of the ET_B subtype, with the estimated amount of ET_B receptors = 385 ± 58 fmol/mg protein[77]. A preliminary study from our laboratories indicated that the proportions of ET_A and ET_B receptors in human bronchial smooth muscle from non-asthmatic and asthmatic lung was about 88% ET_B: 12% ET_A[78]. However, it appears that the relative regional distribution of ET receptor subtypes in the pulmonary system is species-dependent. For example, in porcine pulmonary tissues, binding studies, examining the displacement of $[^{125}I]$-ET-1 binding with receptor subtype-selective ligands, indicated that the proportions of $ET_A:ET_B$ receptors in bronchus appeared to be about 70:30 whereas, in lung parenchyma it was the reverse[79]. Autoradiographic analysis supported the differential predominance of the ET receptor subtypes in porcine pulmonary tissues, with the ET_A receptor prominent in the bronchi and vasculature, and the ET_B receptor more abundant in the parenchyma[79]. Recently, using the novel ET_B-selective radioligand, $[^{125}I]$-BQ-3020, autoradiographic studies in porcine lung revealed significant binding to parenchyma, parasympathetic ganglia, pulmonary and submucosal plexuses, but minimal binding to circular smooth muscle layers or airway epithelium. Interestingly, the binding of $[^{125}I]$-BQ-3020 in blood vessels paralleled the acetylcholinesterase activity suggesting that the ET_B receptors in blood vessels may be located on parasympathetic nerves[80]. More recently, autoradiographic data have revealed that in rat tracheal smooth muscle, ET_A and ET_B receptors exist in approximately equal numbers[81]. In contrast, ovine tracheal smooth muscle contained an almost homogeneous population of ET_A receptors[82,83].

In addition, there is growing data from functional studies in support of ET receptor subtypes in the pulmonary system. Maggi and co-workers comprehensively explored the activity of members of the ET and sarafotoxin family and peptide analogs in isolated tissues including guinea-pig airways, and based on these studies they proposed the existence of ET receptor subtypes[84-86]. They reported that the hexapeptide ET-(16–21) was a full agonist in guinea-pig bronchus but was without effect in rat aorta, whereas ET-1 effectively contracted both tissues. Based on these findings they provisionally designated the proposed ET receptor subtypes as ET_A (representing the *a*orta) and ET_B (for *b*ronchus)[85]. Based on a comparison of the relative contractile activities of ET-1, ET-2 and ET-3, in addition to their ability to cause cross-sensitization, it was proposed that distinct ET receptors mediate contraction in guinea-pig pulmonary artery and trachea[87].

More direct and definitive evidence for ET receptor subtypes in the pulmonary system has been provided utilizing selective ligands, in particular, sarafotoxin S6c the ET_B-selective agonist[88] and recently identified peptide ET_A-selective antagonists such as the cyclic pentapeptide BQ-123[89] and FR 139317[90]. Utilizing these experimental tools functional evidence was provided initially for distinct ET receptors in guinea-pig pulmonary artery and rat aorta (ET_A-subtype) compared with guinea-pig trachea and trachea (non-ET_A, probably ET_B)[91,92]. In human bronchus non-ET_A (ET_B?) receptors predominated in mediating the ET-1-induced contraction whereas in human pulmonary artery contraction was mediated *via* the ET_A receptor[93]. In addition, this study demonstrated regional differences in the relative distribution of ET_A and non-ET_A receptors in guinea-pig airways. Interestingly, evidence was provided for different receptors mediating ET-1-induced contraction (non-ET_A) and mediator release in human bronchus (ET_A)[93]. In rat perfused lungs ET-1-induced PGI_2 release was antagonized by BQ-123 and was therefore ET_A receptor-mediated[94].

It will continue to be important in the future to determine the receptor subtypes mediating the effects of ET-1 in the pulmonary system. The availability of selective ET_B receptor antagonists will assist greatly in this endeavor.

BIOLOGICAL EFFECTS OF THE ETs IN THE PULMONARY SYSTEM

Although to data research has focused on the bronchospastic activity of the ETs, information is accumulating on their effects in cells and systems other than airway smooth muscle. Outlined below is a review of the known effects of the ETs in the different components of the pulmonary system, with emphasis on information that may be pertinent to a potential pathophysiological role (Figure 16.4).

IN VITRO EFFECTS

Constrictor activity

Airway smooth muscle

The ETs are potent (EC_{50}s = approximately 1–30 nM) and effective bronchoconstrictor agents in isolated airway smooth muscle preparations from a variety of species including humans[56,57,62,84,85,93,95,96]. The contraction is relatively slow to develop, is well-maintained and also only slowly reversed by washing. A correlation between the density of ET-1 binding sites and contractile effects of ET-1 in human, rat and guinea-pig preparations was reported[57]. In human bronchus ET-1 is more potent than ET-2 or ET-3[56,62,96]. ET-1-induced contraction of human bronchus, similar to several other species but in contrast to guinea-pig trachea[96], is not modulated by cyclooxygenase products[62,96,98]. In addition, early studies provided evidence that the ET-1 induced response is not mediated by extracellular Ca^{2+} influx *via* voltage-

Pulmonary diseases 261

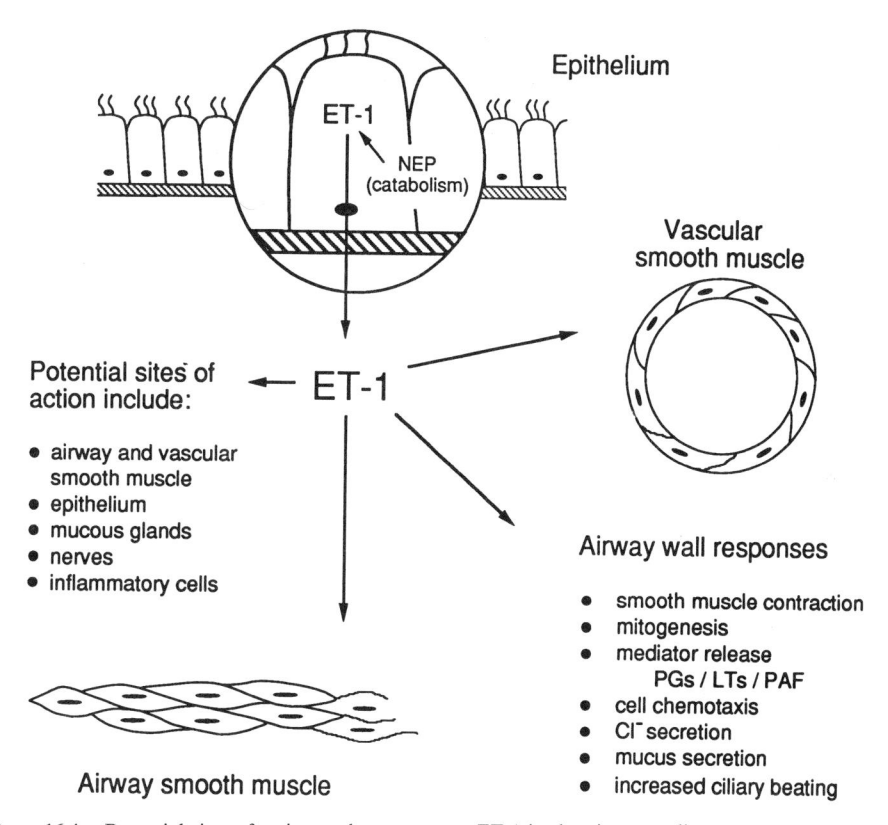

Figure 16.4. Potential sites of action and responses to ET-1 in the airway wall.

sensitive channels[56,62,98]. However, more recent evidence indicates that a component of the response to ET-1 in human bronchus was mediated by activation of voltage-sensitive Ca^{2+} channels[99]. In cultured human bronchial smooth muscle it was proposed that ET-1 produces mobilization of intracellular Ca^{2+} by stimulation of the phosphatidylinositol pathway *via* activation of a receptor (molecular weight of about 70,000 from affinity cross-linking experiments) which is coupled to a pertussis toxin-insensitive G protein. In addition, there is influx of extracellular Ca^{2+} *via* a dihydropyridine-insensitive membrane channel which may contribute to a maintained rise in tone in human bronchial smooth muscle[100].

There is conflicting information as to whether ET-1 produces contraction of guinea-pig trachea in part *via* release of secondary mediators. For example, based on the direct measurement of mediator release and/or the effects of receptor antagonists, a role for PAF[101], histamine[102-104] and thromboxane[105,106] has been proposed. In contrast, similar studies provided no evidence for a significant contribution of histamine, thromboxane, peptidoleukotrienes, acetylcholine or tachykinins to ET-1-induced contraction[97,107]. It has been reported that under some conditions ET-1 will produce relaxation of guinea-pig thrachea; there is conflicting information regarding whether this response is modulated by the airway epithelium[108,109].

Pulmonary vascular smooth muscle

The ETs also potently contract isolated human pulmonary artery and vein, and there is conflicting information on whether they are more potent bronchoconstrictor or vasoconstrictor agents[56,58,62]. The response to ET-1 in human pulmonary artery appears to be mediated predominantly if not solely via ET_A-receptor activation[93]. In guinea-pig pulmonary artery evidence was provided for ET-1 and ET-2, on the one hand, and ET-3, on the other, producing contraction by interacting with distinct receptors[110]. ET-1 potently contracted rat pulmonary artery ($EC_{50} = 1.3$ nM) and pulmonary vein ($EC_{50} = 0.6$ nM)[111]. In the same study in perfused lungs, ET-1 increased microvascular pressure and produced edema which was proposed to be due to venoconstriction.

Airway epithelium

ET-1 increased the negativity of transepithelial potential difference in ferret trachea; the effects on epithelial ion transport were not examined[112]. Furthermore, ET-1 (10^{-10} M–10^{-6} M), but not ET-2 or ET-3, stimulated the potential difference and short-circuit current in canine tracheal epithelium. It was proposed that this translated into a selective increase in Cl^- secretion, with no effect on Na^+ absorption, via a mechanism which was partially dependent on the release of cyclooxygenase products[113]. Leikauf and co-workers also demonstrated an ET-1-induced increase in short-circuit current in canine tracheal epithelium ($EC_{50} = 2.2$ nM) which was reduced by indomethacin. In addition, they reported that ET-1 increased mucosal net ^{36}Cl flux, but had no effect on ^{22}Na flux, stimulated [^3H]-arachidonate release from membrane phospholipids and increased intracellular Ca^{2+} and cAMP accumulation[114]. However, in contrast to Satoh and colleagues, they reported that ET-2 ($EC_{50} = 7.2$ nM) and to a lesser extent ET-3 ($EC_{50} = 10.4$ nM), also increased short-circuit current. In addition to stimulating short circuit current and Cl- secretion, ET-1 potently increased ciliary beat frequency ($EC_{50} = 3$ nM) in canine cultured tracheal epithelium; both effects were attenuated by indomethacin[115]. Relatively high concentrations of ET-1 ($0.1 \mu M$–$10 \mu M$) stimulated the release of several prostanoids from [^3H]-arachidonic acid-labeled cultured feline tracheal epithelial cells[116]. Although several studies indicated few ET receptors localized to the airway epithelial (*vide supra*), Wu and co-workers revealed two saturable binding sites for [^{125}I]-ET-1: $K_d = 35.2$ pM and $B_{max} = 15.0$ fmol/10^7 cells for higher affinity site and $K_d = 205.9$ pM and $B_{max} = 35.0$ fmol/10^7 cells for lower affinity site[116]. Tschirhart and co-workers have also detected two binding sites for ET-1 in guinea-pig airway epithelium, with ET-3 able to interact with both sites[60]. The above data indicates that the ETs exert several effects in airway epithelium, which contains many specialized cell types which are thought to play a key role in airway inflammation in addition to pulmonary physiology and pathophysiology.

Mucous glands

Immunoreactive ET-1 and ET-1 mRNA was found in human nasal mucosal tissue, primarily in the venous sinusoids and to a lesser extent small muscular arteries.

[^{125}I]-ET-1 binding sites were also detected in submucosal glands, venous sinusoids and small muscular arterioles[117]. In addition to the presence of ET in the vascular endothelium and serous cells, ET-1, and also ET-2, but not ET-3, stimulated serous and mucous cell secretion. However, high concentrations of ET-1 and ET-2 (0.1 µM–10 µM) were needed to increase lactoferrin and mucous glycoprotein release[117]. Similarly, high concentrations ($\geqslant$0.1 µM) of ET-1 increased prostanoid production in human cultured nasal mucosa[118]. ET-1 (1 nM–1 µM) increased glycoconjugate secretion from feline tracheal isolated glands but decreased secretion from tracheal explants[119]. In ferret trachea ET-1 was without effect on serous cell secretion, and actually inhibited phenylephrine- or methacholine-induced secretion[112].

Smooth muscle and fibroblast proliferation

ET-1 potently ($pD_2 = 9.82$) but modestly increased rabbit cultured tracheal smooth muscle proliferation[39]. This mitogenic activity was proposed to mediate *via* a pertussis toxin-sensitive G-protein-linked mechanism and by thromboxane release. ET has been shown to be mitogenic for Swiss 3T3 fibroblasts[120]. This may have relevance to the structural changes observed in asthma, which include increased numbers of fibroblasts that may be associated with increased thickness of the collagen layer in the asthmatic airways[121]. ET-1, and also ET-3, induced chemotaxis and replication of fibroblasts obtained from rat pulmonary arteries[122]. Again the effects on replication were small (maximum of 30% above control), and also they occurred in much higher concentrations (>10 nM) than those which induced chemotaxis (1 pM–0.1 µM). It was proposed that this may be relevant to the characteristic vascular remodeling in pulmonary hypertension. ET-1 and ET-3 produced concentration-dependent mitogenesis of human pulmonary artery smooth muscle cells *via* an ET_A-receptor-mediated mechanism[123]. ET-1 (1 nM–3 nM) generally stimulated DNA synthesis and proliferation of pig pulmonary artery smooth muscle cells, although under some conditions there was a paradoxical inhibitory effect[124].

Mediator release

ET-1 stimulates thromboxane A_2 release from perfused guinea-pig lung[52]. However, there is conflicting information on the ability of ET-1 to directly stimulate mediator release from inflammatory cells. For example, although ET_A receptors were detected on murine bone marrow-derived mast cells, their stimulation did not induce histamine release[15]. Furthermore, ET-1 did not stimulate the release of histamine or the peptidoleukotrienes from guinea-pig trachea[107] or human bronchus[98], although increased release of various prostanoids from guinea-pig trachea was noted[107]. In contrast, it was reported that ET-1 markedly and potently stimulated histamine release from guinea-pig pulmonary but not peritoneal mast cells, with an $EC_{50} = 0.05$ nM, which was similar to the affinity for [^{125}I]-ET-1 (about 0.08 nM)[104]. In rats, intravenous administration of ET-1 increased the levels of 15-HETE in BAL fluid and the generation of oxygen radicals in BAL cells[125]. In addition, ET-1 (10 nM) stimulated 15-lipoxygenase activity in lung homogenates. High concentrations of ET-1 ($\geqslant$0.1 µm) increased prostanoid production in human cultured nasal mucosa[118]. ET-1 (1 nM–

10 nM) stimulated thromboxane and PGD_2, but not histamine, release from cells obtained from BALs in canine airways[126].

Microvascular permeability

ET-1 (10 nM) increased microvascular permeability in perfused rat lungs *via* a mechanism which required the presence of both leukocytes and plasma components other than complement[127]. Several other studies in guinea-pig and rat perfused lungs reported that ET-1 induced pulmonary edema, although there is conflicting information regarding the contribution of prostanoids to the response[59,111,128,129]. In rabbit perfused lung ET-1 produced a potent, concentration-dependent pulmonary vasoconstriction, *via* a mechanism which was proposed to involve extracellular Ca^{2+} influx and activation of protein kinase C[130]. It was hypothesized that in rat and guinea-pig lung ET-1 causes lung edema largely through a hydrostatic mechanism rather than directly increasing vascular permeability; for example, ET-1 did not affect albumin fluxes across cultured bovine pulmonary artery or microvessel endothelial cell monolayers or increase lung protein leak index in rats *in vivo*[111,128]. In blood-perfused rather than physiological salt solution-perfused lungs ET-1 produced little edema[111,131].

Other cells

ET-1 (1 nM–1 µM) was reported to stimulate human blood monocyte chemotaxis[132], although another study failed to demonstrate ET-1-induced stimulation of human peripheral blood monocyte chemotaxis, adhesion or superoxide production[133]. ET-1 increased arachidonic acid and thromboxane release from guinea-pig alveolar macrophages, with a maximum effect at 1 nM[134], and at a concentration of 1 µM increased superoxide production, intracellular Ca^{2+} levels and protein phosphorylation in human alveolar macrophages[135].

IN VIVO EFFECTS

Actions on bronchoconstrictor tone

There are no reports of administration of the ETs to human airways *in vivo* although several studies have explored the effects of the ETs following challenge to animals. Intravenous (i.v.) or aerosol administration of ET-1 to guinea-pigs elicits maintained bronchoconstriction which appears to be mediated to a significant extent by an indirect mechanism involving the release of secondary mediators, predominantly thromboxane but also including PAF[136–139]. However, the extent to which secondary mediators contribute to ET-1-induced bronchoconstriction is dependent upon the route of administration[59,136–138,140]. The bronchospasm induced by i.v. administration of ET-1 in guinea-pigs was not associated with a change in the number of circulating PMNs or platelets, suggesting that the response was independent of these circulating cells[139]. ET-1 induced bronchospasm was not affected by Ca^{2+}-channel inhibitors, but was potentiated by hexamethonium or propranolol, suggesting a modulatory influence of the autonomic nervous system[137,138]. It was noted that there was an increase in the responsiveness of aerosol-sensitized and antigen-exposed guinea-pigs to the bronchoconstrictor effects of ET-1, perhaps due to a change in the proteolytic activity in the airway epithelium which normally metabolizes the peptide[141,142]. ET-1 administration also elicits bronchospasm in dog[143], rat[144] and sheep[145].

Aerosolized or i.v. ET-1 failed to induced airway hyperreactivity in guinea-pigs[45,138,146]. However, a low concentration of aerosolized ET-1 (1 pM), which was without direct effect on pulmonary function, increased the bronchospasm induced by aerosol administration of histamine[147]. Intravenous infusion of ET-1 (2 nmol/day) *via* the jugular vein for 6 days did not alter the responsiveness of guinea-pigs to the bronchoconstrictor effects of acetylcholine[148].

Actions on vasomotor tone

In cats, i.v. ET-1, ET-2 and ET-3 elicited pulmonary and systemic vasodilation; the former but not the latter was decreased by the K^+-channel antagonist, glibenclamide[149]. In the rat pulmonary circulation ET-1 produced both vasoconstriction and vasodilation; ET-1 was less potent at eliciting vasoconstriction in the pulmonary than in the systemic circulation, and the pulmonary vasodilation may involve ATP-sensitive K^+-channels and be modulated by the release of EDRF[129,150].

Other *in vivo* effects

Intravenous ET-1 increased microvascular permeability in rats in various tissues, including bronchi, *via* a mechanism which was sensitive to the ET_A receptor antagonist, BQ-123, suggesting it was ET_A receptor-mediated[151]. However, intravenous administration of ET-1 to guinea-pigs did not increase lung permeability, produce epithelial damage or elicit inflammatory cell influx into the alveolar or vascular walls or the bronchial epithelium[138]. Similarly, aerosolized ET-1 did not alter the levels of eosinophils in guinea pig lung samples, 4 or 24 hours after challenge[45], and infusion of ET-1 (2 nmol/day) to guinea pigs *via* the jugular vein for 6 days did not induce histological changes in the lung or cause infiltration of inflammatory cells[148].

POTENTIAL PATHOPHYSIOLOGICAL ROLE

The ETs can only be confidently implicated in the pathophysiology of pulmonary disorders after the following standard criteria have been fulfilled: 1) pathways for the synthesis, release and metabolism of the ETs must be present in the airways; 2) when administered exogenously the ETs must mimic several, if not all, of the features of the disease; 3) the levels of the ETs must be elevated in disease states, with a correlation between the amounts of ETs and the severity of the disease; 4) drugs which inhibit the release and/or antagonize the biological effects of the ETs must ameliorate the symptoms of the disease(s) of interest. Many of the aspects of the criteria outlined in 1)–3) have been fulfilled, at least for asthma and pulmonary hypertension. However, the most important criteria, the clinical testing of the therapeutic utility of selective ET receptor antagonists or ECE inhibitors in pulmonary disorders is several years from complete assessment. Nevertheless, there is increasing evidence, largely from preclinical experiments, in support of a potential pathophysiological role for the ETs in several diseases of the pulmonary system. This information is summarized below with emphasize on asthma and pulmonary hypertension, the two diseases which have been the major focus of research and interest.

Asthma

The first publication on the effects of ET-1 in the pulmonary system reported that it potently contracted isolated guinea-pig trachea and it was hypothesized that ET-1 may be involved in the pathogenesis in asthma[95,152]. The potent bronchoconstrictor activity of ET-1 was subsequently extended to human bronchus, supporting its potential candidacy as an important mediator in asthma. However, asthma is recognized as a chronic inflammatory disorder associated with several characteristic pathologies in the pulmonary system in addition to bronchospasm. These features include airway hyperreactivity, muscus hypersecretion, mucus gland and airway smooth muscle cell hyperplasia, sub-epithelial fibrosis, inflammatory cell infiltration and activation, increased bronchial microvascular permeability and edema, and epithelial cell damage and desquamation. There is some, albeit limited data on the effects of ETs on the pathophysiological aspects of asthma other than bronchoconstriction (see above) and these are summarized in Table 16.1.

The most interesting and relevant observations on a potential role of the ETs in asthma comes from preliminary studies in asthmatics which suggested that there is increased synthesis and release of ET in their airways compared with control individuals. For example, in the first study in humans, Nomura and co-workers reported that in the one asthmatic patient examined there was a 6-fold elevation in the levels of immunoreactive ET (ir-ET) in bronchoalveolar lavage (BAL), from 0.05 to 0.3 pg/ml, during what was termed the "bronchospastic phase" of a status asthmaticus attack[153]. There have been no further reports on the ET levels in airways during

Table 16.1. Features of asthma pathophysiology potentially associated with endothelin

Asthma	Endothelin
Increased bronchial tone	+++
Mucus hypersecretion	+/−
Airway hyperresponsiveness	+/−
Airway smooth muscle hyperplasia	+
Epithelial damage	−
Bronchial edema	+/−
Inflammatory cell influx	−
Inflammatory cell activation	+/−
Associated with increased ir-ET in the bronchialepithelium and in BAL fluid	+

+ = stimulatory effect; − = no effect or inhibitory influence; BAL = bronchoalveolar lavage. This table was adapted from Hay et al., Trends Pharmacol. Sci., **14**, 29–32, 1993.

asthmatic attacks. However, in another, more comprehensive, study by Mattoli and co-workers the levels of ET in BALs of six asthmatics (0.25 ± 0.05 pg/ml) was about 4-fold higher than in five control subjects (0.06 ± 0.02 pg/ml) or five chronic bronchitics (0.08 ± 0.03 pg/ml)[154]. In contrast, there was no difference between the three groups in the amounts of ET in the peripheral venous blood samples. It was hypothesized that the increased BAL levels of ET represent increased local production in the bronchial mucosa, and were not a consequence of any changes in microvascular permeability. Furthermore, ET levels decreased to control values, concomitant with an improvement in lung function, after 15-day treatment with inhaled β-agonists and oral corticosteroids. It was proposed that the ET samples contained ET-1 and ET-3, but not ET-2. Another study by the same group of researchers revealed that bronchial epithelial cells obtained by bronchoscopy from six patients who had symptomatic asthma expressed preproendothelin-1 mRNA and released significant quantities of ET-1 into the supernatant (the range was 12–40 pg/ml/10^6 cells over a 48 hr period)[155]. The release of ET-1, but not the levels of preproendothelin-1 transcripts, was markedly attenuated by hydrocortisone (1 µM). Epithelial cells from five control, non-asthmatic individuals did not contain preproendothelin-1 mRNA and release of ET-1 could not be detected. In addition, only a few cells in two out of five chronic bronchitic patients expressed preproendothelin 1 mRNA and only in one sample was a measurable amount of ET-1 released into the supernatant over 48 hours.

The most extensive study on ET-1 in asthmatic subjects was conducted by Springall and co-workers who performed a comparative immunohistochemical analysis of ET-1 expression in endobronchial biopsies from 17 asthmatic patients, covering a broad clinical spectrum, and 11 atopic and non-atopic healthy controls. It was observed that there was markedly increased incidence of the expression of ET in airway epithelium, and also the vascular endothelium, of asthmatics (detected in 11 out of 17) compared with non-asthmatic controls (detected in 1 out of 11)[156]. In the asthmatic individuals, no correlation was evident between positive staining for ET-1 and such parameters as degree of airflow obstruction, level of bronchial responsiveness, atopy or corticosteroid therapy. No ir-ET-1 was seen in the airway smooth muscle.

Recently, in a study measuring ET amounts in patients with nocturnal worsening of asthma, the mean serum levels of ET-1 significantly decreased with time during the evening from 9.2 ± 2.1 pg/ml at 2000 h to 6.2 ± 1.7 pg/ml at 0400 h in 9 asthmatic individuals, whereas there was no change in mean serum levels in 6 controls (7.3 ± 2.2 pg/ml and 7.2 ± 2.4 pg/ml at 2000 h and 0400 h, respectively)[157]. Thus, and in contrast to their hypothesis, there was no significant difference between asthmatic and non-asthmatic patients. Interestingly, for all individuals there was a significant correlation between the percent predicted FEV_1 and the BAL levels of ET-1 at 0400 h. It was proposed that ET-1 may act locally on the airway smooth muscle and that it may be localized in tissue in a bound state during overnight exacerbations of asthma.

These intriguing but preliminary data need to be followed up and the question of "cause or effect?" remains far from answered. Thus, considerable work, in particular using isolated human tissues and in the clinical setting, has still to be conducted before a definitive link can be established between the ETs and the pathophysiology of asthma.

Pulmonary hypertension

Pulmonary hypertension is generally a progressively deteriorating condition which is characterized by an increase in vascular tone and vasoreactivity and enhanced proliferation of smooth muscle cells, resulting in a marked elevation in pulmonary vascular resistance, which leads to right-heart failure and death. There may be increased recruitment of myofibroblasts into the intima and "muscularization" of pulmonary arteries[158]. The mechanisms underlying pulmonary hypertension remain largely a mystery. Pulmonary hypertension was the first pulmonary disorder in which preliminary evidence was presented to implicate ET in its pathogenesis. Thus, not long after the first publication on ET-1 it was reported that plasma levels of ET were elevated (about 6-fold) in four patients with pulmonary hypertension; controls: 0.26 ± 0.24 pg/ml, n = 14; pulmonary hypertension: 1.52 ± 0.45; $P < 0.001$[159]. Since this first publication, there have been several reports confirming the elevation in plasma endothelin levels in this disease[160-164]. For example, in 7 children with pulmonary hypertension there was a significant increase in plasma ir-ET-1 compared to controls (12.3 ± 3.4 pg/ml versus 3.6 ± 0.7 pg/ml). Furthermore basal ir-ET-1 correlated with the degree of increase in mean pulmonary artery pressure during acute hypoxia[162]. There was no difference in the levels of ir-ET-1 between controls and individuals with chronic cardiopulmonary disorders without pulmonary hypertension. In another study in patients up to 12 years of age there was an incremental increase in ir-ET levels in samples taken from sites from the right ventricle to the pulmonary artery in patients with pulmonary hypertension compared to those with congenital heart defects without hypertension. This increase correlated with the pulmonary artery pressure[161].

In addition to the above studies measuring the plasma levels of ET, the tissue levels of ET-1 (as assessed by analyzing for immunoreactivity and mRNA) was markedly enhanced in patients with various causes of pulmonary hypertension compared with controls, in which ET was rarely detected in endothelial cells[165]. The ET-1-like immunoreactivity was predominant in endothelial cells of pulmonary arteries with medial thickening and intimal fibrosis and the increased ET-1 mRNA was expressed primarily at sites of ET-1-like immunoreactivity. It was noted that there was a strong correlation between the extent of ir-ET-1 and pulmonary vascular resistance in patients with plexogenic pulmonary arteriopathy, but not individuals with secondary pulmonary hypertension.

The ETs have been shown in various studies to be potent constrictors of isolated pulmonary blood vessels from various species including humans[56,58,62]. In addition *in vivo* experiments indicate potent vasoconstrictor properties in the pulmonary vasculature[166,167]. Further support for a potential significant role of the ETs in pulmonary hypertension may lie in their recognized potent mitogenic properties in various systems including vascular smooth muscle[4,120,168,169]. For example, in relation to this disorder, ET-1 and ET-3, but not sarafotoxin S6c, produced concentration-dependent mitogenesis of human pulmonary artery smooth muscle cells, *via* a mechanism which was sensitive to BQ-123 and, thus, appeared to be ET_A-receptor-mediated[123]. This observation may be relevant to the characteristic vascular remodeling and smooth muscle cell proliferation associated with many forms of pulmonary hypertension[170]. Thus, in addition to several reports of an elevation in ET levels in pulmonary hypertension, the ETs are able to produce two key features of pulmonary hypertension, namely vasoconstriction and enhanced proliferation of vascular smooth muscle cells. However, it remains to be determined clinically whether ET contributes directly to the pathogenesis of the disorder or whether the elevated levels of ET are merely markers of the disease, for example, an indicator of endothelial cell damage or dysfunction.

The possibility remains that the elevated levels of ET in the plasma of patients with pulmonary hypertension may reflect decreased clearance or uptake rather than enhanced production and release[160,162]. However, following a study assessing the plasma ir-ET levels in samples from several loci in the cardiopulmonary circulation it was concluded that the increased amounts of ir-ET in patients with pulmonary hypertension were due to enhanced production of ir-ET in the pulmonary circulation[161]. The mechanism and stimulus for the increase in release of ET is not known but may be a consequence of abnormal hemodynamic forces such as high high pressure or enhanced blood flow which may stimulate ET release from endothelial cells. For example, shear stress was demonstrated to increase ET production from cultured endothelial cells[171]. In contrast, ET has been shown to exert vasodilator properties including in the pulmonary system[166], and it is possible that ET exerts a beneficial spasmolytic effect in pulmonary hypertension.

There is experimental evidence in animals supporting a role for ET-1 in the genesis and maintenance of pulmonary hypertension. For example, an increase in ET-1 mRNA expression was detected in rats with idiopathic pulmonary hypertension[172]. In addition, ET-1 and ET-3 induced chemotaxis and replication of fibroblasts obtained from rat pulmonary arteries, suggesting a role in vascular remodeling, although, high concentrations of the ETs were required to produce their modest mitogenic effects[122]. Furthermore, ET-1 (1 nM–3 nM) stimulated DNA synthesis and proliferation of pig pulmonary artery smooth muscle cells[124].

Other pulmonary disorders

Using immunohistochemical and *in situ* hybridization techniques ET immunoreactivity and mRNA were detected in the majority of surgical specimens of various lung tumors, in particular squamous cell carcinoma and adenocarcinoma; ET expression was also detected in adjacent tissues. Based on its synthesis and storage in lung tumors it was hypothesized that ET may be involved in their growth and/or differentiation[173]. Note, ET is located in the pulmonary endocrine cells and airway epithelium and endothelium of several species including humans[10,12,13]. In humans, expression was highest in the developing lung and lowest in adult lung. Accordingly, it was speculated that ET may be important in promoting or regulating cellular growth in lung development[13].

In lung tissue from patients with cryptogenic fibrosing alveolitis (CFA), a fatal condition of unknown cause which is characterized by inflammation, type II pneumocyte and fibroblastic proliferation, and collagen deposition, there was markedly increased expression of ET-1, most notably in airway epithelium and type II pneumocytes, compared with control tissue and tissues from patients with focal fibrosis[173]. Enhanced ET-1-like immunoreactivity and mRNA was also noted in pulmonary vascular endothelial cells, especially in samples from patients with pulmonary hypertension. It was hypothesized that ET-1 may be involved in the pathogenesis of CFA and associated pulmonary hypertension, in particular in the characteristic ultrastructural changes. Furthermore, there was a correlation between the expression of ET-1 and the histological parameters of the disease and it was suggested that ET-1 may be an appropriate marker for disease activity. Another study by the same group detected expression of ET-1 in alveolar epithelial cells of patients with pulmonary fibrosis, but rarely in patients with pulmonary hypertension without fibrosis[165]. Another group reported that in two patients with cystic fibrosis and one with CFA ir-proendothelin-1 and ir-proendothelin-3, but not ir-proendothelin-2, was detected in airway epithelial, whereas immunoreactivity for the three isoforms was localized in submucosal glands; no control samples were analyzed[175]. In support of the synthesis of both ET-1 and ET-3 in airway epithelium, the release of ET-1 and ET-3 from canine and porcine cultured airway epithelial cells[34], and presence of ET-1 and ET-3 mRNA by *in situ* hybridization in rat airway epithelium[12] has been demonstrated. An increase in ET levels in sheep plasma and pulmonary lymph was detected during endotoxin shock. The increase in circulating ET was thought to be due to endotoxin-induced endothelial cell injury[176].

Based on the increased plasma levels of endothelin noted following intravenous administration of ovalbumin in actively and passively sensitized guinea-pigs it was speculated that the ETs may be involved in the pulmonary insufficiency and peripheral circulatory collapse which develops during anaphylactic shock[177].

CONCLUSIONS/THE FUTURE

It is clear that much less is known regarding the effects and potential pathophysiological role of the ETs in the pulmonary compared with the cardiovascular system. However, information describing multiple effects of the ETs, in particular ET-1, in different cells in the respiratory tract is accumulating. Although it is too early to ascribe a role for the ETs in the pathophysiology of pulmonary disorders, the preliminary data, especially in relation to asthma and pulmonary hypertension, are intriguing. Thus far, research has centered largely on a comprehensive analysis of the contractile effects of ET-1 both *in vitro* and *in vivo*. In relation to asthma, a chronic inflammatory disorder, it is important that future studies should focus more on effects of ET on parameters other than bronchoconstriction e.g., influence on nerves, inflammatory cell function, also the effects of chronic exposure on smooth muscle and fibroblast proliferation. Another important area of research will be the elucidation and classification of the ET receptor subtypes mediating these effects. To date, the most convincing evidence and scientific rationale for a pathophysiological role for ET is in pulmonary vascular diseases such as pulmonary hypertension. The unequivocal testing of the pathophysiological role of the ETs in pulmonary disorders requires the clinical evaluation of potent and selective receptor antagonists for the various ET receptor subtypes. It is anticipated that these studies will be conducted in the not-too-distant future, as information is becoming available on compounds which may possess the appropriate pharmacological profile for evaluation in the clinic.

References

1. Yanagisawa, M., Kurihara, H., Kimura, S., Tomobe, Y., Kobayashi, M., Mitsui, Y. et al. (1988) A novel potent vasoconstrictor peptide produced by vascular endothelial cells. *Nature*, **332**, 411–415.
2. Yanagisawa, M. and Masaki, T. (1989) Endothelin, a novel endothelium-derived peptide. *Biochemical Pharmacology*, **38**, 1877–1883.
3. Yanagisawa, M. and Masaki, T. (1989) Molecular biology and biochemistry of the endothelins. *Trends in Pharmacological Sciences*, **10**, 374–378.
4. Masaki, T. and Yanagisawa, M. (1992) Physiology and pharmacology of endothelins. *Medicinal Research Reviews*, **12**, 391–421.
5. Kitamura, K., Tanaka, T., Kata, J., Eto, T. and Tanaka, K. (1989) Regional distribution of immunoreactive endothelin in porcine tissue: abundance in inner medulla of kidney. *Biochemical and Biophysical Research Communications*, **161**, 348–352.
6. Matsumoto H., Suzuki, N., Onda, H. and Funjo, M. (1989) Abundance of endothelin-3 in rat intestine, pituitary gland and brain. *Biochemical and Biophysical Research Communications*, **164**, 74–80.
7. Yoshimi, H., Hirata, Y., Fukuda, Y., Kawano, Y., Emori, T., Kuramochi, M. et al. (1989) Regional distribution of immunoreactive endothelin in rats. *Peptides*, **10**, 805–808.
8. Pernow, J., Hemsén A. and Lundberg, J. M. (1989) Tissue specific distribution, clearance and vascular effects of endothelin in the pig. *Biochemical and Biophysical Research Communications*, **161**, 647–653.
9. Nunez, D. J. R., Brown, M. J., Davenport, A. P., Neylon, C. B., Schofield, J. P. and Wyse, R. K. (1990) Endothelin-1 mRNA is widely expressed in porcine and human tissues. *Journal of Clinical Investigation*, **85**, 1537–1541.
10. Rozengurt, N., Springall, D. R., and Polak, J. M. (1989) Localization of endothelin-like immunoreactivity in airway epithelium or rats and mice. *Journal of Pathology*, **160**, 5–8.
11. Rennick, R. E., Loesch, A. and Burnstock, G. (1992) Endothelin, vasopressin, and substance P like immunoreactivity in cultured and intact epithelium from rabbit trachea. *Thorax*, **47**, 1044–1049.
12. MacCumber, M. W., Ross, C. A., Glaser, B. M. and Snyder, S. H. (1989) Endothelin: visualization of mRNA by *in situ* hybridization provides evidence for local action. *Proceedings of the National Academy of Sciences*, **86**, 7285–7289.
13. Giaid, A., Polak, J. M. Gaitonde, V., Hamid, Q. A., Moscoso, G., Legon, S. et al. (1991) Distribution of endothelin-like immunoreactivity and mRNA in the developing and adult human lung. *American Journal Respiratory Cell and Molecular Biology*, **4**, 50–58.
14. Ehrenreich, H., Anderson, R. W., Fox, C. H., Rieckmann, P., Hoffman, G. S., Travis, W. D. et al. (1990) Endothelins, peptides with potent vasoactive properties, are produced by human macrophages. *Journal of Experimental Medicine*, **172**, 1741–1748.
15. Ehrenreich, H., Burd, P. R., Rotten, M., Hültner, L., Hylton, J. B., Garfield, M. et al. (1992) Endothelins belong to the assortment of mast cell-derived and mast cell-bound cytokines. *The New Biologist*, **4**, 147–156.
16. Inoue, A., Yanagisawa, M., Kimura, S., Kasuya, Y., Miyauchi, T., Goto, K. et al. (1989) The human endthelin family: three structurally and pharmacologically distinct isopeptides predicted by three separate genes. *Proceedings of the National Academy of Sciences USA*, **86**, 2863–2867.
17. Emori, T., Hirata, Y., Ohta, K., Shichiri, M., Shimokado, K. and Marumo, F. (1989) Concomitant secretion of big endothelin and its C-terminal fragment from human and bovine endothelial cells. *Biochemical and Biophysical Research Communications*, **162**, 217–223.
18. Sawamura, T., Kimura, S., Shinmi, O., Sugita, Y., Yanagisawa, M. and Masaki, T. (1989) Analysis of endothelin related peptides in culture supernatant of porcine aortic endothelial cells: evidence for biosynthetic pathway of endothelin-1. *Biochemical and Biophysical Research Communications*, **162**, 1287–1294.
19. Miyauchi, T., Yanagisawa, M., Tomizawa, T., Sugishita, Y., Suzuki, N. Funino, M. et al. (1989) Increased plasma concentration of endothelin-1 and big endothelin-1 in acute myocardial infarction. *Lancet*, **2**, 53–54.
20. Kashiwabara, T., Inagaki, Y., Ohta, H., Iwamatsu, A., Nomizu, M., Morita, A. et al. (1989) Putative precursors of endothelin have less vasoconstrictor activity *in vitro* but a potent pressor effect *in vivo*. *FEBS Letters.*, **247**, 73–76.
21. Kimura, S., Kaysuya, Y., Sawamura, T., Shinmi, O., Sugita, Y., Yanagisawa, M. et al. (1989) Conversion of big endothelin-1 to 21-residue endothelin-1 is essential for expression of full vasoconstrictor activity: structure-activity relationships of big endothelin-1 *Journal of Cardiovascular Pharmacology*, **13 (Suppl 5)**, S5–S7.
22. Leak, L. V. (1989) In *Electron Microscopy in Human Medicine* edited by J. V. Johannessen, vol. 5, pp. 87–154, New York: McGraw-Hill.
23. Hexum, T. D., Hoeger, C., Rivier, J. E. Baird, A., and Brown, M. R. (1990) Characterization of

endothelin secretion by vascular endothelial cells. *Biochemical and Biophysical Research Communications*, **167**, 294–300.
24. Opgenorth, T. J., Wu-Wong, J. R. and Shiosaki, K. (1992) Endothelin-converting enzymes. *FASEB Journal.*, **6**, 2653—2659.
25. Takaoka, M., Shiragami, K., Fujino, K., Miki, K., Miyake, Y., Yasuda, M. *et al.* (1991) Phosphoramidon-sensitive endothelin converting enzyme in rat lung. *Biochemistry International*, **25**, 697–704.
26. Sawamura, T., Shinmi, O., Kishi, N., Sugita, Y., Yanagisawa, M., Goto, K. *et al.* (1993) Characterization of phosphoramidon-sensitive metalloproteinases with endothelin-converting enzyme activity in porcine lung membrane. *Biochemica et Biophysica Acta*, **1161**, 295–302.
27. Takahashi, M., Matsushita, Y., Iijima, Y. and Tanzawa K. (1993) Purification and characterization of endothelin-converting enzyme from rat lung. *Journal of Biological Chemistry*, **268**, 21394–21398.
28. Ishikawa, S., Tsukada, H., Yuasa, H., Fukue, M., Wei, S., Onizuka, M. *et al.* (1992) Effects of endothelin-1 and conversion of big endothelin-1 in the isolated perfused rabbit lung. *Journal of Applied Physiology*, **72**, 2387–2392.
29. Pons, F., Touvay, C., Lagente, V., Mencia-Huerta, J. M. and Braquet, P. (1992) Involvement of a phosphoramidon-sensitive endopeptidase in the processing of big endothelin-1 in the guinea-pig. *European Journal of Pharmacology*, **217**, 65–70.
30. Vemulapalli, S., Rivelli, M., Chiu, P. J. S., del Prado, M. and Hey, J. A. (1992) Phosphoramidon abolishes the increases in endothelin-1 release induced by ischemia-hypoxia in isolated perfused guinea pig lungs. *Journal of Pharmacology and Experimental Therapeutics*, **262**, 1062–1069.
31. Wu-Wong, J. R., Budzik, G. P., Devine, E. M. and Opgenorth, T. J. (1990) Characterization of endothelin converting enzyme in rat lung. *Biochemical and Biophysical Research Communications*, **171**, 1291–1296.
32. Watanabe, T. and Yokosawa, H. (1992) The generation of big-endothelin (1–22) (endothelin-valine) from big-endothelin in the soluble fraction of porcine lung. *Biochemistry International*, **27**, 1–8.
33. Wypij, D. M., Nichols, J. S., Novak, P. J., Stacy, D. L., Berman, J. and Wiseman, J. S. (1992) Role of mast cell chymase in the extracellular processing of big-endothelin-1 to endothelin-1 in the perfused rat lung. *Biochemical Pharmacology*, **43**, 845–853.
34. Black, P. N., Ghatei, M. A., Takahashi, K., Bretherton-Watt, D., Krausz, T., Dollery, C. T. *et al.* (1989) Formation of endothelin by cultured airway epithelial cells. *FEBS Letters*, **255**, 129–132.
35. Mattoli, S., Mezzetti, M., Riva, G., Allegra, L. and Fasoli, A. (1990) Specific binding of endothelin on human bronchial smooth muscle cells in culture and secretion of endothelin-like material from bronchial epithelial cells. *American Journal of Respiratory Cell and Molecular Biology*, **3**, 145–151.
36. Ninomiya, H., Uchida, Y., Ishii, Y., Nomura, A., Kameyama, M., Saotome, M. *et al.* (1991) Endotoxin stimulates endothelin release from cultured epithelial cells of guinea-pig trachea. *European Journal of Pharmacology*, **203**, 299–302.
37. Endo, T., Uchida, Y., Matsumoto, H., Suzuki, N., Nomura, A., Hirata, F. *et al.* (1992) Regulation of endothelin-1 synthesisin cultured guinea pig airway epithelial cells by various cytokines. *Biochemical and Biophysical Research Communications*, **186**, 1594–1599.
38. Rennick, R. E., Milner, P. and Burnstock, G. (1993) Thrombin stimulates release of endothelin and vasopressin, but not substance P, from isolated rabbit tracheal epithelial cells. *European Journal of Pharmacology*, **230**, 367–370.
39. Noveral, J. P., Rosenberg, S. M., Anber, R. A., Pawlowksi, N. A. and Grunstein, M. M. (1992) Role of endothelin-1 in regulating proliferation of cultured rabbit airway smooth muscle cells. *American Journal of Physiology*, **263**, L317–L324.
40. Hay, D. W. P. (1989) Guinea-pig tracheal epithelium and endothelin. *European Journal of Pharmacology*, **171**, 241–246.
41. Vijayaraghavan, J., Scicli, A. G., Carretero, O. A., Slaughter, C., Moomaw, C. and Hersh, L. B. (1990) The hydrolysis of endothelins by neutral endopeptidase 24.11 (Enkephalinase). *Journal of Biological Chemistry*, **265**, 14150–14155.
42. Fagny, C., Michel, A., Léonard, I., Berkenboom, G., Fontaine, J. and Deschodt-Lanckman, M. (1991) *In vitro* degradation of endothelin-1 by endopeptidase 24.11 (Enkephalinase) *Peptides*, **12**, 773–778.
43. Di Maria, G. U., Katayama, M., Borson, D. B. and Nadel, J. A. (1992) Neutral endopeptidase modulates endothelin-1-induced airway smooth muscle contraction in guinea-pig trachea. *Regulatory Peptides*, **39**, 137–145.
44. Noguchi, K., Fukuroda, T., Ikeno, Y., Hirose, H., Tsukada, Y., Nishikibe, M. *et al.* (1991) Local formation and degradation of endothelin-1 in guinea pig airway tissues. *Biochemical and Biophysical Research Communications*, **179**, 830–835.
45. Boichot, E., Pons, F., Lagente, V., Touvay, C., Mencia-Huerta, J.-M. and Braquet, P. (1991) Phosphoramidon potentiates the endothelin-1-induced bronchopulmonary response in guinea-pigs. *Neurochemistry International*, **18**, 477–479.

46. McKay, K. O., Black, J. L. and Armour, C. L. (1992) Phosphoramidon potentiates the contractile response to endothelin-3, but not endothelin-1 in isolated airway tissue. *British Journal of Pharmacology*, **105**, 929–932.
47. Yamaguchi, T., Kohrogi, H., Kawano, O., Ando, M. and Araki, S. (1992) Neutral endopeptidase inhibitor potentiates endothelin-1-induced airway smooth muscle contraction. *Journal of Applied Physiology*, **73**, 1108–1113.
48. Fagny, C., Michel, A., Nortier, J. and Deschodt-Lanckman, M. (1992) Enzymatic degradation of endothelin-1 by activated human polymorphonuclear neutrophils. *Regulatory Peptides*, **42**, 27–37.
49. Koseki, C., Imai, M., Hirata, Y., Yanagisawa, M. and Masaki, T. (1989) Autoradiographic distribution in rat tissues of binding sites for endothelin: a neuropeptide? *American Journal of Physiology*, **256**, R858–R866.
50. Shiba, R., Yanagisawa, M., Miyauchi, T., Ishii, Y., Kimura, S., Uchiyama, Y., et al. (1989) Elimination of intravenously injected endothelin-1 from the circulation of the rat. *Journal of Cardiovascular Pharmacology*, **13 (Suppl 5)**, S98–S101.
51. Sirviö, M.-L., Metsärinne, K., Saijonmaa, O. and Fyhrquist, F. (1990) Tissue distribution and half-life of ^{125}I-endothelin in the rat: importance of pulmonary clearance. *Biochemical and Biophysical Research Communications*, **167**, 1191–1195.
52. De Nucci, G., Thomas, R., D'Orleans-Juste, P., Antunes, E., Walder, C., Warner, T. D. et al. (1988) Pressor effects of circulating endothelin are limited by its removal in the pulmonary circulation and by the release of prostacyclin and endothelium-derived relaxing factor. *Proceedings of the National Academy of Sciences USA*, **85**, 9797–9800.
53. Rimar, S. and Gillis, C. N. (1992) Differential uptake of endothelin-1 by the coronary and pulmonary circulations. *Journal of Applied Physiology*, **73**, 557–562.
54. Ray, S. G., McMurray, J. J., Morton, J. J. and Dargie, H. J. (1992) Circulating endothelin is not extracted by the pulmonary circulation in man. *Chest*, **102**, 1143–1144.
55. Power, R. F., Wharton, J., Zhao, Y., Bloom, S. R. and Polak, J. M. (1989) Autoradiographic localization of endothelin-1 binding sites in the cardiovascular and respiratory systems. *Journal of Cardiovascular Pharmacology*, **13 (Suppl 5)**, S50–S56.
56. Hemsén, A., Franco-Cereceda, A., Matran, R., Rudehill, A. and Lundberg, J. M. (1990) Occurrence, specific binding sites and functional effects of endothelin in human cardiopulmonary tissue. *European Journal of Pharmacology*, **191**, 319–328.
57. Henry, P. J., Rigby, P. J., Self, G. J., Preuss, J. M. and Goldie, R. G. (1990) Relationship between endothelin-1 binding site densities and constrictor activities in human and animal airway smooth muscle. *British Journal of Pharmacology*, **100**, 786–792.
58. Brink, C., Gillard, V., Roubert, P., Mencia-Huerta, J. M., Chabrier, P. E., Braquet, P. et al. (1991) Effects and specific binding sites of endothelin in human lung preparations. *Pulmonary Pharmacology*, **4**, 54–59.
59. Pons, F., Touvay, C., Lagente, V., Mencia-Huerta, J. M. and Braquet, P. (1991) Comparison of the effects of intra-arterial and aerosol administration of endothelin-1 (ET-1) in the guinea-pig isolated lung. *British Journal of Pharmacology*, **102**, 791–796.
60. Tschirhart, E. J., Drijfhout, J. W., Pelton, J. T., Miller, R. C. and Jones, C. R. (1991) Endothelins: Functional and autoradiographic studies in guinea pig trachea. *Journal of Pharmacology and Experimental Therapeutics*, **258**, 381–387.
61. Turner, N. C., Power, R. F., Polak, J. M., Bloom, S. R. and Dollery, C. T. (1989) Endothelin-induced contractions of tracheal smooth muscle and identification of specific endothelin binding sites in the trachea of the rat. *British Journal of Pharmacology*, **98**, 361–366.
62. McKay, K. O., Black, J. L. and Armour, C. L. (1991) The mechanism of action of endothelin in human lung. *British Journal of Pharmacology*, **102**, 422–428.
63. Bolger, G. T., Liard, F., Krogsrud, R., Thibeault, D. and Jaramillo, J. (1990) Tissue specificity of endothelin binding sites. *Journal of Cardiovascular Pharmacology*, **16**, 367–375.
64. Masuda, Y., Miyazaki, H., Kondoh, M., Watanabe, H., Yanagisawa, M., Masaki, T. et al. (1989) Two different forms of endothelin receptors in rat lung. *FEBS Letters*, **257**, 208–210.
65. Takayanagi, R., Ohnaka, K., Takasaki, C., Ohashi, M. and Nawata, H. (1991) Multiple subtypes of endothelin receptors in porcine tissues: characterization by ligand binding, affinity labeling and regional distribution. *Regulatory Peptides*, **32**, 23–37.
66. Arai, H., Hori, S., Aramori, I., Ohkubo, H. and Nakanishi, S. (1990) Cloning and expression of a cDNA encoding an endothelin receptor. *Nature*, **348**, 730–732.
67. Sakurai, T., Yanagisawa, M., Takuwa, Y., Miyazaki, H., Kimura, S., Goto, K. et al. (1990) Cloning of a cDNA encoding a non-isopeptide-selective subtype of the endothelin receptor. *Nature*, **348**, 732–735.
68. Sakamoto, A., Yanagisawa, M., Sakurai, T., Takuwa, Y., Yanagisawa, H. and Masaki, T. (1991) Cloning

and functional expression of human cDNA for the ET$_B$ endothelin receptor. *Biochemical and Biophysical Research Communications*, **178**, 656–663.
69. Masaki, T., Kimura, S., Yanagisawa, M. and Goto, K. (1989) Molecular and Cellular mechanism of endothelin regulation. *Circulation*, **80**, 219–233.
70. Martin, E. R., Brenner, B. M. and Ballermann, B. J. (1990) Heterogeneity of cell surface endothelin receptors. *Journal of Biological Chemistry*, **265**, 14044–14049.
71. Samson, W. K., Skala, K. D., Alexander, B. D. and Huang, F.-L. S. (1990) Pituitary site of action of endothelin: selective inhibition of prolactin release *in vitro*. *Biochemical and Biophysical Research Communication*, **169**, 737–743.
72. Karne, S., Jayawickreme, C. K. and Lerner, M. R. (1993) Cloning and characterization of an endothelin-3 specific receptor (ET$_C$ Receptor) from *Xenopus laevis* dermal melanophores. *Journal of Biological Chemistry*, **268**, 19126–19133.
73. Kondoh, M., Miyazaki, H., Uchiyama, Y., Yanagisawa, M., Masaki, T. and Murakami, K. (1991) Solubilization of two types of endothelin receptors, ET$_A$ and ET$_B$, from rat lung with retention of binding activity. *Biomedical Research*, **12**, 417–423.
74. Kozuka, M., Ito, T., Hirose, S., Lodhi, K. M. and Hagiwara, H. (1991) Purification and characterization of bovine lung endothelin receptor. *Journal of Biological Chemistry*, **266**, 16892–16896.
75. Hagiwara, H., Nagasawa, T., Lodhi, K. M., Kozuka, M., Ito, T. and Hirose, S. (1992) Affinity chromatographic purification of bovine lung endothelin receptor using biotinylated endothelin and avidin-agarose. *Journal of Chromatography*, **597**, 331–334.
76. Lippton, H. L., Hauth, T. A., Cohen, G. A. and Hyman, A. L. (1993) Functional evidence for different endothelin receptors in the lung. *Journal of Applied Physiology*, **75**, 38–48.
77. Hagiwara, H., Nagasawa, T., Yamamoto, T., Lodhi, K. M., Ito, T., Takemura, N. et al. (1993) Immunochemical characerization and location of endothelin ET$_B$ receptor. *Journal of Applied Physiology*, **264**, R777–R783.
78. Goldie, R. G., Henry, P. J., Self, G. J., Knott, P. G., Luttmann, M. and Hay, D. W. P. (1994) Endothelin receptor subtype distribution, density and function in human isolated asthmatic and non-diseased bronchus. *American Journal of Respiratory and Critical Care Medicine*, **149**, A472.
79. Nakamichi, K., Ihara, M., Kobayashi, M., Saeki, T., Ishikawa, K. and Yano, M. (1992) Different distribution of endothelin receptor subtypes in pulmonary tissues revealed by the novel selective ligands BQ-123 and [Ala^{1,3,11,15}]ET-1. *Biochemical and Biophysical Research Communications*, **182**, 144–150.
80. Kobayashi, M., Ihara, M., Sato, N., Saeki, T., Ozaki, S., Ikemoto, F. et al. (1993) A novel ligand, [^{125}I]BQ-3020, reveals the localization of endothelin ET$_B$ receptors. *European Journal of Pharmacology*, **235**, 95–100.
81. Henry, P. J. (1993) Endothelin-1 (ET-1)-induced contraction in rat isolated trachea: involvement of ET$_A$ and ET$_B$ receptors and multiple signal transduction systems. *British Journal of Pharmacology*, **110**, 435–441.
82. Noguchi, K., Ishikawa, K., Yano, M., Ahmed, A., Cortes, A., Hallmon, J. et al. (1992) An endothelin (ET)$_A$ receptor antagonist, BQ-123, blocks ET-1 induced bronchoconstriction and tracheal smooth muscle (TSM) contraction in allergic sheep. *American Review of Respiratory Disease*, **145**, A858.
83. Goldie, R. G., Grayson, P. S. and Henry, P. J. (1993) Endothelin-1 (ET-1)-induced contraction of ovine tracheal smooth muscle is mediated via ET$_A$ receptors. *American Review of Respiratory Disease*, **147**, A182.
84. Maggi, C. A., Giuliani, S., Patacchini, R., Rovero, P., Giachetti, A. and Meli, A. (1989) The activity of peptides of the endothelin family in various mammalian smooth muscle preparations. *European Journal of Pharmacology*, **174**, 23–31.
85. Maggi, C. A., Giuliani, S., Patacchini, R., Santicioli, P., Rovero, P., Giachetti, A. et al. (1989) The C-terminal hexapeptide, endothelin-(16–21), discriminates between different endothelin receptors. *European Journal of Pharmacology*, **166**, 121–122.
86. Maggi, C. A., Giuliani, S., Patacchini, R., Santicioli, P., Giachetti, A. and Meli, A. (1990) Further studies on the response of the guinea-pig isolated bronchus to endothelins and sarafotoxin S6b. *European Journal of Pharmacology*, **176**, 1–9.
87. Cardell, L. O., Uddman, R. and Edvinsson, L. (1992) Evidence for multiple endothelin receptors in the guinea-pig pulmonary artery and trachea. *British Journal of Pharmacology*, **105**, 376–380.
88. Williams, Jr., D. L., Jones, K. L., Pettibone, D. J., Lis, E. V. and Clineschmidt, B. V. (1991) Sarafotoxin S6c: an agonist which distinguishes between endothelin receptor subtypes. *Biochemical and Biophysical Research Communications*, **175**, 556–561.
89. Ihara, M., Noguchi, K., Saeki, T., Fukuroda, T., Tsuchida, S., Kimura, S. et al. (1991) Biological profiles of highly potent novel endothelin antagonists selective for the ET$_A$ receptor. *Life Sciences*, **50**, 247–255.
90. Sogabe, K., Nirei, H., Shoubo, M., Nomoto, A., Henmi, K., Notsu, Y. et al. (1992) A novel endothelin receptor antagonist: studies with FR 139317. *Japanese Journal of Pharmacology*, **58**, 105P.

91. Hay, D. W. P. (1992) Pharmacological evidence for distinct endothelin receptors in guinea-pig bronchus and aorta. *British Journal of Pharmacology*, **106**, 759–761.
92. Cardell, L. O., Uddman, R. and Edvinsson, L. (1993) A novel ET_A-receptor antagonist, FR 139317, inhibits endothelin-induced contractions of guinea-pig pulmonary arteries, but not trachea. *British Journal of Pharmacology*, **108**, 448–452.
93. Hay, D. W. P., Luttmann, M. A., Hubbard, W. C. and Undem, B. J. (1993) Endothelin receptor subtypes in human and guinea-pig pulmonary tissues. *British Journal of Pharmacology*, **110**, 1175–1183.
94. D'Orléans-Juste, P., Télémaque, S., Claing, A., Ihara, M. and Yano, M. (1992) Human big-endothelin-1 and endothelin-1 release prostacyclin via the activation of ET_1 receptors in the rat perfused lung. *British Journal of Pharmacology*, **105**, 773–775.
95. Uchida, Y., Ninomiya, H., Saotome, M., Nomura, A., Ohtsuka, M., Yanagisawa, M. et al. (1988) Endothelin, a novel vasoconstrictor peptide, as potent bronchoconstrictor. *European Journal of Pharmacology*, **154**, 227–228.
96. Advenier, C., Sarria, B., Naline, E., Puybasset, L. and Lagente, V. (1990) Contractile activity of three endothelins (ET-1, ET-2 and ET-3) on the human isolated bronchus. *British Journal of Pharmacology*, **100**, 168–172.
97. Hay, D. W. P. (1990) Mechanism of endothelin-induced contraction in guinea-pig trachea: comparison with rat aorta. *British Journal of Pharmacology*, **100**, 383–392.
98. Hay, D. W. P., Hubbard, W. C. and Undem, B. J. (1993) Endothelin-induced contraction and mediator release in human bronchus. *British Journal of Pharmacology*, **110**, 392–398.
99. Hay, D. W. P., Luttmann, M. A. and Goldie, R. G. (1994) Calcium (Ca^{2+}) Translocation mechanisms mediating endothelin-1 (ET-1)-and sarafotoxin S6c (S6c)-induced contractions in isolated human bronchus. *American Journal of Respiratory and Critical Care Medicine*, **149**, A1083.
100. Mattoli, S., Soloperto, M., Mezzetti, M. and Fasoli, A. (1991) Mechanisms of calcium mobilization and phosphoinositide hydrolysis in human bronchial smooth muscle cells by endothelin 1. *American Journal of Respiratory Cell and Moleculr Biology*, **5**, 424–430.
101. Battistini, B., Sirois, P., Braquet, P. and Filep, J. G. (1990) Endothelin-induced constriction of guinea-pig airways: role of platelet-activating factor. *European Journal of Pharmacology*, **186**, 307–310.
102. Ninomiya, H., Uchida, Y., Saotome, M., Nomura, A., Ohse, H., Matsumoto, H. et al. (1992) Endothelins constrict guinea pig tracheas by multiple mechanisms. *Journal of Pharmacology and Experimental Therapeutics*, **262**, 570–576.
103. Nomura, A., Nimoniya, H., Saotome, M., Ohse, N., Ishi, Y., Uchida, Y., et al. (1990) Multiple mechanisms of bronchoconstrictive responses to endothelin-1. *Journal of Vascular Medicine and Biology*, **2**, 199.
104. Uchida, Y., Ninomiya, H., Sakamoto, T., Lee, J. Y., Endo, T., Nomura, A. et al. (1992) ET-1 released histamine from guinea pig pulmonary but not peritoneal mast cells. *Biochemical and Biophysical Research Communication*, **189**, 1196–1201.
105. Filep, J. G., Battistini, B. and Sirois, P. (1990) Endothelin induces thromboxane release and contraction of isolated guinea-pig airways. *Life Sciences*, **47**, 1845–1850.
106. Filep, J. G., Battistini, B. and Sirois, P. (1991) Pharmacological modulation of endothelin-induced contraction of guinea-pig isolated airways and thromboxane release. *British Journal of Pharmacology*, **103**, 1633–1640.
107. Hay, D. W. P., Hubbard, W. C. and Undem, B. J. (1993) Relative contributions of direct and indirect mechanisms mediating endothelin-induced contraction of guinea-pig trachea. *British Journal of Pharmacology*, **110**, 955–962.
108. White, S. R., Hathaway, D. P., Umans, J. G., Tallet, J., Abrahams, C. and Leff, A. R. (1991) Epithelial modulation of airway smooth muscle response to endothelin-1. *American Review of Respiratory Disease*, **144**, 373–378.
109. Filep, J. G., Battistini, B. and Sirois, P. (1993) Induction by endothelin-1 of epithelium-dependent relaxation of guinea-pig trachea *in vitro*: role for nitric oxide. *British Journal of Pharmacology*, **109**, 637–644.
110. Cardell, L. O., Uddman, R. and Edvinsson, L. (1991) Two functional endothelin receptors in guinea-pig pulmonary arteries. *Neurochemistry International*, **18**, 4, 571–574.
111. Rodman, D. M., Stelzner, T. J., Zamora, M. R., Bonvallet, S. T., Oka, M., Sato, K. et al. (1992) Endothelin-1 increases the pulmonary microvascular pressure and causes pulmonary edema in salt solution but not blood-perfused rat lungs. *Journal of Cardiovascular Pharmacology*, **20**, 658–663.
112. Webber, S. E., Yurdakos, E., Woods, A. J. and Widdicombe, J. G. (1992) Effects of endothelin-1 on tracheal submucosal gland secretion and epithelial function in the ferret. *Chest*, **101**, 63S–67S.
113. Satoh, M., Shimura, S., Ishihara, H., Nagaki, M., Sasaki, H., Takishima, T. (1992) Endothelin-1 stimulates chloride secretion across canine tracheal epithelium. *Respiration*, **59**, 145–150.

114. Plews, P. I., Abdel-Malek, Z. A., Doupnik, D. A. and Leikauf, G. D. (1991) Endothelin stimulates chloride secretion across canine tracheal epithelium. *American Journal of Physiology*, **261**, L188–L194.
115. Tamaoki, J., Kanemura, T., Sakai, N., Isono, K., Kobayashi, K. and Takizawa, T. (1991) Endothelin stimulates ciliary beat frequency and chloride secretion in canine cultured tracheal epithelium. *American Journal of Respiratory Cell and Molecular Biology*, **4**, 426–431.
116. Wu, T., Rieves, R. D., Larivee, P., Logun, C., Lawrence, M. G. and Shelhamer, J. H. (1993) Production of eicosanoids in response to endothelin-1 and identification of specific endothelin-1 binding sites in airway epithelial cells. *American Journal of Respiratory Cell and Molecular Biology*, **8**, 282–290.
117. Mullol, J., Chowdhury, B. A., White, M. V., Ohkubo, K., Rieves, R. D., Baraniuk, J. et al. (1993) Endothelin in human nasal mucosa. *American Journal of Respiratory Cell and Molecular Biology*, **8**, 393–402.
118. Wu, T., Mullol, J., Rieves, R. D., Logun, C., Hausfield, J., Kaliner, M. A. et al. (1992) Endothelin-1 stimulates eicosanoid production in cultured human nasal mucosa. *American Journal of Respiratory Cell and Molecular Biology*, **6**, 168–174.
119. Shimura, S., Ishihara, H., Satoh, M., Masuda, T., Nagaki, N., Sasaki, H. et al. (1992) Endothelin regulation of mucus glycoprotein secretion from feline tracheal submucosal glands. *American Journal of Physiology*, **262**, L208–L213.
120. Takuwa, N., Takuwa, Y., Yanagisawa, M., Yamashita, K. and Masaki, T. (1989) A novel vasoactive peptide endothelin stimulates mitogenesis through inositol lipid turnover in Swiss 3T3 fibroblasts. *Journal of Biological Chemistry*, **264**, 7856–7861.
121. Brewster, C. E. P., Howarth, P. H., Djukanovic, R., Wilson, J., Holgate, S. T. and Roche, W. R. (1990) Myofibroblasts and subepithelial fibrosis in bronchial asthma. *American Journal of Respiratory Cell and Molecular Biology*, **3**, 507–11.
122. Peacock, A. J., Dawes, K. E., Shock, A., Gray, A. J., Reeves, J. T. and Laurent, G. J. (1992) Endothelin-1 and endothelin-3 induce chemotaxis and replication of pulmonary artery fibroblasts. *American Journal of Respiratory Cell and Molecular Biology*, **7**, 492–499.
123. Zamora, M. A., Dempsey, E. C., Walchak, S. J. and Stelzner, T. J. (1993) BQ123, an ET_A receptor antagonist, inhibits endothelin-1-mediated proliferation of human pulmonary artery smooth muscle cells. *American Journal of Respiratory Cell and Molecular Biology*, **9**, 429–433.
124. Janakidevi, K., Fisher, M. A., Del Vecchio, P. J., Tiruppathi, C., Figge, J. and Malik, A. B. (1992) Endothelin-1 stimulates DNA synthesis and proliferation of pulmonary artery smooth muscle cells. *American Journal of Physiology*, **263**, C1295–C1303.
125. Nagase, T., Fukuchi, Y., Jo, C., Teramoto, S., Uejima, Y., Ishida, K. et al. (1990) Endothelin-1 stimulates arachidonate 15-lipoxygenase activity and oxygen radical formation in the rat distal lung. *Biochemical and Biophysical Research Communications*, **168**, 485–489.
126. Ninomiya, H., Yu, X. Y., Hasegawa, S. and Spannhake, E. W. (1992) Endothelin-1 induces stimulation of prostaglandin synthesis in cells obtained from canine airways by bronchoalveolar lavage. *Prostaglandins*, **43**, 401–411.
127. Helset, E., Kjaeve, J. and Hauge, A. (1993) Endothelin-1-induced increases in microvascular permeability in isolated, perfused rat lungs requires leukocytes and plasma. *Circulatory Shock*, **39**, 5–20.
128. Horgan, M. J., Pinheiro, J. M. B. and Malik, A. B. (1991) Mechanism of endothelin-1-induced pulmonary vasoconstriction. *Circulation Research*, **69**, 157–164.
129. Raffestin, B., Adnot, S., Eddahibi, S., Macquin-Mavier, I., Braquet, P. and Chabrier, P. E. (1991) Pulmonary vascular response to endothelin in rats. *American Journal of Physiology*, **70**, 567–574.
130. Mann, J., Farrukh, I. S. and Michael, J. R. (1991) Mechanisms by which endothelin 1 induces pulmonary vasoconstriction in the rabbit. *Journal of Applied Physiology*, **71**, 410–416.
131. Barnard, J. W., Barman, S. A., Adkins, W. K., Longenecker, G. L. and Taylor, A. E. (1991) Sustained effects of endothelin-1 on rabbit, dog, and rat pulmonary circulations. *American Journal of Physiology*, **261**, H479–H486.
132. Achmad, T. H. and Rao, G. S. (1992) Chemotaxis of human blood monocytes toward endothelin-1 and the influence of calcium channel blockers. *Biochemical and Biophysical Research Communications*, **189**, 994–1000.
133. Bath, P. M. W., Mayston, S. A. and Martin, J. F. (1990) Endothelin and PDGF do not stimulate peripheral blood monocyte chemotaxis, adhesion to endothelium, and superoxide production. *Experimental Cell Research*, **187**, 339–342.
134. Millul, V., Lagente, V., Gillardeaux, O., Boichot, E., Dugas, B., Mencia-Huerta, J.-M. et al. (1991) Activation of guinea pig alveolar macrophages by endothelin-1. *Journal of Cardiovascular Pharmacology*, **17 (Suppl 7)**, S233–S235.
135. Haller, H., Schaberg, T., Lindschau, C., Lode, H. and Distler, A. (1991) Endothelin increases $[Ca^+]_i$, protein phosphorylation, and $O_2^- \cdot$ production in human alveolar macrophages. *American Journal of Physiology*, **261**, L478–L484.

136. Payne, A. N. and Whittle, B. J. R. (1988) Potent cyclo-oxygenase-mediated bronchoconstrictor effects of endothelin in the guinea-pig in vivo. *European Journal of Pharmacology*, **158**, 303–304.
137. Lagente, V., Chabrier, P. E., Mencia-Huerta, J.-M. and Braquet, P. (1989) Pharmacological modulation of the bronchopulmonary action of the vasoactive peptide, endothelin, administered by aerosol in the guinea-pig. *Biochemical and Biophysical Research Communications*, **158**, 625–632.
138. Macquin-Mavier, I., Levame, M., Istin, N. and Harf, A. (1989) Mechanisms of endothelin-mediated bronchoconstriction in the guinea pig. *Journal of Pharmacology and Experimental Therapeutics*, **250**, 740–745.
139. Touvay, C., Vilain, B., Pons, F., Chabrier, P.-E., Mencia-Huerta, J. M. and Braquet, P. (1990) Bronchopulmonary and vascular effect of endothelin in the guinea pig. *European Journal of Pharmacology*, **176**, 23–33.
140. Lueddeckens, G., Becker, K., Rappold, R. and Förster, W. (1991) Influence of aminophylline and ketotifen in comparison to the lipoxygenase inhibitors NDGA and esculetin and the PAF antagonists WEB 2107 and BN 52021 on endothelin-1 induced vaso- and bronchoconstriction. *Prostaglandins, Leukotrienes and Essential Fatty Acids*, **44**, 155–158.
141. Boichot, E., Lagente, V., Mencia-Huerta, J. M. and Braquet, P. (1990) Effect of phosphoramidon and indomethacin on the endothelin-1 (ET-1) induced bronchopulmonary response in aerosol sensitized guinea pigs. *Journal of Vascular Medicine and Biology*, **2**, 206.
142. Boichot, E., Carré, C., Lagente, V., Pons, F., Mencia-Huerta, J. M. and Braquet, P. (1991) Endothelin-1 (ET-1) and bronchial hyperresponsiveness in the guinea-pig. *Journal of Cardiovascular Pharmacology*, **17 (Suppl 7)**, S329–S331.
143. Uchida, ., Hamada, M., Kameyama, M., Ohse, H., Nomura, A., Hasegawa, S. et al. (1992) ET-1 induced bronchoconstriction in the early phase but not late phase of anesthetized dogs is inhibited by indomethacin and ICI 198615. *Biochemical and Biophysical Research Communications*, **183**, 1197–1202.
144. Matsuse, T., Fukuchi, Y., Suruda, T., Nagase, T., Ouchi, Y. and Orimo, H. (1990) Effect of endothelin-1 on pulmonary resistance in rats. *Journal of Applied Physiology*, **68**, 2391–2393.
145. Abraham, W. M., Ahmed, A., Cortes, A., Spinella, M. J., Malik, A. B. and Anderson, T. T. (1993) A specific endothelin-1 antagonist blocks inhaled endothelin-1-induced bronchoconstriction in sheep. *Journal of Applied Physiology*, **74**, 2537–2542.
146. Lagente, V., Boichot, E., Mencia-Huerta, J. and Braquet, P. (1990) Failure of aerosolized endothelin (ET-1) to induce bronchial hyperreactivity in the guinea pig. *Fundamentals in Clinical Pharmacology*, **4**, 275–280.
147. Kanazawa, H., Kurihara, N., Hirata, K., Fujiwara, H., Matsushita, H. and Takeda, T. (1992) Low concentration endothelin-1 enhanced histamine-mediated bronchial contractions of guinea pigs in vivo. *Biochemical and Biophysical Research Communications*, **187**, 717–721.
148. Pons, F., Boichot, E., Lagente, V., Touvay, C., Mencia-Huerta, J. M. and Braquet, P. (1992) Role of endothelin in pulmonary function. *Pulmonary Pharmacology*, **5**, 213–219.
149. Lippton, H. L. Cohen, G. A., McMurtry, I. F. and Hyman, A. I. (1991) Pulmonary vasodilation to endothelin isopeptides in vivo is mediated by potassium channel activation. *Journal of Applied Psycology*, **70**, 947–952.
150. Hasunuma, K., Rodman, D. M., O'Brien, R. F. and McMurty, I. F. (1990) Endothelin 1 causes pulmonary vasodilation in rats. *American Journal of Physiology*, **259**, H48–H54.
151. Filep, J. G., Sirois, M. G., Földes-Filep, É., Rousseau, A., Plante, G. E., Fournier, A. et al. (1993) Enhancement by endothelin-1 of microvascular permeability via the activation of ET_A receptors. *British Journal of Pharmacology*, **109**, 880–886.
152. Hay, D. W. P., Henry, P. J. and Goldie, R. G. (1993) Endothelin and the respiratory system. *Trends in Pharmacological Studies*, **14**, 29–32.
153. Nomura, A., Uchida, Y., Kameyama, M., Saotome, M., Oki, K. and Hasegawa, S. (1989) Endothelin and bronchial asthma. *Lancet*, **2** (8665), 747–748.
154. Mattoli, S., Soloperto, M., Marini, M. and Fasoli, A. (1991) Levels of endothelin in the bronchoalveolar lavage fluid of patients with symptomatic asthma and reversible airflow obstruction. *Journal of Allergy and Clinical Immunology*, **88**, 376–384.
155. Vittori, E., Marini, M., Fasoli, A., De Franchis, R. and Mattoli, S. (1992) Increased expression of endothelin in bronchial epithelial cells of asthmatic patients and effect of corticosteroids. *American Review of Respiratory Disease*, **146**, 1320–1325.
156. Springall, D. R., Howarth, P. H., Counihan, H., Djukanovic, R., Holgate, S. T. and Polak, J. M. (1991) Endothelin immunoreactivity of airway epithelium in asthmatic patients. *Lancet*, **337**, 697–701.
157. Kraft, M., Beam, W. R., O'Brien, R. F. and Martin, R. J. (1993) Blood and bronchoalveolar lavage endothelin-1 levels in nocturnal asthma. *American Review of Respiratory Disease*, **147**, A978.
158. Heath, D., Smith, P., Gosney, J., Mulcahy, D., Fox, K., Yacoub, M. et al. (1987) The pathology of the early and late stages of primary pulmonary hypertension. *British Heart Journal*, **58**, 204–213.

159. Cernacek, P. and Stewart, D. J. (1989) Immnoreactive endothelin in human plasma: marked elevations in patients in cardiogenic shock. *Biochemical and Biophysical Research Communications*, **161**, 562–567.
160. Stewart, D. J., Levy, R. D., Cernacek, P. and Langleben, D. (1991) Increased plasma endothelin-1 in pulmonary hypertension: marker or mediator of disease? *Annals of Internal Medicine*, **114**, 464–469.
161. Yoshibayashi, M., Nishioka, K., Nakao, K., Saito, Y., Matsumura, M., Ueda, T. et al. (1991) Plasma endothelin concentrations in patients with pulmonary hypertension associated with congenital heart defects. *Circulation*, **84**, 2280–2285.
162. Allen, S. W., Chatfield, B. A., Koppenhafer, S. A., Schaffer, M. S., Wolfe, R. R. and Abman, S. H. (1993) Circulating immunoreactive endothelin-1 in children with pulmonary hypertension. *American Review of Respiratory Disease*, **148**, 519–522.
163. Cacoub, P., Dorent, R., Maistre, G., Nataf, P., Carayon, A., Piette, J. C. et al. (1993) Endothelin-1 in primary pulmonary hypertension and the Eisenmenger syndrome. *American Journal of Cardiology*, **71**, 448–450.
164. Chang, H., Wu, G-J., Wang, S-M. and Hung, C-R. (1993) Plasma endothelin levels and surgically correctable pulmonary hypertension. *Annals of Thoracic Surgery*, **55**, 450–458.
165. Giaid, A., Yanagisawa, M., Langleben, D., Michel, R. P., Levy, R., Shennib, H. et al. (1993) Expression of endothelin-1 in the lungs of patients with pulmonary hypertension. *New England Journal of Medicine*, **328**, 1732–1739.
166. Lippton, H. L., Hauth, T. A., Summer, W. R., and Hyman, A. L. (1989) Endothelin produces pulmonary vasoconstriction and systemic vasodilation. *Journal of Applied Physiology*, **66**, 1008–1012.
167. Minkes, R. K., Bellan, J. A., Saroyan, R. M., Kerstein, M. D., Coy, D. H., Murphy, W. A. et al. (1990) Analysis of cardiovascular and pulmonary responses to endothelin-1 and endothelin-3 in the anesthetized cat. *Journal of Pharmacology and Experimental Therapeutics*, **253**, 1118–1125.
168. Komuro, I., Kurihara, H., Sugiyama, T., Takaku, F. and Yazaki, Y. (1988) Endothelin stimulates c-*fos* and c-*myc* expression and proliferation of vascular smooth muscle cells. *FEBS Letters*, **238**, 249–252.
169. Hirata, Y., Takagi, Y., Fukuda, Y. and Marumo, F. (1989) Endothelin is a potent mitogen for rat vascular smooth muscle cells. *Atherosclerosis*, **78**, 225–228.
170. Wagenvoort, C. A. (1981) Grading of pulmonary vascular lesions – a reappraisal. *Histopathology*, **5**, 595–598.
171. Yoshizumi, M., Kurihara, H., Sugiyama, T., Takaku, F., Yanagisawa, M., Masaki, T. et al. (1989) Hemodynamics shear stress stimulates endothelin production by cultured endothelial cells. *Biochemical and Biophysical Research Communications*, **161**, 859–864.
172. Stelzner, T. J., O'Brien, R. F., Yanagisawa, M., Sakurai, T., Sato, K., Webb, S. et al. (1992) Increased lung endothelin-1 production in rats with idiopathic pulmonary hypertension. *American Journal of Physiology*, **262**, L614–L620.
173. Giaid, A., Hamid, Q. A., Springall, D. R., Yanagisawa, M., Shinmi, O., Sawamura, T. et al. (1990) Detection of endothelin immunoreactivity and mRNA in pulmonary tumors. *Journal of Pathology*, **162**, 15–22.
174. Giaid, A., Michel, R. P., Stewart, D. J., Sheppard, M., Corrin, B. and Hamid, Q. (1993) Expression of endothelin-1 in lungs of patients with cryptogenic fibrosing alveolitis. *Lancet*, **341**, 1550–54.
175. Marciniak, S. J., Plumpton, C., Barker, P. J., Huskisson, N. S. and Davenport, A. P. (1992) Localization of immunoreactive endothelin and proendothelin in the human lung. *Pulmonary Pharmacology*, **5**, 175–182.
176. Morel, D. R., Lacroix, J. S., Hemsen, A., Steinig, D. A., Pittet, J-F. and Lundberg, J. M. (1989) Increased plasma and pulmonary lymph levels of endothelin during endotoxin shock. *European Journal of Pharmacology*, **167**, 427–428.
177. Filep, J. G., Télémaque, S., Battistini, B., Sirois, P. and D'Orléans-Juste, P. (1993) Increased plasma levels of endothelin during anaphylactic shock in the guinea-pig. *European Journal of Pharmacology*, **239**, 231–236.

17 Endothelin: Role in Endocrine Disorders

Elena I. Barengolts

Department of Medicine, Section of Endocrinology (M/C 787), University of Illinois College of Medicine at Chicago, 820 South Wood Street, Chicago, IL 60612, USA

INTRODUCTION

In 1988 Yanagisawa, *et al.*[1] isolated and characterized a peptide from the supernatant of porcine endothelial cell culture that was named endothelin (ET). This factor is now designated as ET-1 and is the most potent vasoconstricting agent presently known[1,2]. Subsequently the three separate genes were identified in many mammalian species, including humans, encoding for three peptides ET-1, ET-2, and ET-3. The three isoforms of endothelin peptides consist of 21 amino acids, ET-1 differs from ET-2 by two amino acids and from ET-3 by six amino acids.[1-3] ET-1 is derived from endothelial cells and is a predominant form found in circulation, ET-2 is of undetermined origin but is structurally identical to murine vasoactive intestinal constrictor (VIC), and ET-3 is of neural origin and plays an important role in neurotransmission. The ETs found in humans share structural and functional characteristics with rat and mouse isoforms and with sarafotoxin-S6b peptide, isolated from the venom of the snake *Atractaspis engaddensis*. ET-1 is derived from a 203-amino acid precursor (preproET-1), that yields an inactive 39-amino acid pro- or "big" ET-1 (after proteolytic cleavage), which is converted to ET-1 by ET-converting enzyme, a metalloproteinase. ET-3 is similarly derived from 224-amino acid preproET-3 reduced to a 42-amino acid "big"-ET-3 (Ref. 4–7 for review).

The actions of ETs are mediated by receptors, presently designated as ET_A, ET_B, and ET_C[4-8]. These receptors belong to the family of G protein-coupled calcium-mobilizing receptors[9,10]. ET_A has a higher affinity for ET-1 and ET-2 than ET-3, is predominantly distributed in smooth muscle and causes vasoconstriction[9]. ET_B has an equipotent affinity for all three ET isopeptides, is mainly found in endothelial cells, and its major pharmacological action is release of endothelium-derived relaxing factor (EDRF) and eicosanoids[10]. The ET_A and ET_B but not ET_C receptors had been cloned and characterized. The ET_C receptor is suggested to have high affinity for ET-3, predominantly distributed in pituitary cells, and involved in inhibition of prolactin secretion[7,8]. Activation of ET receptors stimulates release of Ca^{2+} from intracellular

Table 17.1 Endothelin (ET) concentration in biological fluids[a]

Fluid	N	ET concentration (pmol/ml)	Reference
Plasma	116	0.5 – 3.5	12, 97
Urine	12	2.1 ± 0.3	12
CSF[b]	7	0.1 ± 0.1	11
Breast milk	16	6.8 ± 1.6	12
Saliva	15	2.0 ± 0.2	12
Amniotic fluid[c]	27	7.5 ± 3.6	13
Seminal fluid[d]	8	838.6 ± 236.5	14

[a]Results are Mean ± SEM; N = number of subjects. To convert ET values to pg/ml, multiply by 2.49; [b]CSF = cerebrospinal fluid; [c]Amniotic fluid was sampled at 16 weeks of gestation, the levels increased (42.8 ± 12.4 pmol/ml, n = 8, p < 0.001) during the third trimester; [d]The cross-reactivity of "big" ET-1 in this assay was 38%.

stores in a manner similar to that of typical calcium-mobilizing receptors, leading to a multitude of cell- and tissue-specific responses[4-7]. The major response to intracellular calcium accumulation in endocrine tissues is hormone secretion.

As a family endothelins have a distinct profile of activities including vasoconstricting, mitogenic, and secretagogue, and modulate function of a multitude of cell types[4-7]. The ETs are found in biological fluids, including plasma[11,12] cerebrospinal fluid[11], urine[12], breast milk[12], saliva[12], amniotic[13], and seminal fluid[14] (Table 17.1). ETs and their receptors are demonstrated to coexist in many tissues of the body[4-8]. Thus, the endothelins have the potential to act via endocrine as well as autocrine and/or paracrine mechanisms.

Variety of endocrine tissues have capability to synthesize and secrete endothelins. The presence of immunoreactive ETs (ir-ETs) was found in the paraventricular and supraoptic nuclei of the hypothalamus, the anterior and posterior lobes of pituitary gland[7], in the adrenals[15], ovaries[16], thyroid[17], and parathyroid cells[18]. Synthesis of ETs is demonstrated *in vivo* by the expression of ET genes and *in vitro* by release of ETs in culture medium[4-7].

Endocrine effects of ETs were demonstrated *in vitro* and *in vivo*. ETs have a wide variety of actions in endocrine system. Functions of virtually all endocrine tissues were shown to be influenced by ETs. ETs were as potent as GnRH in stimulating release of LH, and as important as dopamine in modulating secretion of prolactin from pituitary cells in culture[19]. Vasopressin and oxytocin secretion from pituitary was enhanced by ETs[20]. ETs stimulated release of aldosterone[21] and catecholamines[22] from adrenals, and modulated secretion of thyroglobulin[23], parathyriod hormone[24], progesterone[25], and testosterone[26]. *In vivo* administration of ET-1 increased circulating levels of vasopressin, adrenocorticotropin (ACTH), norepinephrine, epinephrine, renin, aldosterone, and atrial natriuretic peptide in conscious dogs and rats[27,28] (Table 17.2). Circulating ET levels are elevated in various pathological states including hypertension, ischemic heart disease, renal failure, and diabetes[29-31].

Table 17.2 Distribution of ETs, ET receptors and effects of ET on hormone secretion

Organ	ET-1[a]	ET-3[a]	Receptors	Effects on hormones: in vitro	in vivo
Hypothalamus	<5	20	ET$_A$	↑AVP, ↑SP	↑AVP
Pituitary	53	190	ET$_A$, ET$_B$	↓PRL, ↑LH[b] ↑AVP	↑ACTH ↑AVP, ↑OT
Thyroid	1.5	?	?	↓TG	?
Parathyroid			ET$_A$, ET$_B$	↓PTH	?
Pancreas	390	11	?	?	?
Adrenal	120	12	ET$_A$, ET$_B$[c]	↑ALDO, ↑F ↑NE, ↑Epi	↑ALDO ↑NE, ↑Epi
Ovaries	2.8	?	ET$_B$	↓P/↑P, ↑E, ↑T	?
Testes	570	7.7	ET$_A$	↑T	?

[a]Results are ir-ETs measured in rat organs and expressed as means in pg/g wet tissue; [b]FSH and TSH are mildly increased, GH and ACTH are unaffected; [c]Adrenal medulla contains only ET$_B$; Hormonal abbreviations and details are given in the text. SP, substance P; TG, thyroglobulin; F, cortisol; P, progesterone; E, estradiol; T, testosterone; ↑, increased secretion; ↓, descreased secretion.

This review focuses on physiological and pathophysiological roles of ETs in endocrine system and their possible relevance in pathogenesis of some endocrine diseases.

PITUITARY

The presence of ir-ET, endothelin mRNA, and ET receptors was detected in human pituitary gland examined postmortem. Pituitary contained the highest concentration of ir-ET compared with six other regions of the central nervous system studied, including brain stem, cerebral cortex, hypothalamus, cerebellum, basal ganglia, and spinal cord[32]. Similar distribution of ir-ET was found in the rat[33]. Levels of the peptides in pituitary extracts were in picograms per gm of tissue range.

The ET-3 was the main endothelin of pituitary. Stimulation of cultured pituitary cells by insulin-like growth factor-I (IGF-I) resulted in preferential release of ET-3 vs. ET-1[34]. Pituitary contained predominantly ET-3 and a small amount of ET-1 and "big" ET as analyzed by fast protein liquid chromatography[20,32,35]. In the rat, while ET-1 was minimally present in hypothalamo-pituitary system, ET-3 was present in relatively large amount in anterior lobe (4.1 ± 0.9 ng ET-3/mg protein), neuro-intermediate lobe (5.6 ± 1.8 ng ET-3/mg protein), and hypothalamic median eminence (20 ± 3.3 ng ET-3/mg protein), exceeding the amount present in abdominal aorta (0.35 ± 0.04 ng ET-3/mg protein)[20]. In hypothalamus ETs were present in the paraventricular and supraoptic nuclei of the magnocellular neurons. In posterior pituitary ETs were at least partially colocalized with vasopressin (AVP) and oxytocin (OT), as demonstrated by in vivo studies[36] and in vitro double immunogold staining[37].

The presence of [I^{125}]ET binding sites in hypothalamus, anterior, and posterior pituitary lobes was shown by autoradiography and affinity binding studies using hypothalamic tissue, pituitary fragments, dispersed pituitary cells, and pituitary cell membranes[32,33,38,39]. The discrepancy exists between the demonstration of binding sites with higher affinity for ET-1 than ET-3[38,39] and the finding that the main pituitary ET is ET-3. Thus, it was suggested that ET pituitary receptor is different from the cloned ET_A and ET_B receptors and was proposed to be designated ET_C[8]. The existence of multiple classes of ET receptors in the pituitary was supported by the finding of two classes of binding sites, high and low affinity, in the human pituitary postmortem. Scatchard analysis of binding data showed dissociation constants and binding capacities of $K_d = 0.059 \pm 0.002$ nM and $B_{max} = 418 \pm 63$ fmol/mg protein as well as $K_d = 0.652 \pm 0.103$ nM and $B_{max} = 1,717 \pm 200$ fmol/mg protein[32].

Regulation of ETs secretion from the rat pituitary cells by various growth factors showed that ET-3 secretion was stimulated by insulin, IGF-I, and IGF-II but inhibited by transforming growth factor β (TGFβ). The ET-1 secretion was stimulated by TGFβ but slightly reduced by IGFs[34].

Several systems were employed to study hypothalamo-pituitary effects of ETs. *In vitro* two systems were used: 1) the static culture of dispersed pituitary cells and 2) dynamic perifusion of pituitary cells, where pituitary cells were loaded onto a column which was perfused with various culture mediums at a pre-determined rate, and medium was collected and analyzed at various intervals[19,39]. *In vivo* intravenous[19] or intracerebroventricular (ICV) administration of ETs was used; ICV injections were given to either anesthetized or conscious animals. The latter technique involved implantation of an indwelling canulae into the third ventricle couple of weeks before experiment and placement of canulae in the external jugular vein to allow injections and blood sample drawing in unrestrained animals without confounding effects of anesthesia[28,40].

Endocrine responses known to be elicited by ETs in the hypothalamo-pituitary system include the release of substance P from the rat hypothalamus and pituitary *in vitro*[41]; the release of AVP from perifused hypothalamic fragments[42], and the modification of secretion of pituitary hormones[19,43,44].

Regulation of prolactin (PRL) secretion

The most prominent effect of ETs in the anterior pituitary is regulation of prolactin secretion. The predominant and long-lasting effect was inhibitory as demonstrated by *in vitro* studies[19,45-48]. The inhibition was observed in cells obtained from either female or male rats suggesting gender-independent effect[19]. Analysis of static culture of dispersed pituitary cells showed that the inhibitory effect of endothelin was dose and time dependent[19,45-47]. Dynamic incubation of perifused pituitary cells demonstrated a biphasic response of lactotrophs of ET exposure. The initial response was stimulation of PRL secretion which was transitory and was followed by a sustained but reversible inhibition of PRL release[19]. The minimum effective dose for ETs inhibitory effect was in physiological relevant range. Circulating ET levels in the rats and humans are in the low picogram per ml plasma range, and levels of the peptides in pituitary and hypothalamic extracts are in picograms per tissue range. Of the three ETs tested, ET-2 demonstrated the highest potency, 1 pM of ET-2 inhibited PRL secretion from cultured pituitary cells for four hours. The minimal effective doses for PRL inhibition were as follows: ET-1 – 0.1 nM, ET-2 – 1 pM, ET-3 – 6.25 nM. The ETs effective doses were comparable to Dopamine doses, the minimal effective Dopamine dose in the same culture system was 25 nM[46]. The duration of lactotrophs inhibition by ETs was long-lasting with the maximum inhibition of PRL secretion occurring after 12 hours of pituitary cells exposure to ET-3[45].

The mechanisms of ETs inhibitory effect on PRL secretion are not known but appear to mimic those of Dopamine (DA). Although the receptors for Dopamine and ET are different and ligand-specific, the postreceptor signal transduction involves similar pathways. Dopamine activates the specific anterior pituitary receptor, D_2, and triggers a complex spectrum of intracellular signals including stimulation of pertussis-sensitive G protein, suppression of adenylate cyclase, increase in K^+ conductance, regulation of protein kinase C (PKC), and inhibition of Ca^{2+} entry. The result is a decrease in the level of intracellular calcium ion and a decline in PRL secretion[49,50]. The activation of ET receptor in lactotrophs, like in other cells, was linked to G protein and, down the signaling pathway, to PKC[5,51]. It was shown that the ETs inhibitory effect on lactotrophs was independent of D_2 or voltage-sensitive (nifedipine-sensitive) calcium channels, but was suppressed by pertussis toxin (PTX) and staurosporine[19,46,51]. The pertussis toxin is an inhibitor of G protein. Of several PTX sensitive G proteins G_k and/or G_i were suggested to be involved. Activation of these proteins results in an increase in K^+ conductance and a decrease in adenylate cyclase activity, respectively. Staurosporine is an inhibitor of protein kinase C. The substrates for PKC in lactotrophs have not been identified, but activation of these substrates, which may include cytoplasmic phosphorylated proteins or membrane-bound phospholipids, may lead to depletion of intracellular Ca^{2+} and attenuation of PRL secretion[46] (Figure 17.1).

The initial stimulation of PRL secretion by ETs was probably nonspecific. It required higher doses of ETs than doses needed for inhibitory effect (10–100 nM vs. 0.1 nM, respectively), it was transitory, and suppressed by nifedipine blockade of calcium channels[19,46,47]. There is probably no physiological significance in transient

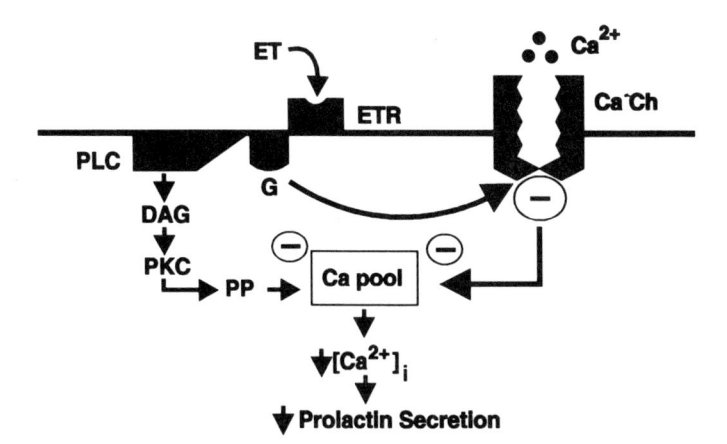

Figure 17.1. Intracellular pathways for the inhibitory effects of endothelin (ET) on prolactin (PRL) secretion in lactotrophs. G, G protein; ETR, ET receptor; PLC, phospholipase C; DAG, 1,2 diacylglycerol; PKC, protein kinase C; PP, phosphorilated proteins; CaCh, calcium channel; $[Ca^{2+}]_i$, calcium ion.

PRL stimulation by ETs since the doses required for this effect are significantly higher than ET levels present in circulation or locally in the pituitary gland.

Physiological importance of ET-mediated lactotrophs' inhibition may be significant. Several factors are involved in inhibition of PRL secretion under various conditions[47,49]. Dopamine, a hypothalamic neurotransmitter, is the major PRL-inhibiting factor (PIF). Some of the other PIFs identified to date include γ-aminobutiric acid (GABA) of hypothalamic origin; gonadotropin-releasing hormone-associated peptide; and PRL itself acting via a short feedback loop[49]. Dopamine is the only PIF used clinically. The similarities between Dopamine and ETs mechanisms of action may prove to be of clinical significance, and ET or its agonist may be employed in hyperprolactinemic states in the future.

Regulation of luteinizing hormone (LH) release

Regulation of LH secretion is the second most prominent effect of ET in the anterior pituitary. The ETs (ET-1 and ET-3) stimulated LH secretion from pituitary cells harvested from random cycle or oophorectomized female rats, and exposed to ETs in static cultures or during dynamic perifusion[19,43,51,53]. The minimal stimulatory dose of ET-1 was 1 nM in perifused pituitary cells[37,53] and the EC_{50} value for ET-3 was 4 nM in dispersed pituitary cells[45]. The maximal stimulatory effect for ET-3 was reached at 100 nM concentration after 4 hours of incubation[45].

Comparison of ET-1 and gonadotropin-releasing hormone (GnRH), showed that GnRH and ET-1 induced comparable secretion of LH during short term incubation but GnRH was a more potent stimulus than ET-1 during long term incubation of pituitary cells in culture[19,51]. GnRH, a 10 amino acid hypothalamic peptide, is a principal stimulator of LH and follicle-stimulating hormone (FSH) secretion from the pituitary gland[54]. There was no synergism or antagonism between GnRH and ET-stimulated LH release[19,43]. Concomitant incubation of cells with GnRH and ET-3 did not affect the values for LH secretion compared with those observed when each agent was used alone in static or dynamic cultures[19]. Sequential exposure of pituitary cells to ET-1 and GnRH showed that GnRH-treated cells recovered their full $[Ca^{2+}]_i$ and secretory responses to ET-1 within 30 minutes. The ET-1-treated cells became refractory to further stimulation with ET-1 and demonstrated either attenuated or enhanced $[Ca^{2+}]_i$ and LH responses to GnRH dependinng on the duration of exposure to ET-1 and the following recovery period. Although the complete picture is not clear, the data indicated that GnRH and ET post-receptor signaling pathways may be similar but capacities to generate, maintain, and reinitiate the calcium signal may be different[43,51].

The mechanisms of ET effects on LH release resemble those of GnRH. Each agonist activated its specific receptor but both receptors belong to the class of calcium-mobilizing receptors that activated G protein and subsequently diacylglycerol and inositol phosphates[39,51,54]. The postreceptor events for both agonists involved mobilization of intracellular calcium probably from endoplasmic reticulum (ER), since oscillatory $[Ca^{2+}]_i$ responses induced by ET-1 and GnRH were affected by thapsigargin, an inhibitor of calcium-sequestering ER-associated Ca^{2+}-ATPase[55]. The observed refractoriness of gonadotrophos to prolonged or repetitive stimulation with

ET had been explained by two possible mechanisms: internalization of ET receptor-ligand complex, similar to the response seen in vascular smooth muscle, and/or depletion of $[Ca^{2+}]_i$ pool as suggested for GnRH-induced desensitization[39,43]. ET may also play a role as a permissive factor regulating responsiveness of gonadotrophs to other hormones. It was observed that low, subthreshold concentrations of ET-1 can evoke a rapid oscillation of the $[Ca^{2+}]_i$ in gonadotrophs without producing hormone release[39,51,53].

Physiological significance of ET-stimulated LH release remains unclear. ET may be a non-specific stimulator of LH secretion due to its calcium-mobilizing effect or it may have an important role in normal LH responses, since its mechanism of action closely resembles that of GnRH. ET-3 may be important for normal ovulation. The ET-stimulated LH secretion was gender-specific, found in pituitary cells obtained from female and not male rats[19]. This observation suggests that ET-3 may play a role in female sexual function, specifically in preovulatory LH surge, mechanism of which involves GnRH stimulation of LH secretion. Also, even though both LH and FSH secretion are dependent on intracellular calcium mobilization, LH and FSH secretions were affected differently by ETs[45].

Regulation of thyrotropin (TSH), growth hormone (GH), and ACTH secretion

The data on TSH and GH regulation by ETs are controversial. TSH secretion was either not affected by ET-3[19], or was stimulated during prolong exposure of pituitary cells to ET-3 with maximal effect reached to 100 nM concentration of ET-3 (EC_{50} = 8.5 nM) after 48 hours of incubation[45]. By contrast, ET-1 (100 nM) induced significant but transitory stimulation of TSH secretion[51]. Similar to the data on TSH, GH was either not affected[19,45] or was significantly but transitory stimulated when pituitary cells were exposed to perifusion with high doses of ET-1 (100 nM)[51].

ACTH secretion was not affected by ET-1 in either static or dynamic pituitary cultures[45,51]. In vivo, centrally (ICV) administered ET-3 increased plasma ACTH level in dose dependent manner, suggesting possible ET involvement in stimulation of hypothalamo-pituitary-adrenal axis[28]. Thus, ET may play a role in hormonal responses to stress. It is widely distributed in the brain, and influences ACTH as well as cortisol, and catecholamine release[35,27,28,56].

Comparison of the responsiveness of different pituitary cells to ET-1 in culture showed different times and amplitudes of the maximal responses of individual hormones. Prolactin was suppressed, glycoprotein hormones (LH, FSH, and TSH) were stimulated, and GH and ACTH were unresponsive[45,51] (Figure 17.2). Thus, ET may play a role of a specific regulator of some anterior pituitary hormones (PRL and LH) and operate as a nonspecific permissive factor for others (FSH, TSH, GH, and ACTH).

In vivo studies using subcutaneous or IV injections were mostly non-productive being explained by inability of ETs to cross blood-brain barrier[2,53,56]. This phenomenon, however, may be explained by the short exposure of pituitary cells to ETs. In culture the maximum responses were observed after 4–48 hours of incubation[50]. When ET-1 was infused IV at a rate 14 nM/min for 45 minutes, glucose utilization measured

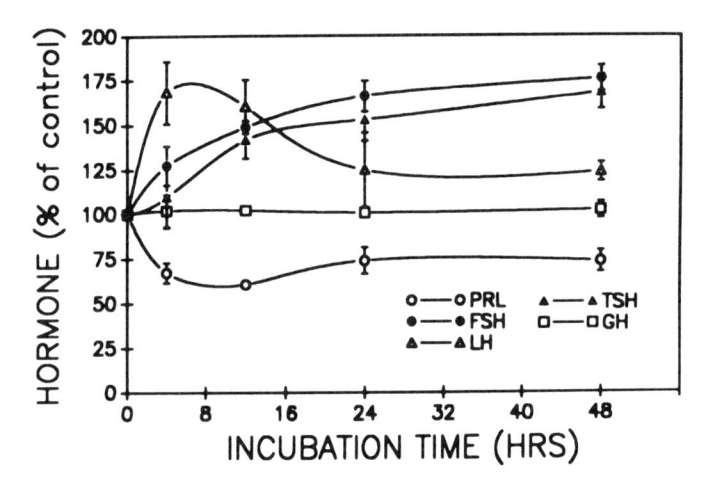

Figure 17.2. Effects of 100 nM ET-3 on the secretion of PRL, GH, LH, FSH and TSH from pituitary cell cultures as a function of incubation time. The ordinate represents the changes in hormone concentration expressed as percentage of untreated control cells. [Reproduced with permission from the publisher, Ref. 45].

by quantitative [^{14}C]deoxyglucose autoradiography was increased by 106% in rat anterior pituitary lobes. Glucose metabolism was also increased in the anterior (+75%) and posterior pituitary (+92%) after ICV injection of ET-1 (9 pM). Metabolic activation of anterior pituitary by centrally given ET was inhibited by ICV pretreatment with the calcium channel blocker, nimodipine, suggesting the requirement for extracellular calcium for ET-mediated effects[57]. These results are in agreement with *in vitro* studies and confirm that ET, indeed, may have physiological significance for pituitary function regulation.

Regulation of vasopressin (AVP) and oxytocin (OT) release

In vitro, ET-1 stimulated the release of AVP from the perifused rat hypothalami[42] and both ET-1 and ET-3 potentiated AVP secretion from pituitary neural lobes[36]. *In vivo*, intravenous infusion of pressor doses of ET increased AVP plasma levels in conscious[27] and anesthetized[58,59] dogs. The ICV injection of ET-3 increased blood pressure as well as plasma AVP and OT levels in conscious rabbits[60] and rats[20,40], in dose-dependent manner. Preinjection of brain natriuretic peptide (BNP) (a 26 amino acid peptide with structural and functional homology to atrial natriuretic polypeptide) attenuated central ET-3-induced pressor response[28] and AVP secretion[40]. Similarly, ET-induced pressor response was abolished by pretreatment with hexamethonium and AVP antagonist, indicating that central ET may elevate blood pressure through sympathetic nervous system activation and AVP secretion[61]. Also, the ICV administration of ET-3 inhibited water drinking stimulated by dehydration, hyperosmotic challenge, and angiotensin II (ANG-II)[20].

The ET effects in posterior pituitary were mediated via subfornical organ (SFO), the forebrain circumventricular organ devoided of blood-brain barrier. Systemic administration of ET-1 (50–100 pM) to anesthetized rats induced exitatory responses in AVP and OT-secreting neurons, and this effect was abolished in rats with destroyed subfornical organ[44]. The SFO had high density binding sites for ET and contained efferent axons extending to both paraventricular (PVN) and supraoptic (SON) nuclei of hypothalamus[28,44,56]. The SFO neurons were responsive to circulating ET-1[44]. At intracellular level mechanisms of ET-stimulated AVP release from neurosecretory endings in posterior pituitary were different from signaling pathway documented for anterior pituitary. These mechanisms did not involve mobilization of intracellular calcium and were linked to activation of phospholipase A_2 and arachidonic acid pathway[36].

Thus, available data suggest that ETs may be important in central regulation of blood pressure and fluid and electrolyte homeostasis, and this role of ET is supported by similarities between actions of ET and AVP as well as ET and ANG-II[20,28].

ADRENALS

In adrenals, similar to pituitary, ir-ETs and ET receptors have been identified[15,21,36,56,62]. De novo ET synthesis by adrenal tissue was proved by gene expression found in human adrenal cortical cells. The messenger RNAs encoding for preproET-1 and preproET-3 (2.3 kb and 2.8 kb in sizes, respectively) were demonstrated by Northern blot analysis of poly(A)$^+$ RNa from normal adrenal cortex[15]. In medulla ET- converting enzyme was identified in the chromaffin granules, suggesting that these cells synthesize ET[63].

Two types of receptors have been identified in adrenal tissue. Adrenal cortex expressed ET_A and ET_B[15,21] while adrenal medulla expressed only ET_B receptors[64,65]. In human adrenal cortex scatchard analysis of competitive binding data using [^{125}I]ET-1 showed the presence of a single class of high-affinity binding sites for ET-1 with the apparent dissociation constant (K_d) of 65 pM and maximal density of binding (B_{max}) of 60 fmol/mg protein. The presence of both ET_A and ET_B receptors was evident by the expression of two distinct bands of 4.3 and 4.8 kb by Northern blot analysis, corresponding to the sizes of ET_A and ET_B mRNA, respectively.[15] In adrenal medulla binding sites with K_d of 230 pM and B_{max} of 44 fmol/mg protein for ET-1 as well as K_d of 145 pM and B_{max} of 74 fmol/mg protein for ET-3 were demonstrated. Although no molecular studies are available the receptor was identified as ET_B by its equal affinity for the ET isoforms[64].

Regulation of aldosterone (ALDO) secretion

Aldosterone secretion was stimulated by ET-1 in rabbit[66], calf[21], rat[67,68], and human[69] zona glomerulosa (ZG) cells in cultures, and in perifused frog adrenal slices[70] in dose-dependent manner. The minimum concentration required for a significant change in ALDO was 10 fM for ET-2 and ET-3, and 0.1 pM for ET-1 in rat ZG cells[67,68]. The ET-1 EC_{50} for human adrenal cells was 36 pM[69]. ET-1 also significantly magnified the stimulatory effect of ACTH on ALDO secretion[67]. *In vivo* systemic administration of pressor doses of ET-1 increased plasma ALDO[27,58], and *de novo* ALDO synthesis was evident by the finding of ZG hypertrophy on adrenal gland histological examination[71]. The proliferogenic effects of ET on ZG were confirmed by the 9-fold increase in the mitotic index (% of metaphase-arrested cells) in the rat ZG after subcutaneous ET-1 infusion (0.2 μg/kg/hr for 7 days). This effect was additive for combined infusion of ET-1 and ACTH (20-fold) while ACTH alone produced a 13-fold increase in mitotic index. ET-1 effects compared well with the effects of other known ZG proliferogenic factors, angiotensin II and AVP. Infusion of ANG-II and AVP (30 pM/min × 24 h for both) raised mitotic index 9-fold and 10-fold, respectively, but the effects of ET-1 and ANG-II or AVP were not additive[72]. Electron microscopy demonstrated that enhanced circulating ALDO level was accompanied by the increase in the volume of mitochondrial compartment and the proliferation of endoplasmic reticulum, two organelles in which the enzymes of steroid synthesis are contained[71].

Mechanisms of ET effects in adrenals were similar to adrenal effects of ANG-II and AVP as well as ET action in other tissues. Binding to specific receptors was followed by activation of phospholipase C and increase in cytosolic $[Ca^{2+}]_i$. By contrast, ACTH acted via phospholipase A and was calcium independent, explaining the additive effects of ET and ACTH on induction of steroidogenesis[52,73].

Regulation of cortisol secretion

Cortisol (corticosterone in the rat and rabbit) secretion was either not affected[67,69,71] or stimulated in dose-dependent manner by all three ETs in rat[74,75] and human[74] cells in culture, as well as in perfused frog adrenal slices[70]. In intact adrenal perfused with ACTH, cortisol secretion was increased and was accompanied by significant increase in ET-1 release[74]. Hinson et al.[74] found that there was fundamental difference in functions and properties of adrenal tissue *in vitro* and *in vivo* and proposed to explain it by the presence of intraglandular mediator. Various stimuli, including AVP, OT, calcitonin-gene-related peptide, VIP, histamine, were shown to have no effect on adrenal cell culture but stimulated cortisol release from intact adrenal gland. For example, histamine was shown to have no effect on adrenal cells in culture, yet it stimulated steroidogenesis and ET secretion by intact perfused adrenal gland[74]. ANG-II was required in significantly higher concentrations to stimulate steroidogenesis by cell culture than by the intact adrenal gland[76]. By contrast, systemic ET-1 administration at a rate that minimally elevated blood pressure (less that 10 mHg) decreased adrenal blood flow and cortisol secretion in conscious calves[77].

The controversial results produced by *in vitro* and *in vivo* studies suggested that ET may differently regulate cortisol secretion depending on ET concentrations and whether ET acted in paracrine or endocrine fashion. ET was proposed to play a role of an intraglandular signal transducer that mediated the effects of various agents on adrenal zona fasciculata. ET was among only a few agents, including ACTH and melanocyte stimulating hormone (αMSH), that stimulated zona fasciculata *in vitro*[74]. Since ET was released by the gland in response to ACTH stimulation and it had a potent stimulatory effect on adrenocortical cells, ET may indeed act as an intraglandular signal transducer and explain variable effects observed with the same agents in cultured cells and in the intact adrenal gland. Alternatively, since ACTH induces vasodilation and ET causes vasoconstriction, ET may act by decreasing blood flow and cortisol secretion, providing a feedback mechanism for ACTH action[77].

Regulation of catecholamine (CA) secretion

Both norepinephrine (NE) and epinephrine (Epi) were released from cultured chromaffin cells stimulated by ET-1. The dose-response relationship showed EC_{50} of about 1 nM for both norepinephrine and epinephrine. The release was synergistic with acetylcholine-evoked secretion of catecholamines and additive with the calcium-channel stimulator[22,78]. The absence of the response from chromaffin cells in some studies[79] was suggested to be explained by high levels of NE and Epi in control cultures due to high sensitivity of chromaffin cells to non-specific stimuli. *In vivo*, central (ICV) administration of ET-3 (40 pM) elevated plasma CA levels, and this increase was prevented by ICV injection of brain natriuretic peptide[28].

There is controversy over mechanisms of ET effects in chromaffin cells. The secretagogue effects of ET-1 was calcium-dependent. These effects were attenuated by chelation of extracellular calcium, inhibited by calcium-channel blockers, and were additive with the calcium channel enhancer, BAY K 8644[22,78]. Contrary to the calcium-dependent effects of ET in other tissues, however, the total inositol phosphate content of chromaffin cells was not affected by high concentration (10 nM) of either ET-1 or ET-3[64]. One of the inositol phosphates, inositol 1,3,4,5,6-pentakiphosphate (IP_5) was rapidly and transiently increased in cultured chromaffin cells under ET stimulation, and this ET effect was independent of extracellular calcium. The significance of this observation was unclear, since IP_5 does not have a role as a second messenger as do other inositol phosphates, but rather suggested to play a role of "housekeeping" inositol polyphosphate. Alternatively, ET may stimulate CA production *in vivo* by causing vasoconstriction and reduced blood flow in tissues resulting in acidosis, a stimulus known to evoke secretion of CA[80].

ET content in pheochromocytoma, neuroblastoma and adrenal cortical adenoma

The attempts to reveal pathophysiological significance of ETs for adrenal pathology are evident by the studies of adrenal cortical adenoma, neuroblastoma, and pheochromocytoma.

Pheochromocytoma is a tumor of chromaffin cells of adrenal medulla. It presents in a variety of fashions but the most common presenting feature is hypertension. All symptoms and signs of pheochromocytoma are due to production of CA by the tumor. Vasoactive peptides that are produced by this tumor include neuropeptide Y and calcitonin gene-related peptide. ET-1 was measured in tumor tissue and plasma of 12 patients with pheochromocytomas. There were no significant differences in ET-1 concentrations among three groups of tested tissues. ET-1 levels ranged 62–253 fmol/gm wet tissue (gwt) in pheochromocytoma, 66–132 fmol/gwt in primary aldosteronism, and 71-120 fmol/gwt in normal adrenal glands. Plasma ET-1 levels in the patients with pheochromocytoma were also not significantly different from normotensive controls, 1.4 ± 0.9 fmol/ml and 1.0 ± 0.4 fmol/ml, respectively. In six of 12 pheochromocytomas, however, ET-1 values were higher than 132 fmol/gwt (the upper value of the control tissues). No correlations were made between ET-1 concentrations and the patients' symptoms and signs or presence of hemorrhages and/or necrosis in the tumors.[62]

Neuroblastoma is a tumor arising from the neuroblast of the neural crest analogous to phenochromocytoma originating from phenochromoblast of the neural crest. Like pheochromocytoma, neuroblastoma produces NE and Epi but usually it presents as nonfunctional tumor localized in the posterior mediastinum and abdomen. One study that evaluated the presence of ET receptors in neuroblastoma cell line revealed a single class of high affinity binding sites with the characteristics of an ET_A receptor[65].

The study of tissue from three aldosterone-producing adenomas from the patients with primary aldosteronism demonstrated concomitant expression of two isopeptides (ET-1 and ET-2) and two receptor subtypes (ET_A and ET_B) similar to their expression in adjacent normal cortex. Comparison of Northern blots of tumor and normal tissue showed greater expression of ET-1 mRNA in adenomatous than in normal tissue, while ET-3 mRNA was expressed equally[15].

Since ET has secretagogue and mitogenic properties[81–83] it may play a role as a local regulator of tumor growth and CA and ALDO secretion but to date pathogenetic significance of ETs for adrenal hormone-secreting adenomas remains unclear.

OVARIES

The ET concentration was high (2.79 ± 0.51 ng/g ovarian wet weight) in ovarian homogenates from mature rats[84]. The ir-ET was also identified in porcine and human follicular fluid[16,85]. The ET-1 level in porcine follicular fluid aspirated from small (1–2 mm), medium (3–5 mm), and large (6–11 mm) follicles was 9.4 ± 1.1 pg/ml, 12.2 ± 1.1 pg/ml, and 14.2 ± 1.8 pg/ml, respectively. These levels were within 0.42 to 0.62-fold of the porcine plasma level ($22.7 + 3.1$ pg/ml)[16].

There is *in vitro* and *in vivo* evidence of intraovarian *de novo* ET synthesis. ET-1 was secreted by porcine granulosa cells[16] and by rat luteal cells[86] in culture. In granulosa cells ET secretory rate was lower in the presence of LH than in the absence of LH: 4.9 ± 1.2 vs. 56 ± 9.3 pg/10^6 cellsxh, respectively[16]. When immature rats were primed by sequential injections of pregnant mare's serum gonadotropin and human chorionic gonadotropin (hCG), ET-1 measured in extracts from corpora lutea was significantly higher 7 days than it was 4 days after hCG injection: 17.04 ± 0.89 vs. 9.23 ± 0.32 pg/ovary, respectively[86]. Also there was higher concentration of ET-1 in ovarian vein than in ovarian artery[86].

Local direct auto/paracrine action of ET was supported by the presence of ET receptors on granulosa cells[85]. The presence of a single class of high affinity (apparent K_d 0.59 nM) binding sites was demonstrated using ^{125}I-labelled ET-1 as radioligand. The receptor was identified as ET_B type by equal affinity of ET-1 and ET-3 and by molecular weight (M_r) of 46.5 kD, which accords with 46.9 kD, the M_r of ET_B receptor[10].

Physiological role of ET is suggested by ET involvement in regulation of ovarian steroidogenesis and development of the follicle. Follicular development is a complex process regulated by multiple endocrine and paracrine factors. FSH and LH are actively involved in follicular development, supporting early and late stage of follicular preovulatory maturation, respectively. After ovulation, luteinization of granulosa cells occurs predominantly under the influence of gonadotropines. Involvement of intraovarian factors in the process of luteinization was suggested by spontaneous luteinization of granulosa cells *in vitro*. Follicular fluid from porcine, bovine, rat, and human follicles inhibited secretion of progesterone from cultured granulosa cells and follicular luteinization. These data pointed to the presence of yet unidentified "luteinization inhibitor"[87]. Accumulated data on intraovarian ET implicate it as a possible inhibitor of luteinization of granulosa cells, thus allowing normal development and maturation of the follicle. Treatment with ET-1 was inhibitory to the FSH-supported[25,88] (early follicular development) and LH-supported[16] (late follicular development) accumulation of progesterone in a dose-dependent manner in rat[25] and porcine[16,88] granulosa cells in culture. ET-1 was very effective with a median inhibitory dose ranging from 20 pM to 50 pM[16,25] and a maximal inhibitory effect of 90% at the 1 nM dose level[25]. ETs also inhibited LH-stimulated morphologic transformation of granulosa cells[16] and did not stimulate DNA synthesis even at high concentration (10 µM), despite increasing DNA polymerase α activity[84].

Evaluation of function of progesterone-forming enzymes revealed that ET-1 was a potent inhibitor of cholesterol side-chain cleavage and 3β-hydroxysteroid dehydrogenase (HSD)/isomerase (76% and 47% inhibition, respectively) and a potent stimulator of 20α-HSD and 5α-reductase (3.6 and 1.7-fold stimulation, respectively) with no significant changes in 3α-HSD activity. Thus, ET-1 inhibited the activities of enzymes concerned with progesterone formation, including rate-limiting enzyme of progesterone secretion, HSD, while enhancing the activities of enzymes concerned with progesterone degradation[25].

ET-mediated inhibition of progesterone synthesis was contradictory to the data demonstrating ET-1 and ET-3 stimulation of ovarian steroidogenesis. ET-1 and ET-3 produced dose-dependent increase in ovarian progesterone, testosterone, and 17β-estradiol in both static and dynamic cultures with a predominant stimulation of progesterone[85,89]. ET-1 stimulated ovarian steroid production more effectively than ET-3 but doses required for these effects were two powers higher than those needed for inhibitory effects of ET. The stimulation of progesterone secretion required the minimum effective dose of ET-1 40 nM and ET-3 4 nM[89] while inhibitory effects were associated with minimum ET-1 dose 5 pM[16].

Mechanisms of inhibitory and stimulatory effects of ETs on progesterone synthesis were found to be different. Inhibitory effects involved accretion of intracellular calcium and decreased cAMP production[16,88] while stimulatory effects were associated with either no effect or an increase in cAMP[85,89]. The accumulation of inositol phosphates and increased intracellular $[Ca^{2+}]_i$, suggested linkage of ET-1 receptor to G protein and phospholipase C as observed in other ET target cells. A common intracellular signal for hormone action in the ovary is cAMP accumulation and stimulation of protein kinase A. Basal cAMP accumulation was not affected by ET-1 but FSH-stimulated cAMP production was completely suppressed[88]. Similarly, LH-stimulated but not basal cAMP production was suppressed by ETs in a dose-dependent manner with an EC_{50} of 50 pM for all three peptides[16].

Additional potential effect of ET in the ovary may be inhibition of meiosis in primordial follicle. Meiosis is initiated in oocyte during fetal life but is sustained in early prophase until it is reinitiated by LH surge about 30–48 hours before ovulation. If oocyte is removed from the follicle, meiosis occurs spontaneously *in vitro* but is prevented by addition of follicular fluid to the culture. The small polypeptide produced by granulosa cells was suggested to act as oocyte maturation inhibitor[87]. The role of intracellular calcium and possibly ET in oocyte development is suggested by the recent observations of development of bovine oocyte[90] and surf clam oocyte[91] *in vitro*. Supporting this hypothesis is the finding that urinary extracts from pregnant women, inhibiting mouse oocyte maturation *in vitro*, contained a protein of small molecular weight of approximately 2,000 Da[92] which is close to ET M_r of 2,492 Da[4].

Mechanism of dual action of ET on ovarian tissue is probably related to different intraovarian levels of ET in follicular and luteal phases. ET concentration in luteal tissue[86] was higher than in follicular homogenates[84]. It may be hypothesized that low ovarian concentration of ET in follicular phase is associated with inhibition of progesterone synthesis, granulosa cell luteinization, and oocyte maturation. In luteal phase, higher concentration of ET may be induced by vascularization of corpus luteus. The observed stimulation of steroidogenesis by ET may then be explained by either non-specific ET effect (as it was suggested for prolactin) or by specific effects of higher levels of ET (Figure 17.3).

There is limited data on regulation of intraovarian ET secretion. ET-releasing activity was observed in porcine follicular fluid. The reversed phase HPLC identified this activity as activin A and TGFβ. TGFβ was 10-fold more potent than activin A in stimulation of ET release from bovine aortic endothelial cells[93]. Activins are two dimers of the β-subunits of inhibin, $β_Aβ_B$ and $β_Aβ_A$ present in follicular fluid and able to stimulate FSH release without affecting the secretion of LH. Other substances present in follicular fluid and known to stimulate ET production include angiotensin-II and IGFs[87].

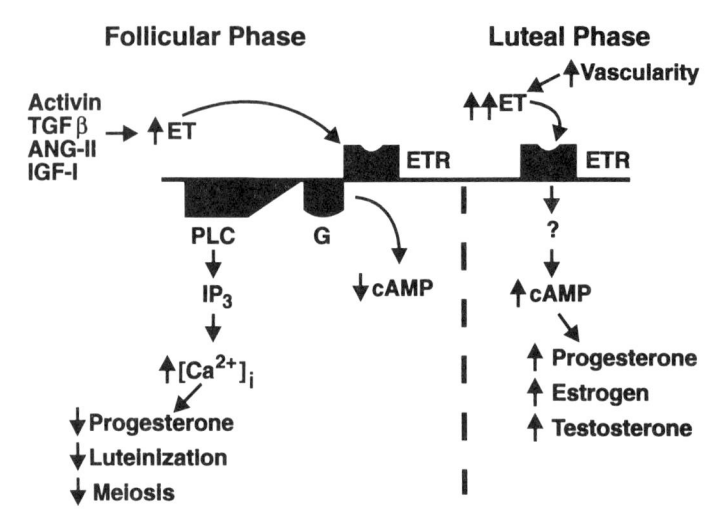

Figure 17.3. Endothelin (ET) effects in the ovaries. In follicular phase, ET supresses progesterone synthesis via mobilization of inracellular Ca^{2+} and decreased cAMP. In luteal phase, signaling may be switched to cAMP accumulation and subsequent stimulation of steroidogenesis. Abbreviations are as in Figure 17.1. IP_3, 1,4,5 inositol trisphosphate.

Pathophysiological significance of intraovarian ET is unclear. It only may be speculated that importance of ET for normal follicular growth, development and maturation suggests ET possible pathogenetic role in disorders of ovarian function including luteal phase defect, polycystic ovarian disease, and premature ovarian failure.

TESTES

Testes function as an exocrine gland by forming sperm in spermatogenic cells and as an endocrine gland by producing androgen in Leydig cells. Immunoreactive ET-1 was abundantly present in rat testes (570 pg/g wet weight)[35] and in human seminal fluid (500–5000 pg/ml) but ET-1 gene (preproET-1) was not expressed in human sperm[14]. The ET receptor was identified in Leydig and peritubular myoid cells in testes[94,95]. Single class high affinity binding sites in rat testicular membranes had an apparent K_d of 0.35 ± 0.06 nM and B_{max} of 250 ± 62 fmol/mg protein. The comparison of affinities for ET isopeptides suggested that the receptor was of ET_A type. Autoradiography localized these receptors in peritubular myoid cells and interstitial Leydig cells[94]. High affinity binding sites for ET-1 with K_d and B_{max} of 1 nM and 59 fmol/10^6 cells, respectively, were also found in the transformed murine Leydig cell line, MA-10[95]. These cells originally derived from spontaneous Leydig cell tumor, retain many of the differentiated functions of normal Leydig cells. MA-10 cells are deficient in 17α-hydroxylase/17–20-lyase, and thus, progesterone, not testosterone is the major steroid secreted into the medium[95].

ET effects on testicular steroidogenesis strikingly resemble responses of ovarian hormones to ET. ET-1 and ET-3 stimulated basal and hCG-induced testosterone secretion by purified rat Leydig cells when relatively low (10 pM) doses were used for incubation[26]. ET-1, however, induced biphasic response in progesterone production by Leydig cell line MA-10. While low concentrations of ET-1 (1–10 pM) inhibited progesterone production, high ET-1 concentrations (0.1 nM–1 µM) promoted steroidogenesis by MA-10 cells[95]. Mechanism of this dual action is unclear but may be due to various signal transduction systems, including involvement of extracellular calcium and protein kinase C[26,95].

Potential of ET as a growth factor for Leydig cells was evaluated but, similar to the observation in ovarian granulosa cells, replication of MA-10 cells was not affected by ET[95]. ET increased the transcriptional activators *c-fos* and *c-myc*, and stimulated DNA synthesis in vascular smooth muscle cells[81]. Although ET-1 enhanced proto-oncogene expression (*c-jun* and *c-myc*), mitosis did not occur in Leydig cells[95].

Physiological role of ET in testes and seminal fluid may be concerned with ET function as a regulator of steroidogenesis and smooth muscle contractor, and potentially as a modulator of mitosis and/or meiosis. Smooth muscle contraction is important for sperm transport through male and female reproductive tracts. Since ET_A was found on smooth muscle[1] and testicular myoid cells[94], and ET was shown to stimulate uterine contractions[96], ET importance for sperm transport seems plausible. Pathophysiological role of ET may also be related to its involvement in spermatozoa maturation and transport. Casey *et al.*[14] found that ET in seminal fluid of men with oligospermia (947 ± 87 pg/ml, n = 9), defined as less than 20×10^6 sperm/ml ejaculate, and azoospermia (806 ± 242 pg/ml, n = 3) was lower than in men with normal semen analysis (2,088 ± 589 pg/ml, n = 8). Because of small number of samples there was no statistical differences between groups, and there was no specific reference to sperm motility. Idiopathic oligospermia is the most common cause of male infertility but little is known about its pathogenesis and no definitive treatment is available. Until further studies are done association between ET concentration in seminal fluid and male infertility may only be presumed speculative.

Sex-associated differences in circulating ET

Sex-associated variation in circulating ET levels may be an explanation for different predisposition to atherogenesis and cardiovascular disease between men and women. Comparison of ET levels measured by RIA between healthy men, women, pregnant women, male-to-female, and female-to-male transsexuals showed that ET was higher (p < 0.01) in men (5.9 ± 1.2 pg/ml) than in women (4.17 ± 0.67 pg/ml). ET levels were lower in pregnant women (2.19 ± 0.73 pg/ml) than in age-matched nonpregnant controls (4.17 ± 0.67 pg/ml) (p < 0.01). To assess changes in ET plasma levels with sex hormone therapy, ET was measured before and 4 months after hormone use. In 12 male-to-female transsexuals treated with estradiol and the progestational agent cyproterone acetate, ET levels decreased from 8.1 ± 3.0 to 5.1 ± 2.0 pg/ml (p < 0.01). In 13 female-to-male transsexuals treated with testosterone, ET levels increased from 6.2 ± 1.1 to 7.8 ± 1.2 pg/ml (p < 0.01)[97] (Figure 17.4). Estrogen was shown to confer protection from coronary heart disease. Risk of coronary heart disease in postmenopausal women treated with estrogen was decreased by 40%. This protective effect was explained by estrogen modification of plasma lipoproteins and ability of estrogen to alter vascular responses[98]. The importance of estrogen-endothelin interaction at vascular wall was supported by recent observation that 17β-estradiol attenuated vasoconstrictor effect of ET on coronary arterioles *in vitro*[99].

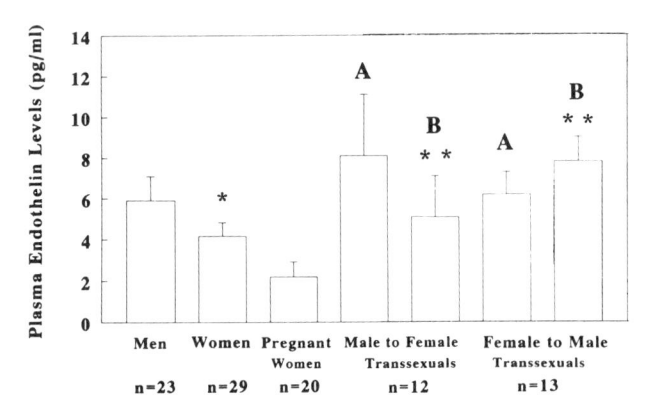

Figure 17.4. Sex-associated variations in circulating ET levels. A, before and B, after four months of hormone use (estradiol and cyproterone acetate were used in males, testosterone was used in females). Reconstructed based on data from ref. 97. * p < 0.01 vs. men and pregnant women; ** p < 0.01 vs. A.

THYROID

Immunoreactive ET was detected in rat and porcine thyroid glands at concentrations 1.5 and 0.75 pg/mg wet weight, respectively. Immunohistochemical study localized ir-ET-1 within epithelial follicular cells with strong immunoreactivity present in inclusions within these cells. In procine gland ir-ET-1 was also present in smooth muscle cells of large blood vessels[17]. Primary human thyroid cells derived from human thyroids with various histopathologic diagnoses released ET into culture medium where its concentration ranged from undetectable to 35 fM/10^{-5} cells[100]. Specific high affinity receptors for ET were found on human thyrocytes derived from multinodular goiter, colloid nodule, follicular adenoma, and normal tissue[23,100]. TGFβ and TSH dose-dependently stimulated ET binding to thyroid cells. Coincubation of cells with TGFβ increased the number of receptors without changing their affinity while TSH did not influence either number of affinity of the receptors[100].

ET was involved in regulation of thyroid growth and function. ET-1 (0.1 nM) inhibited thyroglobulin release from human thyroid cell culture after 6 days of incubation and this effect was cAMP and cGMP independent[23]. ET inhibited TSH-induced iodine metabolism in porcine thyroid cells in culture via interaction with ET receptor[101]. Cell growth was not affected in primary human thyroid cell culture[23]. In thyroid epithelial cell line (FRTL5 cells) ET-1 alone had no effect on DNA synthesis but caused a transient increase in c-fos mRNA levels and stimulated IGF-I induced DNA synthesis and cell proliferation. ET-1 reduced DNA synthesis stimulated by TSH. This inhibitory effect was completely reversed by a C-kinase inhibitor, H-7, suggesting that the effect of ET-1 was at least in part mediated by C-kinase dependent pathway[101].

Studies on regulation of ET secretion in thyroid cells found that TSH stimulated ET synthesis, while TGFβ stimulated both synthesis and secretion. Two of 12 cell lines derived from human thyroids responded to TGFβ treatment with increased ET secretion into the medium. In responsive thyrocytes, TSH did not affect ET release into the medium but stimulated perinuclear region where ET was localized by immunostaining studies. If perinuclear intracellular ir-ET represents precursors of secretory form of ETs, these results suggest that TSH regulated ET synthetic while TGFβ regulated synthetic and secretory pathways[100].

In vivo studies showed that in hyperthyroid but not hypothyroid rats plasma ET-1 levels were increased and the population of ET receptors in the pituitary was decreased. The rats were made thyrotoxic by daily administration of thyroxine and developed signs of hyperthyroidism, including decreased rate of gain of body weight, increased serum T_3 and T_4 concentrations, elevated blood pressure and heart rate, as compared to untreated controls. It was suggested that in hyperthyroid rats ET-1 production was stimulated leading to higher plasma ET-1 which in turn produced downregulation of ET receptors in the pituitary[102]. The origin of ET in the induced hyperthyroid state was unclear. ET was not present in culture medium of cells derived from one gland with Graves' disease[100]. However, gene expression of TGFβ was found to be higher in thyroid tissue from patients with Graves' disease than in patients with nontoxic goiter[103], and TGFβ can stimulate ET secretion from cultured thyroid cells[100] and endothelial cells[83]. It may be speculated that ET secretion by endothelial cells was stimulated by thyroid hormones. Since both thyroid hormones and ET increase the sensitivity of peripheral vascular α-adrenoreceptors, and ET is a potent vasoconstrictor, high circulating ET levels may contribute to cardiovascular complications of hyperthyroidism as it was observed in vivo studies in rats[102]. Whether ET may contribute to the development of hyperthyroidism or elevated ET level is a consequence of hyperthyroid state is unknown. Endothelial cells were shown to stimulate proliferation of human thyrocytes from normal and Graves' thyroid glands, and ET was suggested to be involved[103]. Autoimmunity is implicated in pathogenesis of Graves' disease, the most common cause of human hyperthyroidism[104]. ET may be a trophic factor for immune system[105], and may play a role in pathogenesis of hyperthyroidism and/or its complications.

Paracrine and/or autocrine actions of ET may play a role in "euthyroid sick syndrome". This syndrome defines conditions with abnormal thyroid hormone values (most commonly low T_4 and/or low T_3 states) in nonthyroidal illnesses and no intrinsic thyroid disease[106]. The pathogenesis of this syndrome is unclear but multiple factors have been implicated. It may only be speculated that, since ET was shown to be elevated in severely ill patients[107] and ET decreased thyroglobulin synthesis and inhibited TSH-induced iodine metabolism in vitro[101], ET may be involved in abnormal thyroid function in some disease states.

The presence of ET in extracts from nontoxic goiter may be interpreted as a possibility that ET may be important in pathogenesis of nontoxic goiter. ET secretion by thyrocytes was modified by TSH and TGFβ[100]. ET inhibited the stimulatory effects of TSH on DNA synthesis and follicular cell proliferation, and suppressed TSH-induced iodine metabolism[101]. TSH is a stimulator but TGFβ is shown to be an inhibitor for thyroid cell growth[103]. Even though this interpretation would be purely conjectural, it may be speculated that ET may play a role in pathogenesis of nontoxic goiter similar to the role suggested for TGFβ.

PARATHYROID

ET-1 gene transcripts (preproET-1, 2.3 kb) as well as ir-ET-1 synthesis and secretion have been demonstrated in rat, bovine and human parathyroid glands[18,24]. Immunocytochemistry and Northern blot analysis of poly(A)$^+$ RNA localized ET-1 in epithelial but not capillary endothelial cells of parathyroid glands[18]. Both ET_A and ET_B receptors were found in parathyroid tissue by binding and gene expression studies with identified mRNA sizes of 4.3 kb for ET_A and 4.8 kb for ET_B receptors, respectively[18,24,108]. ET_A receptors were more prevalent and found on both epithelial and endothelial cells[18,108]. Scatchard analysis of high affinity binding sites for ET-1 on human parathyroid cells revealed the apparent K_d of 62 ± 18 pM and B_{max} of 77 ± 15 fmol/mg protein[24].

Basal PTH secretion from dispersed human adenoma cells was inhibited by ET-1 in dose-dependent manner ($ET_{50} = 80$ pM) and more potently than by ET-3 ($EC_{50} = 5$ nM)[24]. Mechanisms of ET action in parathyroid endothelial cells were similar to those observed in other ET responsive cells. In clonal parathyroid endothelial cells ET-1 but not ET-3 induced phospholipase C activation, as shown by the increase in inositol 1,4,5-trisphosphate ($EC_{50} = 0.11 \pm 0.24$ nM) and increased cytosolic $[Ca^{2+}]_i$

by mobilizing intracellular and extracellular calcium. Growth of these cells was not affected by ET-1 in wide range of concentrations[108]. In parathyroid epithelial cells involvement of phospholipase C pathway in ET effects was also demonstrated[18]. Synthesis of ET-1 by parathyroid cells *in vitro* was regulated by calcium[18] as well as atrial natriuretic peptide and brain natriuretic peptide[109]. Physiologically important role of ET as an autocrine/paracrine regulator for parathyroid gland was supported not only by the presence of ET gene transcripts and ET receptors in parathyroid tissue but also by observation that approximate EC_{50} value (80 pM) of ET-1 for inhibition of PTH secretion was comparable to that of the apparent K_d (62 pM) of ET-1 receptors[24].

ET may be relevant for pathogenesis of hypertension complicating primary hyperparathyroidism. Hypertension is frequently observed in patients with primary hyperparathyroidism, and parathyroidectomy in these patients alleviates hypertension[110]. Hypertension in these patients and in spontaneously hypertensive rats[111], however, showed no relationship to intact PTH levels and PTH *per se* was shown to cause vasodilation and a decrease in blood pressure[112]. It may be speculated that the hypertensive factor (which is not PTH) identified in parathyroid glands of spontaneously hypertensive rats[111] may be related to peptides of endothelin family. ET caused vasoconstriction *in vitro*[1] and elevated blood pressure *in vivo*[27,58,59], and preproET-1 mRNA was identified in tissues obtained from patients with hyperparathyroidism (2 adenomas, 2 hyperplasias)[24]. It only may be hypothesized that ET pays a role in hypertension associated with primary hyperparathyroidism since PTH-induced hypercalcemia as well as stimulation of renin, aldosterone and norepinephrine release can also contribute to an elevation of blood pressure in this condition[110].

DIABETES MELLITUS

Controversy exists in the reports of plasma levels of ir-ET in patients with diabetes mellitus (DM). The ir-ET was significantly higher ($p < 0.005$) in a group of 100 DM patients (1.88 ± 0.12 pmol/l), including 16 patients with insulin-dependent (IDDM) and 84 patients with non-insulin-dependent diabetes (NIDDM) compared with 19 healthy controls (0.54 ± 0.05 pmol/l)[31]. By contrast the mean plasma ir-ET-1 in a group of 25 patients with NIDDM (1.70 ± 0.16 pg/ml, about 0.68 ± 0.06 pmol/l) was not significantly different from healthy subjects (1.42 ± 0.31 pg/ml, about 0.57 ± 0.12 pmol/l)[113]. Sensitivity and coefficients of variation were similar in both studies and cannot account for differences in the results. Lower ir-ET concentrations perhaps may be explained by lower blood pressure in patients used in Kanno et al. study[113] (Figure 17.5). There was, however, no significant correlation between plasma ir-ET and blood glucose, blood pressure, urinary microalbumin, incidence of background retinopathy or duration of DM[31]. ET is metabolized in the lung and kidney and excreted in the urine. Urinary concentration and daily excretion of ET was not different between patients with DM (6.9 ± 1.0 pmol/day, $n = 13$) and normal subjects (8.0 ± 0.9 pmol/day, $n = 5$). Analysis of urinary ir-ET by HPLC showed two components which may represent metabolites of ET and/or ET precursors[114].

The rat models were not helpful in resolving controversial results on circulating ET in DM patients. Plasma concentrations of ir-ET in rats with dexamethasone-induced

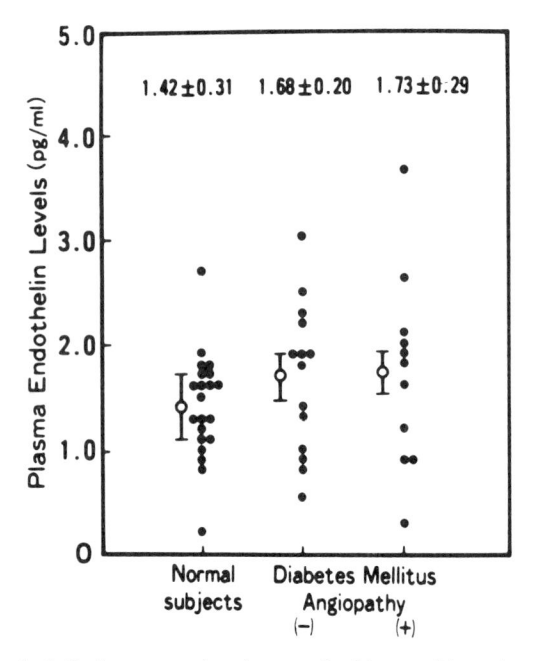

Figure 17.5. Plasma endothelin-1 concentrations in normal subjects and in patients with diabetes mellitus with or without angiopathy (mean ± SE). [Reproduced with permission from the publisher, Ref. 113].

DM (3.13 ± 0.28 pmol/l) were significantly higher than in controls (1.33 ± 0.18 pmol/l), while ir-ET levels in rats with streptozotocin-induced DM and in rats treated with both dexamethasone and streptozotocin were undetectable (<0.5 pmol/l)[115].

ET acting in endocrine or paracrine/autocrine fashion may potentially contribute to the development of diabetes complications. Although, differences between plasma ir-ET-1 levels in patients with and without angiopathy did not reach statistical significance and number of patients was small, ET plasma levels were higher in patients with background retinopathy, cerebral or coronary artery disease and patients treated with anti-hypertensive medications than in the other diabetic patients[31,113].

Hyperglycemia is a major cause of diabetic micro- and macroangiopathy, although pathogenesis of vascular complications is not well understood. The findings implicating ET as one of the factors involved in accelerated atherosclerosis in patients with DM include observation that hyperglycemia increased secretion of ET-1 from vascular endothelial cells[116], the presence of ET receptors on vascular smooth muscles, and mitogenic and constricting effects of ET on vascular smooth muscle[1,117]. ET may play a role in the development of retinopathy. ET was secreted by cultured endothelial cells obtained from bovine retinal microvessels and ET receptors were present on associated pericytes. Since pericytes play supportive and muscle-like role in retinal capillaries, downregulation of ET receptors and/or loss of pericytes may result in retinal vasodilation observed in diabetic retinopathy[118]. Importance of ET in the evolution of diabetic nephropathy, including renal vasoconstriction and hypertrophy, is suggested by ET secretion by renal epithelial cells[119], the presence of ET receptors in the kidney[56,120], and mitogenic effect of ET on glomerular mesangial cells[121].

Endocrine disorders 299

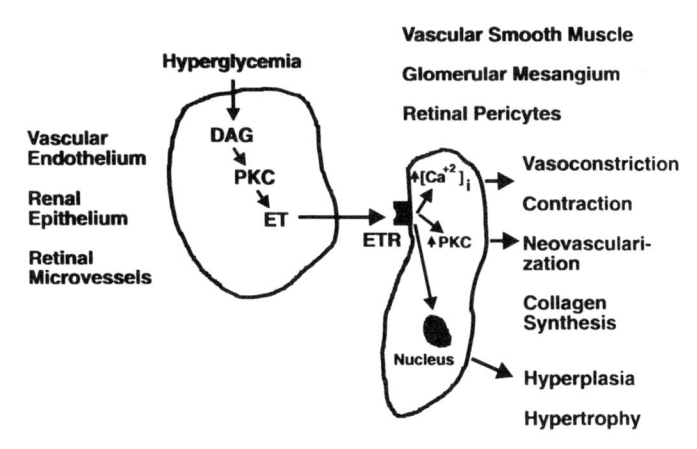

Figure 17.6. Hypothetical contribution of endothelin (ET) to diabetes mellitus complications. Hyperglycemia-induced ET secretion results in vasoconstriction, cell contraction, neovascularization, collagen synthesis, hyperplasia, and hypertrophy of target cells.

Diabetic angiopathy is, undoubtedly, multifactorial in origin, and ET may be contributing to its development. In endothelial cells hyperglycemia was shown to induce diacylglycerol (DAG) synthesis which was followed by activation of PKC[122,123]. In ET target cells, PKC was activated as part of ET receptor → G protein → phospholipase C → DAG → PKC signaling pathway.[5] PKC was also shown to mediate ET effects by downregulation of ET receptors and by stimulation of ET synthesis[124]. PKC activity was increased while density of low affinity ET receptors was decreased in glomeruli isolated from rats with streptozotocin-induced DM compared to control rats. Infusion of PKC inhibitor (1-(6-isoquinolinesulfonyl)piperazine) normalized PKC activity and receptor density in diabetic rats[125]. Thus, potentially vicious cycle may develop with hyperglycemia-induced sequential activation of DAG, PKC, ET, and again PKC, perpetuating progression of angiopathy in diabetes (Figure 17.6).

BONE

Important physiological role of ET in bone metabolism was suggested by *in vitro* and *in vivo* studies. ET was shown to be secreted by at least one type of cells present in bone marrow[126] and may be secreted by endothelial cells abundant at this location. ET receptor of ET_A type was identified on cultured osteoblastic cells from rat calvariae[127]. ET stimulated bone formation[128] and inhibited bone resorption[129]. The ET effects in osteoblasts were mediated via phospholipase C and intracellular calcium[127]. The intracellular calcium and cAMP are two secondary messengers in osteoblasts that mediate effects of various factors on bone[130]. The cAMP mediates osteoblast-dependent bone resorption[131] and inhibits osteoblast proliferation[132]. Calcium inhibits osteoblast-dependent bone resorption[131] and antagonizes effects of cAMP on osteoblast proliferation[132]. Since ET utilizes calcium as a secondary messenger[5] and was shown to induce proliferation of osteoblasts[127], it is reasonable to suggest that ET may inhibit osteoclastic bone resorption by increasing intracellular calcium in osteoblasts. Additionally, osteoclast motility was directly suppressed by ET *in vitro*[129]. *In vivo* infusion of ET-1 into the tibial nutrient artery of mongrel dogs resulted in marked vasoconstriction and dose-related increase in bone perfusion pressure without concomitant changes in systemic arterial pressure[133]. ET-related actions, including regulation of bone turnover and mediation of effects of other known calciotropic factors[134], suggest its role in metabolic bone disease such as osteoporosis. In addition, ET vasoconstriction properties may be important in avascular necrosis of bone, condition pathogenetically related to bone ischemia[133].

SUMMARY

Few clinical studies make it difficult to assess ET role in endocrine diseases. Marked vascularization of endocrine organs with specialized vascular beds (portal circulation of pituitary[135], sinusoids of adrenal cortex[136], *etc.*) suggests important interaction between vascular and endocrine tissues. Ubiquitous distribution of ETs and their receptors in endocrine system make them uniquely suited for an important regulatory role. Potent actions and pleiotropic interactions of ETs at systemic and local levels are involved in hormonal synthesis and secretion as well as hormone effects on target organs. Vascular, mitogenic, and paracrine/autocrine effects of ET were all demonstrated in endocrine tissues. Practically in all areas tested, ET proved to be an important regulatory peptide. ET is implicated in growing number of pathological conditions. Myocardial infarction[29,137] and hypertension[137] were most intensively studied[138]. ET secreting tumor has been described[139]. ET role in Raynoud's syndrome[140], Takayasu's arteritis[141], Buerger's disease[141], diabetes mellitus[31] has been proposed. Although clinical implications for endocrine conditions suggested in this review remain at present primarily conjectural, *in vitro* and *in vivo* animal studies demonstrate that ET may contribute to pathogenesis of many endocrine diseases.

References

1. Yanagisawa, M., Kurihara, H., Kimura, S., Tomobe, Y., Kobayashi, M., Yakaki, Y. *et al.* (1988) A novel potent vasoconstrictor pertide produced by vascular endothelial cells. *Nature*, **332**, 411–415.
2. Yanagisawa, M., Inove, A. I., Ishikawa, T., Kasuya, T., Kimura, S., Kumagaye, S. I., *et al.* (1988) Primary structure, synthesis, and biological activity of rat endothelin, an endothelium-derived vasconstrictor. *Proceedings of the National Acadamy of Sciences*, **85**, 6964–6967.
3. Inoue, A., Yanagisawa, M., Kimura, S., Kasuya, Y., Miyauchi, Y., Goto, K. *et al.* (1989) The human endothelin family: three structurally and pharmacologically distinct isopeptides predicted by three separate genes. *Proceedings of the National Acadamy of Sciences*, **86**, 2863–2867.
4. Gulati, A. and Srimal, R. C. (1992) Endothelin mechanisms in the central nervous system: A target for drug development. *Drug Development Research*, **26**, 361–387.
5. Simonson, M. and Dunn, M. (1990) Cellular signaling by peptides of the endothelin gene family. *FASEB Journal*, **4**, 2989–3000.
6. Vane, J., Anggard, E., Botting, R. (1990) Regulatory functions of the vascular endothelium. *New England Journal of Medicine*, **323**, 27–36.
7. Stojilkovic, S. and Catt, K. (1992) Neuroendocrine actions of endothelins. *Trends in Pharmacological Sciences*, **13**, 385–391.
8. Masaki, T. (1991) Tissue specificity of the endothelin-induced responses. *Journal of Cardiovascular Pharmacology*, **17 (Suppl 7)**, S1–S4.

9. Arai, H., Hori, S., Aramori, I., Ohkubo, H., Nakanishi, S. (1990) Cloning and expression of a cDNA encoding an endothelin receptor. *Nature*, **348**, 730–732.
10. Sakurai, T., Yanagisawa, M., Takuwa, Y., *et al.* (1990) Cloning of a cDNA encoding a non-isopeptide-selective subtype of the endothelin receptor. *Nature*, **348**, 732–735.
11. Yamaji, T., Johshita, H., Ishibashi, M., Takaku, F., Ohno, H., Suzuki, N., *et al.* (1990) Endothelin family in human plasma and cerebrospinal fluid. *Journal of Clinical Endocrinology and Metabolism*, **71**, 1611–1615.
12. Lam, H., Takahashi, K., Ghatei, M., Warrens, A., Rees, A., Bloom, S. (1991) Immunoreactive endothelin in human plasma, urine, milk, and saliva. *Journal of Cardiovascular Pharmacology*, **17 (Suppl 7)**, S390–S393.
13. Raboni, S., Folli, M., Bresciani, D., Modena, A., Merialdi, A., Berbinschi, A., Ketelslegers, J. (1991) Amniotic endothelin increases during pregnancy. *American Journal of Obstetetrics and Gynecology*, **164**, 237.
14. Casey, M., Byrd, W., and McDonald, P. (1992) Massive amounts of immunoreactive endothelin in human seminal fluid. *Journal of Clinical Endocrinology and Metabolism*, **74**, 223–225.
15. Imai, T., Hirata, Y., Eguchi, S., Kanno, K., Ohta, K., Emori, T., *et al.* (1992) Concomitant expression of receptor subtype and isopeptide of endothelin by human adrenal gland. *Biochemical and Biophysical Research Communications*, **183**, 1115–1521.
16. Iwai, M., Hasegawa, M., Taii, S., Sagawa, N., Nakao, K., Imura, H., *et al.* (1991) Endothelin inhibit luteinization of cultured porcine granulosa cells. *Endocrinology*, **129**, 1909–1914.
17. Colin, II, Berbinschi, A., Denef, J., Ketelslegers, J. (1992) Detection and identification of endothelin-1 immunoreactivity in rat and porcine thyroid follicular cells. *Endocrinology*, **130**, 544–546.
18. Fujii, Y., Moreira, J., Orlando, C., Maggi, M., Aurbach, G., Brandi, M., and Sakaguchi, K. (1991) Endothelin as an autocrine factor in the regulation of parathyroid cells. *Proceedings of the National Academy of Sciences*, **88**, 4235–4239.
19. Samson, W., Skala, K., Alexander, B., Huang, F. (1991) Possible neuroendocrine actions of endothelin-3. *Endocrinology*, **128**, 1465–1473.
20. Samson, W., Skala, K., Alexander, B., and Huang, F. (1991) Hypothalamic Endothelin: Presence and effects related to fluid and electrolyte homeostasis. *Journal of Cardiovascular Pharmacology*, **17 (Suppl 7)**, S346–S349.
21. Cozza, E., Gomez-Sanchez, C., Foecking, M. and Chiou, S. (1989) Endothelin binding to cultured calf adrenal zona glomerulosa cells and stimulation of aldosterone secretion. *Journal of Clinical Investigation*, **84**, 1032–1035.
22. Boarder, M. and Marriott, D. (1991) Endothelin-1 stimulation of noradrenaline and adrenaline release from adrenal chromaffin cells. *Biochemical Pharmacology*, **41**, 521–526.
23. Jackson, S., Tseng, Y., Lahiri, S., Burman, K. and Wartofsky, L. (1992) Receptors for endothelin in cultured human thyroid cells and inhibition of endothelin of thyroglobulin secretion. *Journal of Clinical Endocrinology and Metabolism*, **75**, 388–392.
24. Eguchi, S., Hirata, Y., Imai, T., Kanno, K., Akiba, T., Sakamoto, A., *et al.* (1992) Endothelin receptors in human parathyroid gland. *Biochemical and Biophysical Research Communications*, **184**, 1448–1455.
25. Tedeschi, C., Hazum, E., Kokia, E., Ricciarelli, E., Adashi, E., Payne, D. (1992) Endothelin-1 as a luteinization inhibitor: Inhibition of rat granulosa cell progesterone accumulation via selective modulation of key steroidogenic steps affecting both progesterone formation and degradation. *Endocrinology*, **131**, 2476–2478.
26. Conet, D., Questino, P., Pillo, S., Nordio, M., Isidori, A., Romanelli, F. (1993) Endothelin stimulates testosterone secretion by rat leydig cells. *Journal of Endocrinology*, **136**, R1–R4.
27. Goetz, K., Wang, B., Madwed, J., Zhu, J., and Leadley, R. Jr. (1988) Cardiovascular, renal, and endocrine responses to intravenous endothelin in conscious dogs. *American Journal of Physiology*, **255**, R1064–R1068.
28. Makino, S., Hashimoto, K., Hirasawa, R., Hattori, T., Kageyama, J. and Ota, Z. (1990) Central interaction between endothelin and brain natriuretic peptide on pressor and hormonal responses. *Brain Research*, 117–121.
29. Lerman, A., Edwards, B., Hallett, J., Heublein, D., Sandberg, S., and Burnett, J. Jr. (1991) Circulating and tissue endothelin immunoreactivity in advanced atherosclerosis. *New England Journal of Medicine*, **325**, 997–1001.
30. Koyama, H., Tabata, T., Nishzawa, Y., Inoue, T., Morii, H., Yamaji, T. (1989) Plasma endothelin levels in patients with uraemia. *Lancet*, **1**, 991–992.
31. Takahashi, K., Ghatei, M., Lam, H., O'Halloran, D., Bloom, S. (1990) Elevated plasma endothelin in patients with diabetes mellitus. *Diabetologia*, 306–310.
32. Takahashi, K., Ghatei, M., Jones, P., Murphy, Journal., Lam, H. C., O'Halloran, D., and Bloom S. (1991) Endothelin in human brain and pituitary gland: presence of immunoreactive endothelin,

endothelin messenger ribonucleic acid, and endothelin receptors. *Journal of Clinical Endocrinology and Metabolism*, 693–699.
33. Takahashi, K., Ghatei, M., Jones, P., Murphy, J., Lam, H.-C., O'Halloran, D. J and Bloom, S. (1991) Endothelin in human brain and pituitary gland: Comparison with rat. *Journal of Cardiovascular Pharmacology*, **17 (Suppl 7)**, S101–S103.
34. Matsumoto, H., Suzuki, N., Shiota, K., Inoue, K., Tsuda, M. and Fujino, M. (1990) Insulin-like Growth Factor-I stimulates endothelin-3 secretion from rat anterior pituitary cells in primary culture. *Biochemical and Biophysical Research Communications*, **172**, 661–668.
35. Matsumoto, H., Suzuki, N., Onda, H., and Fujino, M. (1989) Abundance of endothelin-3 in rat intestine, pituitary gland and brain. *Biochemical and Biophysical Research Communications*, **164**, 74–80.
36. Ritz, M.-F., Stuenkel, E., Dayanithi, G., Jones, R., and Nordmann, J. (1992) Endothelin regulation of neuropeptide release from nerve endings of the posterior pituitary. *Proceedings of the National Academy of Sciences*, **89**, 8371–8375.
37. Nakamura, S., Naruse, M., Naruse, K., Shioda, S., Nakai, Y., Uemura, H. (1993) Colocalization of immunoreactive endothelin-1 and neurohypophysial hormones in the axons of the neural lobe of the rat pituitary. *Endocrinology*, **132**, 530–533.
38. Samson, W. K. (1992) The endothelin-A receptor subtype transduces the effects of the endothelins in the anterior pituitary gland. *Biochemical and Biophysical Research Communications*, **187**, 590–595.
39. Stojilkovic, S., Balla, T., Fukuda, S., Cesnjaj, M., Merelli, F., Krmanovic, L., and Catt, K. J. (1992) Endothelin ET_A receptors mediate the signaling and secretory actions of endothelins in pituitary gonadotrophs. *Endocrinology*, **130**, 465–474.
40. Makino, S., Hashimoto, K., Hirasawa, R., Hattori, T., Ota, Z. (1992) Central interaction between endothelin and brain natriuretic peptide on vasopressin secretion. *Journal of Hypertension*, **10**, 25–28.
41. Calvo, J., Gonzalez, R., DeCarvalho, L., Takahashi, K., Kanse, S. M., Hart, G. R., Ghatei, M. M., and Bloom, S. R. (1990) Release of substance P from rat hypothalamus and pituitary by endothelin. *Endocrinology*, **126**, 2288–2295.
42. Shichiri, M., Hirata, Y., Kanno, K., Ohta, K., Emori, T., Marumo, F. (1989) Effect of endothelin-1 on release of arginine-vasopressin from perifused rat hypothalamus. *Biochemical and Biophysical Research Communications*, **163**, 1332–1337.
43. Stojilkovic, S., Iida, T., Cesnjaj, M., Catt, K. (1992) Differential actions of endothelin and gonadotropin-releasing hormone in pituitary gonadotrophs. *Endocrinology*, **131**, 2821–2828.
44. Wall, K. and Ferguson, A. (1992) Endothelin acts at the subfornical organ to influence the activity of putative vasopressin and oxytocin-secreting neurons. *Brain Research*, **586**, 111–116.
45. Kanyicska, B., Burris, T., Freeman, M. (1991) Endothelin-3 inhibits prolactin and stimulates LH, FSH and TSH secretion from pituitary cell culture. *Biochemical and Biophysical Research Communications*, **174**, 338–343.
46. Samson, W. and Skala, K. (1992) Comparison of the pituitary effects of the mammalian endothelins: Vasoactive intestinal inhibitor of prolactin secretion. *Endocrinology*, **130**, 2964–2970.
47. Dymshitz, J., Laudon, M., Ben-Jonathan, N. (1992) Endothelin-induced biphasic response of lactotrophs cultured under different conditions. *Neuroendocrinology*, **55**, 724–729.
48. Samson, W., Skala, K., Alexander, B., Huang, F.-L., Gomez-Sanchez, C. (1992) A prolactin release inhibiting activity isolated from neurointermediate lobe extracts is an endothelin-like peptide. *Regulatory Peptides*, 103–112.
49. Lamberts, S. W. J. and McLeod, R. M. (1990) Regulation of prolactin secretion at the level of the lactotroph. *Physiology Review*, **70**, 279–318.
50. DeLa Escalera, G. M. and Weiner, R. I. (1992) Dissociation of dopamine from its receptor as a signal in the pleiotropic hypothalamic regulation of prolactin secretion. *Endocrinology Reviews*, **13**, 241–255.
51. Stojilkovic, S., Iida, T., Merelli, F. and Catt, K. (1991) Calcium signaling and secretory responses in endothelin-stimulated anterior pituitary cells. *Molecular Pharmacology*, **39**, 762–770.
52. Buris, T., Kanyicska, B. and Freeman, M. (1991) Inhibition of prolactin secretion by endothelin-3 is pertussis toxin-sensitive. *European Journal of Pharmacology*, **198**, 223–225.
53. Stojilkovic, S. S., Merelli, F., Iida, T., Krsmanovic, L., Catt, K. J. (1990) Endothelin stimulation of cytosolic calcium and gonadotropin secretion in anterior pituitary cells. *Science*, **248**, 1663–1666.
54. Naor, Z. (1990) Signal transduction mechanisms of Ca^{2+} mobilizing hormones: The case of gonadotropin-releasing hormone. *Endocrine Reviews*, **11**, 326–353.
55. McArdle, C. A. and Poch, A. (1992) Dependence of gonadotropin-releasing hormone-stimulated luteinizing hormone-release upon intracellular Ca^{2+} pools is revealed by desensitization and thapsigargin blockade. *Endocrinology*, **130**, 3567–3574.
56. Koseki, C., Imai, M., Hirata, Y., Yanagisawa, M., and Masaki, T. (1989) Autoradiographic distribution in rat tissues of binding sites for endothelin: A neuropeptide? *American Journal of Physiology*, **256**, R858–R866.

57. Gross, P. M., Wainman, D. S. and Espinosa, F. J. (1991) Differentiated metabolic stimulation of rat pituitary lobes by peripheral and central endothelin-1. *Endocrinology*, **129**, 1110–1112.
58. Miller, W. L., Redfield, M. M., and Burnett, J. C. Jr. (1989) Integrated cardiac, renal and endocrine actions of endothelin. *Journal of Clinical Investigation*, **83**, 317–320.
59. Ota, K., Kimura, T., Shoji, M., Inoue, M., Sato, K., Ohta, M., Yamamoto, T., Tsunoda, K., Abe, K., and Yoshinaga, K. (1992) Interaction of ANP with endothelin on cardiovascular, renal, and endocrine function. *American Journal of Physiology*, **262**, E135–E141.
60. Matsumura, K., Abe, I., Tsuchihashi, T., Tominaga, M., Kobayashi, K., Fujishima, N. (1991) Central effect of endothelin on neurohormonal responses in concious rabbits. *Hypertension*, **17**, 1192–1196.
61. Kawano, Y., Yoshida, K., Yoshimi, H., Kuramochi, M., Omae, T. (1989) The cardiovascular effect of intracerebroventricular endothelin in rats. *Journal of Hypertension*, **7 (Suppl. 6)**, S22–S23.
62. Sone, M., Totsune, K., Yakahashi, K., Ohneda, M., Itoi, K., K., Murakami, O., Miura,Y., Mouri, T., and Yoshinaga, K. (1991) Immunoreactive endothelin in pheochromocytomas. *Journal of Cardiovascular Pharmacology*, **17 (Suppl 7)**, S427–S429.
63. Sawamura, T., Kimura, S., Shinmi, O., *et al*. (1990) Purification and characterization of putative endothelin converting enzyme in bovine adrenal medulla: evidence for a cathepsin D-like enzyme. *Biochemical and Biophysical Research Communications*, **168**, 1230–1236.
64. Wilkes, L. C. and Boarder, M. R. (1991) Characterization of the endothelin binding site on bovine adrenomedullary chromaffin cells: comparison with vascular smooth muscle cells. Evidence for receptor heterogeneity. *Journal of Pharmacology and Experimental Therapeutics*, **256**, 628–633.
65. Wilkes, L. C. and Boarder, M. R. (1991) Characterization of endothelin receptors on a human neuroblastoma cell line: evidence for the ET_A subtype. *British Journal of Pharmacology*, **104**, 750–754.
66. Morishita, R., Higaki, J. and Ogihara, T. (1989) Endothelin stimulates aldosterone biosynthesis by dispersed rabbit adreno-capsular cells. *Biochemical and Biophysical Research Communications*, **160**, 628–632.
67. Mazzocchi, G., Malendowicz, L. K. and Nussdorfer, G. G. (1990) Endothelin-1 acutely stimulates the secretory activity of rat zona glomerulosa cells. *Peptides*, **11**, 763–765.
68. Hinson, J. P., Kapas, S., Teja, R. and Vinson G. P. (1991) Effect of the endothelins on aldosterone secretion by rat zona glomerulosa cells *in vitro*. *Journal of Steroid Biochemistry and Molecular Biology*, **40**, 437–439.
69. Zeng, Z.-P., Naruse, M., Guan, B.-J., Naruse, K., Sun, M.-L., Zang, M.-F., Demura, H. and Shi, Y.-F. (1992) Endothelin stimulates aldosterone secretion *in vitro* from normal adrenocortical tissue, but not adenoma tissue, in primary aldosteronism. *Journal of Clinical Endocrinology and Metabolism*, **74**, 874–878.
70. Delarue, C., Delton, I., Fiorini, F., Homo-Delarche, F., Fasolo, A., Braquet, P. and Vaudry, H. (1990) Endothelin stimulates steroid secretion by frog adrenal gland *in vitro*: Evidence for the involvement of prostaglandins and extracellular calcium in the mechanism of action of endothelin. *Endocrinology*, **127**, 2001–2008.
71. Mazzocchi, G., Rebuffat, P., Meneghelli, V., Malendowicz, L., Kasprzak, A. and Nussdorfer, G. (1990) Effects of prolonged infusion with endothelin-1 on the function and morphology of rat adrenal cortex. *Peptides*, **11**, 767–772.
72. Mazzocchi, G., Malendowicz, L. K., Meneghelli, V., and Nussdorfer, G. (1992) Endothelin-1 stimulates mitotic activity in the zona glomerulosa of the rat adrenal cortex. *Cytobios*, **69**, 91–96.
73. Woodcock, E. A., Little, P. J. and Tanner, J. K. (1990) Inositol phosphate release and steroidogenesis in rat adrenal glomerulosa cells. *Biochemical Journal*, **271**, 791–796.
74. Hinson, J. P., Vinson, G. P., Kapas, S. and Teja, R. (1991) The role of endothelin in the control of adrenocortical function: stimulation of endothelin release by ACTH and the effects of endothelin-1 and endothelin-3 on steroidogenesis in rat and human adrenocortical cells. *Journal of Endocrinology*, **128**, 275–280.
75. Hinson, J. P., Vinson, G. P., Kapas, S. and Teja, R. (1991) The relationship between adrenal vascular events and steroid secretion: the role of mast cells and endothelin. *Journal of Steroid Biochemistry and Molecular Biology*, **40**, 1–3, 381–389.
76. Hinson, J. P., Vinson, G. and Whitehouse, B. J. (1988) Effects of dietary sodium restriction on peptides stimulation of aldosterone secretion by the isolated perfused rat adrenal gland *in situ*: a report of exceptional sensitivity to angiotensin II amide. *Journal of Endocrinology*, **119**, 83–88.
77. Jones, C. T., Edwards, A. V. and Bloom, S. R. (1990) The effect of changes in adrenal blood flow on adrenal cortical responses to adrenocorticotrophin in conscious calves. *Journal of Physiology*, **429**, 377–386.
78. Ohara-Imaizumi, M. and Kumakura, K. (1991) Dynamics of the secretory response evoked by endothelin-1 in adrenal chromaffin cells. *Journal of Cardiovascular Pharmacology*, **17 (Suppl 7)**, S156–S158.

79. Rasmussen, K. and Printz, M. (1989) Depolarization potentiates endothelin-induced effects on cytosolic calcium in bovine adrenal chromaffin cells. *Biochemical and Biophysical Research Communications*, **165**, 1, 306–311.
80. Sasakawa, N., Nakaki, T. and Kato, R. (1990) Stimulus-responsive and rapid formation of inositol pentakisphosphate in cultured adrenal chromaffin cells. *Journal of Biological Chemistry*, **265**, 29, 17700–17705.
81. Komuro, I., Kurihara, H., Sugiyama, T., Takaku, F., Yazaki, Y. (1988) Endothelin stimulates *c-fos* and *c-myc* expression and proliferation of vascular smooth muscle cells. *FEBS Letters*, **238**, 249–252.
82. Simonson, M., Wann, S., Mene, S., Dubyak, P., Kester, G., Nakazato, Y., Sedor, J. and Dunn, M. (1989) Endothelin stimulates phospholipase C, Na^+/H^+ exchange, *c-fos* expression, and mitogenesis in rat mesangial cells. *Journal of Clinical Investigation*, **83**, 708–712.
83. Shichiri, M., Hirata, Y., Nakajima, T., Ando, K., Imai, T., Yanagisawa, M., Masaki, T., Marumo, F. (1991) Endothelin-1 is an autocrine/paracrine growth factor for human cancer cell line. *Journal of Clinical Investigation*, **87**, 1867–1871.
84. Usuki, S., Otani, S., Goto, K., Matsumoto, H., Suzuki, N., Yanagisawa, M. and Masaki, T. (1991) Endothelin induces DNA polymerase $\propto$ activity in ovaries of hypophysectomized estrogen-treated immature rats. *Hormone and Metabolic Research*, **23**, 621–622.
85. Kamada, S., Kubota, T., Hirata, Y., Taguchi, M., Eguchi, S., Marumo, F. and Aso, T. (1992) Direct effect of endothelin-1 on the granulosa cells of the porcine ovary. *Journal of Endocrinology*, **134**, 59–66.
86. Usuki, S., Suzuki, N., Matsumoto, H., Yanagisawa, M. and Masaki, T. (1991) Endothelin-1 in luteal tissue. *Molecular and Cellular Endocrinology*, **80**, 147–151.
87. Tonetta, S. A. and DiZerga, G. S. (1989) Intragonadal regulation of follicular maturation. *Endocrine Reviews*, **10**, 205–229.
88. Flores, J., Quyyumi, S., Leong, D. and Veldhuis, J. (1992) Actions of Endothelin-1 on swine ovarian (granulosa) cells. *Endocrinology*, **131**, 1350–1358.
89. Usuki, T., Saitoh, T., Suzuki, N., Kitada, C., Goto, K. and Masaki, T. (1991) Endothelin-1 and endothelin-3 stimulate ovarian steroidogenesis. *Journal of Cardiovascular Pharmacology*, **17 (Suppl 7)**, S256–259.
90. Collas, P., Fissore, R., Robi, J., Sullivan, E. and Barnes, F. (1992) Electrically induced calcium elevation, activation, and parthenogenetic development of bovine oocytes. *Molecular Reproduction and Development*, **34**, 212–223.
91. Dube, F. (1992) Thapsigargin induces meiotic maturation in surfa clam oocytes. *Biochemical and Biophysical Research Communications*, **189**, 79–84.
92. Sakakibara, R., Sakai, K., Sakurai, Y., Kohnoura, T., Ishiguro, M. (1993) Factor in urinary extracts from pregnant women that inhibits mouse oocyte maturation *in vitro*. *Molecular Reproduction and Development*, **34**, 101–106.
93. Brown, M., Vaughan, J., Walsh, J., Jimenez, L., Hexum, T., Baird, A. Vale, W. (1990) Endothelin releasing activity in calf serum and porcine follicular fluid. *Biochemical and Biophysical Research Communications*, **173**, 807–815.
94. Sakaguchi, H., Kozuka, M., Hirose, S., Ito, T., Hagiwara, H. (1992) Properties and localization of endothelin-1-specific receptors in rat testicles. *American Journal of Physiology*, **263**, R15–R18.
95. Ergul, A., Glassberg, M., Majercik, M. and Puett, D. (1993) Endothelin-1 promotes steroidogenesis and stimulates protooncogene expression in transformed murine Leydig cells. *Endocrinology*, **132**, 2, 598–603.
96. Borges, R., Von Grafenstein, H. and Knight, D. (1989) Tissue selectivity of endothelin. *European Journal of Pharmacology*, **1652**, 223–230.
97. Polderman, K., Stehouwer, C., VanKamp, G., Dekker, G., Verheught, F. and Gooren, L. (1993) Influence of sex hormones on plasma endothelin levels. *Annals of Internal Medicine*, **118**, 429–432.
98. Stamper, M. and Colditz, G. (1991) Estrogen replacement therapy and coronary heart disease: a quantitative assessment of the epidemiologic evidence. *Preventive Medicine*, **20**, 47–63.
99. Nuno, D. and Lamping, K. (1993) Constriction of coronary microvessels to endothelin is attenuated by 17 β-estradiol *in vitro*. *FASEB Journal*, **7**, A559.
100. Tseng, Y.-C., Lahiri, S., Jackson, S., Burman, K. and Wartofsky, L. (1993) Endothelin binding to receptors and endothelin production by human thyroid follicular cells: effects of transforming growth factor-β and tyrotropin. *Clinical Endocrinology and Metabolism*, **76**, 1, 156–161.
101. Miyakawa, M., Tsushima, T., Isozaki, O., Demura, H., Shizume, K., Arai, M. (1992) Endothelin-1 stimulates *c-fos* mRNA expression and acts as a modulator on cell proliferation of rat FRTL5 thyroid cells. *Biochemical and Biophysical Research Communications*, **184**, 231–238.
102. Rebello, S., Thompson, E. and Gulati, A. (1993) Endothelin mechanisms in altered thyroid states in the rat. *European Journal of Pharmacology*, **237**, 9–16.
103. Grubeck-Loebenstein, B., Buchan, R., Sadeghi, G., Kissonerghis, M., Londei, M., Turner, M., Pirich, K.,

Roka, R., Niederle, B., Kassal, H., Waldhausl, W. and Feldman, M. (1989) Transforming growth factor beta regulates thyroid growth. Role in pathogenesis of nontoxic goiter. *Journal of Clinical Investigation*, **83**, 764–770.

104. McKenzie, J. M. and Zakarija, M. (1989) Hyperthyroidism. *In Endocrinology*, edited by DeGroot, L. J., Philadelphia, W. B. Saunders Co, pp. 646–682.
105. Millul, V., Legente, V., Gillardeaux, O., Bichot, E., Bugas, B., Mencia-Huerta, J., Bereziat, G., Braquet,P., Masliah, J. (1991) Activation of guinea pig alveolar macrophages by endothelin-1. *Journal of Cardiovascular Pharmacology*, **17 (Suppl 7)**, S233–235.
106. Wartofsy, L. and Burman, K. D. (1982) Alterations in thyroid function in patients with systemic illness: the "euthyroid sick syndrome". *Endocrine Reviews*, **3**, 164–217.
107. Cernacek, P. and Stewart, D. J. (1989) Immunoreactive endothelin in human plasma: marked elevations in patients in cardiogenic shock. *Biochemical and Biophysical Research Communications*, **161**, 562–567.
108. Tanini, A., Failli, P., Maggi, M., Franceschelli, F., Frediani, U., Becherini, L., Giotti, A., Ruocco, C., Brandi, M. (1993) Effects of endothelin-1 on bovine parathyroid cells. *Biochemical and Biophysical Research Communications*, **193**, 59–66.
109. DeFeo, M., Bartolini, O., Orlando, C., Maggi, M., Serio, M., Pines, M., Hurwitz, S., Fujii, Y., Sakaguchi, K., Aurbach, G. and Brandi, M. (1991) Natriuretic peptide receptors regulate endothelin synthesis and release from parathyroid cells. *Proceedings of the National Academy of Sciences*, **88**, 6496–6500.
110. Resnick, L. M. (1989) *Endocrine mechanisms in hypertension*. eds. Laragh, J., Brenner, B. M. & Kaplan, N. M., New York, Raven, pp. 265–286.
111. Pang, P. and Lewanczuk, R. (1989) Parathyroid origin of a new circulating hypertensive factor in spontaneously hypertensive rats. *American Journal of Hypertension*, 898–902.
112. Mok, L., Nickols, G., Thompson, J. and Cooper, C. (1989) Parathyroid hormone as a smooth muscle relaxant. *Endocrine Reviews*, **10**, 420–436.
113. Kanno, K., Hirata, Y., Shichiri, M., and Marumo, F. (1991) Plasma endothelin-1 levels in patients with diabetes mellitus with or without vascular complication. *Journal of Cardiovascular Pharmacology*, **17 (Suppl 7)**, S475–S476.
114. Totsune, K., Sone, M., Takahashi, K., Ohneda, M., Itoi, K., Murkami, O., Saito, T., Mouri, T. and Yoshinaga, K. (1991) Immunoreactive endothelin in urine of patients with and without diabetes mellitus. *Journal of Cardiovascular Pharmacology*, **17 (Suppl 7)**, S423–S424.
115. Takahashi, K., Suda, K., Lam, H.-C., Ghatei, M. and Bloom, S. (1991) Endothelin-like immunoreactivity in rat models of diabetes mellitus. *Journal of Endocrinology*, **130**, 123–127.
116. Yamauchi, T., Ohnaka, K., Takayanagi, R., Umeda, F. and Nawata, H. (1990) Enhanced secretion of endothelin-1 by elevated glucose levels from cultured bovine aortic endothelial cells. *FEBS Letters*, **267**, 16–18.
117. Nakaki, T., Nakayama, M., Yamamoto, S. and Kato, R. (1989) Endothelin-mediated stimulation of DNA synthesis in vascular smooth muscle cells. *Biochemical and Biophysical Research Communications*, **158**, 880–883.
118. Takahashi, K., Brooks, R., Kanse, S., Ghatei, M., Kohner, E., Bloom, S. (1989) Production of endothelin 1 by cultured bovine retinal endothelial cells and presence of endothelin receptors on associated pericytes. *Diabetes*, **38**, 1200–1202.
119. Shichiri, M., Hirata, Y., Emori, T., Ohta, K., Nakajima, T., Sato, K., Sato, A., Marumo, F. (1989) Secretion of endothelin and related peptides from renal epithelial cell lines. *FEBS Letters*, **253**, 203–206.
120. Kohzuki, M., Johnson, C. I., Chai, S. Y., Casley, D. J., Mendelsohn, F. A. (1989) Localization of endothelin receptors in rat kidney. *European Journal of Pharmacology*, **160**, 193–194.
121. Simonson, M., Wann, S., Mene, P., Dubryak, G., Kester, M., Nakazato, Y., Sedor, J., Dunn, M. (1989) Endothelin stimulates phospholipase C, Na^+/K^+ exchange, *c-fos* expression, and mitogenesis in rat mesangial cells. *Journal of Clinical Investigation*, **83**, 708–712.
122. Lee, T.-S., Saltsman, K., Ohashi, H., King, G. (1989) Activation of protein kinase C by elevation of glucose concentration: proposal for a mechanism in the development of diabetic vascular complications. *Proceedings of the National Acadamy of Sciences*, **86**, 5141–5145.
123. Craven, P., and DeRubertis, F. (1989) Protein kinase C is activated in glomeruli from streptozotocin diabetic rats. Possible mediation by glucose. *Journal of Clinical Investigation*, **83**, 1667–1675.
124. Emori, T., Hirata, Y., Ohta, K., Kanno, K., Eguchi, S., Imai, T., Shichiri, M., Marumo, F. (1991) Cellular mechanism of endothelin-1 release by angiotensin and vasopressin. *Hypertension*, **18**, 165–170.
125. Awazu, M., Parker, R., Harvie, B., Ichikawa, I. and Kon, V. (1991) Down-regulation of endothelin-1 receptors by protein kinase C in streptozotocin diabetic rats. *Journal of Cardiovascular Pharmacology*, **17 (Suppl 7)**, S500–S502.
126. Ehrenreich, H., Burd, P., Rottem, M., Hultner, L., Hylton, J., Garfield, M., Coligan, J., Metcalfe, D., Fauci, A. (1992) Endothelins belong to the assortment of mast cell-derived and mast cell-bound cytokines. *New Biologist*, **4**, 147–156.

127. Takuwa, Y., Masaki, Y. and Yamashita, K. (1990) The effects of the endothelin family peptides on cultured osteoblastic cells from rat calvariae. *Biochemical and Biophysical Research Communications*, **170**, 998–1005.
128. Takuwa, Y., Ohue, Y., Takuwa, N., Yamashita, K. (1989) Endothelin-1 activates phospholipase C and mobilizes Ca^{2+} from extra- and intracellular pools in osteoblastic cells. *American Journal of Physiology*, **257**, E797–E803.
129. Alam, A., Gallagher, A., Shankar, V., Ghatei, M., Datta, H., Huang, C., Moonga, B., Chambers, T., Bloom, S., Zaidi, M. (1992) Endothelin inhibits osteoclastic bone resorption by a direct effect on cell motility: implications for the vascular control of bone resorption. *Endocrinology*, **130**, 3617–3624.
130. Radan, G. and Martin, T. G. (1981) Role of osteoblasts in hormonal control of bone resorption – a hypothesis. *Calcified Tissue International*, **33**, 349–351.
131. Herrmann-Erlee, M. P. M. and Meer, J. M. (1974) The effects of dibutyryl cyclic AMP, aminophylline and propranolol on PTE-induced bone. *Endocrinology*, **94**, 424–434.
132. Yamaguchi, D., Hahn, T., Beeker, T., Kleeman, C., Maullem, S. (1988) Relationship of cAMP and calcium messenger systems in prostaglandin-stimulated UMR-106 cells. *Journal of Biological Chemistry*, **263**, 10745–10753.
133. Brinker, M., Lippton, H., Cook, S., Hyman, A. (1990) Pharmacological regulation of the circulation of bone. *Journal of Bone and Joint Surgery*, **72**, 964–975.
134. Lee, S. K. and Stern, P. H. (1993) Enhancement of parathyroid hormone induced calcium signals by endothelin-1 pretreatment. *Journal of Bone and Mineral Research*, **8**, S186.
135. Riskind, P. N. and Martin, J. B. (1989) Functional anatomy of the hypothalamic-anterior pituitary complex. *In Endocrinology*, ed. by DeGroot, L. J., Philadelphia, W. B. Saunders Co. pp. 97–107.
136. Vinson, G., Pudney, J., Whitehouse, B. (1985) The mammalian adrenal circulation and the relationship between adrenal blood flow and steroidogenesis. *Journal of Endocrinology*, **105**, 285–294.
137. Naruse, M., Kawana, M., Hifumi, S., Naruse, K., Yoshihara, I., Oka, T., Kato, Y., Monzen, C., Kurimoto, F., Ohsumi, K., Hosoda, S., Demura, H. (1991) Plasma immunoreactive endothelin, but not thrombomodulin, is increased in patients with essential hypertension and ischemic heart disease. *Journal of Cardiovascular Pharmacology*, **17 (Suppl 7)**, S471–S474.
138. Lerman, A., Hildebrand, F., Margulies, K. O'Murchu, B., Perrella, M., Heublein, D., et al. (1990) Endothelin: a new cardiovascular regulatory peptide. *Mayo Clinic Proceedings*, **65**, 1441–1455.
139. Yokokawa, K., Tahara, H., Kohno, M., Murakawa, K., Yasunari, K., Nakagawa, K., et al. (1991) Endothelin-secreting tumor. *Journal of Cardiovascular Pharmacology*, **17 (Suppl 7)**, S398–S401.
140. Kanno, K., Hirata, Y., Emori, T., Ohta, K., Shichiri, M., Shinohara, S., et al. (1991) Endothelin and Raynaud's Phenomenon. *American Journal of Medicine*, **90**, 130–131.
141. Kanno, K., Hirata, Y., Numano, F., Emori, T., Ohta, K., Shichiri, M., Marumo, F. (1990) Endothelin-1 and vasculitis. *Journal of the American Medical Association*, **264**, 2868.

18 Endothelin: Role in Obstetrics and Gynecological Disorders

Annie L. Wrobel Eis, Murray D. Mitchell* and Leslie Myatt

Department of Obstetrics and Gynecology, University of Cincinnati College of Medicine, 231 Bethesda, Cincinnati, OH 45267, USA

*Department of Obstetrics and Gynecology, University of Utah Medical Center, 50 North Medical Drive, Salt Lake City, UT, 84132, USA

INTRODUCTION

Endothelin (ET), a 21 amino acid peptide, originally isolated from the supernatant of porcine aortic endothelial cells[1] has been shown to be a very potent vasoconstrictive agent throughtout the entire body. Subsequently, a family of 21 amino acid peptides, ET-1, ET-2 and ET-3, which are coded for by three separate genes[2] was described. Each peptide contains two intrachain disulfide bridges with ET-2 and ET-3 differing from ET-1 by two or six amino acids, respectively. A 2.3 kb preproendothelin-1 messenger RNA[3] and a separate 2.3 kb preproendothelin-3 mRNA[2] produce 203 and 224 amino acid prepro ETs as their primary gene products. Prepro ETs are then cleaved by a dibasic pair-specific endopeptidase[3] to their respective 39[3] and 42[4] amono acid pro or big ETs. Big ETs are converted into their 21 amino aacid bioactive forms by a putative endothelin converting enzyme. ET-1 converting enzyme has been characterized[5] as a membrane-bound, neutral metalloendopeptidase; however, big ET-1 and big ET-3 may each be converted by a separate but similar enzyme, as the conversion of big ET-3 by this enzyme was only one-ninth that of big ET-1. The ETs were found to be structurally similar to sarafotoxin-S6b, a snake venom produced by the burrowing asp[6] and murine vasoactive intestinal constrictor (VIC)[7] which also share most of their biological characteristics.

Despite the fact that ETs have a short half-life in plasma ($t_{1/2} = 1.9$ min) with high regional plasma clearance, their actions are very persistent, lasting 30 minutes in the splanchnic circulation and up to two hours in the renal circulation[8]. This persistent vasoconstriction, in contrast to the short half-life, is most likely due to the irreversible binding of the ETs to receptor sites, resulting in continuous stimulation of smooth muscle contractile mechanisms[9]. In addition to being the most potent vasoconstrictor discovered to date, the ETs also possess other properties such as oxytocic action on the uterus[10], stimulation of the release of peptide hormones[11], EDRF and eicosanoids[12-14] and mitogenic activity in several different cell types[15-18].

To date, two distinct high-affinity subtypes of ET receptors, each serving different functions, have been cloned. Both belong to the superfamily of rhodopsin-like receptors, have seven transmembrane domains and are coupled to a G protein. They have been classified according to their different affinities for the three ET peptides and by their different tissue distributions. The ET_A receptor, which shows a higher specificity for ET-1 and ET-2 than for ET-3, may be the vascular smooth muscle receptor[19]. The ET_B receptor which is non-isoform specific, is coupled through a G protein to phospholipase C, leading to a transient increase in intracellular free calcium[20]. This subtype is not found in vascular smooth muscle. Although the precise physiological relationship between ETs and their two receptor subtypes has not yet been described, it is thought that vasoconstriction may be mediated by ET-1 binding to ET_A receptors located on vascular smooth muscle cells. ET_B receptors, which may be localized on endothelial cells, may be responsible for the release of endothelial derived relaxing factor (EDRF) and prostacyclin[21] both of which oppose the vasoconstrictive action of ET.

Endothelins are present throughout the uteroplacental and fetal-placental vasculatures. Its own vasoactive nature and ability to interact with other vasoactive compounds makes it an ideal candidate as a vascular regulatory element in these circulations. Due to its highly vasoconstrictive nature, ET is also a natural suspect in the etiology of pregnancy-induced vascular disease states, such as hypertension and preeclampsia and in cases of fetal hypoxia and intrauterine growth retardation (IUGR). Since ETs are such persistent and potent contractile agents, and are found througout gestational tissues and amniotic fluid, it is widely speculated that it may function as an oxytocic agent in the uterus during labor. There may also be a role for ET in regulatory mechanisms during the menstrual cycle[22] and it has been postulated that ET may be involved in dysfunctional uterine bleeding[23].

To provide a background for discussing the role of ET in obstetrics and gynecological disorders, this review will first discuss the presence of ET in gestational and uterine tissues and will then examine its putative physiologic/pathophysiologic roles in gestation, parturition and the menstrual cycle.

ENDOTHELIN IN THE PLACENTA

In light of the fact that the placental vasculature lacks autonomic innervation[24,25], vascular resistance must be determined by humoral factors or by paracrine/autocrine mechanisms. Compounds such as the ETs, whether circulating through the blood stream or produced locally, are ideal candidates as regulators of vascular tone in the feto-placental circulation.

Localization and identification of endothelin protein

Immunohistochemistry (IHC) has been used to localize immunoreactive ET (IR-ET) within term placental tissues. However, as most of the ET antibodies used were non-isoform specific, the results of these studies are somewhat contradictory. The presence of IR-ET in endothelial cells lining fetal vessels throughout the entire placental vasculature has been reported[26-28], the latter group using an ET-1 specific antibody, confirmed that ET-1 is the isoform present in these vessels. IR-ET is also present in umbilical cord arteries and veins[26]. Immunogold electron microscopy of umbilical cord sections using a nonisoform specific ET antibody preabsorbed with either ET-1, ET-2 or ET-3 revealed the presence of IR-ET-1 and 2 but not ET-3 in the cytoplasm of epithelial cells and primitive fibroblasts. The staining was diffuse throughout the cytoplasm and not associated with organelles or membranes, suggesting a local synthesis of ET and a constitutive pathway for its release[29]. Hemsen et al [26] reported the presence of IR—ET in squamous and cuboidal epithelium of umbilical cord and placental amnion, but not chorion. While van Papendorp et al.[27] found no IR-ET in amnion nor in chorion using IHC, they did find large quantities of IR-ET by radioimmunoassay (RIA) of separate homogenates of amnion and chorion tissues, with the concentration of IR-ET being significantly higher in amnion than chorion or placenta. No change was seen in localization or tissue content of IR-ET before or after labor. IR-ET is also reported to be localized by IHC in the cytoplasm of decidual stromal cells in the basal maternal plate of the placenta and in retained decidual stromal cells attached to the chorion[27].

Further attempts to identify the IR-ET isoforms present in placental tissues using reverse-phase high-pressure liquid chromatography (RP-HPLC), have also given conflicting results. Whereas Benigni et al.[30] reported that extracted human placental tissue homogenates at term appeared to produce equivalent amounts of big ET-1, ET-2, and ET-3, but little ET-2, Hemsen et al.[26] detected high levels of IR-ET in umbilical cord vessels, amniotic membranes and placenta at term, most of which eluted with ET-1 or oxidized ET-1, but none of which eluted with big ET-1, ET-2, ET-3 nor big ET-3. Using very specific antibodies against ET-1-(ET-2) or ET-3 in a sensitive enzyme immunoassay (EIA), Onda et al.[4] detected IR-ET-3 in tissue homogenates from term placenta but 20-fold higher concentrations of IR-ET-1. The reason for these contradictory results is not known, however ET-1 seems to be the dominant isoform found in the placenta. Endothelin-1 has also been detected by RP-HPLC in conditioned medium from primary cultures of human decidual cells, but not trophoblast cells of early (6–8 week) pregnancies and the expression of mRNA for preproET-1 has been demonstrated, also in decidua but not trophoblast, by Northern blot analysis. Decidual cells were also shown to possess functional ET_A receptors[31].

Expression and regulation of endothelin mRNA

Messenger RNA's encoding for preproET-1 and preproET-3 are transcribed and expressed in human term placenta[3,4]. Human umbilical vein endothelial cells (HUVEC) in culture express a 2.3 kb preproET mRNA which is identical in size to that reported for human term placenta[30]. Avascular human amnion was found to express preproET-1 mRNA and to synthesize and release IR-ET-1[32]. Amnion cells in mono-layer culture were found to retain the ability to express the preproET gene[33]. However, expression of preproET mRNA was not found in term chorion, villous trophoblast, nor in myometrium or decidua[33]. This is contradictory to findings of IR-ET, detected by RIA, in chorion and by IHC in term decidua and the reported presence of IR-ET-1 and preproET-1 mRNA in first trimester decidual cells in culture. It is known why preproET-1 mRNA appears to be expressed in decidual cells of early, but not term pregnancies, but suggests that ET-1 may be acting as a decidual cell mitogen early in gestation[31].

A number of substances have been shown to regulate the expression of the preproET message and/or the synthesis of the ET protein in gestational tissues. Phorbol myristate acetate, a protein kinase C activator, elicited a dose-dependent increase in IR-ET-1 release from first trimester decidual cells in culture, while H7, a protein kinase C inhibitor, significantly attenuated this effect[31]. In primary HUVEC cultures, the calcium ionophores ionomycin and A-23187 caused concentration-dependent inhibition of ET production, while the calcium channel blockers verapamil and nifedipine had no consistent effects[34]. HUVEC ET production is regulated in an inverse manner by intracellular calcium concentrations, suggesting a negative feedback from mediators of ET actions on cells. Physical trauma generally increased the mean production of IR-ET-1 and 2, while oxidant damage to HUVEC resulted in a decrease in IR-ET production[34]. These findings suggest that elevated levels of ET in conditions such as pregnancy induced hypertension (PIH) may represent endothelial cell activation rather than endothelial cell damage. A number of agents commonly present in amniotic fluid, including epidermal growth factor (EGF), interleukin-1 (IL-1), and tumor necrosis factor-α (TNF-α), stimulate preproET mRNA levels and IR-ET production by human amnion cells in primary monolayer culture; in addition, the induction of preproET mRNA by these agents is super-induced upon simultaneous treatment of the cells with cycloheximide, an inhibitor of protein synthesis[33]. In HUVEC, which show a higher basal level of preproET mRNA than amnion cells, treatment with IL-1, TNF-α, and EGF did not stimulate preproET mRNA, but inhibition of protein synthesis did lead to increased levels of preproET mRNA[32]. In addition to suggesting that ET production may be differentially regulated in different tissues, these findings suggest that protein synthesis dependent mechanisms may be very important in maintaining low levels of preproET mRNA in amnion tissue and in regulating its transcription[32].

Placental endothelin receptors

Two types of ET receptor are found in the placenta. On the basis of their different affinities for various ETs these appear to be the ET_A subtype in the umbilical cord and chorionic plate vessels and the ET_B subtype in the villous vasculature[26,35]. Controversy still exists with respect to the molecular weight and properties of these receptors, perhaps due to the wide variety of methods used to study them. Although it is agreed that there is only a single class of ET binding site in placental villous membrane preparations, a variety of molecular weights have been reported. These range from 32–40 kDa[36-39], 50–55 kD[38,39], 200 kDa[39] and 340 kDa[36]. The 50 kDa molecular weight corresponds most closely to that reported for the cloned ET_A and ET_B receptors[19,20]. The lower reported molecular weights may correspond to proteolytic breakdown products of the receptor protein, while the higher reported molecular weights are probably due to oligomerization of the receptor protein subunits and/or to divalent cations complexed to the receptor[37,39]. Reported dissociation constants (K_d)

for the placental membrane receptor against ET-1 range from 24–57 pM[13,35,37,39,40] or from 80–106 pM in the presence of added divalent cations[25,29]. Maximal density of binding (B_{max}) ranged from 93–600 fmol/mg protein[13,26,35,39,40]. Half-maximal inhibition of binding (IC_{50}) ranged from 80–140 pM and association half time from 20–30 minutes[35,40]. In the placental villous membrane preparation, K_ds for ET-2, ET-3, sarafotoxin-S6b and VIC were similar to those reported for ET-1 for the placental membrane receptor, with the big ETs having a much lower affinity[13,35]. The properties of the umbilical cord and chorionic plate vessel receptor are similar to those in the placental membranes except for a K_d closer to 45 pM for ET-1[35] and a three-fold lower affinity for ET-3[25,35]. This lower affinity for ET-3 indicates that this receptor is of the ET_A subtype.

Fischli et al.[40] and Kalina and Löffler[39] found that divalent cations, especially Mn^{2+}, significantly alter the binding properties of placental ET receptors by increasing the maximal binding, the time required to reach equilibrium binding and the B_{max}, while decreasing K_d. In contrast, Nakajo et al.[36] report that neither divalent nor monovalent cations have any effect on the binding properties of placental ET receptors. The ET receptors are very specific for ET or ET-like peptides. They have no affinity for several other vasoactive agents[35,40].

ENDOTHELIN IN MATERNAL AND FETAL PLASMA

It has been suggested[41] that ET may act as a circulating hormone during pregnancy and labor in both fetal and maternal circulations; however, circulating plasma ET concentrations are not high enough to produce physiological effects, which may be due to the fact that ETs have a very short half-life in plasma. It is possible that ET may be produced locally at high enough concentrations to have autocrine/paracrine physiological effects. Reported ET concentrations varies with respective antibody used in the RIA, thus they will be reported here as approximate ranges. The concentration of IR-ET in maternal plasma increases during gestation from 2–6 pM (non-pregant) to 3–12 pM at term[41–43], although others report no such increase[30,44,45]. Maternal plasma ET concentration falls shortly after birth, suggesting that it is of placental origin[41,42]. Maternal urinary excretion of ET-1 is also significantly increased during gestation from approximately 3 pg/mg creatinine (non-pregnant) to 20 pg/mg creatinine during the third trimester[30].

Umbilical cord plasma has a much higher IR-ET concentration (3–25 pM) than does maternal plasma. It is possible that the stress of delivery can stimulate increased production of ET in gestational tissues. Some studies[41–43,46], but not all[44,45], report higher IR-ET levels in the umbilical artery and/or vein after vaginal versus non-laboring cesarean delivery. There was no significant difference in cord plasma IR-ET concentration between pre-term and full-term infants, but an increase in IR-ET-1 was found in cord venous plasma from vaginally delivered infants complicated by asphyxia, over that of non-asphyxiated infants[46]. Cord venous plasma ET-1 concentrations were also elevated in hypoxia (pH < 7.3) but not normoxic (pH > 7.3) infants[47]. Interestingly, ET concentrations in the umbilical cord vessels are reported to increase following the onset of fetal breathing[45].

ENDOTHELIN IN AMNIOTIC FLUID

Reported concentrations of IR-ET in amniotic fluid range from 10–77 pM[32,41,42,45], which is higher than is found in both fetal and maternal plasma. Since the amniotic membrane was found to contain preproET mRNA and to secrete the ET protein, it has been suggested to be one tissue source of amniotic fluid ET[32]. It is not known whether amnion-derived ET-1 can cross fetal membranes to reach the myometrium and exert an oxytocic effect. Endothelin-1 in intrauterine tissues may exert a paracrine effect to mediate peptide hormone release, as it does in the pituitary[11], or it may effect fluid transfer across the fetal membranes. In studies using amnion alone or intact amnion/chorion/decidua mounted in Ussing chambers[48], ^{125}I-labeled ET-1 added to either the fetal or maternal side, was not found to cross either membrane preparation appreciably (Table 18.1). Most of the radio labeled ET-1 remained bound to the membrane, even after repeated washing. Endothelin-1 did not influence the movement of tritiated H_2O across the membranes using this system (Table 18.2).

Elevated levels of IR-ET in amniotic fluid have been found to be associated with certain pregnancy-related disorders. Women in preterm labor with associated intra-uterine bacterial infections had higher amniotic fluid levels of IR-ET-1 and 2 than did those without infection[49]. Cytokines such as interleukin-1$_\beta$ (IL-1$_\beta$) are produced by human decidua in response to bacterial products and IL-1$_\beta$ is found in the amniotic fluid of women with preterm labor and amniotic infection[49]. It has been shown that

Table 18.1 Permeability of fetal membranes to ^{125}I endothelin

	Permeability coefficient ($cm/sec \times 10^{-5}$)
Amnion	3.34 ± 0.79
Amnion/Chorion/Decidua	2.43 ± 0.68

Mean ± SE (n = 5).

Table 18.2 The effect of endothelin on permeability to tritiated water

	Permeability coefficient ($cn/sec \times 10^{-4}$)	
	Fetal → Maternal	Maternal → Fetal
Fetal Endothelin	n = 6	n = 5
Control	1.26 ± 0.21	0.90 ± 0.07
+ Endothelin 10^{-8} M	1.25 ± 0.10	0.98 ± 0.15
Maternal Endothelin	n = 15	n = 15
Control	1.12 ± 0.18	0.83 ± 0.16
+ Endothelin 10^{-9} M	0.96 ± 0.10	0.94 ± 0.09

Mean ± SE.

IL-1$_\beta$ can increase ET production by amnion[50]. Increased ET levels might then alter prostaglandin levels[51] which could trigger premature labor. Amniotic fluid ET levels were also shown to be elevated in some cases of IUGR[52], which raises the possibility that ET might contribute to the pathogenesis of gestational disorders associated with vasomotor control.

ACTIONS OF ENDOTHELIN IN GESTATIONAL TISSUES

Placental growth and development

The placenta is a highly vascularized organ which rapidly grows and develops in a comparatively short period of time. Proliferation of the fetal vascular bed and surrounding stroma is essential for placental growth. Since ET is a known mitogen of several different cell types, it may serve a similar function in the growth and development of placental tissues. Fant et al.[53] used placental fibroblast cells to explore potential growth-regulatory functions of ET-1 in the human placenta. Endothelin-1 was found to stimulate DNA synthesis in placental fibroblasts in a dose-dependent manner and ET-1 acted synergistically with insulin-like growth factor I (IGF-I). Endothelin-1 also stimulated phosphoinositide turnover (accompanied by a 2–3 fold increase in intracellular calcium), IGF binding proteins and the secretion of IGF-II. PreproET-1 mRNA was found to be significantly increased in placental tissue at term versus early in gestation. Endothelin-1 synthesis may, therefore, be developmentally regulated by the placenta and may serve in an autocrine/paracrine manner to regulate placental growth.

Fetal-placental vascular tone

There is a wealth of evidence to date supporting an active role for ETs in modulating fetal-placental vascular tone. Immunoreactive ET is found in placental tissues as are the corresponding preproET mRNAs and functional receptors. It has been shown that the synthesis and release of IR-ET in cultured HUVEC is polar[54]. HUVEC were cultured on acellular amniotic membranes, thereby simulating a luminal (apical) and abluminal (basolateral) vessel surface. Intact endothelium was found to be a major barrier to the diffusion of ET-1, with only 6.5% of unilaterally added ET-1 crossing. The secretion of ET-1 was polar with 80% of synthesized ET-1 found in the basolateral compartment which corresponds to the location *in vitro* of smooth muscle cells. Thrombin (10 units/ml) caused a 2-fold increase in ET-1 production, but did not change the distribution; whereas dexamethasone (10^{-7} M) influenced the polarity of ET-1 secretion towards the basolateral compartment without affecting the total amount produced, nor the permeability of endothelial monolayers for ET-1. The different vascular sensitivity to luminally and adventitially applied ET-1[55] together with differential secretion of ET-1 towards its site of action in the underlying smooth muscle is evidence supporting a local paracrine role for ET-1 in the placental vasculature.

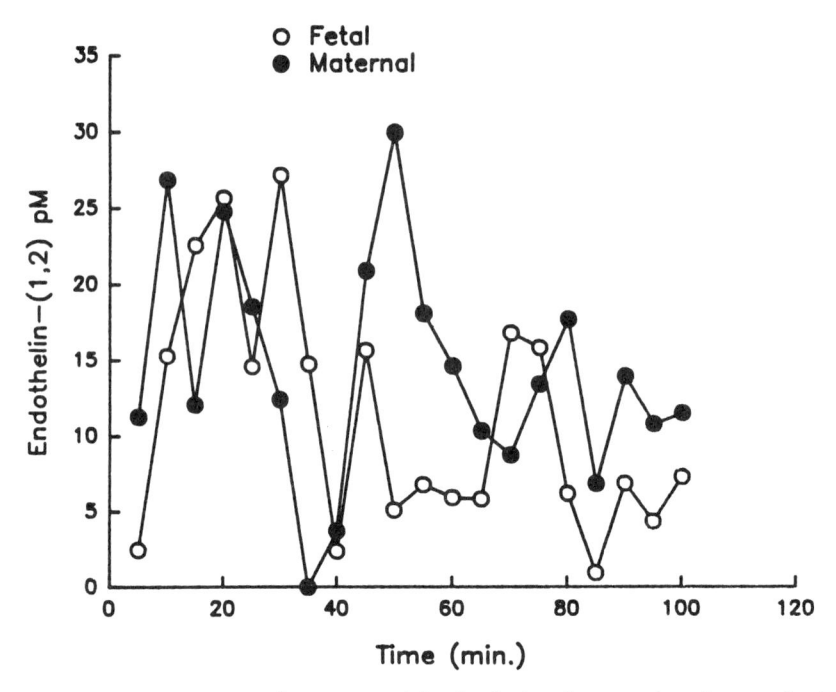

Figure 18.1. Endothelin concentrations measured in the fetal and maternal perfusates of a human placental cotyledon perfused *in vitro*. Flow rates are 4 ml/min (fetal) and 10 ml/min (maternal).

Immunoreactive ET could be measured in both the maternal (2–4 fmol/ml[56] and fetal (6–7 fmol/ml[56] or 0.8 ± 0.6 fmol/min/g[57]) effluents of the dually perfused placental cotyledon *in vitro* at concentrations similar to those found in maternal plasma during pregnancy. Endothelin appears to be released into maternal and fetal circulations in a pulsatile manner[56], with a periodicity of 15–30 min, which appeared to be synchronous in both circulations (Figure 18.1). Perfusion experiments have also been used to examine the actions of ET on the placental villous vascular bed. ET-1 and ET-3 were found to be potent long-lasting (45–60 min)[58] vasoconstrictors in the placenta at concentrations between 10^{-11} and 10^{-6} M[13,57–59]. The relative potencies of the ET's and other substances which are known placental vasoconstrictors are ET-1 > U46619 (thromboxane A_2 mimetic) > ET-3 > prostaglandin $F_{2\alpha}$ ($PGF_{2\alpha}$)[57]. Big ET-1 was also shown to increase placental perfusion pressure with approximately one-tenth the potency of ET-1; however, big ET-1 always elicited transient vasodilation before constriction[59]. Phosphoramidon, a neutral metalloprotease inhibitor, inhibited the vasoconstrictor effect of big ET-1, indicating that ET converting enzyme is present in the fetal-placental circulation. As ET receptors have been shown to have much lower affinity for big ET than for ET itself, the conversion of big ET-1 to ET-1 may be necessary in order for it to exert its effect.

In some vasculatures, endothelin action has been shown to be mediated by thromboxane release and subsequent action of specific receptors[60,61] although other studies have demonstrated effects independent of thromboxane[62]. During ET-1-induced vasoconstriction of the placental cotyledons, perfusate thromboxane concentrations increased with increasing concentrations of ET-1[13]. However, when values were corrected for reduced perfusate flow rate due to increased vasoconstriction[58], thromboxane release was shown to *decrease* in a dose-dependent fashion. A similar decrease in the release of 6-keto prostaglandin $F_{1\alpha}$ (6-keto $PGF_{1\alpha}$), a prostacyclin metabolite, was reported. Inhibition of thromboxane synthesis by dazoxiben did not affect ET-1 action in the perfused fetal-placental vasculature nor did blocking of the thromboxane receptor with SQ29548, thereby indicating that the action of ET-1 in the placental vasculature appears to be direct and not mediated by thromboxane[58]. The vasoconstrictor effects of both ET and thromboxane in the perfused placental cotyledon were significantly attenuated by nitric oxide (NO), the endothelial-derived relaxing factor[63]. Since NO is released in response to vasoconstriction by ET-1 and U46619, there is evidence that ET-1 interacts with other vasoactive agents in the control of placental vascular tone. Prostaglandins are thought to have important roles in the regulation of uteroplacental[64,65] and fetal-placental[66] hemodynamics. ET-1 (10^{-11}–10^{-7} M) significantly increased the rate of biosynthesis of 6-keto $PGF_{1\alpha}$ and prostaglandin E_2 (PGE_2) in HUVEC. Prostaglandin E_2 production was decreased in amnion cells incubated with ET-1, while PGE_2 and $PGE_{2\alpha}$ production by decidual cells was unaffected[51]. Although ET-1 can cause changes in cellular PG production of gestational tissues, it has been reported that endothelin-induced changes in renal and cardiovascular functions in the rat are not affected by inhibition of PG synthesis using the cyclooxygenase inhibitors meclofenamate and indomethacin[67].

The action of ET was also studied in umbilical cord and chorionic plate vessels. Isolated umbilical arteries and veins *in vitro* were constricted by threshold levels of 10–100 pM ET-1[26]. Veins appeared to be slightly more sensitive than arteries. The contractile effects were persistent even with repeated rinsing of the vessels. In the same preparation $PGF_{2\alpha}$ was about three orders of magnitude less potent as a vasoconstrictor and neuropeptide Y was only effective at micromolar concentrations. Endothelin-3 at concentrations as high as 10^{-7} M did not constrict umbilical vessels. This is in agreement with the observation that these vessels contain the ET_A receptor subtype. Vessels of the umbilical cord, chorionic plate and villous tree contracted similarly in response to ET-1[68]. Arterial vessels were ten times more sensitive to ET-1 than to 5-hydroxytryptamine (5-HT) and venous vessels were ten times more sensitive to ET-1 than their corresponding arteries. The vasoconstrictor effect of ET-1 is more pronounced on placental veins than on arteries, which appears to be opposite to and may be related to the relative synthesis of NO by these vessels. Endothelin may assist in closing down the umbilical circulation at brith. Although, unlike 5-HT, the umbilical arteries are not super-sensitized to the action of ET-1 at the higher O_2 tensions present during birth[68], the concentration of ET-1 found in fetal cord blood plasma is greatly increased at the onset of fetal breathing [45]. It is felt that, since umbilical veins are more responsive to ET-1 than are arteries, increased levels of ET-1 may be an essential factor in the closure of the umbilical venous circulation at birth. It appears that the placental vessels can both produce and react to the ETs as vasoconstrictors and as stimulators or inhibitors of other vasoactive compounds. As the effects of ETs are so long-lasting and potent, it is likely that they do not act as acute regulators of fetal-placental vascular resistence, but rather act in a local paracrine manner to help maintain overall vascular homeostasis.

PATHOPHYSIOLOGY OF ENDOTHELIN IN OBSTETRICS

Pregnancy induced hypertension (PIH) is defined as a blood pressure of 140/90 mmHg on two occasions six hours apart after the twentieth week of gestation, or an increase of 30 mmHg systolic or 15 mmHg diastolic over preexisting values. Preeclampsia is PIH with concurrent proteinuria and edema. Other symptoms of preeclampsia can include activation of the coagulation cascade, hypersensitivity to pressor agents, arterial vasospasm and hemolysis of red blood cells. Preeclampsia is a major cause of maternal and fetal morbidity and mortality and is thought to be a state of endothelial cell dysfunction. While it is unlikely that ET is the cause of PIH and preeclampsia, it may contribute to the pathophysiology of these conditions.

Many studies[69-74], but not all[75-77] have shown that plasma ET levels are increased in preeclamptic women as compared to normotensive pregnant women. These elevated concentrations were still not high enough to cause systemic physiological effects; however, subthreshold concentrations of ET may increase sensitivity to other vasoconstrictors such as norepinephrine and 5-HT[78-79]. Some reports indicate that increased plasma ET levels correlate to the severity of the disease[73,80] or strongly correlate[69,81-83] to increased urinary uric acid and proteinuria and to reduced creatine clearance. The elevated ET levels in preeclampsia return to normal within 48 hours post partum, which corresponds to the prompt post partum disappearance of the clinical symptoms of this disorder[71,82]. Elevated plasma ET levels are most likely secondary to the onset of preeclampsia[82,84]. Increased ET-1 levels could not be detected in second trimester blood samples from women who later developed preeclampsia in their third trimester[82].

Most of the maternal and fetal morbidity in preeclamptic pregnancies results from vasospasm and ischemia[82]. Local release of ET from vascular endothelium is thought to cause vasospasm in the uterine and umbilical arteries[85]. Elevated ET levels in preeclamptic pregnancies have been associated with umbilical artery spasm which may contribute to intrauterine growth retardation (IUGR) and asphyxia of the fetus[86]. ET concentration is also increased in the uterine venous plasma of preeclamptic subjects and may contribute to reduced uteroplacental blood flow[75]. An increase in atrial natriuretic peptide (ANP) has been correlated with increased ET levels in preeclampsia[87], especially in cases of preeclampsia with associated vasospasm[85]. Like ET, plasma ANP levels in preeclampsia fall to normal shortly after birth[87], indicating that ANP may be released as a compensatory mechanism against endothelin-induced vasospasm.

Increased plasma levels of ET are not always associated with PIH, but are almost always associated with impaired renal function[83]. Endothelin was shown to act directly on the rat kidney causing hemodynamic, diuretic and natriuretic responses which were increased upon inhibition of cyclooxygenase and counteracted by treatment with ANP[88]. Increased levels of ET may also contribute to platelet aggregation and clot formation, as preproET mRNA is increased in response to thrombin stimulation[75].

A putative role for ET in preeclampsia was questioned by Benigni et al.[77] who found that the concentration of ET-1 in preeclamptic plasma, the expression of placental preproET-1 mRNA and big ET-1 and ET-1, 2, 3 protein production did not differ from that of normotensive subjects. Urinary excretion of ET was decreased in preeclamptic as compared to normotensive pregnant subjects and this decrease was due to increased renal breakdown of ET rather than to decreased protein production.

ENDOTHELIN IN THE UTERUS

Introduction: the menstrual cycle

Human menstruation consists of a series of events involving the decline in the ovarian steroids 17β-estradiol and progesterone following by the shedding most of the endometrial lining and its eventual replacement. The uterine vascular changes leading to menstruation were described by Markee[89]. A regression in the endometrial growth cycle which proceeds the onset of menstruation by 2–6 days occurs during the late secretory phase. This involves stromal edema followed by a marked decrease in endometrial tissue volume which are both temporally associated with the decline in plasma estrogen and progesterone. During this event spiral arteries become more coiled, causing blood stasis within these vessels. These vessels then become highly constricted for periods up to 24 hours, after which bleeding occurs in dilated spiral arterioles. Thus, we can see that intense vasoconstriction of uterine spiral arterioles proceeds the onset of menstrual bleeding. Likewise, the cessation of menstrual bleeding was found to involve basal arteriolar constriction rather than formation of a platelet-fibrin plug[90]. A potent vasoconstrictor such as ET must therefore be involved in these processes. It has been hypothesized[91] that ET-1 secreted by endometrial stromal cells comes in contact with the adventitial surface of endometrial spiral arteries where it causes these vessels to constrict during the premenstrual phase of an infertile ovulatory cycle. Because the ETs are also cell mitogens, there is also the possibility that they could be involved in tissue regeneration following menstrual shedding. Although the definitive roles of ET in uterine biology have not been unequivocably elucidated, its presence in and actions on uterine tissues are undergoing examination.

Localization and regulation of endothelin protein and mRNA

Immunohistochemical localization of IR-ET in the uterus has been demonstrated by some investigators[92,93] but not by others[94] and the localization of IR-ET reportedly changes during the different phases of the menstrual cycle. Cameron et al.[92] reported IR-ET in the cytoplasm of glandular epithelium and vascular endothelium of endometrium and myometrium during the proliferative and secretory phases of the menstrual cycle. The most intense staining was at the endometrial-myometrial junction. Others[93] have reported finding low levels of IR-ET staining in endometrial stromal cells throughout the menstrual cycle. Strong staining was found in luminal epithelium during the secretory phase and in glandular epithelium during the late-secretory phase. Immunoreactive ET has also been demonstrated in the endometrium of rabbit uterus[95]. Changes in the staining pattern due to treatment with ovarian steroids were observed. Epithelial cells were positively stained for IR-ET in immature rabbits, whereas the stromal cells surrounding the glandular epithelium were positively stained in animals treated with estrogen alone or sequentially with estrogen and progesterone.

Messenger RNA for both ET-1 and ET-3 is found in human endometrium throughout the menstrual cycle[22]. A greater expression of preproET mRNA was found in tissue from the premenstrual-menstrual phase as compared to that found in the proliferative or early- and mid-secretory phases[96]. PreproET-1 mRNA has also been found in endometrial stroma and glandular epithelial cells in culture[96] and the protein was secreted into the culture medium. Endothelin-1 production by these cells was stimulated by TGF_β and $IL-1_\alpha$.

Uterine endothelin receptors

In the non-pregnant uterus, binding sites for all three ET isoforms were found to have a similar gross anatomical distribution[97]. There was a higher density of binding sites found in the endometrium than in the myometrium, wth the highest density being found at the junction of these two tissues. The highest densities of binding sites were localized to glandular epithelial cells, with a lower density found in myometrium and vascular smooth muscle. All three isoforms of ET could compete for these binding sites. A study comparing non-pregnant and pregnant human uterine tissues[94] reports no clear pattern of structural distribution of binding sites in non-pregnant uterus and a high density of binding sites in myometrium and vascular smooth muscle in pregnant uterus. This finding seems to indicate that ETs may be involved in labor and in the regulation of vascular tone. In the non-pregnant uterine artery, binding sites were found in the *tunica muscularis* smooth muscle layer[98]. The ET_A receptor subtype seems to be the most predominant form found in the uterus[99,100]. One study which included uterine endometrial tissues from all phases of the menstrual cycle[22] found that the ET_A receptor subtype is present in endometrium throughout the menstrual cycle and is the only type found during the proliferative phase. During the secretory and menstrual phases, the ET_B receptor subtype is also present, thus the ratio of ET_A and ET_B receptor subtype in the endometrium changes throughout the menstrual cycle. It is felt that the different physiologic actions of the ETs in the uterus may be mediated by this change in receptor ratio.

Regulation of endothelin in uterine tissues

The cyclic nature of IR-ET and ET receptor localization suggests a differential regulation, possibly by ovarian steroids. In the rabbit myometrial membrane preparation[95] ET receptors are stimulated in a dose-dependent manner by 17β-estradiol (0.2–200 µg/Kg × 4 days), which was completely counteracted by sequential treatment with progesterone (5 mg/Kg × 4 days). Incubation of uterine myocytes in culture with 17β-estradiol did not, however, increase ET receptor density. Divalent cations Ca^{2+} and Mg^{2+} enhance ET binding to both myometrial cell preparations and cultured cells.

There is evidence[91] that progesterone regulates enkephalinase, a metalloendopeptidase which catalyzes the degradation of ETs, enkephalins, ANP, substance P and other small bioactive peptides. Enkephalinase is present with relatively high specific activity in the stromal cells of human endometrium. Specific activity of enkephalinase is positively correlated to the rise and decline of progesterone levels throughout the menstrual cycle and appears to be directly regulated through action of progesterone via the progesterone receptor. Thus, the highest specific activity is present during the midluteal phase of the menstrual cycle and during pregnancy when ET activity is expected to be low, and lowest during the late secretory phase when ET activity should be highest.

Actions of endothelin in the uterus

Endothelin may regulate utero-placental blood flow. Endothelin produced vasoconstrictor effects in small uterine arteries from pregnant women *in vitro*[101]. The effects of ET were three times as powerful and 70-fold as potent as those produced by noradrenaline in parallel experiments. Endothelin produces potent, slow and long-lasting contractions in isolated uterine arteries and veins[102], whereas neuropeptide Y did not affect uterine artery and only triggered spontaneous contraction in uterine veins at high concentrations.

Uterine smooth muscle is also affected by ET. Endothelin stimulates contractile effects in myometrial strips from pregnant women with a similar force and frequency to those produced by oxytocin in the same tissue[103]. Endothelin and oxytocin were found to modulate Ca^{2+}, each through its own receptor[104]. Endothelin promotes contraction in the myometrium by effecting an increase in intracellular Ca^{2+}, thus increasing myosin light chain phosphorylation[105]. It can stimulate Ca^{2+} influx and Ca^{2+} release from intracellular stores. Like oxytocin, endothelin in likely an important modulator of uterine contractility.

Endothelin was shown[14] to stimulate the release of $PGF_{2\alpha}$ but not PGE_2 in tissue explants from proliferative but not secretory endometrium. This appears to occur through activation of the phospholipase A_2 and PtdIns (4, 5) P_2-specific phospholipase C by ET, which results in the generation of $PGF_{2\alpha}$ and other second messengers[106]. These second messengers may be involved in the control of the endometrial vascular bed and/or in cell proliferation.

Summery: roles of endothelin in the uterus

In summary, there exists impressive, albeit circumstantial, evidence that the ETs are important regulators during the menstrual cycle. They have been shown to contract uterine vessels more effectively than other known vasoactive agents tested. There appears to be a cyclic variation of ET message, protein and receptor density and location throughout the menstrual phases. Endothelin seems to be present at the right time and location in the uterus to be involved in vascular constriction leading to the onset and cessation of menstrual bleeding. Appropriate mechanisms for up or down regulation of this compound and its receptors are also evident. In addition, ET is a known mitogen in many cell types and can activate phospholipase A and phospholipase C to produce $PGF_{2\alpha}$ and other second messengers which could be involved in cell proliferation during the proliferative phase of the menstrual cycle when endometrial tissue regeneration is occurring.

Endothelins are likely modulators of uterine contractility. They produce long-lasting contractions in myometrial smooth muscle. Endothelin receptor density is higher in vascular smooth muscle and myometrium in pregnant uterus than in non-pregnant uterus. Endothelins can also stimulate intracellular Ca^{2+} influx and release from intracellular stores, thereby increasing myosin light chain phosphorylation. Endothelins are likely regulators of uterine blood flow for many of the same reasons. Uterine vessels of all sizes are responsive to endothelin and it has been shown to be a more effective contractile agent of uterine vessels than many other known vasoactive agents tested. Functional ET receptors are present on the smooth muscle layer of uterine vessels. The fetal-placental vasculature has been shown to be similarily regulated by ET.

ENDOTHELINS IN UTERINE PATHOPHYSIOLOGY

If endothelins do indeed play a regulatory role in normal menstrual bleeding, they could just as readily be involved in dysfunctional uterine bleeding[23]. There is as yet no evidence to support this theory, but there is evidence of aberrant endothelin production in a number of disease states such as cardiogenic shock[107], Crohn's disease[108], hemolytic uremic syndrome[109] and preeclampsia (see this review), to name a few. It is possible that a misregulation of endothelin during the menstrual cycle could lead to excessive or untimely uterine bleeding.

Many of the other putative pathophysiologic roles of endothelins have been discussed previously in this review, as they relate mainly to pregnancy. Briefly, elevated ET levels have been found in pregnant women with intrauterine infection who deliver prematurely. In this case, bacterial cytokines may stimulate excessive production of ET by amnion and/or other gestational tissues which could act on the uterus to stimulate contraction leading to preterm delivery of the infant. Chronic or acute reduction in uterine blood flow will, in turn, affect the placental circulation. Poor utero-placental circulation is likely to produce infants with hypoxia or asphyxia. Umbilical plasma ET levels are elevated in babies born with these conditions. Endothelin concentration is elevated in plasma from preeclamptic women, especially in cases involving vasospasm of the uterine and umbilical arteries. Infants with IUGR and asphyxia are most likely to result from these pregnancies.

References

1. Yanagisawa, M., Kurihara, H., Kimura, S., Tomobe, Y. Kobayashi, M., Yazaki, Y., et al. (1988) A Novel Potent Vasoconstrictor Peptide Produced by Vascular Endothelial Cells. *Nature*, **322**, 411–415.
2. Inoue, A., Yanagisawa, M., Kimura, S., Kasuya, Y., Miyauchi, Y., Goto, K., et al. (1989) The Human Endothelin Family: Three Structurally and Pharmacologically Distinct Isopeptides Predicted by Three Separete Genes. *Proceedings of the National Academy of Sciences*, **86**, 2863–2867.
3. Itoh, Y., Yanagisawa, M., Ohkubo, S., Kimura, C., Kosaka, T., Inoue, A., et al. (1988) Cloning and Sequence Analysis of DNA Encoding the Precursor of a Human Endothelin: Identity of Human and Porcine Endothelin. *FEBS Letters*, **231**, 440–444.

4. Onda, H., Ohkubo, S., Ogi, K., Kosaka, T., Kimura, C., Matsumoto, B., et al. (1990) One of the Endothelin Gene Famly Endothelin 3 Gene, is Expressed in the Placenta. *FEBS Letters*, **26**, 327–330.
5. Okada, K., Miyazaki, Y., Takakada, J., Matsuyama, K., Yamaki, T., and Yano, M. (1990) Conversion of Big Endothelin-1 by Membrane-Bound Metalloendopeptidase in Cultured Bovine Endothelial Cells. *Biochemical and Biophysical Research Communications*, **171**, 1192–1198.
6. Sokolovsky, M. (1991) Endothelins and Sarafotoxins: Physiological Regulation, Receptor Subtypes and Transmembrane Signalling, *Trends in Biochemical Sciences*, **16**, 261–264.
7. Saida, K., Mitsui, Y., and Ishida, N. (1989) A Novel Peptide, Vasoactive Intestinal Contractor, of a New (Endothelin) Peptide Family. *Journal of Biological Chemistry*, **264**, 14613–14616.
8. Lundberg, J. M., Ahlborg, G., Hemsén, A., Nisell, H., Lunell, N-O., Pernow, J., et al. (1991) Evidence for Release of ET-1 in Pigs and Humans. *Journal of Cardiovascular Pharmacology*, **17 (Suppl. 7)**, S350–S353.
9. Yanagisawa, M., and Masaki, T. (1989) Molecular Biology and Biochemistry of the Endothelins. *Trends in Pharmacological Science*, **10**, 374–378.
10. Kozuka, M., Ito, T., Hirose, S., Takahashi, K., Hagiwara H. (1989) Endothelin Induces Two Types of Contractions of Rat Uterus: Phasic Contractions by Way of Voltage-Dependent Calcium Channels and Developing Contractions Through a Second Type of Calcium Channel. *Biochemical and Biophysical Research Communications*, **159**, 317–323.
11. Samson, W. K., Skala, K. D., Alexander, B. D., and Huang, F-L. S. (1990) Pituitary Site of Action of Endothelin: Selective inhibition of Prolactin Release *In Vitro*. *Biochemical and Biophysical Research Communications*, **169**, 737–743.
12. DeNucci, G., Thomas, R., D'Orleans-Juste, P., Antunes, E. Walden, C., Warner, T. D., et al. (1988) Pressor Effects of Circulating Endothelin are Limited by its Removal in Pulmonary Circulation and Release of Prostacyclin and Endothelium-Derived Relaxing Factor. *Proceedings of the National Academy of Science*, **85**, 9797–9800.
13. Wilkes, B. M., Mento, P. F., Hollander, A. M., Maita, M. E., Sung, S., and Girardi, E. P. (1990) Endothelin Receptors in Human Placenta: Relationship to Vascular Resistance and Thromboxane Release. *American Journal of Physiology*, **258**, E864–E870.
14. Cameron, I. T., Davenport, A. P., Brown, M. J., and Smith, S. K. (1991) Endothelin-1 Stimulates Prostaglandin $F_{2\alpha}$ Release from Human Endometrium. *Prostaglandins Leucotrienes and Essential Fatty Acids*, **42**, 155–157.
15. Hirata, Y., Yoshimi, H., Takata, S., Watanabe, T. X., Kumagai S., Nakajima, K., et al. (1988) Cellular Mechanism of Action by a Novel Vasoconstrictor Endothelin in Cultured Rat Vascular Smooth Muscle, *Biochemical and Biophysical Research Communications*, **154**, 868–875.
16. Simonson, M. S., Wann, S., Mené, P., Dubyak, G. R., Kester, M., Nakazato, Y., et al. (1989) Endothelin Stimulates Phospholipase C, Na^+/H^+ Exchange, *c-fos* Expression, and Mitogenesis in Rat Mesangial Cells. *Journal of Clinical Investigation*, **83**, 708–712.
17. Takuwa, N., Takuwa, Y., Yanagisawa, M., Yamashita, K., and Masaki, T. (1989) A Novel Vasoactive Peptide Endothelin Stimulates Mitogenesis Through Inositol Lipid Turnover in Swiss 3T3 Fibroblasts. *Journal of Biological Chemistry*, **264**, 7856–7861.
18. Shichiri, M., Hirata, Y., Nakajima, T., Ando, K., Imai, T., Yanagisawa, M., et al. (1991) Endothelin-1 is an Autocrine/Paracrine Growth Factor for Human Cancer Cell Lines. *Journal of Clinical Investigation*, **87**, 1867–1871.
19. Arai, H., Hori, S., Aramori, I., Ohkubo, H. and Nakanishi, S. (1990) Cloning and Expression of a cDNA Encoding an Endothelin Receptor. *Nature*, **348**, 730–732.
20. Sakurai, T., Yanagisawa, M., Takuwa, Y., Miyazaki, H., Kimura, S., Goto, K., et al. (1990) Cloning of a cDNA Encoding a Non-Isopeptide Selective Subtype of the Endothelin Receptor. *Nature*, **348**, 732–735.
21. Vane, J. (1990) Endothelins Come Home to Roost. *Nature*, **348**, 673.
22. O'Reilly, G., Charnock-Jones, D. S., Davenport, A. P., Cameron, I. T., and Smith, S. K. (1992) Presence of Messenger Ribonucleic Acid for Endothelin-1, Endothelin-2 and Endothelin-3 in Human Endometrium and a Change in the Ratio of ET_A and ET_B Receptor Subtype Across the Menstrual Cycle. *Journal of Endocrinology and Metabolism*, **75**, 1545–1549.
23. Mitchell, M. D. (1992) Endothelins in Dysfunctional Uterine Bleeding. In *Steroid Hormones in Uterine Bleeding*, edited by Alexander, N. J. and d'Arcangues, K. pp. 193–200. American Association for the Advancement of Science.
24. Spivak, M. (1943) On the Presence or Absence of Nerves in the Umbilical Vessels of Man and Guinea Pig. *Anatomical Record*, **85**, 85–109.
25. Reilly, F. D. and Russell, P. T. (1977) Neurohistochemical Evidence Supporting an Abscence of Adrenergic and Cholinerigic Innervation in the Human Placenta and Umbilical Cord. *Anatomical Record*, **188**, 277–286.

26. Hemsen, A., Gillis, C., Larsson, O., Haegerstand, A. and Lundberg, J. M. (1991) Characterization, Localization and Actions of Endothelins in Umbilical Vessels and Placenta of Man. *Acta Physiologica Scandinavica*, **143**, 395–404.
27. van Papendorp, C. L., Cameron, I. T., Davenport, A. P., King, A., Barker, P. J., Huskisson, N. S., et al. (1991) Localization and Endogenous Concentration of Endothelin-Like Immunoreactivity in Human Placenta. *Journal of Endocrinology*, **131**, 507–511.
28. Wilkes, B. M., Susin, M. and Mento, P. F. (1993) Localization of Endothelin-1-Like Immunoreactivity in Human Placenta. *Journal of Histochemistry and Cytochemistry*, **41**, 535–541.
29. Gu, J., Pinheiro, J. M. B., Yu, C-Z., D'Andrea, M., Muralidharan, S. and Malik, A. (1991) Detection of Endothelin-Like Immunoreactivity in Epithelium and Fibroblasts of the Human Umbilical Cord. *Tissue and Cell*, **23**, 437–444.
30. Benigni, A., Gaspari, F., Orisio, S., Bellizi, L., Amuso, G., Frusca, T., et al. (1991) Human Placenta Expresses Endothelin Gene and Corresponding Protein is Excreted in Urine in Increasing Amounts During Normal Pregnancy. *American Journal of Obstetrics and Gynecology*, **164**, 844–848.
31. Kubota, T., Kamata, S., Hirata, Y., Eguchi, S., Imai, T., Marumo, F., et al. (1992) Synthesis and Release of Endothelin-1 by Human Decidual Cells. *Journal of Clinical Endocrinology and Metabolism*, **75**, 1230–1234.
32. Casey, M. L., Word, R. A. and MacDonald, P. C. (1991) Endothelin-1 Gene Expression and Regulation of Endothelin mRNA and Protein Biosynthesis in Avascular Human Amnion: Potential Source of Amniotic Fluid Endothelin. *Journal of Biological Chemistry*, **266**, 5762–5768.
33. Sunnergren, K. P., Word, R. A., Stambrook, J. f., MacDonald, P. C. and Casey, M. L. (1990) Expression and Regulation of Endothelin Precursor mRNA in Avascular Human Amnion. *Molecular and Cellular Endocrinology*, **68**, R7–R14.
34. Mitchell, M. D., Ware Branch, D., LaMarche, S. and Dudley, D. J. (1992) The Regulation of Endothelin Production in Human Umbilical Vein Endothelial Cells: Unique Inhibitory Action of Calcium Ionophores. *Journal of Clinical Endocrinology and Metabolism*, **75**, 666–668.
35. Robaut, C., Mondon, F., Bandet, J., Ferre, F. and Cavero, I. (1991) Regional Distribution and Pharmacological Characterization of [^{125}I] Endothelin-1 Binding Sites in Human Fetal Placental Vessels. *Placenta*, **12**, 55–67.
36. Nakajo, S., Sugiura, M. and Inagami, T. (1990) Native Form of Endothelin Receptor in Human Placental Membranes. *Biochemical and Biophysical Research Communications*, **167**, 280–286.
37. Wada, K., Tabuchi, H., Ohba, R., Satoh, M., Tachibana, Y., Akiyama, N., et al. Purification of an Endothelin Receptor from Human Placenta. *Biochemical and Biophysical Research Communications*, **167**, 251–257.
38. Takasuka, T., Horii, I., Furuichi, Y. and Watanabe, T. (1991) Detection of an Endothelin-1 Binding Protein Complex by Low Temperature SDS-PAGE. *Biochemical and Biophysical Research Communications*, **176**, 392–400.
39. Kalina, B. and Löffler, B-M. (1992) Crosslinking Analysis of an Endothelin Receptor Protein from Human Placenta. *Biochemistry International*, **27**, 735–744.
40. Fischli, W., Clozel, M. and Guilly, C. (1989) Specific Receptors for Endothelin on Membranes from Human Placenta. Characterization and Use in a Binding Assay. *Life Sciences*, **44**, 1429–1436.
41. Iwata, J., Takagi, T., Yamaji, K. and Tanizawa, O. (1991) Increase in the Concentration of Immunoreactive Endothelin in Human Pregnancy. *Journal of Endocrinology*, **129**, 301–307.
42. Usuki, S., Saitoh, T., Sawamura, T., Suzuki, N., Shigemitsu, S., Yanagisawa, M., et al. (1990) Increased Maternal Plasma Concentration of Endothelin-1 During Labor Pain or at Delivery and the Existence of a Large Amount of Endothelin-1 in Amniotic Fluid. *Gynecologic Endocrinology*, **4**, 85–97.
43. Hakkinen, L. M., Vuolteenaho, O. J., Leppaluoto, J. P., and Laatikainen, T. J. (1992) Endothelin in Maternal and Umbilical Cord Blood in Spontaneous Labor and at Elective C/S Delivery. *Obstetrics and Gynecology*, **80**, 72–75.
44. Nakamura, T., Kasai, K., Konuma, S., Emoto, T., Banba, N., Ishikawa, M., et al. (1990) Immunoreactive Endothelin Concentrations in Maternal and Fetal Blood. *Life Sciences*, **46**, 1045–1050.
45. Nisell, H., Hemsén, A., Lunell, N-O., Wolff, K., and Lundberg, M. J. (1990) Maternal and Fetal Levels of a Novel Polypeptide, Endothelin: Evidence for Release During Pregnancy and Delivery. *Gynecological and Obstetrical Investigations*, **30**, 129–132.
46. Isozaki-Fukuda, Y., Kojima, T., Hirata, Y., Ono, A., Sawaragi, S., Sawaragi, I., et al. (1991) Plasma Immunoreactive ET-1 Concentration in Human Fetal Blood. *Pediatric Research*, **30**, 244–247.
47. Hashiguchi, K., Takagi, K., Nakabayashi, M., Takeda, Y., Sakamoto, S. Naruse, M., et al. (1991) Relationship Between Fetal Hypoxia and Et-1 in Fetal Circulation. *Journal of Cardiovascular Pharmacology*, **17 (Suppl. 7)**, S509–S510.
48. Eis, A. W., Mitchell, M. D. and Myatt, L. (1992) Endothelin Transfer and Endothelin Effects on Water Transfer in Human Fetal Membranes. *Obstetrics and Gynecology*, **79**, 411–415.

49. Romero, R., Avila, C. A., Edwin, S. S. and Mitchell, M. D. (1992) Endothelin-1, 2 Levels are Increased in the Amniotic Fluid of Women with Preterm Labor and Microbial Invasion of the Amniotic Cavity. *American Journal of Obstetrics and Gynecology*, **166**, 95–99.
50. Mitchell, M. D., Lundin-Schiller, S. and Edwin, S. S. (1991) Endothelin Production by Amnion and its Regulations by Cytokines. *American Journal of Obstetrics and Gynecology*, **165**, 120–124.
51. Mitchell, M. D., Romero, R. J., Lepara, R., Rittenhouse, L. and Edwin, S. S. (1992) Actions of Endothelin-1 on Prostaglandin Production by Gestational Tissues. *Prostaglandins*, **40**, 627–635.
52. Raboni, S., Folli, M. C., Bresciani, D., Bacchi, Modena, A., and Merialdi, A. (1990) Amniotic Endothelin Increases During Pregnancy. *American Journal of Obstetircs and Gynecology*, **164**, 237.
53. Fant, M. E., Nanu, L. an Word, R. A. (1992) A Potential Role for Endothelin-1 in Human Placental Growth: Interactions with the Insulin-Like Growth Factor Family of Peptides. *Journal of Clinical Endocrinology and Metabolism*, **74**, 1158–1163.
54. Wagner, O. F., Christ, G., Wojta, J., Vierhapper, H., Parzer, S., Nowotny, P. J., et al. (1992) Polar Secretion of Endothelin-1 by Cultured Endothelial Cells. *Journal of Biological Chemistry*, **267**, 16066–16088.
55. Pohl, U. and Busse, R. (1989) Differential Vascular Sensitivity to Luminally and Adventitially Applied Endothelin-1. *Journal of Cardiovascular Pharmacology*, **13 (Suppl 5)**, S188–S190.
56. Myatt, L., Brewer, A., LaMarche, S. and Mitchell, M. D. (1992) Pulsatile Release of Endothelin by the Perfused Human Placenta. In *Proceedings of the Thirty-Ninth Annual Meeting of the Society for Gynecologic Investigation*, San Antonio, TX, Abstract 65, p. 141.
57. Gude, N. M., King, R. G. and Brennecke, S. P. (1991) Endothelin: Release by the Potent Constrictor Effect on the Fetal Vessels of Human Perfused Placental Lobules. *Reproduction, Fertility, and Development*, **3**, 495–500.
58. Myatt, L., Langdon, G., Brewer, A. S. and Brockman, D. E. (1991) Endothelin-1-Induced Vasoconstriction is not Mediated by Thromboxane Release and Action in the Human Fetal-Placental Circulation. *American Journal of Obstetrics and Gynecology*, **165**, 1717–1722.
59. Myatt, L., Brewer, A. S. and Brockman, D. E. (1992) the Comparative Effects of Big Endothelin-1, Endothelin-1 and Endothelin-3 in the Human Fetal-Placental Circulation. *American Journal of Obstetrics and Gynecology*, **167**, 1651–1656.
60. Filep, J. G., Battistini, B. and Sirois, P. (1990) Endothelin Induces Thromboxane release and constriction of Isolated Guinea Pig Airways. *Life Sciences*, **47**, 1845–1850.
61. Takayasu-Okishio, M., Terashita, Z-I. and Kondo, K. (1990) Endothelin-1 and Platelet Activating Factor Stimulate Thromboxane A_2 Biosynthesis in Rat Vascular smooth Muscle Cells. *Biochemical Pharmacology*, **40**, 2713–2717.
62. McKay, K. O., Black, J. L. and Armour, C. L. (1991) The Mechanism of Action of Endothelin in Human Lung. *British Journal of Pharmacology*, **102**, 422–428.
63. Myatt, L., Brewer, A. S., Langdon, G. and Brockman, D. E. (1992) Attenuation of the Vasoconstrictor Effects of Thromboxane and Endothelin by Nitric Oxide in the Human Fetal-Placental Circulation. *American Journal of Obstetrics and Gynecology*, **166**, 224–230.
64. Mitchell, M. D. (1986) Pathways of Arachidonic Acid Metabolism with Specific Application to the Mother and Fetus. *Seminars in Perinatology*, **10**, 242.
65. Parisi, V. M. and Walsh, S. W. (1986) Arachidonic Acid Metabolites and the Regulation of Placental and Other Vascular Tone During Pregnancy. *Seminars in Perinatology*, **10**, 288.
66. Glance, D. G., Elder, M. G. and Myatt, L. (1986) The Actions of Prostaglandins and Their Interactions with Angiotensin II in the Isolated Perfused Human Placental Cotyledon. *British Journal of Obstetrics and Gynecology*, **93**, 488–494.
67. Cao, L. and Banks, R. O. (1990) Cardiorenal Actions of Endothelin, Part II: Effects of Cyclooxygenase Inhibitors, *Life Sciences*, **46**, 585–590.
68. MacLean, M. R., Templeton, A. G. B. and McGrath, J. C. (1992) The Influence of Endothelin-1 on Human Foeto-Placental Blood Vessels: A Comparison with 5-Hydroxytryptamine. *British Journal of Obstetrics and Gynecology*, **106**, 937–941.
69. Clark, B. A., Halvorson, L., Sachs, B. and Epstein, F. H. (1992) Plasma Endothelin Levels in Preeclampsia: Elevation and Correlation with Uric Acid Levels and Renal Impairment. *American Journal of Obstetrics and Gynecology*, **166**, 962–968.
70. Ihara, Y., Sagawa, N., Hasegawa, M., Okagaki, A., Li, M., Inamori, K., et al. (1991) *Journal of Cardiovascular Pharmacology*, **17 (Suppl 7)**, S443–S445.
71. Kamol, K., Sudo, N., Ishibasi, M. and Yamaji, T. (1990) Plasma Endothelin-1 Levels in Patients with Pregnancy-Induced Hypertension. *New England Journal of Medicine*, **323**, 1486–1487.
72. Florijn, K. W., Derkx, F. H. M., Visser, W., Hofman, J. A., Rosmalen, F. M. A., Wallenberg, H. C. S., et al. (1991) Plasma Immunoreactive Endothelin-1 in Pregnant Women with and without Preeclampsia. *Journal of Cardiovascular Pharmacology*, **17 (Suppl 7)**, S446–S448.
73. Dekker, G., Kraayenbrink, A. A., Zeeman, G. and vanKamp, G. J. (1991) Increased Plasma Levels of

the Novel Vasoconstrictor Peptide Endothelin in Severe Preeclampsia. *European Journal of Obstetrics and Gynecology and Reproductive Biology*, **40**, 215–220.
74. Mastrogiannis, D. S., O'Brien, W. F., Krammer, J. and Benoit, R. (1991) Potential Role of Endothelin-1 in Normal and Hypertensive Pregnancies. *Journal of Obststrics and Gynecology*, **165**, 1711–1716.
75. Nisell, H., Wolff, K., Hemsén, A., Lindblom, B., Lunell, N-O. and Lundberg, J. M. (1991) Endothelin, a Vasoconstrictor Important to the Uteroplacental Circulation in Preeclampsia. *Journal of Hypertension*, **9 (Suppl 6)**, S168–S169.
76. Otani, S., Usuki, S., Saitoh, T., Yanagisawa, M., Iwasaki, H., Tanaka, J., *et al.* (1991) Comparison of Endothelin-1 Concentrations in Normal and Complicated Pregnancies. *Journal of Cardiovascular Pharmacology*, **17 (Suppl 7)**, S308–S312.
77. Benigni, A., Orisio, S., Gaspari, F., Frusca, T., Amuso, G. and Remuzzi, G. (1992) Evidence Against a Pathogenic Role for Endothelin in Pre-Eccelampsia. *British Journal of Obstetrics and Gynecology*, **99**, 798–802.
78. Consigny, P. M. (1990) Endothelin-1 Increased Arterial Sensitivity to 5-Hydroxytryptamine. *European Journal of Pharmacology*, **186**, 239–245.
79. Yang, Z., Richard, V., vasSegesser, L., Bauer, E., Schulz, P., Turina, M. and Lüscher, T. F. (1990) Threshold Concentrations of Endothelin-1 Potentiate Contractions to Norepinephrine and Serotonin in Human Arteries. A New Method of Vasospasm. *Circulation*, **82**, 188–195.
80. Nova, A., Sibai, B. M., Barton, J. R., Mercer, B. M. and Mitchell, M. D. (1991) Maternal Plasma Level of Endothelin is Increased in Preeclampsia. *American Journal of Obstetrics and Gynecology*, **165**, 724–727.
81. Florijn, K. W., Derkx, F. H. M., Visser, W., Hofman, H. J. A., Rosmalen, F. M. A., Wallenberg, H. C. S., *et al.* (1991) Elevated Plasma Levels of Endothelin in Pre-Eclampsia. *Journal of Hypertension*, **9 (Suppl 6)**, S166–S167.
82. Taylor, R. N., Varma, M., Teng, N. N. H. and Roberts, J. M. (1990) Women with Preeclampsia Have Higher Plasma Endothelin Levels than Women with Normal Pregnancies. *Journal of Clinical Endocrinology and Metabolism*, **71**, 1675–1677.
83. Kohno, M., Yasunari, K., Murakawa, K-I., Yokokawa, K., Horio, T., Fukui, T., *et al.* (1990) Plasma Immunoreactive Endothelin in Essential Hypertension. *American Journal of Medicine*, **88**, 614–618.
84. Greer, I. A., Leask, R., Hodson, B. A., Dawes, J., Kilpatrick, D. C. and Liston, W. D. (1991) Endothelin Elastase, and Endothelial Dysfunction in Pre-Eclampsia. *The Lancet*, **337**, 558.
85. Lumme, R., Laatikainen, t., Vuolteenaho, O. and Leppaluoto, J. (1992) Plasma Endothelin, Atrial Natriuretic Peptide (ANP) and Uterine and umbilical Artery Flow Velocity Waveforms in Hypertensive Pregnancies. *British Journal of Obstetrics and Gynecology*, **99**, 761–764.
86. Hartikainen-Sorri, A-L., Vuolteenaho, O., Leppäluoto, J. and Ruskoaho, H. (1991) Endothelin in Umbilical Artery Vasospasm. *The Lancet*, **337**, 619.
87. Malee, M. P., Malee, K. M., Azuma, S. D., Taylor, R. N. and Roberts, J. M. (1992) Increase in Plasma Atrial Natriuretic Peptide Concentration Antedate Clinical Evidence of Pre-eclampsia. *Journal of Clinical Endocrinology and Metabolism*, **74**, 1095–1100.
88. Perico, N., Dadan, J., Gabanelli, M. and Remuzzi, G. (1989) Cyclooxigenase Products and Atrial Natriuretic Peptide Modulate Renal Response to Endothelin. *Journal of Pharmacology and Experimental Therapeutics*, **252**, 1213–1220.
89. Markee, J. E. (1940) Menstruation in Intraocular Endometrial Transplants in the Rhesus Monkey. *Contributions to Embryology, Carnegie Institution*, **28**, 219–308.
90. Christiaens, G. C. M. L., Sixma, J. J. and Haspels, A. A. (1980) Morphology of Haemostasis in Menstrual Endometrium. *British Journal of Obstetrics and Gynecology*, **87**, 425–439.
91. Casey, M. L., Smith, J. W., Nagai, K., Hersh, L. B. and MacDonald, P. C. (1991) Progesterone-Regulated Cyclic Modulation of Membrane Metallopeptidase (Enkephalinase) in Human Endometrium. *Journal of Biological Chemistry*, **266**, 23041–23047.
92. Cameron, I. T., Davenport, A. P., van Papendorp, C., Barker, P. J., Huskisson, N. S., Gilmour, R. S., *et al.* (1992) Endothelin-like Immunoreactivity in Human Endometrium. *Journal of Reproduction and Fertility*, **95**, 623–628.
93. Salamonsen, L. A., Buff, A. R., Macpherson, A. M., Rogers, P. A. W. and Findlay, J. K. (1992) Immunolocalization of the Vasoconstrictor Endothelin in Human Endometrium During the Menstrual Cycle and in Umbilical Cord at Birth. *American Journal of Obstetrics and Gynecology*, **167**, 163–167.
94. Svane, D., Larsson, B., Alm, P., Andersson, K-A. and Forman, a. (1993) Endothelin-1: Immunocytochemistry, Localization of Binding Sites, and Contractile Effects in Human Uteroplacental Smooth Muscle. *American Journal of Obstetrics and Gynecology*, **168**, 233–241.
95. Maggi, M., Vanelli, G. B., Peri, A., Brandi, M. L., Fantoni, G., Gianni, S., *et al.* (1991) Immunolocaliza-

tion, Binding, and Biological Activity of Endothelin in Rabbit Uterus: Effect of Ovarian Steroids. *American Journal of Physiology*, **260**, E292–E305.

96. Economos, K., MacDonald, P. C. and Casey, M. L. (1992) Endothelin-1 Gene Expression and Protein Biosynthesis in Human Endometrium: Potential Modulator of Endometrial Blood flow. *Journal of Clinical Endocrinology and Metabolism*, **74**, 14–19.

97. Davenport, A. P., Cameron, I. T., Smith, S. K. and Brown, M. J. (1990) Binding Sites for Iodinated Endothelin-1, Endothelin-2 and Endothelin-3 Demonstrated on Human Uterine Glandular Epithelial Cells by Quantitative High-Resolution Autoradiography. *Journal of Endocrinology*, **129**, 149–154.

98. Bodelsson, G., Sjoberg, N-O. and Stjernquist, M. (1992) Contractile Effect of Endothelin in the Human Uterine Artery and Audioradiographic Localization of its Binding Sites. *American Journal of Obstetrics and Gynecology*, **167**, 745–750.

99. Williams, D. L., Jones, K. L., Colton, C. D. and Nutt, R. F. (1991) Identification of High Affinity Endothelin-1 Receptor Subtypes in Human Tissues. *Biochemical and Biophysical Research Communications*, **180**, 475–480.

100. Kimura, T., Azuma, C., Saji, F., Tokugawa, Y., Takemura, M., Miki, M., et al. (1992) Functional expression of Human Myometrial Endothelin Receptors in *Xenopus laevis* Oocytes. *ACTA Endocrinologica*, **126**, 64–66.

101. Lindblom, B., Lundberg, J. M., Lunell, N-O., Nisell, H., Norén, H. and Wolff, K. (1991) Endothelin-1 a Potent Constrictor of Small Myometrial Arteries of Term Pregnant Women. *Acta Obstetrica Gynecologica Scandanavica*, **70**, 267–270.

102. Fried, G., and Samuelson, U. (1991) Endothelin and Neuropeptide Y are Vasoconstrictors in Human Uterine Blood Vessels. *American Journal of Obstetrics and Gynecology*, **164**, 1330–1336.

103. Word, R. A., Kamm, K. E. and Casey, M. L. (1992) Contractile Effects of Prostaglandins, Oxytocin, and Endothelin-1 in Human Myometrium *In Vitro*: Refractoriness of Myometrial Tissue of Pregnant Women to Prostaglandins E_2 and $E_{2\alpha}$. *Journal of Clinical Endocrinology and Metabolism^2*, **75**, 1027–1032.

104. Maher, E., Bardequez, A., Gardner, J. P., Goldsmith, L., Weiss, G., Mascarina, M., et al. (1991) Endothelin- and Oxytocin-Induced Calcium Signalling in Cultured Human Myometrial Cells. *Journal of Clinical Investigation*, **87**, 1251–1258.

105. Word, R. A., Kamm, K. E., Stull, J. T. and Casey, M. L. (1990) Endothelin Increases Cytoplasmic Calcium and Myosin Phosphorylation in Human Myometrium. *American Journal of Obstetrics and Gynecology*, **162**, 1603–1608.

106. Ahmed, A., Cameron, I. T., Ferriani, R. A. and Smith, S. K. (1992) Activation of Phospholipase A_2 and Phospholipase C by Endothelin-1 in Human Endometrium. *Journal of Endocrinology*, **135**, 383–390.

107. Cernacek, P. and Stewart, D. J. (1989) Immunoreactive Endothelin in Human Plasma: Marked Elevations in Patients in Cardiogenic Shock. *Biochemical and Biophysical Research Communications*, **161**, 5626–5627.

108. Murch, S. H., Braegger, C. P., Sessa, W. C. and MacDonald, T. T. (1992) High Endothelin-1 Immunoreactivity in Crohn's Disease and Ulcerative Colitis. *The Lancet*, **339**, 381–385.

109. Siegler, R. L., Edwin, S. S., Christoffersen, R. D. and Mitchell, M. D. (1991) Endothelin in the Urine of Children with Hemolytic Uremic Syndrome. *Pediatrics*, **88**, 1063–1066.

19 Role of Endothelins in Neonatology

Ravi S. Iyer and Rama Bhat

Department of Pediatrics (M/C 856), University of Illinois at Chicago, 840 S. Wood Street, Chicago, IL 60612, USA

The vascular endothelium synthesizes a number of active substances such as prostacyclin, nitric oxide, endothelin (ET), interleukin, etc. They have various actions including vasodilation (prostacyclin and nitric oxide) and vasoconstriction (ET). Between them they maintain the vascular tone and play a major role in the regulation of blood pressure. Experiments with isolated canine arteries and veins show that hypoxia, transmural pressure and vascular stretch elicits endothelium dependent contraction[1]. Yanagisawa and co-workers isolated the peptide (ET-1) responsible for this contraction[2]. Though ET was originally thought to be synthesized and secreted exclusively by endothelium, later experiments show that it is secreted by a wide variety of tissue cells including kidney, liver, heart, gut, eye, adrenals, central and peripheral nervous systems[3]. Many of the actions of ET are from its vasoactive properties. However, there are also other actions independent of alterations in vascular tone. These actions may be short term (contraction, secretion) or may result in long term adaptive responses (mitogenesis, hypertrophy). ET appears to act both centrally and peripherally to regulate physiological events. The role of ET-1 on the regulation of blood flow to various vascular beds has been studied in adult animal models. However there is very little information on its role in the regulation of immature and mature newborn vascular system. In this review we have attempted to summarize the published studies on ET-1 in the neonatal period.

CARDIOVASCULAR EFFECTS

ET produces a sustained vasoconstriction in the mesentric, pulmonary and coronary arteries of several species, including humans[5,6]. The pulmonary and coronary vasoconstrictor effects of ET are diminished by cyclooxygenase blockade with indomethacin *in vitro* in guinea pigs[7,8]. Its coronary vasoconstrictor action in other species (e.g., pigs) is attenuated only by calcium-channel blockade[9]. In piglets less than 10 days of age, Bradley *et al.* evaluated the circulatory effects of ET in the presence of hypoxia and the extent to which ET action could be modified by indomethacin with cyclooxygenase inhibition *in vivo*[10]. They found a decrease in pulmonary vascular resistance index (PVRI) and increase in coronary blood flow with low dose (100 pmol/kg) intravenous bolus administration of ET. There was no change in coronary vascular resistance or cardiac index. The pulmonary and coronary vascular responses to ET were preserved during hypoxia. Low dose ET moderately increased mean arterial pressure (MAP) and systemic vascular resistance index (SVRI). High dose (1000 pmol/kg) ET mildly decreased PVRI, moderately increased SVRI and markedly decreased coronary blood flow. Left ventricular end-diastolic pressure increased and shortening fraction fell in response to high dose ET. Pretreatment with indomethacin did not significantly alter either the pulmonary or coronay vascular responses to low-dose ET but completely prevented high–dose ET induced coronary vasoconstriction and left ventricular dysfunction. It is possible that cyclooxygenase products are unlikely to exclusively mediate ET-induced vasodilation but may play a role in ET induced vasoconstriction in newborn piglets.

With injection of ET-1 (500 ng/kg) into the pulmonary artery, Krzeski *et al.* found a transient decrease in mean pulmonary artery pressure and a biphasic change (initial decline followed by substantial increase) in pulmonary vascular resistance[11]. They also found in increase in systemic vascular resistance and an initial increase in cardic output followed by a decrease (Table 19.1).

These responses are different from those observed in adult species where a biphasic systemic vascular response with a transient hypotension followed by a prolonged hypertensive phase occurs. The initial phase is due to a decrease in peripheral vascular resistance and a minimal change in cardiac index. These findings indicate a developmental difference in the response of pulmonary circulation to ET-1.

The most striking property of ET-1 is its long lasting vasoconstrictor action[2]. ET-1 has a vasoconstrictor potency 10 times that of angiotensin II. After a single intravenous injection into pithed or chemically denervated rats, the blood pressure was elevated for more than 1 hour. The greatest increases in peripheral resistance by ET-1 occurred in mesenteric, renal and hindquarters vascular beds. ET-1 was quickly eliminated from

Table 19.1 Maximal lowest & highest changes in hemodynamic parameters (mean ± SD) from baseline after administration of endothelin-1 (ET-1, 500 ng/kg) into the pulmonary artery (with permission from Krzeski *et al.*)[11]

	Control value before ET-1 injection	Lowest value after ET-1 injection	Highest value after ET-1 injection	n
AoP	76 ± 15	70 ± 14*	86 ± 16***	6
PAP	22 ± 7	18 ± 5***	22 ± 6	6
CO	0.39 ± 0.12	0.33 ± 0.11***	0.43 ± 0.14*	6
PVR	4,390 ± 1,994	3,826 ± 1,820***	5,875 ± 3,114*	6
SVR	15,692 ± 6,349	Not observed	22,076 ± 9,919**	6
HR	220 ± 46	210 ± 43	206 ± 42	6

n, number of animals.
AoP, aortic blood pressure (mm Hg); PAP, pulmonary artery pressure (mm Hg); CO, cardiac output (L/min); PVR, pulmonary vascular resistance (dyn cm/s^5); SVR, systemic vascular resistance (dyn cm/s^5); HR, heart rate (beats/min).
*$p < 0.05$, **$p < 0.005$, ***$p < 0.001$.

blood stream with 60% disappearing after 1 minute with high uptake in lung, kidney and liver[12]. Recent studies from our laboratory in 7–10 day old piglets showed a plasma half-life of 2.1 ± 0.4 minutes[13]. The potent vasoconstrictor action taken together with raised plasma levels detected in patients with myocardial infraction, pulmonary and essential hypertension may argue for involvement of ET-1 in hypertensive states. Tomobe et al. reported increased sensitivity of renal arterary segments in spontaneously hypertensive rats[14]. We determined ET-1 levels in various brain regions, heart and thoracic aorta of spontaneously hypertensive (SHR) and normotensive Wistar Kyoto (WKY) rats from 1 to 8 weeks of age. In both SHR and WKY rats ET-1 levels in brain areas increased with age. However at 8 weeks of age levels were significantly lower in SHR rats when compared to WKY rats. In the aorta and heart of SHR rats ET-1 levels were significantly higher at 8 weeks of age as compared to WKY rats[15]. An altered expression of ET-1 in the blood vessels and myocardium of SHR rats may be contributing to the onset of hypertension.

ROLE OF ET IN CONSTRICTION OF DUCTUS ARTERIOSUS

Coceani and co-workers have shown that ET-1 is a powerful constrictor of the ductus arteriosus in vitro[16]. They have also shown that ET-1 is formed within the ductus, including the muscle layer[17]. They studied the role of ET-1 in the closure of ductus arteriosus by measuring the in vitro release of the peptide under conditions of oxygenation mimicking the fetal versus neonatal state. They also examined the ability of isolated ductus arteriosus to constrict in the presence of oxygen after treatment with inhibitors of ET synthesis (phosphoramidon) and receptor antagonist (BQ-123)[18]. They found an increase in ET-1 release with increasing concentration of oxygen up to a value mimicking the neonatal condition. Phosphoramidon and BQ-123 inhibited the contraction of the ductus to oxygen. These experiments suggest ET-1 as the effector agent for oxygen in the ductus and may play a critical role in closure of ductus at birth. Further studies are needed to examine the role of ET-1 in the closure of ducts arteriosus.

CEREBRAL MICROCIRCULATION

Armstead et al. studied the response of newborn pig cerebral microcirculation to ET[19]. Pial arterioles were observed directly using a closed cranial window. ET was applied topically. At lower concentrations ET produced an increase in pial arteriolar diameter whereas higher concentration produced a decrease in pial arteriolar diameter. Indomethacin and aspirin blocked the dilator responses and attenuated the constrictor responses. ET also produced concentration-dependent increase in the CSF levels of 6-ketoprostaglandin $F_{1\alpha}$, PGE_2, $PGF_{2\alpha}$ and thromboxane B_2. Thus ET can produce either dilation or constriction of cerebral arterioles in newborn pigs, depending on its concentration. At low concentrations ET appears to mediate vasodilation via prostanoids and at high concentrations produces vasoconstriction. In adult animals mechanisms other than prostaglandin have been described.

Pial vessels are important resistance vessels in the cerebral circulation. The effect of ET with prostanoids in changing the conductance in these vessels could be an important contribution to the regulation of cerebrovascular tone in piglets.

RENAL EFFECTS

The effects of ET on renal function have been well described in adult animals: a bolus injection of ET induced a slow-developing and long-lasting vasoconstriction of afferent and efferent arterioles that led to a dramatic decrease in renal blood flow (RBF) and glomerular filtration rate (GFR)[20,21].

Semama et al. conducted a study on newborn rabbits to evaluate the renal actions of ET[22]. They observed the changes in RBF, GFR, mean blood pressure (MBP), renal vascular resistance (RVR), urine flow rate (V), urinary sodium extraction (UNa) and filtration fraction (FF) with 1 and 5 nmol/kg of ET given as a bolus injection. Lower doses of ET did not induce any changes in MBP but the higher dose (5 nmol/kg) caused an initial fall followed by a gradual but significant increase. The MBP remained elevated for 45 minutes after injection. The initial fall in MBP may be due to the release of nitric oxide induced by exogenous ET[23]. Renal hemodynamics did not change significantly with the injection of 1 nmol/kg of ET. It however significantly increased sodium excretion during second half hour of the experiment. When 5 nmol/kg of ET was injected V, GFR, RBF and FF did not change significantly in the first 30 minutes of the experiment whereas RVR increased by $40 \pm 9\%$ (Table 19.2). In the second 30 minutes GFR and RBF decreased significantly and UNa increased markedly. RVR remained elevated. The diuretic effect of ET is probably due to increased salt excretion or inhibition of arginine vasopressin-stimulated osmotic water permeability in collecting ducts. RVR was markedly elevated by ET injection. As this was not related to the MBP a local action of ET on renal efferent arterioles may be responsible. GFR and RBF did not change despite the high RVR probably because the high BP maintained blood flow and filtration through constricted vessels. A low dose (1 nmol/kg) of ET usually induces severe renal and systemic vasoconstriction in adult models. Failure of such a response in the newborn rabbit may be due to receptor immaturity or interference of counteracting hormones.

Table 19.2. Effects of ET on renal hemodynamics and water and sodium excretion in group 1 (1 nmol/kg) and group 2 (5 nmol/kg) (with permission from Semama et al.)[22]

Group	Period	U_{Na} (μmol·kg^{-1}·min^{-1})	GFR (mL·kg^{-1}·min^{-1})	RBF (mL·kg^{-1}·min^{-1})	RVR (mm Hg·mL^{-1}·kg·min)
1	Control	2.02 ± 0.61	2.13 ± 0.18	20.3 ± 2.1	1.91 ± 0.12
	I	2.71 ± 0.94	2.26 ± 0.22	20.2 ± 2.5	2.03 ± 0.17
	II	3.01 ± 0.90*	1.95 ± 0.22	20.3 ± 3.7	2.13 ± 0.27
2	Control	5.48 ± 1.74	2.17 ± 0.22	21.0 ± 1.8	1.69 ± 0.10
	I	4.93 ± 0.88	2.06 ± 0.18	18.8 ± 1.6	2.35 ± 0.17†
	II	7.24 ± 1.91†	1.95 ± 0.26*	17.7 ± 1.7†	2.16 ± 0.13‡

* $p < 0.05$ significant difference when comparing values with the control period of the same group.
† $p < 0.01$, significant difference when comparing values with the control period of the same group.
‡ $P < 0.001$ significant difference when comparing values with the control period of the same group.

Table 19.3 Mean ± SD in the 100 ng/kg/min ET infusion group

Periods	RBF	RVR	GFR	UV	FE_{Na}	ET-1
Baseline	1.26 ± 0.12	5.76 ± 0.6	0.24 ± 0.02	0.13 ± 0.01	0.4 ± 0.13	24 ± 1
ET-1	0.25 ± 0.17*	39.7 ± 11*	0.05 ± 0.02*	0.03 ± 0.01*	0.3 ± 0.1*	1655 ± 85
60 min	0.91 ± 0.21	7.6 ± 1	0.26 ± 0.02	0.08 ± 0.01	0.25 ± 0.01	17 ± 2

GFR: ml/min/G kidney, RVR: mmHg/ml/min, ET-1: pmol/L, RBF: ml/min/G kidney UV: ml/min, FE_{Na}: % *vs baseline p < 0.005.

We examined the effects of 25, 50 and 100 ng/kg/min of ET-1 infusion on MBP, GFR, RBF, urine volume (UV) and cardiac index (CI) in 7–10 day old piglets. ET-1 produced a dose dependent decrease in CI, RBF, GFR and a 15–17% increase in MBP. These changes returned to 75–80% of baseline by 60 minutes after discontinuation of ET-1. Low dose (25 ng/kg/min) infusion of ET-1 did not result in any changes in systemic or renal hemodynamics (Table 19.3).

Pretreatment with specific ET_A receptor antagonist BQ-123 completely blocked the ET-1 induced systemic and renal hemodynamic changes. Indomethacin pretreatment failed to block any ET-1 induced changes. These results indicate that in piglets renal vascular bed is highly sensitive to ET-1 and its effects are predominantly mediated through ETA receptors[13].

Plasma atrial natriuretic factor (ANF) measured in neonates showed a good correlation with plasma ET-1 levels[24]. ANF may compensate for the effect of ET-1 during the neonatal period, thus reflecting one of the adaptive mechanisms to maintain body sodium and fluid and peripheral vascular resistance during the period of transition from fetal to postnatal life. Endogenous ET may act in concert with renin-aldosterone system to regulate vascular tone and blood pressure during postnatal life.

ENDOTHELIN IN PREGNANCY

ET may act to affect the mechanism of parturition either directly via an action on myometrium or indirectly through modulation of secretion or function of other uterotonic agents. A direct action is highly effective since ET-1 is highly potent in its action to increase intracellular calcium concentrations and phosphorylation of myosin light chain in myometrial smooth muscle cells[25]. ET may stimulate biosynthesis of prostaglandin and indirectly induce uterine contractions[26]. ET-1 is known to be a potent oxytocic agent on rat[27] and human[25] myometrium. ET has been found in the supraoptic and paraventricular nuclei, posterior pituitary and plays a role in the release of vasopressin[28,29]. Stojilkovic et al. demonstrated that ET releases luteinizing hormone (LH) and follicle-stimulating hormone (FSH) from the anterior pituitary cells that respond mostly to gonadotropin releasing hormone[30]. Cultured human breast epithelial cells express the ETmRNA and this is enhanced 20-fold after prolactin stimulation[31.] It is speculated that ET may affect the process of parturition and lacation indirectly via induced oxytocin release.

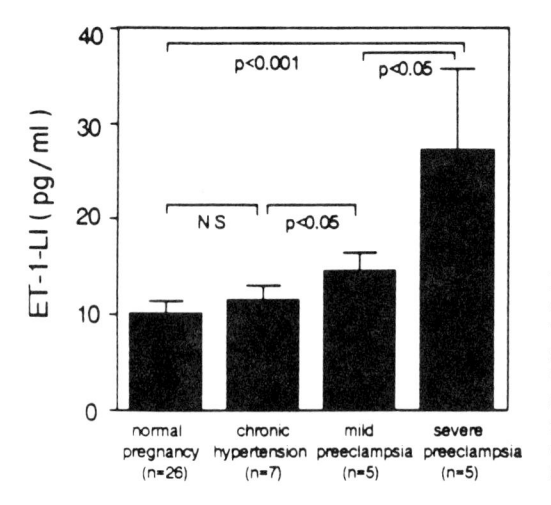

Figure 19.1. Comparison between concentrations of ET-1 in the plasma of normotensive and hypertensive women. ET-1 in the plasma of both mild and severe preeclampsia was significantly higher than in that of normotensive pregnant women with chronic hypertension were not higher than those of normotensive women unless the hypertension was aggravated during pregnancy. (With permission from Ihara et al.)[32].

Ihara and co-workers measured ET-1 material and cord blood at various stages of pregnancy[32.] ET levels did not change significantly throughout normal pregnancy and were comparable to those of non-pregnant women. Levels of ET-1 in umbilical vessels obtained at normal term deliveries were three times higher than maternal levels. In patients with mild and severe pre-eclampsia, the levels of plasma ET-1 were significantly higher than those of normal pregnancy (27.2 ± 8.6 pg/ml and $14.3 + 2.2$ pg/ml). Two pregnant women with DIC had extremely high ET-1 levels which gradually returned to normal with normalization of coagulation process (Figure 19.1).

However Otani and co-workers compared ET-1 concentrations in normal and complicated pregnancies and noted no significant difference in plasma ET-1 concentration between normal and toxemic pregnancy[33.] There was also no correlation between ET-1 concentration, blood pressure or renal functions during toxemic pregnancy. Damage to endothelial cells and disturbance of microcirculation may stimulate the release of ET-1. A decreased clearance of ET-1 from the kidneys of preeclamptic women also may be responsible for high levels of ET-1.

ENDOTHELIN IN THE FETUS

Many factors regulate pulmonary blood flow at the time of birth. The oxygen environment plays an important role, as does the local release of vasoactive substances such as bradykinin, eicosanoids (PGI_2 and PGD_2), EDRF (NO) and ET. ET by itself can stimulate not only secretion of vasodilator substances such as endothelium derived relaxing factor and prostacyclin but also secretion of vasoconstrictor substances such as thromboxane A_2[12]. ET has been demonstrated in late-gestation fetal rat lungs[34] and is vasoactive in the fetus[35,36]. Its physiologic role in the lung is unknown. It has been speculated that ET-1 may contribute to the high pulmonary vascular resistance in the fetus. Kojima et al. studied the changes in blood immunoreactive ET from birth (cord

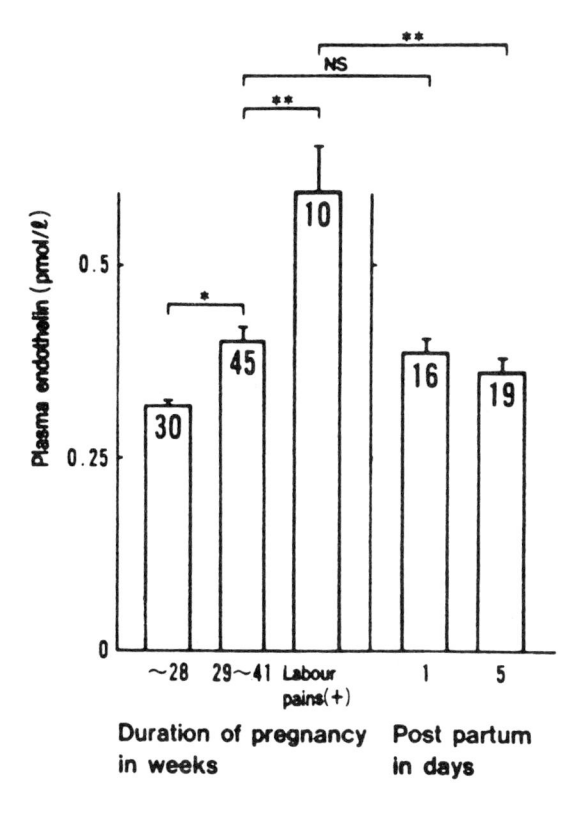

Figure 19.2. Changes in the level of the immunoreactive ET-1 in maternal blood during gestation, labor and in the postpartum. The number in each group indicates the number of samples. *P < 0.05; **P < 0.02 (With permission from Usuki et al.)[47].

blood) through the first month of life[24]. They found plasma irET-1 levels in newborn infants were far greater than those in maternal blood. The highest levels were observed on first day of life (8.7 ± 3.7 pmol/l) which gradually decreased with increasing postnatal age. There was no significant difference in irET-1 levels between preterm and fullterm infants. Adult levels were reached by 7 months of age[37]. This posnatal decline in irET-1 level appears to be delayed in sick infants with persistent pulmonary hypertension.

Haegerstrand et al. studied umbilical cord and mixed blood collected from the vessels immediately after delivery[38]. They found the level of ET like immunoreactivity in fetal blood plasma to be 4–5 times higher than in normal adult human plasma. ET was also shown in umbilical arteries and vein. In vitro studies with circular segments of isolated umbilical vessels showed a dose dependent contraction to ET. These findings suggest a significant contribution of ET towards the constriction of umbilical blood vessels soon after birth. ET has also been shown to induce contractions in fetal stem villous arterial preparations[39] and to cause pressure increases in perfused placental cotyledons[40]. Haugen and Stray-Pedersen studied the effect of ET-1 on the vascular tension in human umbilical arteries and veins perfused in vitro[41]. They also observed a vaoconstrictor response in both vessels, and the responses were clearly dose-dependent. These results further support the role for ET-1 in the regulation of umbilicoplacental blood flow.

Sunnergren et al.[42] recently showed that the avascular amnion but not the chorion, trophoblast or myometrial tissue expressed the messenger RNA for ET-1, and the release of ET by cultured human amnion cells has also been demonstrated[43]. ET is present in human amniotic fluid and the level increases during pregnancy. Highest levels were reported at time of birth[44,45], (Figure 19.2). Experiments done on human amnion and amnion/chorion/decidua *in vitro* showed that ET-1 did not appear to affect transfer of water across fetal membranes[46].

PLASMA ET-1 LEVELS IN NORMAL CHILDREN

Plama ET-1 levels in healthy children show significantly higher values in those less than 3 months of age[48]. After 3 months, plasma ET-1 levels were nearly constant at all ages. The mechanism for this difference is not clear but may explain the physiological pulmonary hypertension observed in normal infants under 3 months of age.

PLASMA ET-1 LEVELS IN SICK NEWBORN

Kojima and co-workers studied irET-1 in sick neonates and compared them with healthy preterm and term newborn babies[49]. Plasma ET-1 levels in preterm infants with respiratory distress syndrome and in infants with asphyxia were significantly higher than those in healthy full term infants through first week of life. Infants with transient tachypnea of newborn had plasma ET-1 levels comparable to those in healthy full term infants whereas it was elevated during first two months of life in infants with bronchopulmonary dysplasia. This suggests that plasma ET-1 may be a specific marker for pulmonary endothelial injury in infants with respiratory distress.

In another study the same group of workers observed urinary ET-1 like immunoreactivity during first week of life in asphyxiated infants with secondary renal dysfunction[50]. In these infants urinary ET-1 concentrations were significantly elevated throughout the first week of life when compared to healthy infants. Fractional excretion of sodium and ET-1 clearance were also more elevated in the sick infants. They observed a good correlation between urinary ET-1 concentration and urinary N acetyl beta D-glucosaminidase index. These results suggest that the origin of urinary ET-1 may be from the renal tissue and that ET-1 may be a nonspecific marker of renal injury in neonates.

Vaginally delivered babies had higher concentration of irET-1 in umbilical venous plasma than those delivered by cesarean section without labor. In vaginally delivered neonates complicated by asphyxia, irET-1 was significantly higher than those who were not asphyxiated. It is likely that birth stress, especially asphyxia, may contribute to the increase in fetal circulating irET-1 levels[51]. Whether ET levels can be used as marker for acute birth asphyxia remains to be proven.

Wong and others studied the effect of intrapulmonary injection of ET-1 (250 ng/kg) at rest and during pulmonary hypertension induced by the infusion of U-46619 (a thromboxane mimic) in lambs less than 1 week old and more than 6 months old[52]. ET-1 did not change the resting pulmonary artery pressure (PAP) in lambs but decreased

Table 19.4 Plasma immunoreactive endothelin-1 levels

	Cord blood (n = 10)	HMD (n = 8)	PPHN (n = 12)	PPHN, ECMO (n = 12)
irET1 (pg/ml)	15.1 ± 4.1	11.8 ± 1.2	21.2 ± 2.0	31.0 ± 4.7*[a][#]

*p < 0.003 compared with cord blood control.
[a]p < 0.002 compared with HMD.
[#]p < 0.05 compared with PPHN, no ECMO.

PAP by 31.2 ± 10.1% during drug induced pulmonary hypertension. In juvenile lambs (> 6 months old) a biphasic response was seen: during pulmonary hypertension, either an decrease or decrease followed by increase in PAP. These effects suggest that the pulmonary hemodynamic effects of ET-1 are dependent on post natal age. In another study, the same group demonstrated that agonists of ET_B receptors decreased PAP without changing systemic arterial pressure[53].

Persistent pulmonary hypertension (PPHN) in the newborn is associated with a wide variety of neonatal cardiopulmonary disorders. The pathophysiology is characterized by variable degrees of remodeling, decreased arterial number and active vasoconstriction. Rosenberg *et al.* measured arterial irET-1 in neonates with PPHN and compared the levels to samples obtained from neonates with hyaline membrane disease (HMD) but without pulmonary hypertension and also umbilical cord samples from normal infants [54]. They also measured irET-1 levels in babies with PPHN who required extracorporeal membrane oxygenation (ECMO) therapy and compared them to those who did not need ECMO. Infants with PPHN were found to have markedly elevated circulating irET-1 levels. Those neonates requiring ECMO therapy had higher irET-1 levels than infants with milder disease (Table 19.4).

In babies treated without ECMO, irET-1 progressively decreased over 3–5 days paralleling clinical improvement. In babies treated with ECMO, irET-1 levels remained elevated during the therapy.

Factor that contribute to enhanced ET-1 production include increased intramural pressure, severe hypoxia, low flow or shear stress and decreased endothelium derived relaxing factor (EDRF) release[55]. The normal pulmonary circulation clears upto 67% of circulating ET-1 in a single passage[12]. Thus low pulmonary blood flow seen in PPHN and ECMO therapy could result in diminished ET-1 clearance. High levels of ET-1 seen in babies with PPHN may directly contribute to the pathophysiology of PPHN or may simply be a marker of the disease severity.

CONCLUSION

ETs are biologically active peptides with many effects and actions on a large variety of tissues. It plays an important role in regulating the vascular tone. Exciting results have been demonstrated in its possible role in parturition, pregnancy induced hypertension and lactation. It is likely that it contributes to umbilicoplacental blood flow, regulation of pulmonary vascular tone in the fetus and could be involved in the pathophysiology of pulmonary hypertension in the newborn. It may also have a role in closure of ductus arteriosus soon after birth. ET has been demonstrated to have important actions on renal and systemic hemodynamics in the young animal. Finally much research still needs to be done on its role in perinatal circulation.

References

1. Rubanyi, G. and Vanhoutte, P. M. (1985) Hypoxia releases a vasoconstrictor substance from canine vascular endothelium. *J Physiol Lond*, **364**, 45–56.
2. Yanagisawa, M., Kurihara, H., Kimura, S., Tombe, Y., Kobayashi, M., Mitsui, Y., Yazaki, Y., Goto, K. and Masaki, T. (1988) A novel potent vasoconstrictor peptide produced by vascular endothelial cells. *Nature Lond*, **332**, 411–415.
3. Lemonnier Degouville A–C, Lippton H. L., Cavero I., Summer W. R. and Hyman A. L. (1989) Endothelin- a new family of endothelium derived peptides with widespread biological properties. *Life Sci*, **45**, 1499–1513.
4. Simonson M. S. (1993) Endothelins: Multifunctional renal peptides. *Physiol Rev*, **73**, 375–411.
5. Chester A., Clarke J., Kauser S., Larkin S., Davies G. and Yacoub M. (1989) Endothelin is a potent constrictor of human coronary arteries *in vitro* (Abstract) *J Am Coll Cardiol*, **13**, 85A.
6. Miyauchi T., Tomoke Y., Yanagisawa M., Sugishita Y., Ito I., Kimura S., Goto K. and Masaki T. (1989) Effects of endothelin, a novel vasoconstrictor peptide, on the isolated human mesenteric arteries (Abstract) *J Am Coll Cardiol*, **13**, 85A.
7. Folta A., Joshua I. G. and Webb R. C. (1989) Dilator actions of endothelin in coronary resistance vessels and the abdominal aorta of the guinea pig. *Life Sci*, **45**, 2627–2635.
8. Penheino J., Horgan M., Everitt J. and Malik A. (1989) Effects of endothelin on pulmonary vascular hemodynamics on guinea pig isolated, perfused lungs. (Abstract) *Pediatr Res*, **25**, 42A.
9. Kasuya Y., Ishikawa T., Yanagisawa M., Kimura S., Goto K., Masaki T. (1989) Mechanism of contraction to endothelin in isolated porcine coronary. *Am J Physiol*, **257**, H1828–H1835.
10. Bradley L. M., Czaja J. F., Goldstein R. E. (1990) Circulatory effects of endothelin in newborn piglets. *Am J Physiol*, **259**, H1613–H1617.
11. Krzeski R., Long W., Katayama H. and Henry W. (1991) Hemodynamic effects of Endothelin-1 in the newborn piglet: influence on pulmonary and systemic vascular resistance. *J Cardiovasc Pharmac*, **17(Suppl 7)**, S322–S325.
12. deNucci G., Thomas R., D'Orleans-Justa P., *et al.* (1988) Pressor effects of circulatory endothelin are limited by its removal in the pulmonary circulation and by the release of prostacyclin and endothelium derived relaxing factor. *Natl Acad Sci USA*, **85**, 9797–9800.
13. Bhat R., John E., Chari G. *et al.* (1993) Endothelin-1, Dose dependent effect on renal function in piglets (Abstract). *Pediatr Res*, **33**, 62A.
14. Tomobe Y., Miyauchi T., Satio A. *et al.* (1988) Effects of endothelin on the renal artery from SHR and WHY rats. *Eur J Pharmacol*, **152**, 373–374.
15. Iyer R. S., Rebello S., Singh G. *et al.* (1994) Endothelin-1 (ET-1) levels in brain and cardiovascular system of hypertensive rats (SHR) and normotensive (WKY) rats during development. *Ped. Res*, **35**, 84A.
16. Coceani F., Armstrong C. and Kelsey L. (1989) Endothelin is a potent constrictor of the lamb ductus arteriosus. *Can J Physiol Pharmacol*, **67**, 902–904.
17. Coceani F. and Kelsey L. (1991) Endothelin-1 release from lamb ductus arteriosus: relevance to post natal closure of the vessel. *Can J Physiol Pharmacol*, **69**, 218–221.
18. Coceani F., Kelsey L., Seidlitz E. (1992) Evidence for an effector role of endothelin in closure of the ductus arteriosus at birth. *Can J Pharmacol*, **70**, 1061–1064.
19. Armstead W. M., Mirro R., Leffer L. W., Busija D. W. (1989) Influence of endothelin on piglet microcirculation. *Am J Physiol*, **275**, H707–H710.
20. Banks R. O. (1989) Cardiovascular and renal effects of endothelin in the dog and in the rat. *Kidney Int*, **35**, 309(Abstr).
21. King A. J., Brenner B. M., Andersen S. (1989) Endothelin: a potent renal and systemic vasoconstrictor peptide. *Am J Physiol*, **256**, F1051–F1058.
22. Semama D. S., Thonney M., Guignard J.–P. and Gouyon J. B. Effects of endothelin on renal function in newborn rabbits. *Ped Res*, **34**, 120–123.
23. Hirata Y., Matsuoka H., Kimura K. *et al.* (1991) Role of endothelin-derived relaxing factor in endothelin induced renal vasoconstriction. *J Cardiovasc Pharmac*, **17(Suppl 17)**, S169–S171.
24. Kojima T., Isozaki-Fukuday, Takedatsu M., Hirata Y., Kobashi Y. (1992) Circulating levels of endothelin and atrial natriuretic factor during postnatal life. *Acta Pediatr*, **81**, 676–7.

25. Word R. A., Kamm K. E., Stull J. T. et al. (1990) Endothelin increases cytoplasmic calcium and myosin phosphorylation in human myometrium. *Am J Obstet Gynecol*, **162**, 1103–1108.
26. Romero R., Avila C., Mitchell M. D. (1990) Endothelin-1 in human parturition. Proceedings of 37th Annual Meeting of Society for Gynecologic Investigation, *St Louis, MO*, **351**, (abstr 510).
27. Hagiwara H., Kozuka M., Ito T., Eguchi S., Hirose S. (1990) Properties of rat uterus endothelin receptors sites. *Biomed Res*, **11**, 93–8.
28. Yoshizawa T., Shinmi O., Giaid A. et al. (1990) Endothelin: a novel peptide in the posterior pituitary system. *Science*, **247**, 462–464.
29. Goetz K. L., Wangg B. C., Madwed J. B. et al. (1988) Cardiovascular, renal and endocrine responses to intravenous endothelin in conscious dogs. *Am J Physiol*, **255**, R1064–R1068.
30. Stojilkovic S. S., Merelli F., Iida T. et al. (1990) Endothelin stimulation of cytosolic calcium and gonadotropin secretion in anterior pituitary. *Science*, **148**, 1663–1666.
31. Baley P. A., Resink T. J., Eppenberger U. et al. (1990) Endothelin messenger RNA and receptors are differentially expressed in cultured human breast epithelial and stromal calls. *J Clin Invest*, **85**, 1320–1323.
32. Ihara Y., Sagawa N., Hasegawa M. et al. (1991) Concentrations of endothelin-1 in materal and umbilical cord blood at various stages of pregnancy. *J Cardiovasc Pharmac*, **17 (Suppl 7)**, S443–S445.
33. Otani S., Usuki S., Satioh T., Yanagisawa M., Iwasaki H., Tanaka J., Suzuki N., Fujino M., Goto K. and Masaki T. (1991) Comparison of endothelin-1 concentrations in normal and complicated pregnancies. *J Cardiovasc Pharmac*, **17 (Suppl 7)**, S308–S312.
34. MacCumber M. W., Ross C. A., Glaser B. M., Snyder S. H. (1989) Endothelin visualization of mRNAs by *in situ* hybridization provides evidence for local action. *Proc Natl Acad Sci USA*, **86**, 7285–7289.
35. Cassin S., Kristova, Davis T., Kadowitz P., Gause G. (1991) Tone dependent responses to endothelin in the isolated perfused fetal sheep pulmonary cirulation *in situ*. *J Appl Physiol*, **70**, 1228–34.
36. Chatfield B. A., McMurtry I. F., Huel S. L., Abman S. H. (1991) Hemodynamic effects of endothelin-1 in ovine fetal pulmonary circulation. *Am J Physiol*, **261**, R182–7.
37. Allen S. W., Chatfield B. A., Koppenhaffer S. L. et al. (1992) Circulating immunoreactive ET-1 and hypoxic pulmonary vasoconstriction in childhood pulmonary hypertension. (Abstract) *Pediatr Res*, **31**, 16A.
38. Haegerstrand A., Hempen A., Gills C., Larsson O. (1989) Endothelin: presence in human umbilical blood vessels high levels in fetal blood and potent constrictor effect. *Acta Physiol Scand*, **137**, 541–542.
39. Svane D., Skajaak, Andersson K–E and Forman A. Effects of endothelin on human uteroplacental arteries. Abstract, VII World Congress of Hypertension in Pregnancy. Perugia, Italy.
40. Wilkes B. M., Mento P. F., Hollander A. M., Maita M. E., Sung S. and Girardi E. P. (1990) Endothelin receptors in human placenta: relationship to vascular resistance and thromboxane release. *Am J Physiol*, **258**, E864–E870.
41. Haugen G. and Stray-Pedersen S. (1991) Effects of endothelin on vascular tension in human umbilical vessels. *Early Human Dev*, **27**, 25–32.
42. Sunnergren K. P., Word A. R., Sambrook J. F., MacDonald P. C., Casey M. L. (1990)Expression and regulation of endothelin precursor mRNA in avascular human amnion. *Mol Cell Endocrinol*, **68**, R7–14.
43. Mitchell M. D., Lundin-Schiller S., Edwin S. (1991) Endothelin production by amnion and its regulation by cytokines. *Am J Obstet Gynecol*, **165**, 120–124.
44. Raboni S., Folli M. C., Bresciani D. (1991) Amniotic endothelin increases during pegnancy (letter). *Am J Obstet Gynecol*, **164**, 237.
45. Iwata I., Takagi T., Yamaji K., Tanizawa O. (1991) Increase in concentration of immunoreactive endothelin in human pregnancy. *J Endocrinol*, **129**, 301–307.
46. Eis A. W., Mitchell M. D., Myatt L. (1992) Endothelin transfer and endothelin effects on water transfer in human fetal membranes. *Obstet Gynecol*, **79**, 411–5.
47. Usuki S., Saitoh T., Sawamma T. et al. (1990) Increased maternal plasma concentration of endothelin-1 during labor pain or on delivery and the existence of large amount of endothelin-1 in amniotic fluid. *Gynecol Endocrinol*, **4**, 9–19.
48. Yoshibayashi M., Nishioka K., Nakao K., Saito Y.,Temma S., Matsumura M., Ueda T., Shirakami G., Imura H. and Mikawa H. (1991) Plasma endothelin levels in healthy children: high values in early infancy. *J Cardiovasc Pharmac*, **17(Suppl 7)**, S404–S405.
49. Kojima T., Isozaki-Fukuda Y., Takedatsu M., Ono A., Hirata Y., Kobayashi Y. (1992) Plasma endothelin-1 like immunoreactivity in neonates. *Eur J of Pediatr*, **151**, 913–915.
50. Kojima T., Isozaki-Fukuda Y., Sasai M., Mirata Y., Matasuzaki S., Kobayashi Y. (1993) Urinary endothelin-1 like immunoreactivity excretion in the newborn period. *Am J Perinatol*, **106**, 220–223.
51. Isozaki-Fukuda Y., Kojima T., Hirata Y., Ono A., Sawaragi S., Sawaragi I., Kobayashi Y. (1991) Plasma immunoreactive endothelin-1 concentration in human fetal blood: its relation to asphyxia. *Pediatr Res*, **30**, 244–247.

52. Wong J., Vanderford P. A., Jeffrey R. *et al.* (1993) Developmental effects of endothelin-1 on pulmonary circulation in the intact sheep (Abstract). *Pediatr Res*, **33**: 71A.
53. Wong J., Winters J. W., Vanderford P. A. *et al.* (1993) ET_B receptor agonists produce potent pulmonary vasodilation in the intact newborn lamb (Abstract). *Pediatr Res*, **33**, 71A.
54. Rosenberg A. A., Kenaugh J., Koppenhafer S. L., Loomis M., Chatfield B. A., Abman S. H. (1993) Elevated immunoreactive endothelin-1 levels in newborn infants with persistent pulmonary hypertension. *J Pediatr*, **123**, 109–114.
55. Rubanyi G. M. (1992) Endothelium derived vasoconstrictor factors: an overview. In: Ryan US. Rubanyi GM, Eds. Endothelial regulation of vascular tone. New York: *Marcel Dekker*, 375–386.

20 Role of Endothelin in Inflammatory Reactions

Maria Das Graças M. O. Henriques and Giles A. Rae*

Department of Physiology and Pharmacodynamics, IOC Oswaldo Cruz Foundation, Av. Brasil, 4365, P.O. Box 926, Rio de Janeiro, 21045-900, RJ, Brazil

Department of Pharmacology, CCB, Federal University of Santa Catarina, Rua Ferreira Lima, 82, Florianópolis, 88015-420, SC, Brazil

INTRODUCTION

Acute inflammation can be broadly defined as the non-specific response of vascularized tissue to the disturbance of its integrity. In response to an insult, the normal function of the tissue is suppressed and a new function is adopted: that of eliminating the damaging agent and restoring the tissue to its former condition. To achieve this, it is necessary to direct elements of the defense system (complement proteins, antibodies, phagocytic cells) to the inflamed area. Thus, inflammation is not a stable but a dynamic process, consisting of an overlapping succession of events. During an inflammatory reaction, mediators can be generated in the blood or by cells to modify either blood vessel function or cellular events[1].

Vascular changes start immediately and develop during the first few hours. They comprise dilatation of the blood vessels with increased blood flow, followed by slowing of the blood, increased vascular permeability and exudation of plasma. The vasodilatation is brought about by various mediators produced by the interaction of the micro-organism with tissue cells (histamine, bradykinin, prostaglandin E_2 and prostaglandin I_2) acting on the small arterioles and pre-capillary sphincters. The increase vascular permeability is regulated by factors which control exudation from the post-capillary venules. The initial phase of increased vascular permeability is also brought about by some mediators (histamine, bradykinin, platelet activating factor) and neutrophil association with the walls of the post-capillary venules contributes to the later, more prolonged phase of increased vascular permeability[2,3]. It was also described that endogenous vasodilator prostaglandins and permeability-increasing mediators act synergistically modulating the oedema formation in certain inflammatory models[4].

The endothelium does not, however, only produce vasodilators. In early 1988, Yanagisawa *et al.* reported that cultured porcine endothelial cells release an extremely potent vasoconstrictor peptide, containing 21 amino acids, which was named endothelin[5]. It soon became clear that endothelin belongs to a family of peptides[6]. Thus, it was renamed endothelin-1 (ET-1), to distinguish it from the other mammalian endothelins ET-2, ET-3 and vasoactive intestinal contractor (The mouse equivalent of ET-2)[7], and sarafotoxins present in venom of the snake Atractaspis engaddensis[8-10].

The discovery of the endothelins immediately stimulated intense research into their pharmacology, cellular distribution, biochemical processing and possible physiopathological roles. This chapter attempts to summarize and interpret the data accumulated on possible roles of endothelins in inflammation. To address this issue in a comprehensive manner, however, it is important to lay down some fundamental aspects of endothelin biosynthesis and release and of the receptors they interact with.

ENDOTHELIN FORMATION AND RELEASE

Mammalian endothelins are synthesized from distinct precursors called preproendothelins, each one encoded by a separated gene[6]. The first step in ET-1 formation involves cleavage of prepro-ET-1 (203 amino acid peptide), by a specific but uncharacterized endopeptidase(s), to originate pro-ET-1 (or big-ET-1). Big-ET-1, a 38–39 amino acid intermediate, is then most likely cleaved by a phosphoramidon-sensitive endopeptidase to yield ET-1[8,11]. The pathways and enzymes involved in ET-2 and ET-3 formation are less clear. Although phosphoramidon has been shown to inhibit conversion of big-ET-2 and big-ET-3 *in vivo*[12], other studies have been unsuccessful[13-15].

Secretion of ET-1 from endothelial cells can be triggered by many stimuli including the vasoconstrictors adrenaline, angiotensin II and arginine-vasopressin[5,16] thrombin[5,17,18], low density lipoproteins[19], shear stress[5,20] and hypoxia[21,22]. Cytokines can also stimulate ET-1 release from endothelium, especially TGFβ, which is particularly potent, TNFα and interferon gamma, but not IL-1β, IL-6 or IL-8[23,24]. However these cytokines can stimulate ET-1 release from cultured airway epithelial cells, as do TNFα, TGFβ and IGF-1[25]. Moreover, rat mesangial cells increase ET-1 production in response to TNFα[26], whereas human amnion cells respond to IL-1α, IL-6 and TNFα with increased synthesis of both ET-1 and/or ET-2[27].

Human macrophages synthesize both ET-1 and ET-3 and their release is enhanced by LPS[28] or by modified low density lipoproteins[29]. Non-activated human polymorphonuclear cells (PMNs) *in vitro* also show rapid phosphoramidon-sensitive conversion of big-ET-1, but ET-1 formation is not altered by activation with the chemotactic peptide FMLP[30]. In fact, FMLP accelerates degradation of ET-1 by a phenylmethylsulfonylfluoride sensitive neutral protease which is insensitive to phosphoramidon[30]. Most of the endothelin converting activity of these cells is cytosolic and consists of an elastase-initiated serine protease cascade which ultimately transforms big-ET-1 into ET-1[31]. Elastase may also be partly responsible for ET-1 degradation.

RECEPTORS FOR ENDOTHELINS

Two distinct receptors for endothelin have been cloned so far and have been named ET_A and ET_B receptors. The ET_A-receptor displays marked affinity for ET-1 and ET-2, but less for ET-3, yielding a rank order of affinities of ET-1 = ET-2 > ET-3[32]. In contrast, the ETB-receptor is non-selective, showing similar affinities for all three peptides[33], however recent evidence suggests that there may be different ET_B-receptor subtypes with super-high affinity for ET-3[34]. Both receptors ET_A and ET_B belong to the seven transmembrane domain G-protein coupled receptor superfamily, and can be distinguished by use of selective agonists and antagonists[35,36].

RELEASE OF MEDIATORS BY ENDOTHELINS

Many effects of endothelins are mediated or modulated by release of vasoactive products, such as NO, eicosanoids, PAF, and others[37]. Release of NO from the endothelium mediates the vasodilator effects of ET-1 and ET-3 in preconstricted rat perfused arterial mesentery[38,39] and porcine pulmonary artery[40]. Also, NO-synthase inhibitors markedly reduce ET-1 induced transient hypotension[41] and dilatation of the pulmonary vasculature in anaesthetized rats[42]. The receptor stimulating NO release appears to be of the ET_B type[43,34]. However, vasodilatation caused by ET-1 in rat perfused hindquarters[44], hypoxic lungs[45] and in cats[46] appears to involve not NO release, but activation of potassium channels.

ET-1 is also a potent releaser of cyclo-oxygenase-derived eicosanoids in several preparations, such as perfused rat and guinea pig lungs[38], rabbit spleen and kidney[47], rat hindquarters[48] and dog kidney[49], possibly by stimulation of ET_A receptors[50]. Eicosanoids can directly mediate some effects of ET-1 in selected vessels[51,52] and modulate the pressor effects of ET-1 in vivo[38,53] and in perfused organs[47]. Bronchoconstriction induced by ET-1, ET-2 and ET-3 in guinea pigs is largely mediated by thromboxane A_2 (TXA_2)[54,55]. Furthermore, ET-1 has been shown to release leukotrienes in guinea pig lung parenchyma[56], but this has not been confirmed in the whole lung[57].

In rat glomerular mesangial cells, ET-1 can trigger release of PAF[58], but pretreatment with PAF antagonists does not modify the pressor effects of ET-1[59,60]. PAF antagonist can, however, reduce the constrictor effect of ET-1 in rat perfused mesentery[61] and aorta[62] and its bronchoconstrictor effect in vivo[63] and in vitro. PAF antagonist also protect mice from the lethal effects of ET-1 [59], but surprisingly, the reverse has also been reported, i.e. that ET-1 protects mice from PAF-induced sudden death[64]. Thus, some effects of ET-1 may be mediated by PAF release (see below).

Endothelins do not have direct pro- or anti-aggregatory effects on blood platelets in vitro[38,65,66] can modulate aggregetion triggered by ADP[66], adrenaline[67], noradrenaline and serotonin[68,69]. In vivo, however, both ET-1 and ET-3 potently inhibit platelet aggregation, possibly by stimulating PGI2 release from the endothelium[70-72]. Both peptides also induce endothelial cells to release tissue-type plasminogen sotivator (an endogenous anti-thrombotic and fibrinolytic substance) and Von Willebrand factor[73,74].

ENDOTHELIN AND MICROVASCULATURE

ET-1 induces profound effects in the microvasculature in vivo. Thus, it is a powerful constrictor of arterioles and venules in rat mesentery[75], in rabbit tenuissimus muscle[76] and ear[77]. However, the effect of ET-1 in the hamster cheek pouch is controversial, some finding only arteriole constriction[76-78], and others a concomitant venular constriction[79]. The peptide is also able to decrease blood flow in rabbit and human skin[78,80].

Endothelins and vascular permeability

Endothelin-1 presents a marked inhibitory effect on vascular permeability which is considered as a consequence of intense local vasoconstriction.

Plasma extravasation induced in rat dorsal skin by carrageenin or by the inflammatory mediators histamine, serotonin, bradykinin and PAF is markedly inhibited by co-injection ET-1[81]. The peptide also blocks the leakage triggered by the vasodilators NO and nitroprusside[81]. Similarly, given intradermally in rabbit dorsal skin together with bradykinin or FMLP, ET-1 blocks the increase extravascular accumulation of radiolabelled albumin potentiated by calcitonin gene-related peptide[82]. Nethertheless, the vasoconstrictor effect of ET-1 could be actually masking an oedematogenic effect of the peptide, because Brain et al.[82] also found ET-1 to cause a flare reaction surrounding the ischaemic area in the human forearm, and others have reported oedema following ET-1 application in this tissue[83].

The inhibitory effects of ET-1 on vascular permeability in rat dorsal skin seems to be mediated by ET_A receptors, as ET-3 is roughly 50-fold less than ET-1 in antagonizing histamine-induced plasma extravasation[84]. A comparable difference in potency between ET-1 and ET-3 is also seen regarding their inhibitory effects in carrageenin-induced rat paw oedema, which is characterized more by a delay in onset of oedema than a true reduction in oedema[84]. Surprisingly, however, neither ET-1 (up to 3 pmoles/site) nor ET-3 (up to 50 pmoles/site) display significant effects against carrageenin-induced pleurisy in rats, another well established model of inflammation[81,84].

In sharp contrast to the findings obtained in rats and rabbits, ET-1 selectively inhibits PAF-induced paw oedema in the mouse, without affecting that caused by bradykinin, histamine, or serotonin[85]. This selective anti-PAF effect of ET-1 in the mouse, which dose-dependent, potent (0.2–0.5 pmol/site) and long-lasting, does not seem to result from microvascular vasoconstriction, as this would also affect oedema induced by other inflammatory mediators. Also in contrast to what is seen in rats[84], in mice ET-1 inhibits paw oedema triggered by zymosan, but not by carrageenin[85]. Nevertheless, the development of carrageenin-induced paw oedema in mice occurs in two phases over 72 h, whereas in rats it reaches a maximum in only 4 h decaying afterwards[86]. Perhaps the efficacy of ET-1 against paw swelling induced by zymosan is also mediated by an anti-PAF effect, as PAF may mediate the inflammatory reaction to this agent[87].

PAF-induced pleural exudation in the mouse is also markedly inhibited by local injection (0.5 pmol/site) of ET-1[85]. The mechanisms involved in this effect are again unclear, but seems to be mediated by ET_A-receptors, because it is blocked by co-administration of the selective ET_A-receptor antagonist BQ-123 (150 pmoles/site), and ET-3 (0.5 pmol/site) causes no effect on PAF-induced pleural exudation (Sampaio, Rai, D'Orleans-Juste and Henriques, manuscript in preparation).

Interestingly, intravenous administration of ET-1 to conscious rats increases plasma extravasation in several organs (or tissues) including heart, trachea and bronchi, stomach, duodenum, spleen, liver, diaphragm and kidney[88-90]. In some tissues this effect of ET-1 can be observed even at doses causing minimal hemoconcentration[88]. Pretreatment with the PAF antagonist BN 52021 reduces ET-1-induced leakage in the lower bronchi, stomach, duodenum, spleen and kidney, but not in trachea or upper bronchi[88-90], thus corroborating reports on participation of PAF in mediating some effects of ET-1 (see previous sections for references). Likewise, the leakage of plasma induced by intravenous ET-1 in bronchi, stomach, duodenum and kidney is also substantially reduced or blocked by pretreatment of rats with the TXA_2-receptor antagonist BM-13505, the TXA_2 synthase inhibitor OKY-046 or the cyclo-oxygenase inhibitor indomethacin[90]. Thus, besides PAF, TXA_2 is another important mediator of this effect of ET-1. May be the participation of PAF in this process involves stimulation of TXA_2 synthesis. It is also noteworthy that, in this same model, big-ET-1 is roughly equipotent to ET-1 in causing a phosphoramidon-sensitive plasma leakage in many, but not all, of these organs, suggesting that the availability of endothelin- converting enzyme(s) in different beds is not homogenous[89].

As topical application of ET-1 inhibits vascular permeability in rat and rabbit skin[81,78], what could be the explanations for this paradoxical pro-inflammatory effect of intravenous ET-1? Perhaps an important reason is that topically applied ET-1 acts locally to reduce blood flow via arteriolar constriction, thus masking any ongoing effect it may have on vascular permeability in the skin. In contrast, given intravenously, the access of ET-1 to extravascular compartments is somewhat restricted by endothelium, and its greater potency as a venoconstrictor[91,92] may lead to an elevation of capillary hydrostatic pressure and subsequently to enhanced transcapillary fluid transfer[93]. Alternatively, these differences could be accounted for if ET-1 had any chemotactic activity for leukocytes, since it would only be effective stimulus when applied topically. However, as mentioned below, there is very little evidence for such an action of ET-1. Interestingly, plasma extravasation induced by ET-1 in the coronary circulation is blocked by selective ETa-receptor antagonist BQ-123[93]. Also, ET-1 promptly increases the permeability of monolayers of bovine endothelial cells cultivated on polycarbonate filters to radioactive albumin[94]. As ET-3 was found to be equally potent in causing this response, this is probably an ET_B-receptor-mediated phenomenon. Therefore, like many inflammatory mediators, ET-1 can increase inter endothelial cell gaps to facilitate plasma protein extravasation via activation of ET_A- and/or ET_B- receptors.

In summary, ET-1 can cause plasma leakage (oedema) by triggering endothelial cell contraction, either directly or indirectly, and/or by increasing the hydrostatic pressure at the capillaries, by way of its venoconstrictor action. On the other hand, ET-1 can also inhibit plasma extravasation by reducing local blood flow. Possibly, the ultimate effect of ET-1 in a particular tissue or organ, whether oedematogenic or anti-oedematogenic, will depend on the balance between these opposing actions. Nethertheless, other yet undetected mechanisms may underlie the marked differences in results obtained with ET-1 in different species and models.

ACTIONS OF ENDOTHELINS ON LEUKOCYTES

Accumulation of leukocytes is an important step in inflammation, triggered by endothelium damage and/or by chemotactic factors generated at the injured site. Leukocyte migration probably starts by margination and rolling of these cells in proximity to the endothelium of post capillary venules. This is followed by firm adhesion of the leukocyte to the endothelium, diapedesis and migration to injured sites, allied to an increased capacity of such cells to phagocytose and kill other cells.

No intravital microscopic studies have yet been reported on the possible effects of endothelin on leukocyte margination and rolling. Nethertheless, ET-1 does not stimulate adhesion of human circulating monocytes to cultured porcine endothelial cells, nor does it modify adhesion or chemotaxis triggered by FMLP[95]. In contrast, another study found ET-1 increases human monocyte chemotaxis in a dose-dependent manner[96].

Guinea pigs given ET-1 intravenously fail to develop any histological signs of lung inflammation[97], but in rat lungs ET-1 increases oxygen radical and 15-lipo-oxygenase product formation, which could indicate leukocyte activation[98]. In human alveolar macrophages ET-1 can directly stimulate superoxide production[99]. Also, though ET-1 alone does not truly activate human neutrophils, it stimulates their aggregation via PAF production[100] and sensitizes then to activation by FMLP, leading to enhanced superoxide generation[101]. In sharp contrast, no changes in superoxide production were seen following exposure of human blood monocytes to ET-1[95]. Moreover, neutrophils taken from dogs after intravenous ET-1 also show unaltered oxygen free radical formation[102].

Also, intradermal injection of ET-1 into rat dorsal skin does not alter PMN cell accumulation *per se* or that stimulated by FMLP[103]. In rabbit dorsal skin, however, ET-1 clearly reduces FMLP-induced PMN infiltration in presence of calcitonin-gene related peptide[78]. There is also conflicting evidence regarding the effects of intravenous ET-1 on circulating leukocyte counts. In guinea pigs, one study failed to detect any changes in total leukocyte numbers[104], but another found a significant reduction[105]. Dogs given intravenous ET-1 also show a decreased number of circulating leukocytes and PMNs[102].

Thus, surprisingly few studies have analyzed possible effects of endothelins on the various aspects of leukocyte activation. Moreover, although some have found ET-1 to cause some signs of leukocyte activation, the results of these studies are often conflicting, even within a same species. Furthermore, it appears reasonable to postulate that some effects of endothelins on leukocyte functions may be secondary to the generation of other mediators. Besides this, the actions of endothelins on leukocytes may be masked by their vasoconstrictor effects. However, considering that some leukocytes, particularly macrophages[28] and PMNs[30,31], are capable of synthesizing ET-1, future studies may well confirm important actions of endothelins on leukocytes during inflammation.

ENDOTHELIN AND PAIN

Considering that endothelins are potent releasers of eicosanoids, including the hyperalgesic prostaglandins PGE1 and PGE2, it is hardly unexpected that these peptides can also induce pain. Indeed, ET-1 causes abdominal constrictions (wriths) when injected intraperitoneally in mice[106,107]. However, it is controversial if this effect is actually mediated by eicosanoids. In one study, the pain triggered by 1 µg/kg of ET-1 was fully blocked by pretreatment with 10 mg/kg (s.c.) indomethacin[106]. In contrast, pretreatment with 1 mg/kg (p.o.) of indomethacin, acetaminophen or ibuprofen, all failed to modify the percentage of mice responding to 0.1 mg/kg of ET-1 whereas morphine was highly effective[108]. ET-2 and ET-3 also cause abdominal constrictions, with potencies not very different from that of ET-1, suggesting that ET_B-receptors contribute to this effect[108]. Furthermore, as big-ET-1 is also potent in causing phosphoramidon-sensitive abdominal constrictions, marked endothelin-converting enzyme activity is present in the peritoneal cavity[108].

Injected locally into the hind paw, ET-1 induces long-lasting hyperalgesia which, unlike that caused by carrageenin, is insensitive to inhibition by indomethacin or guanethidine[106]. Thus, in this model of inflammatory pain, rather than a result of eicosanoid release or stimulation of sympathetic nerves, the hyperalgesic effect of the peptide may well involve direct activation of the nociceptors. In addition to causing hyperalgesic *per se*, ET-1 can also synergize with other hyperalgesic mediators. In the dog knee joint, ET-1 alone causes only a transient incapacitation. However, local injection of a low non-hyperalgesic dose of PGE2, up to two hours after the transient incapacitation produced by ET-1 has subsided, resulted in marked and long-lasting incapacitation[106].

Intradermal injection of ET-1 in the human forearm causes locally an area of intense hotness, accompanied sometimes[106], but not always[78] by wheal formation. The peptide also causes a large flare response surrounding the central pale zone[106,78], itching and hyperalgesia[106]. The later effects show that endothelins can also stimulate nociceptors (and, thus, C-fibers) in humans, either directly or via mast cell degranulation.

In summary, endothelins, or at least ET-1, can cause pain or hyperalgesia in several animal models of inflammatory pain and in humans. Mast cell degranulation and eicosanoid synthesis and release may conribute to ET-1-induced pain in some models. However, the details of the mechanisms underlying the nociceptive properties of endothelins are far from clear.

PATHOPHYSIOLOGICAL SIGNIFICANCE

As mentioned above, endothelins can induce, at least under certain conditions, many signs of inflammation including plasma extravasation, hyperemia and pain. They can also affect leukocyte function and are synthesized by some of these cells. Furthermore, intravenous ET-1 causes fever in rabbits, possibly via stimulation of ET_B-receptors[109]. Finally, it also mimics most acute inflammatory process in that it is a potent co-mitogen which could be potentially important for repair of injured tissue.

There is extensive evidence that circulating levels of ET-1 are raised under conditions of tissue injury[110]. Thus, plasma levels of ET-1 are increased followng major trauma injuries[111], kidney transplant[112,113], acute renal failure[114], abdominal surgery[115] and systemic lupus erythematosus[116]. Also, rats given endotoxin exhibit a pronounced elevation in plasma ET-1 levels[117]. Urine levels of ET-1 are markedly raised in patients with chronic glomerulonephritis[118], and an important role for the peptide in glomerular inflammation has been suggested[119]. Furthermore, treatment of rats with monoclonal ET-1-antibody or with the selective ETA-receptor antagonist BQ-123 protects the kidneys from the tubular necrosis associated with ischemic acute renal failure[120,121]. The content of ET-1 is also strikingly increased in bronchoalveolar fluid of subjects with asthma[122] or undergoing status asthmaticus[123]. Interestingly, treatment of asthmatic patients with corticosteroids or with β-adrenoceptor agonists not only reduced airway obstruction, but also lowered ET-1 content in bronchoalveolar fluid[122]. Carrageenin-induced paw oedema is associated with increased plasma and local tissular levels of ET-1 in rats[124]. ET-1 and ET-3 also are potent inducers of gastric ulcers in the rat[125,126].

As seen for several other putative inflammatory mediators, the fact that endothelins can cause pro-inflammatory effects, and that their levels are increased in plasma and/or other fluids during various inflammatory states or diseases, does not necessarily imply that these peptides play an active role in inflammation. Alternatively, for example, the increased endothelin levels may merely be a consequence, and therefore a marker, of tissue injury. In addition, it is worth bearing in mind that ET-1 is more likely produced to act locally, like mastocyte-derived histamine, in an autocrine and paracrine fashion. Thus, circulating levels of ET-1 may not necessarily reflect its content in injured tissues or sites, except, perhaps, when the lesion is associated with extensive damage of the endothelial cells. Thus, at present, despite the extensive number of studies suggesting possible roles for endothelins in inflammation, a definitive implication remains to be established.

Acknowledgement

This study received support from the Brazilian National Research Council (CNPq).

References

1. Dale, M. M. and Foreman, J. C. (1989) Introduction to the immunology and pathology of host defence mechanisms. In: Textbook of Immunopharmacology, edited by M. M. Dale, et al., pp. 1–16. *Blackwell Scientific Publications*, Oxford, London, Edinburgh.
2. Williams, T. J., Jose, P. J., Forrest, M. J., Wedmore, C. V., and Clough, G. F. (1984) Interactions between neutrophils and microvascular endothelial cells leading to cell emigration and plasma protein leakage. In: *White Cell Mechanisms: Basic Science and Clinical Aspects*, edited by H. J. Meiselman, et al. pp. 195–208. Alan R. Liss, New York.
3. Wedmore, C. V. and Williams, T. J. (1981) Control of vascular permeability by polymorphonuclear leukocytes in inflammation. *Nature*, **289**, 646–650.
4. Williams, T. J. and Peck, M. J. (1977) Role of prostaglandin-mediated vasodilation in inflammation. *Nature*, **270**, 530–532.
5. Yanagisawa, M., Kurihara, H., Kimura, S., Tomobe Y., Kobayashi, M., Mitsui, Y., Yazaki, Y., et al. (1988) A novel potent vasoconstrictor peptide produced by vascular endothelial cells. *Nature*, **332**, 411–415.
6. Inoue, A., Yanagisawa, M., Kimura, S., Kasuya, Y., Miyauichi, T., Goto, K., and Masaki, T. (1989) The human endothelin family: three separate genes. *Proc. Natl. Acad. Sci. USA*, **86**, 2863–2867.
7. Ishida, N., Tsujioka, K., Tomoi, M., Saida, K., and Mitsui, Y. (1989) Differential activities of two distinct endothelin family peptides on ileum and coronary artery. *FEBS Lett.*, **247**, 337–340.
8. Kloog, Y., Ambar, I., Sokolovsky, M., Kochva, E., Wollberg, Z., and Bdolah, A. (1988) Sarafotoxin,

a novel vasoconstrictor peptide: phosphoinositide hydrolysis in rat heart and brain. *Science*, **242**, 268–270.
9. Saida, K., Mitsui, Y., and Ishida, N. (1989) A novel peptide, vasoactive intestinal contractor, of a new (endothelin) peptide family. *J. Biol. Chem.*, **264**, 14613–14616.
10. Masaki, T. and Yanagisawa, M. (1992) Physiology and pharmacology of endothelins. *Med. Res. Rev.*, **12**, 391–421.
11. Opgenorth, T. J., Wu-Wong, J. R., and Shiosaki, K. (1992) Endothelin-converting enzymes. *FASEB J.*, **6**, 2653–2659.
12. Gardiner, S. M., Kemp, P. A., and Bennett, T. (1992) Inhibition by phosphoramidon of the regional haemodynamic effects of proendothelin-2 and -3 in conscious rats. *Br. J. Pharmacol.*, **107**, 584–590.
13. D'Orleans-Juste, P., Telemaque, T., and Claing, A. (1991) Different Pharmacological profiles of big-endothelin-3 and big-endothelin-1 *in vivo* and *in vitro*. *Br. J. Pharmacol.*, **104**, 440–444.
14. Telemaque, T. and D'Orleans-Juste, P. (1991) Presence of phosphoramidon-sensitive endothelin-converting enzyme which converts big-endothelin-1 but not big-endothelin-3, in the rat vas deferens. *Naunym-Schmiedeberg's Archieves of Pharmacology*, **344**, 505–507.
15. Takada, J, Hata, M., Okada, K., Matsuyama, K., and Yano, M. (1992) Biochemical properties of endothelin converting enzyme in renal epithelial lines. *Biochem. Biophys. Res. Commun.*, **182**, 1383–1388.
16. Emori, T., Hirata, Y., Ohta, K., Sichiri, M., and Marumo, F. (1989) Secretory mechanism of immunoreactive endothelin in cultured bovine endothelial cells. Biochem. Biophys. Res. Commmun., **160**, 93–100.
17. Moon, D. G., Horgan, M. J., Andersen, T. T., Krystek Jr., R., Fenton II, J. W., and Malik A. B. (1989) Endothelin-like pulmonary vasoconstrictor peptides release by alfa-trombin. *Proc. Natl. Acad. Sci. USA*, **86**, 9529–9533.
18. D'Orleans-Juste, P., Mitchell, J. A., Wood, E. G., Hecker, M., and Vane, J. R. (1992) Comparison of the release of vasoactive factors from venous and arterial bovine cultured endothelial cells. *Can. J. Physiol. Pharmacol.*, **70**, 687–694.
19. Boulanger, C. M., Tanner, F. C., Bea, M. L., Hahn, A. W. A., Werner, A.,, and Luscher, T. F. (1992) Oxidized low density lipoprotein induces mRNA expression of ET from human and porcine endothelium. *Circ. Res.*, **70**, 1191–1197.
20. Yoshizumi, M., Kurihara, H., Sugiyama, T., Takaku, F., Yanagisawa, M., Masaki, T., and Yasaki, Y. (1989) Haemodynamic shear stress stimulates endothelin production by cultured endothelial cells. *Biochem. Biophys. Res. Commun.*, **161**, 859–864.
21. Kourembanas, S., Marsden, P. A., McQuillan, L. P., and Faller, D. (1991) Hypoxia induces endothelin gene expression and secretion in cultured human endothelium. *J. Clin. Invest.*, **88**, 1054–1057.
22. Shirakami, G., Nakao, K., Saito, Y., Magaribuchi, T., Jougasaki, M., Mukoyama, M., Arai, H. H., Hosoda, K., Suga, S., Ogawa, Y., Yamada, T., Mori, K., and Imura, H. (1991) Acute pulmonary alveolar hypoxia increases lung and plasma endothelin-1 levels in conscious rats. *Life Science*, **48**, 969–976.
23. Kurihara, H., Yoshizumi, M., Sugiyama, T., Takaku, F., Yanagisawa, M., and Masaki, T. (1989) Transforming growth factor-beta stimulates the expression of endothelin mRNA by vascular endothelial cells. *Biochem. Biophys. Res. Commun.*, **159**, 1435–1440.
24. Kanse, S. M., Takahashi, K., Lam, H. C., Rees, A., Warren, J. B., Porta, M., Molinatti, P., Ghatei, M., and Bloom, S. R. (1991) Cytokine stimulated endothelin release from endothelial cells. *Life Science*, **48**, 1379–1384.
25. Endo, T., Uchida, Y., Matsumoto, H., Suzuk, N., Nomura, A., Hirata, F., and Hasegawa, S. (1992) Regulation of endothelin-1 synthesis in cultured guinea-pig airway epithelial cells by various cytokines. *Biochemical and Biophysical Research Communications*, **186**, 1594–1599.
26. Kohan, D. E. and Padilla, E. (1992) Endothelin-1 is an autocrine factor in rat inner medullary collecting duct. *Am. J. Physiol.*, **263**, F607–F612.
27. Mitchell, M. D., Lundin-Schiller, S., and Edwin, S. S. (1991) Endothelin production by amnion and its regulation by cytokines. *Am. J. Gynecol. Obst.*, **165**, 120–124.
28. Ehrenreich, H., Anderson, R. W., Fox, C. H., Rieckmann, P., Hoffman, G. S., Travis, W. D., Coligan, J. E., Kehrl, J. H., and Fauci, A. S. (1990) Endothelins, Peptides with Potent Vesoactive Properties, are Produced by Human Macrophages. *J. Exp. Med.*, **172**, 1741–1748.
29. Martin-Nizard, F., Houssani, H. S., Lestavel-Delattre, S., Duriez, P., and Fruchart, J. C. (1991) Modified low density lipoproteins activate macrophages to secrete immunoreactive endothelin. *FEBS Lett.*, **293**, 127–130.
30. Sessa, W. C., Kaw, S., Hecker, M., and Vane, J. R. (1991) The biosynthesis of endothelin-1 by human polymorphonuclear leukocytes. *Biochem. Biophys. Res. Commun.*, **174**, 613–618.

31. Kaw, S., Hecker, M., and Vane, J. R. (1992) The two-step conversion of big-endothelin-1 to endothelin-1 and degradation of endothelin-1 by subcellular fractions from human polymorphonuclear leukocytes. *Proc. Natl. Acad. Sci. USA*, **89**, 6886–6890.
32. Arai, H., Hori, S., Aramori, I., Ohkubo, H., and Nakanishi, S. (1990) Cloning and expression of a cDNA encoding an endothelin receptor. *Nature*, **348**, 730–732.
33. Sakurai, T., Yanagisawa, M., Takuwa, Y., Miyazaki, H., Kimura, S., Goto, K., and Masaki, T. (1990) Cloning of an cDNA encoding a non-isopeptide-selective subtype of the endothelin receptor. *Nature*, **348**, 732–735.
34. Hirata, F., Emori, T., Eguchi, S., Kanno, K., Imai, T., Ohta, K., and Marumo, F. (1993) Endothelin receptor subtype B mediates synthesis of nitric oxide by cultured bovine endothelial cells. *J. Clin. Invest.*, **91**, 1367–1373.
35. Sakurai, T., Yanagisawa, M., and Masaki, T. (1992) Molecular characterization of endothelin receptor. *TIPS*, **13**, 103–108.
36. Miller, R. C., Pelton, J. T., and Huggins, J. P. (1993) Endothelins – from receptors to medicine. *TIPS*, **14**, 54–60.
37. Hyslop, S. and de Nucci, G. (1992) Vasoactive mediators released by endothelins. *Pharmacol. Res.*, **26**, 223–242.
38. de Nucci, G., Thomas, R., D'Orleans-Juste, P., Antunes, E., Walder, C., Warner, T. D., and Vane, J. R. (1988) Pressor effects of circulatig endothelin are limited by its removal in the pulmonary circulation and by release of prostacyclin and endothelium-derived relaxing factor. *Proc. Natl. Acad. Sci. USA*, **85**, 9797–9800.
39. Warner, T. D., de Nucci, G., and Vane, J. R. (1989) Rat endothelin is a vasodilator in the isolated perfused mesentery of the rat. *Eur. J. Pharmacol.*, **159**, 325–326.
40. Namiki, A., Hirata, Y., Ishikawa, M., Moroi, M., Aikawa, J. and Machii, K. (1992) Endothelin-1 and endothelin-3-induced vasorelaxation via common generation of endothelium-derived nitric oxide. *Life Science*, **50**, 677–682.
41. Whittle, B. J., Payne, A. N., and Espluges, J. V. (1989) Cardiopulmonary and gastric ulcerogenic actions of endothelin-1 in the guinea pig and rat. *J Cardiovasc Pharmacol*, **13** (suppl. 5), S103–S107.
42. Raffestein, B., Adnot, S., Eddahibi, A., Macquin-Mavier, I., Braquet, P., and Chabrier, P. E. (1991) Pulmonary vascular response to endothelin in rats. *J. Appl. Physiol.*, **70**, 567–574.
43. Warner, T. D., Mitchell, J. A., de Nucci, G., and Vane, J. R. (1989) Endothelin-1 and endothein-3 release EDRF from isolated perfused arterial vessels of the rat and rabbit. *J Cardiovasc Pharmacol*, **13 (Suppl 5)**, S85–S88.
44. Gardiner, S. M., Compton, A. M., Bennett, T., Palmer, R. M. J., and Moncada, S. (1989) N- monomethyl-L-arginine does not inhibit hindquarters vasodilator action of endothelin-1 in conscious rats. *Eur. J. Pharmacol.*, **171**, 237–240.
45. Hasunuma, K., Rodman, D. A., O'Brien, R. F., and McMurty, I. F. (1990) Endothelin-1 causes pulmonary vasodilation in rats. *Am. J. Physiol.*, **259**, H48–H54.
46. Lippton, H., Cohen, G. A., McMurty, I. F., and Hyman, A. (1991) Pulmonary vasodilation to endothelin isopeptides *in vivo* is mediated by potassium channel activation. *J. Appl. Physiol.*, **70**, 947–952.
47. Rae, G. A., Trybulec, M., de Nucci, G., and Vane, J. R. (1989) Endothelin-1 Releases Eicosanoids from Rabbit Isolated Perfused Kidney and Spleen. *J Cardiovasc Pharmacol*, **13 (Suppl 5)**, S89–S92.
48. Katoh, K., Mizuno, K., Haga, H., and Fugushi, S. (1990) Low-dose endothelin stimulates release of prostaglandin I2 from isolated perfused hindlegs in the rat. *Res. Commun. Chem. Pathol. Pharmacol.*, **69**, 187–195.
49. Miura, K., Yukimura, T., Yamashita, Y., Shimmen, T., Okumura, M., Yamanaka, S., Imanishi, M., and Yamamoto, M. (1991) Renal and femoral vascular responses to endothelin-1 in dogs: role of prostaglandins. *J. Pharmacol. Exp. Ther.*, **256**, 11–17.
50. D'Orleans-Juste, P., Telemaque, T., Claing, A., Ihara, A., Ihara, M., and Yano, M. (1992) Human big-endothelin-1 and endothelin-1 release prostacyclin via the activation of ET1 receptors in the rat perused lung. *Br. J. Pharmacol.*, **105**, 773–775.
51. Folta, A., Joshua, I. G., and Webb, R. C. (1989) Dilator actions of endothelin in coronary resistance vessels and the abdominal avita of the guinea pig. *Life Science*, **45**, 2627–2635.
52. Armstead, W. M., Mirro, R., Lffer, C. W., and Busija, D. W. (1989) Influence of endothelin on piglet cerebral microcirculation. *Am. J. Physiol.*, **257**, H707–H710.
53. Miura, K., Yukimura, T., Yamashita, Y. Shimmen, T., Okumura, M., Imanshi, M., and Yamamoto, M. (1989) Endothelin stimulates the renal production of prostaglandin E2 and I2 in anesthetized dogs. *Eur. J. Pharmacol.*, **170**, 91–93.
54. Payne, A. and Whittle, B. J. R. (1988) Potent cyclo-oxygenase-mediated broncho-constrictor effects of endothelin in the guinea-pig *in vivo*. *Eur. J. Pharmacol.*, **158**, 303–304.

55. Pons, F., Touvay, C., Lagente, V., Mencia-Huerta, J. M., and Braquet, P. (1991) Comparison of intra-arterial and aerosol administration of endothelin-1 in the guinea-pig isolated lung. *Br. J. Pharmacol.*, **102**, 791–796.
56. Filep, J. G., Battistini, B., and Sirois, P. (1991) Pharmacological modulation of endothelin-induced contraction of guinea-pig isolated airways and thromboxane release. *Br. J. Pharmacol.*, **103**, 1633–1640.
57. Pons, F. Loquet, C., Touvay, C., Roubert, P., Chabrier, J. M., Mencia-Huerta, J. M., and Braquet, P. (1991) Comparison of the bronchopulmonary and pressor activities of endothelin isoforms ET-1, ET-2 and ET-3 and characterization of their binding sites in guinea pig lung. *Am. Rev. Respir. Dis.*, **143**, 294–300.
58. Lopez-Farre, A., Gomez-Garre, D., Bernabew, F., and Lopez-Novoa, J. M. (1991) A role for endothelin in the maintenance of post-ischaemic renal failure in the rat. *J. Physiol*, **444**, 513–522.
59. Terashita, I., Shibouta, Y., Imura, H., Iwasaki, K., and Nishikawa, K. (1989) Endothelin-induced sudden death and the possible involvement of platelet-activating factor (PAF). *Life Science*, **45**, 1191–1198.
60. Le Monnier de Gouville, A. C., Mondot, S., Lippton, H., Hyman, A., and Cavero, I. (1990) Hemodynamic and pharmacological evaluation of the vasodilator effect of endothelin-1 in rats. *J. Pharmacol. Exp. Ther.*, **252**, 300–311.
61. Korose, I., Miura, S., Suematsu, M., Fukumura, D., Nagata, H., Sekizuka, E., and Tsuchiya, M. (1991) Involvement of platelet-activating factor in endothelin-induced vascular smooth muscle cell contraction. *J Cardiovasc Pharmacol*, **17 (Suppl 7)**, S279–S283.
62. Reynolds, E. E. and Mok, L. L. S. (1990) Role of thromboxane A2/prostaglandin H2 receptor in the vasconstrictor response of rat aorta to endothelin. *J. Pharmacol. Exp. Ther.*, **252**, 915–921.
63. Lagente, V., Chabrier, P. E., Mencia-Huerta, J. M., and Braquet, P. (1989) Pharmacological modulation of the bronchopulmonary action of the vasoactive peptide, endothelin, administered by aerosol in the guinea-pig. *Biochem. Biophys. Res. Commun.*, **158**, 625–632.
64. Ettiene, A., Pannetier, M. C., Soulard, C., and Braquet, P. (1990) Effects of endothelin on the lethality induced by platelet-activating factor or endotoxin in mice. *Circ. Shock*, **32**, 77–81.
65. Edlund, A. and Wennamlm, A (1990) Endothelin does not affect aggregation of human platlets. *Clin. Physiol.*, **10**, 585–590.
66. Ohlstein, E. H., Storer, B., Nambi, P., Given, M., and Lippton, H. (1990) Endothelin and platelet function. *Thromb. Res.*, **57**, 967–974.
67. Matsumoto, Y., Ozaki, Y., Kariya, T., and Kume, S. (1990) Potentiating effects of endothelin on platelet activation induced by epinephrine and ADP. *Biochem. Pharmacol.*, **40**, 909–914.
68. Yang, Z., Richard, V., Von Segesser, L., Bauer, E., Stuiz, P., Turina, M., and Luscher, T. (1990) Threshold concentrations of endothelin-1 potentiate concentrations to norepinephrine and serotonin in human arteries. A new mechanism of vasopasm? *Circulation*, **82**, 188–197.
69. Pietraszek, M. H., Takada, Y., and Takada, A. (1992) Endothelins inhibit serotonin-induced platelet aggregetion via a mechanism involving protein kinase C. *Eur. J. Pharmacol.*, **219**, 289–293.
70. Thiemermann, C., Lidbury, P. S., Thomas, D. S., and Vane, J. R. (1988) Endothelin inhibits *ex vivo* platelet aggregation in the rabbit. *Eur. J. Pharmacol.*, **158**, 181–182.
71. Thiemermann, C., Lidbury, P. S., Thomas, D. S., and Vane, J. R. (1989) Endothelin-1 releases prostacyclin and inhibits *ex vivo* platelet aggregation in the anesthetized rabbit. *J Cardiovasc Pharmacol*, **13 (Suppl 5)**, S138–141.
72. Lidbury, P. S., Thiemermann, C., Thomas, D. S., and Vane, J. R. (1989) Endothelin-3: selectivity as an anti-aggregatory peptide *in vivo*. *Eur. J. Pharmacol.*, **166**, 335–338.
73. Korbut, R. P., Libdury, P. S., Thomas, G. R., and Vane, J. R. (1989) Fibrinolytic activity of endothelin-3. *Thromb. Res.*, **55**, 797–803.
74. Pruis, J. and Emeis, J. J. (1990) Endothelin-1 and -3 induce the release of tissue plasminogen activator and Von Willebrand factor from endothelial cells. *Eur. J. Pharmacol.*, **187**, 105–112.
75. Fortes, Z. B., de Nucci, G., and Garcia-Leme, J. (1989) Effect of endothelin-1 on arterioles and venules *in vivo*. *J Cardiovasc Pharmacol*, **13 (Suppl 5)**, S200–S201.
76. Ohlen, A., Raud, J., Hedqvist, P., and Wiklund, N. (1989) Microvascular effects of endothelin in the rabbit tenuissimus muscle and hamster cheek pouch. *Microvasc. Res.*, **37**, 115–118.
77. Randall, M. D., Edwards, D. H., and Griffith, T. M. (1990) Activities of endothelin-1 in the vascular network of the rabbit ear: a microangiographic study. *Br. J. Pharmacol.*, **101**, 781–788.
78. Brain, S. D., Crossman, D. C., Buckley, T. L., and Williams, T. J. (1989) Endothelin-1: demonstration of potent effects on the microvascular of human and other species. *J Cardiovasc Pharmacol*, **13 (Suppl 5)**, S147–S149.
79. Borie, M. P., Conoso, V., Fournier, A., Pierre, S. St., and Huidobro-Toro, J. P. (1990) Endothelin reduces microvascular blood flow by acting on arterioless and venules of the hamster cheek pouch. *Eur. J. Pharmacol.*, **190**, 123–133.

80. Brain, S. D., Tippins, J. R., and Williams, T. J. (1988) Endothelin induces potent microvascular constriction. *Br. J. Pharmacol.*, **95**, 1005–1007.
81. Chander, C. L., Moore, A. R., Dessa, F. M., Howat, D., and Willoughby, D. A. (1988) The local modulation of vascular permeability by endothelial cell derived products. *J. Pharm. Pharmacol.*, **40**, 745–746.
82. Brain, S. D., Crossman, D. C., Buckley, T. L., and Williams, T. J. (1989) Endothelin-1: demonstration of potent effects on the microvascular of human and other species. *J Cardiovasc Pharmacol*, **13 (Suppl 5)**, S147–149.
83. Dahlof, B., Gustafsson, D., Hedner, T., Jern, S., and Hansson, L. (1990) Regional haemodynamic effects of endothelin-1 in rat and man: unexpected adverse reaction. *J. Hypert*, **8**, 811–817.
84. Chander, C. L., Howat, D. W., Moore, A. R., Colville-Nash, P. R., Desa, F. M., Braquet, P., and Willoughby, D. A. (1990) Comparison of endothelin-1 and -3 on models of inflammation. *Agents and Actions*, **29**, 1/2, 27–29.
85. Henriques, M. G. M. O., Rae, G. A., Cordeiro, R. S. B., and Williams, T. J. (1992) Endothelin-1 inhibits PAF-induced paw oedema and pleurisy in the mouse. *Br. J. Pharmacol.*, **106**, 579–582.
86. Henriques, M. G. M. O., Weg, V. B., Martins, M. A., Silva, P. M. R., Fernandes, P. D., Cordeiro, R. S. B., and Vargaftig, B. B. (1990) Differential inhibition by two hetrazepine PAF antagonists of acute inflammation in the mouse. *Br. J. Pharmacol.*, **99**, 164–168.
87. Martins, M. A., Silva, P. M. R., Castro-Faria-Neto, H. C., Bozza, P. T., Dis, P. M. L. F., Lima, M. C. R., Cordeiro, R. S. B., and Vargaftig, B. B. (1989) Pharmacological modulation of PAF-acether-induced pleurisy in rats and its relevance for the inflammation by zimosan. *Br. J. Pharmacol.*, **96**, 363–371.
88. Filep, J. G., Sirois, M. G., Rousseau, A., Fournier, A., and Sirois, P. (1991) Effects of endothelin-1 on vascular permeability in the conscious rat: interaction with platelet-activating factor. *Br. J. Pharmacol.*, **104**, 797–804.
89. Lehoux, S., Plante, G. E., Sirois, M. G., Sirois, P., and D'Orleans-Juste, P. (1992) Phosphoramidon blocks big-endothelin-1 but not endothelin-1 enhancement of vascular permeability in the rat. *Br. J. Pharmacol.*, **107**, 996–1000.
90. Sirois, M. G., Filep, J. G., Rousseau, A., Fournier, A., Plante, G. E., and Sirois, P. (1992) Endothelin-1 enhances vascular permeability in conscious rats: role of thromboxane A2. *Eur. J. Pharmacol.*, **214**, 119–125.
91. D'Orleans-Juste, P., Finet, M., de Nucci, G., and Vane, J. R. (1989) Pharmacology of endothelin-1 in isolated vessels: effect of nicardipine, methylene blue, hemoglobin and gossypol. *J. Cardiovasc Pharmacol*, **13 (Suppl 5)**, S19–S22.
92. Warner, T. D. (1990) Simultaneous perfusion of rat isolated superior arterial and venous beds – comparison of their vasoconstrictor and vasodilator responses to agonists. *Br. J. Pharmacol.*, **99**, 427–436.
93. Filep, J. G., Foldes-Filep, E., Rousseau, A., Fournier, A., Sirois, P., and Yano, M. (1992) Endothelin-1 enhances vascular permeability in the rat heart through the ETa receptor. *Eur. J. Pharmacol.*, **219**, 343–344.
94. Farmer, P. Kawagushi, T. Sirois, M. G. D'Orleans-Juste, P., Sirois, P. (1993) Endothelin-1 and -3 increase albumin permeability in monolayers of bovine aortic endothelial cells, *Abstracts of the Meeting on Cells and Cytokines in Pulmonary Inflammation*, Paris (in Press).
95. Bath, P. M. W., Mayston, S. A., and Martin, J. F. (1990) Endothelin and PDGF do not stimulate peripheral blood monocyte chemotaxis, adhesion to endothelium and superoxide production. *Exp. Cell Res.*, **187**, 339–342.
96. Achmad, T. H. and Rao, G. S. (1992) Chemotaxis of human blood monocytes toward endothelin-1 and the influence of calcium channel blockers. *Biochem. Biophys. Res. Commun.*, **189**, 994–1000.
97. Macquin-Mavier, I., Levame, M., Istin, N., and Harf, A. (1989) Mechanisms of endothelin-mediated bronchoconstriction in the guinea pig. *J. Pharmacol. Exp. Ther.*, **250**, 740–745.
98. Nagase, T., Fukuchi, Y., Jo, C., Teramoto, S., Uejima, Y., Ishida, K., Shimizu, T., and Orimo, H. (1990) Endothelin-1 stimulates arachidonate 15-lipoxygenase activity and oxygen radical formation in the rat distal lung. *Biochem. Biophys. Res. Commun.*, **168**, 485–489.
99. Haller, H., Schaberg, T., Lindschau, C., Lode, H., and Distler, A. (1991) Endothelin increases $[Ca^{2+}]^i$, proteinphosphorylation, and O2-production in human alveolar macrophages. *Am. J. Physiol.*, **261**, 4478–4484.
100. Gomez-Garre, D., Guerra, M., Gonzalez, E., Lopez-Farre, A., Riesco, A., Caramelo, C., Escanero, J., and Egido, J. (1992) Aggregation of human polymorphonuclear leukocytes by endothelin' role of platelet-activating factor. *Eur. J. Pharmacol.*, **224**, 167–172.
101. Ishida, N., Takeshige, K., and Minakami, S. (1990) Endothelin-1 enhances superoxide generation of human neutrophils stimulated by the chemotactic peptide N-formyl-methionyl-leucyl-phenyl-alanine. *Biochem. Biophys. Res. Commun.*, **173**, 496–500.

102. Prasad, K., Lee, P., and Kalra, L. (1991) Influence of endothelin on cardiovascular function oxygen free radicals and blood chemistry. *Am. Heart. J.,* **121**, 179–190.
103. Chander, C. L., Moore, A. R., Desa, F. M., Howat, D. W., and Willoughby, D. A. (1989) Anti-Inflammatory Effects of Endothelin-1. *J Cardiovasc Pharmacol,* **13 (Suppl 5)**, S218–S219.
104. Touvay, C., Villain, B., Pons, F., Chabrier, P. E., Mencia-Huerta, J. M., and Braquet, P. (1990) Bronchopulmonary and vascular effect of endothelin in the guinea-pig. *Eur. J. Pharmacol.,* **176**, 23–33.
105. Schumacher, W. A., Steinbacher, T. E., Allen, G. T., and Ogletree, M. L. (1990) Role of thromboxane receptor activation in the bronchospastic response to endothelin. *Prostaglandins,* **40**, 71–79.
106. Ferreira, S. H., Romitelli, M., and de Nucci, G. (1989) Endothelin-1 participation in overt and inflammation pain. *J Cardiovasc Pharmacol,* **13 (Suppl 5)**, S220–S222.
107. Raffa, R. B., Schupsky, J. J., Martinez, R. P., and Jacoby, H. I. (1991) Endothelin-1-induced nociception. *Life Science,* **49**, PL61–PL65.
108. Raffa, R. B. and Jacoby, H. I. (1991) Endothelin-1, -2 and -3 directly and big-endothelin-1 indirectly elicit an abdominal constriction response in mice. *Life Science,* **48**, PL85–PL90.
109. Koshi, T. Edano, T., Arai, K., Suzuki, C., Ehara, M., Hirata, M., Ohkuchi, M., and Okabe, T. (1992) Pyrogenic action of endothelin in conscious rabbit. *Biochem. Biophys. Res. Commun.,* **186**, 1322–1328.
110. Battistini, B., D'Orleans-Juste, P., and Sirois, P. (1993) Enodthelins: circulating plasma levels and presence in other biological fluids. *Lab. Invest.,* (in press).
111. Koller, J., Mair, P., Wieser, C., Pomarolli, A., Puschendorf, B., and Harold, M. (1991) Endothelin and big endothelin concentrations in injured patients. *N. Engl. J. Med,* **321**, 1518.
112. Berbinschi, A. and Ketelslegers, J. M. (1989) Endothelin in urine. *Lancet,* **2**, 46.
113. Watschinger, B., Vychytil, A., Schuller, M., Hartter, E., Traind, E., and Pohanka, E. (1991) The pathophysiologic role of endothelin in acute vascular rejection after renal transplantation. *Transplantation,* **52**, 743–746.
114. Tomita, K., Ujiie, K., Nakanishi, T., Tomura, S., Matsuda, O., Ando, K., Sichiri, M., Hirata, Y., and Marumo, F. (1989) Plasma endothelin levels in patients with acute renal failure. *N. Engl. J. Med,* **321**, 1127.
115. Saito, T., Yanagisawa, M., and Miyauchi, T. (1989) Endothelin in human circulating blood: effects of major surgical stress. *Jpn. J. Pharmacol.,* **49**, 215P.
116. Julkunen, H., Saijonmaa, O., Gronhagen-Riska, C., Teppo, A. M., and Fyhrquist, F. (1991) Raised plasma concentrations of immunoreactive endothelin in systemic lupus erythematosus. *Ann. Rheum. Dis.,* **50**, 526–527.
117. Sugiura, M., Inagami, T., and Kon, V. (1989) Endotoxin stimulates endothelin-release *in vivo* and *in vitro* as determined by ratio-immunoassay. *Biochem. Biophys. Res. Commun.,* **161**, 1220–1227.
118. Ohta, K., Hirata, Y., Sichiri, M., Kanno, K., Emori, T., and Tomita, K. (1991) Urinary excertion of endothelin in patients with renal disease. *Kidney Int.,* **39**, 307–311.
119. Simonson, M. S. and Dunn, M. J. (1991) Endothelin peptides: possible role in glomerular inflammation. *Lab. Invest.,* **64**, 1–4.
120. Shibouta, Y., Suzuki, N., Shino, A., Matsumoto, H., Terashita, I., Kondo, K., and Nishikawa, K. (1990) Pathophysiological role of endothelin in acute renal failure. *Life Science,* **46**, 1611–1618.
121. Mino, N., Kobayashi, M., Nakajima, A., Amano, H., Shimamoto, K., Watanable, K., Yano, M., and Ikemoto, F. (1992) Protective effect of a selective endothelin receptor antagonist, BQ-123, in ischemic acute renal failure in rats. *Eur. J. Pharmacol.,* **221**, 77–83.
122. Matolli, S., Soloperto, M., Marini, M., and Fasoli, A. (1991) Levels of endothelin-1 in the bronchoalveolar lavage fluid of patients with symptomatic asthma and reversible airflow obstruction. *J. Allery Clin. Immunol.,* **88**, 376–384.
123. Nomura, A., Uchida, Y., Kameyama, M., Saotome, M., Oki, K., and Hasegawa, S. (1989) Endothelin in bronchial asthma. *Lancet,* **2**, 747–748.
124. Bertelli, A., Clerico, A, Chicca, A., Giovannini, L., Gorio, A., and Romano, M. A. (1992) Role of endothelin-1 in carrageenin-induced inflammation. *Int. J. Tiss. Reactions,* **14**, 225–230.
125. Whittle, B. J. R., Lopez-Belmonte, J., and Rees, D. D. (1989) Modulation of the vasodepressor actions of acetylcholine, bradykinin, substance P and endothelin in the rat by a specific inhibitor of nitric oxide formation. *Br. J. Pharmacol.,* **98**, 646–652.
126. Wallace, J. L., Keenan, C. M., MacNaughton, W. K., and MacKnight, G. W. (1989) Comparison of the effects of endothelin-1 and endothelin-3 on the rat stomach. *Eur. J. Pharmacol.,* **167**, 41–47.

21 Pathophysiological Roles of Endothelin in the Liver

Namiki Izumi*, Fumiaki Marumo, and Chifumi Sato[†‡]

Second Department of Internal Medicine and [†]Division of Health Science
Tokyo Medical and Dental University, 5-45 Yushima 1-chome, Bunkyo-ku, Tokyo 113, Japan
*Division of Gastroenterology, Department of Internal Medicine, Musashino
Red-Cross Hospital, Musashino-shi, Tokyo 180, Japan

INTRODUCTION

Endothelin (ET) is a potent vasoconstrictor peptide purified from the culture supernatant of procine aortic endothelial cells[1]. Recently, besides its vasoconstrictor and pressor actions, many biological actions have been reported in nonvascular tissues including the liver. Plasma concentrations of ET have been measured in hepatic disorders, and its pathological roles have been suggested. In the present article, physiological roles and pathological implications of ET in the liver have been summarized.

RELEASE OF ENDOTHELIN IN THE LIVER

The regional distribution of ET was studied in rat tissue extracts by radioimmunoassay, and a significant amount of ET was detected in the liver[2].

Intravenous administration of endotoxin stimulated arterial ET-like immunoreactivity in the pig[3]. The main portion of the increased ET-like immunoreactivity collected during endotoxemia was shown to be identical to the synthetic ET-1 and big ET by chromatographic characterizations. The stimulation of ET-release by endotoxin *in vivo* and *in vitro* was reported by Sugiura *et al.* as determined by radioimmunoassay[4]. In the rat model, endotoxin (30 mg/kg i.v. over 15 min.) augmented plasma ET-1 levels by sevenfold and ET-3 levels by twofold, while both ET-1 and ET-3 levels in liver lymph were increased by twofold[5]. ET release was also examined *in vitro* using cultured guinea pig sinusoidal endothelial liver cells[6]. A time-dependent release of immunoreactive ET from the cells was observed during the first 12 hours, which was inhibited by cyclohexamide, an inhibitor of protein synthesis.

[‡]Correspondence to Chifumi Sato, M.D.

The mechanisms of the increased ET production by endothelin have been studied *in vivo* and *in vitro*. Human tumor necrosis factor-alpha (TNF-a), a putative mediator of endotoxin shock, enhanced plasma levels of ET-1 and ET-3[5]. Pretreatment of rats with indomethacin significantly attenuated endotoxin-induced increases in plasma ET-1 and ET-3 levels, suggesting that eicosanoids may be involved in the release of ET by endotoxin[5]. *In vitro*, transforming growth factor beta (TGF-β) increased the release of ET from cultured guinea pig sinusoidal endothelial liver cells in a dose dependent manner with a maximum effect at 1 nM[6]. Kupffer-cell conditioned media also augmented the release of ET from the cells, while endotoxin itself did not significantly alter the release of ET. These findings suggest that endotoxin enhances ET production by stimulating Kupffer cells to produce cytokines that increase ET production from sinusoidal endothelial cells.

It is not known to what extent the increase in plasma ET levels by endotoxin could be attributable to the enhanced production of ET in the liver. The production of ET by sinusoidal endothelial liver cells, however, may play an important role through an autocrine mechanism or a paracrine mechanism since other liver cells such as hepatocytes and fat-storing cells have been shown to express ET receptors and to respond to ET as mentioned below.

REMOVAL OF ENDOTHELIN IN THE LIVER

The elimination of intravenously injected ET-1 from the circulation was examined in the rat by Shiba *et al.*[7]. Following the bolus injection of ^{125}I-ET-1 (30 pmol/kg), the radioactivity decayed rapidly from plasma with a half-life of 7 min. Similar results were reported by Anggard *et al.*, in which more than 60% of the injected radiolabelled ET-1 and ET-3 (app. 0.2 pmol/animal) was removed in the first minuted in the rat, and the highest uptake of the radioactivity was observed in the lung, kidneys, and liver[8]. The rapid disappearance of ET-1 from the blood stream is mostly due to the removal of he peptide by parenchymal tissues. Autoradiographic localization of ET-1 was examined in the rat after intravenous administration of ^{125}I-ET-1, and the highest enrichment of the radioactivity was again found in the liver, as well as in the lung, kidneys, adrenal gland, and heart[9]. Therefore, the liver seems to be an important organ for the removal of the circulating ET-1. This is further suggested by the findings in patients who underwent liver transplantation. Kraus *et al.* reported a marked nonpersisting rise in big-ET and ET-1 during the anhepatic period, followed by a decrease in mean concentrations immediately after allograft reperfusion[10], suggesting that the liver may play a major role in the removal of circulating ET-1 from the blood stream.

ENDOTHELIN RECEPTORS IN THE LIVER

Organ distributions and biological characteristics of ET receptors are described elsewhere in this book. In the present chapter, we describe ET receptors in the liver.

The recent extensive studies have shown that there exists multiple subtypes of ET receptors. Four different ET-1 receptor binding affinites have been reported in crude microsomal fractions of various tissues from dogs[11]. Although ET-1 binding receptors in the liver are mostly high affinity sites (Kd_{50} 50 pM, B_{max} 200 fmol/mg of protein), very low affinity receptors (Kd_{50} 4 nM) have also been detected. More recently, high affinity binding sites for ET-1 were also identified on rat liver plasma membranes (K_d 32 pM, B_{max} 1084 fmol/mg of protein)[12].

In human livers, the ligand selectivity of ET-1 and ET-3 binding sites has been examined[13]. ET-3 displaces the ^{125}I-ET-1 with nearly the same affinity as ET-1 in the liver. The B_{max} value for ^{125}I-ET-3 (0.3 pmol/mg of protein) is 83% of that for ^{125}I-ET-1 in human liver membranes. These findings are in contrast with those obtained in arterial membranes where the B_{max} for ^{125}I-ET-3 is only 12% of that for ^{125}I-ET-1, suggesting the presence of different subclasses of ET receptors between liver plasma membranes and arterial membranes.

A cDNA encoding non-selective type (ET_B) of ET receptors has recently been isolated from a human liver cDNA library[14]. The isolated cDNA encodes a protein of 442 amino acid residues which are 88% identical to that rat ET_B receptor but only 64% to that of the bovine ET_A receptor. The receptor contains a proline-rich extracellular N-terminal region with seven transmembrane segments. which are characteristics of the G protein-coupled receptor superfamily[14].

ET binding sites were also examined in non-parenchymal cells in the liver. After intravenous administration of ^{125}I-ET-1 to the rat, silver grains, which indicate ET-1 binding sites, were observed on fat-storing cells in the sinusoid of the liver[15]. The ^{125}I-ET-1 binding was also observed on sinusoidal endothelial cells, Kupffer cells, and microvilli of hepatocytes[16]. The grain density of fat-storing cells was threefold higher than that of Kupffer cells and 18-fold than that of hepatocytes. The injected ^{125}I-ET-1 was gradually internalized into the cytoplasm of fat-storing cells and often associated with multivesicular bodies[16].

Intracellular distribution of ET-1 receptors was analyzed in rat liver cells, and the specific binding to Golgi cisternae and nuclei in addition to plasma membranes was observed[17]. The presence of ET-1 receptors on the Golgi cisternae may suggest that they are glycosylated within the cisternae or there exists a recycling pathway in hepatocytes[17]. In human livers, ET-1 and ET-3 binding sites are present in plasma membranes, whereas ET-2 binding sites are observed in a compartment associated with mitochondria fractions[18].

PHYSIOLOGICAL EFFECTS ON THE LIVER

Hepatic circulation

In the perfused rat liver, ET-3 induced sustained vasoconstriction of portal vasculature in a concentration-dependent manner with EC_{50} of 1 nM[19]. The hepatic vasoconstriction induced by ET-3 infusion was inhibited when Ca^{2+} was removed from the perfusion medium[19]. In contrast, in the dog, the hepatic arterial vascular response to the intra-arterial injection of ET-1 was characterized by vasodilatation at doses of 50 pM or less, and was biphasic at doses higher than 200 pM, consisting of an initial increase in the flow (vasodilatation) with a short duration followed by a prolonged reduction in the flow (vasoconstriction)[20]. Intra-portal injection of ET-1 increased the portal perfusion pressure, indicating an increase in portal inflow resistance[20].

Intravenous injection of ET-1 or ET-3 (2 nmol/kg) reduced hepatic blood flow in the rat as determined by a laser-Doppler blood meter, and the decrease in hepatic blood flow induced by ET-3 was significant compared to that by ET-1[21]. The decrease in hepatic blood flow due to ET-1 was slightly inhibited by the pretreatment with BQ-123, an ET_A receptor antagonist, but it has no effect on the decrease due to ET-3. These results suggest that the decrease in hepatic blood flow is induced mainly by ET-3 via non-ET_A receptors, presumably ET-3 selective receptors (ETc) that are not inhibited by BQ-123.

The same group reported that the pretreatment with indomethacin, an inhibitor of biosynthesis of prostaglandins, significantly inhibited the decrease in hepatic blood flow elicited by ET-3, while indomethacin failed to inhibit the decrease in hepatic blood flow by ET-1[22]. These findings suggest that ET-1 decreases hepatic blood flow through its direct effects, while arachidonic acid metabolism may be involved in the reduction of hepatic blood flow induced by ET-3.

Since fat-storing cells have been shown to express ET receptors [15,16], these cells may contribute to changes in hepatic blood flow by modulating sinusoidal perfusion pressures.

Glycogenolysis and Ca^{2+} mobilization

ET has been reported to show a direct effect on hepatocytes, especially in terms of glycogenolysis. Using the perfused rat liver, Gandhi et al. demonstrated that ET-3 induced hepatic glycogenolysis and increased oxygen consumption[19]. The hepatic glycogenolysis was partially inhibited when Ca^{2+} was removed from the perfusion medium. They also showed that ET-3 stimulated the metabolism of inositol phospholipids in hepatocytes and Kupffer cells. Similar results for ET-1 were also described[19].

Utilizing primary cultured rat hepatocytes, Serradeil-Le Gal et al. reported that ET-1 at doses less than 1 nM induced a rise in cytosolic free Ca^{2+} and glycogenolysis whereas it has no effect on cAMP production[12]. A 1.8-fold increase in glycogen phosphorylase a was observed at 1 pM ET-1 with an EC_{50} of 0.03 pM. They have concluded that ET-1 behaves as a typical Ca^{2+} mobilizing hormone in the liver[12]. Furthermore, using isolated perfused rat livers in a non-recirculating system, Roden et al. reported that ET-1 (0.5–10 nM)-induced hepatic glucose release was accompanied by a decrease in hepatic glycogen contents, but ET-1 affected neither hepatic lactate nor cAMP releases[23].

From these results, it is suggested that ET-1 stimulates hepatic glycogenolysis via cAMP-independent mechanisms that lead to the elevation of intracellular Ca^{2+}.

PATHOLOGICAL ROLES OF ENDOTHELIN IN HEPATIC DISORDERS

Vascular permeability

Concerning whether ET increases vascular permeability in the liver, conflicting results have been reported. Filep et al. reported that vascular permeability of the liver was not affected by intravenous bolus injection of ET-1 (0.1–2 nmol/kg)[24]. Lehonx et al., however, reported that vascular permeability in the liver was enhanced by 20% after intravenous injection of ET-1 (400 pmol/kg)[25]. The latter also reported that vascular permeability was increased dose-dependently by big-ET-1 injection, and that the increase in vascular permeability was induced following the conversion of big-ET-1 to ET-1. The difference in the ET-1 dosage used in those studies may be a possible reason for the discrepancy.

Endothelin in hepatic disorders and its clinical implications

Five independent groups have so far presented data concerning plasma levels of ET in patients with hepatic disorders. In four of the five, plasma ET concentrations have been shown to be elevated in patients with liver cirrhosis, especially in those with ascites. Gulberg et al. measured plasma ET-3 concentrations, which were three times higher in patients with liver cirrhosis than normal control subjects[26]. We reported that plasma ET-1 levels, measured by ELISA using a monoclonal antibody, were significantly elevated in cirrhotic patients with ascites (Figure 21.1)[27]. Plasma ET-1 showed a significant negative correlation with creatinine clearance (Figure 21.2), and plasma ET-1 levels were significantly higher in patients with endotoxemia than in those without. From these findings, we have postulated that ET-1, which is released by endotoxin, may be involved in renal dysfunction in liver cirrhosis. These findings were further supported by two other studies. Moore et al. observed that patients with hepatorenal syndrome had markedly elevated plasma concentrations of ET-1 and

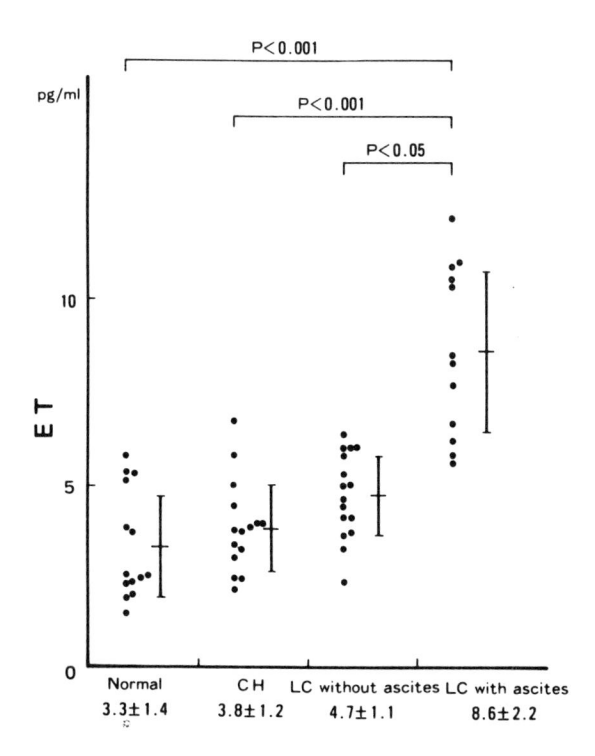

Figure 21.1. Plasma endothelin concentrations (ET) in normal controls and in patients with chronic hepatitis (CH), cirrhosis (LC) without ascites, and cirrhosis with ascites. (From ref. 27 with modifications)

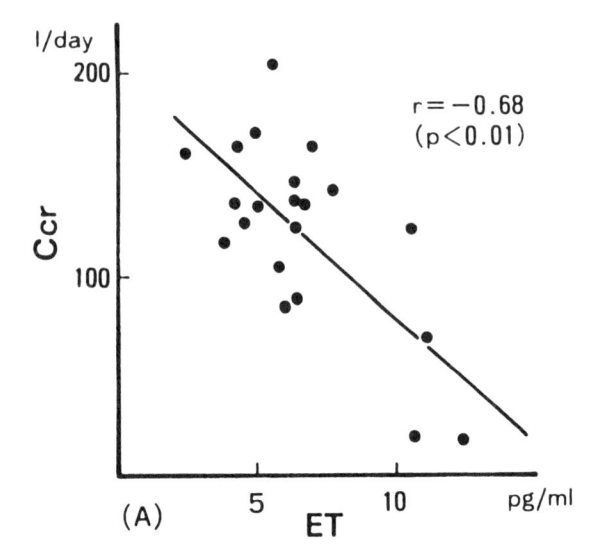

Figure 21.2. In patients with liver cirrhosis, plasma concentrations of endothelin are negatively correlated with creatinine clearance. (From ref. 27 with modifications)

ET-3[28]. They proposed a hypothesis that ET-1 and ET-3 play a role in the pathogenesis of hepatorenal syndrome. Increased plasma ET levels in patients with liver cirrhosis was also confirmed by Uemasu et al.[29]. On the other hand, no elevation[30] or a decrease[31] in plasma ET-1 concentrations in patients with liver cirrhosis was reported by the other group. Precise reasons for the discrepancy are unknown, but the difference in anti-RT-1 antibody utilized in those studies may be incriminated in the discrepancy.

Pernow et al. demonstrated in pig experiments that the arterial elevated plasma ET during endotoxemia correlated significantly with renal vasoconstriction[3]. They suggested that the ET released by endotoxin might be involved as a mediator of renal vasoconstriction. Claria et al. reported that the bolus injection of ET (100 and 600 pmol/kg) induced an increase in the mean arterial pressure, decreases in the renal plasma flow and the glomerular filtration rate in both control rats and cirrhotic rats with ascites[32]. Interestingly, they found that the high-dose of ET induced a reduction in $U_{Na}V$ in control rats while it produced marked natriuresis in cirrhotic rats. ET significantly increased plasma aldosterone, atrial natriurtic peptide, and renin activity in both groups. From these studies, it is suggesting that ET may inhibit tubular sodium reabsorption in cirrhotic rats.

Liver transplantation and endothelin

Lerman et al. reported the elevated plasma ET concentration and the increased mean arterial pressure during the first week after orthotopic liver transplantation[33]. The increase in plasma ET concentrations during the first week after orthotopic liver transplantation has also been confirmed by Textor et al.[34] and Kraus et al.[10]. As mentioned above, the latter study showed marked rises in plasma big-ET and ET-1 during the anhepatic period, followed by decrease in mean concentrations immediately after allograft reperfusion[10], suggesting that the liver may play a major role in the removal of circulatng ET-1.

SUMMARY

From the recently established results, ET has been shown to be a potent agonist in the liver, and also it has been clarified that ET has a wide variety of pathological implications in extra-hepatic manifestations in hepatic disorders. Precise mechanisms, i.e., intra-cellular second messenger system, and other biological effects besides vasoconstriction and glycogenolysis in the liver remain to be examined, and association of ET in the pathogenesis of extra-hepatic complications in hepatic disorder should be examined.

References

1. Yanagisawa, M., Kurihara, H., Kimura, S., Tombe, M., Kobayashi, Y., Mitsui, Y., Yazaki, Y., Goto, K., Masaki, T. (1988) A novel potent vasoconstrictor peptide produced by vascular endothelial calls. *Nature*, 332, 411–415.
2. Yoshimi, H., Hirata, Y., Fukuda, Y., Kawano, Y., Emori, T., Kuramochi, M., Omae, T., Marumo, F. (1989) Regional distribution of immunoreactive endothelin in rats. *Peptides*, 10, 805–808.
3. Pernow, J., Hemsen, A., Hallen, A., Lundberg, J. M. (1989) Release of endothelin-like immunoreactivity in relation to neuropeptide Y and catecholamines during endotoxin shock and asphyxia in the pig. *Acta Physiol. Scand.*, 140, 311–322.
4. Sugiura, M., Inagami, T., Kon, V. (1989) Endotoxin stimulates endothelin-release *in vivo* and *in vitro* as determined by radioimmunoassay. *Biochem. Biophys. Res. Commun.*, 161, 1220–1227.
5. Vemulapalli, S., Chin, P. J. S., Rivelli, M., Foster, C. J., Sybertz, E. J. (1991) Modulation of circulating endothelin levels in hypertension and endotoxemia in rats. *J. Cardiovasc. Pharmacol.*, 18, 895–903.
6. Rieder, H., Ramadori, G., Meyer zum Buschenfelde, K. H. (1991) Sinusoidal endothelial liver cells *in vitro* release endothelin- Augmentation by transformating growth facter β and Kupffer cell-conditioned media. *Klin. Wochenschr.*, 69, 387–391.
7. Shiba, R., Yanagisawa, M., Miyauchi, T., Ishii, Y., Kimura, S., Uchiyama, Y., Masaki, T., Goto, T. (1989) Elimination of intravenously injected endothelin-1 from the circulation of rat. *J. Cardiovasc. Pharmacol.*, 13 (Suppl 5), S98–S101.
8. Anggard, E., Gatlon, S., Rae, G., Thomas, R., McLoughlin, L., Nucci, G., Vane, J. R. (1989) The fate of radionated endothelin-1 and endothelin-3 in the rat. *J. Cardiovasc. Pharmacol.*, 13 (Suppl 5), S46–S49.
9. Neuser, D., Steinke, W., Theiss, G., Stasch, J. P. (1989) Autoradiographic localization of [^{125}I] endothelin-1 and [^{125}I] atrial natriuretic peptide in rat tissue: A comparative study. *J. Cardiovasc. Pharmacol.*, 13 (Suppl 5), S67–S73.
10. Kraus, T., Mehrabi, A., Klar, E., Mathias, D., Otto, G., Herfath, C. (1992) Peri and postoperative plasma kinetics of big endothelin and endothelin 1/2 after liver transplantation. *Transpl. Proc.*, 24, 2569–2571.
11. Loffer, B. M., Lohrer, W. (1991) Different endothelin receptor affinities in dog tissues. *J. Receptor Res.*, 11, 293–298.
12. Serradeil-Le Gal, C., Jouneaux, C., Sandiez-Bueno, A., Raufaste, D., Rache, B., Prenaux, A. M., Maffrand, J. P., Cobbold, P. H., Hanoune, J., Lotersztajn, S. (1991) Endothelin action in rat liver. Receptors, free Ca^{2+} oscillations, and activation of glycogenolysis. *J. Clin. Invest.*, 87, 133–138.
13. Takayangi, R., Ohnaka, K., Takasaki, C., Ohashi, M., Nawata. H. (1991) Multiple subtypes of endothelin receptors in human and porcine tissues: Characterization by ligand binding, affinity labeling, and regional distribution. *J. Cardiovasc. Pharmacol.*, 17 (Suppl 7), S127–S130.
14. Nakamuta, M., Takayanagi, R., Sakai, Y., Sakamoto, S., Hagiwara, H., Mizuno, T., Saito, Y., Hirose, S., Yamamoto, M., Nawata, H. (1991) Cloning and sequencing of a cDNA encoding human non–selective type of endothelin receptor. *Biochem. Biophys. Res. Commun.*, 177, 34–39.
15. Furuya, S., Naruse, S., Nakayama, T., Furuya, K., Norihara, K. (1991) Localization of [^{125}I]endothelin-1 in rat tissues observed by electron-microscopic radioautography. *J. Cardiovasc. Pharmacol.*, 17 (Suppl 7), S452–S454.

16. Furuya, S., Naruse, S., Nakayama, T., Norihara, K. (1992) Binding of ^{125}I-endothelin-1 to fat-storing cells in rat liver revealed by electron microscopic radioautography. *Anat. Embryol.* **185**, 97–100.
17. Hocher, B., Christoph, R., Johannes, H., Peter, G., Christian, B. (1992) Intracellular distribution of endothelin-1 receptors in rat liver cells. *Biochem. Biophys. Res. Commun.* **184**, 498–503.
18. Loffler, B. M., Kalina, B., Kurze, H. (1991) Partial characterization and subcellular distribution patterns of endothelin-1, -2 and -3 binding sites in human liver. *Biochem. Biophys. Res. Commun.*, **181**, 840–845.
19. Gandhi, C. R., Stephenson, K., Olson, M. S. (1990) Endothelin, a potent peptide agonist in the liver. *J. Biol. Chem.*, **265**, 17432–17435.
20. Withrington, P. G., de Nucci, G., Vane, J. R. (1989) Endothelin-1 causes vasoconstriction and vasodilation in the blood perfused liver of the dog. *J. Cardiovasc. Pharmacol.*, **13 (Suppl 5)**, S209–S210.
21. Kurihara, T., Akimori, M., Kurokawa, K., Ishiguro, H., Yokoyama, I., Hirayama, Y., Ihara, M., Yano, M. (1992) ET-1 sensitive reduction of tissue blood flow in rat liver. *Life Sci.*, **511**, 101–106.
22. Kurihara, T., Akimori, M., Kurokawa, K., Ishiguro, H., Niimi, A., Maeda, A., Shigemoto, M., Yamashita, K., Yokoyama, I., Hirayama, Y., Ihara, M., Yano, M (1992) Relationship between endothelin and thromboxane A2 in rat liver microcirculation. *Life Sci.*, **51**, 281–285.
23. Roden, M., Vierhapper, Liener, H., K., Waldhausl, W. (1992) Endothelin-1-stimulated glucose production *in vitro* in the isolated perfused rat liver. *Metabolism*, **41**, 290–295.
24. Filep, J. G., Sirois, M. G., Rousseau, A., Fournier, A., Sirois, P. (1991) Effect of endothelin-1 on vascular permeability in the conscious rat: interactions with platelet-activating factor. *Br. J. Pharmacol.*, **104**, 797–804.
25. Lehoux, S., Plante, G. E., Sirois, M. G., Sirois, P., D'Orleans-Juste, P. (1991) Phosphoramidon blocks big-endothelin-1 but not endothelin-1 enhancement of vascular permeability in the rat. *Br. J. Pharmacol.*, **107**, 996–1000.
26. Gulberg, V., Gerbes, A. L., Vollmar, A. M., Paumgartner, G. (1992) Endothelin-3 like immunoreactivity in plasma of patients with cirrhosis of the liver. *Life Sci.*, **51**, 1165–1169.
27. Uchihara, M., Izumi, N., Sato, C., Marumo, F. (1992) Clinical significance of elevated serum endothelin concentration in patients with liver cirrhosis. *Hepatology*, **16**, 95–99.
28. Moore, K., Wendon, J., Frazer, M., Karani, J., Williams, R., Bard, K. (1992) Plasma endothelin immunoreactivity in liver disease and the hepatorenal syndrome. *N. Engl. J. Med.*, **327**, 1774–1778.
29. Uemasu, J., Matsumoto, H., Kawasaki, H. (1992) Increased plasma endothelin levels in patients with liver cirrhosis. *Nephron (Letter)*, **60**, 380.
30. Veglio, F., Pinna, G., Melchio, R., Rabbia, F., Panarelli, M., Schavone, D., Mulatero, P., Chandussi, L., (1992) Hormonal aspects of the relation of liver cirrhosis to essential hypertension. *Clin. and Exper. Hyper.-Theory and Practice*, **A14**, 889–903.
31. Vegligo, F., Pinna, G., Melchio, R., Rabbia, F., Panarelli, M., Gagliardi, B., Chiandussi, L. (1992) Plasma endothelin levels in cirrhotic subjects. *J. Hepatol.*, **15**, 85–87.
32. Claria, J., Jimenez, W., Arroyo, V., Castro, A., Asbert, M., Ross, J., Rivera, F., Rodes, J. (1991) Doses of endothelin have natriuretic effects in conscious rats with cirrhosis and ascites. *Kidney Int.*, **30**, 182–187.
33. Lerman, A., Click, R. L., Narr, B. J., Weisner, R. H., Krom, R. A. F., Textor, S. C., Burnett Jr., J. C. (1991) Elevation of plasma endothelin associated with systemic hypertension in humans following orthotopic liver transplantation. *Transplantation*, **51**, 646–650.
34. Textor, S. C., Wilson, D. J., Lerman, A., Romero, J. C., Burnett, J. C., Weisner, R., Dickson, E. R., Krom, R. A. F. (1992) Renal hemodynamics, urinary eicosanoids, and endothelin after liver transplantation. *Transplantation*, **54**, 74–80.

22 The Role of Endothelin in Skeletal Homeostasis

Mone Zaidi, Michael Pazianas, Vijai S. Shankar, Olugbenga A. Adebanjo, Ali Zaidi and Christopher L.-H. Huang

The Bone Research Unit, Department of Biochemical Medicine, St. George's Hospital Medical School, London SW17 0RE, UK

* The Physical Laboratory, University of Cambridge, Dawning Street, Cambridge CB2 3EG, UK

INTRODUCTION

It has become increasingly clear that the vascular endothelium acts, not merely as a passive barrier between the blood and tissue components, but also as a local regulator through the humoral agents which its cells release. Osteoclasts, the bone resorbing cells, occur in close proximity to vascular endothelial cells, particularly in the "cutting cones" of cortical bone. Endothelial cells are also found in abundance in bone marrow. Endothelial cells products such as endothelin, nitric oxide (NO) and reactive oxygen species are now known to affect the activity of osteoclasts as well as bone-forming osteoblasts[1]. It is therefore important to understand the regulatory functions of endothelin in osseous tissue and its possible role in bone metabolism.

CELLULAR BIOLOGY OF BONE

The mechanical integrity of the skeleton is preserved by the continued remodelling of bone. The cells responsible for this tightly coupled lifelong process are bone-forming osteoblasts and bone-resorbing osteoclasts. The initial event in the resorptive episode is an increased osteoclast activity the precise mechanism of which is unclear. However, recent evidence has suggested the involvement of focal adhesion and *c-src* kinases in osteoclast activation. The next stage of resorption represents the formation of specialized structures, namely the "ruffled border" and "clear zone". The former comprises finger-like cytoplasmic and membrane projections, whilst the latter is an area subadjacent to ruffled border cytoplasm that contains cytoskeletal elements, but no organelles. The third stage results in the attachment of the clear zone to the bone substrate. This creates a unique microcompartment into which resorptive enzymes and protons are secreted for the subsequent resorption of bone. Completion of the resorptive episode results in osteoclast detachment and retraction. The latter occurs via a cell surface receptor, the calcium receptor, that is activated by the calcium ions generated as a result of hydroxyapatite dissolution. Resorption is closely followed by

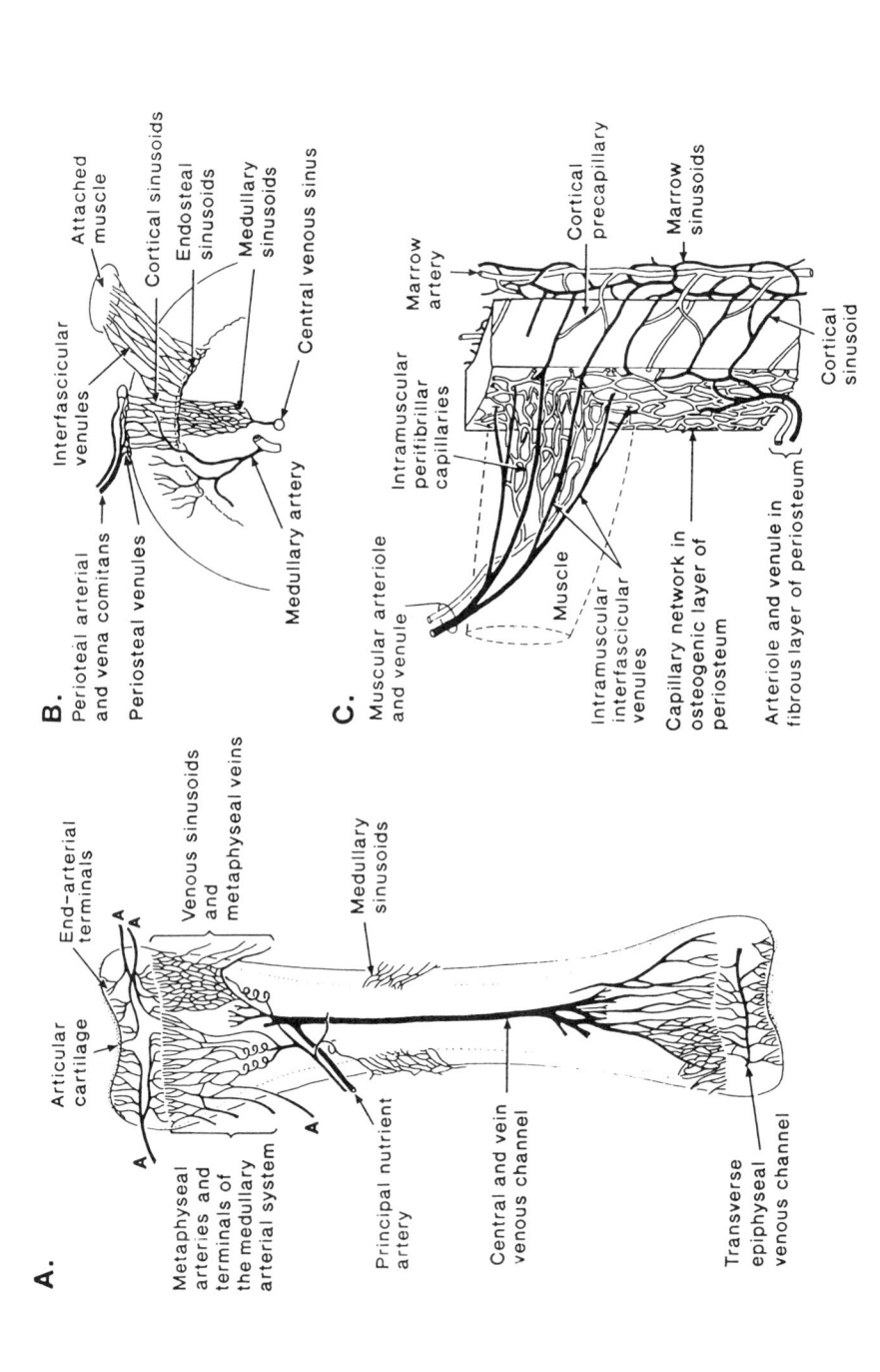

Figure 22.1 (A, B, C). Anatomy of the circulation in long bone longitudinal (A), cross section (B) and three dimensional section (C). [Adopted from M. Brooks "An anatomy of the osseous circulation" in Bone, Clinical and Biochemical News and Reviews 1986; 3:32–34].

bone formation. This starts with the accumulation of osteoblasts at the resorption bay or "pit" created by the osteoclast. The cavity is initially refilled with collagen resulting in an osteoid seam. The next stage is dominated by mineralization of this laid down osteoid.

It is thought that both local and hormonal factors interact in complex ways to precisely balance bone formation and resorption. These include hormones such as parathyroid hormone, 1, 25-dihydroxyvitamin D and calcitonin, as well as short-range messengers including Ca^{2+} itself, and small molecules released from osteoblasts and endothelial cells. Recent studies have allowed the isolation and short-term culture of osteoclasts, thus enabling a better understanding of how these factors act and interact. For further details the reader is referred to a recent review on the subject[2].

VASCULAR SUPPLY OF BONE

Bone is a highly vascularized tissue (Figure 22.1). Wide varieties of bones through a large range of animal exhibit similar patterns of vascular supply[3]. In the diaphysis of long bones, this begins with a single piercing nutrient artery which then breaks up into ascending and descending arteries. The nutrient artery ultimately supplies the greater part of the vascular requirements of both the complex and the marrow of the diaphysis. Sub-branches then extend to the bone extremities. However, successive branchings do not give rise to the muscular arterioles that normally function as resistance vessels in other tissues. Instead, small 250 μm arteries abruptly give rise to terminal vessels. These are made up only of an endothelium surrounded by a single layer of non-muscular cells. These terminal branches, reducing from 30 to 5 μm in diameter feed into the functional vascular lattice of both cortex and marrow.

The bone marrow capillaries (or sinusoids) are fenestrated endothelial tubes with a variable diameter of 15 to 30 μm. They lack basement membranes and their cells are held together by junctional complexes. The capillary walls thus normally permit the passage of blood cells from their extravascular site of development in haemopoietic marrow through the intercellular endothelial fenestrae into the circulating blood. The cortex in the shaft of a long bone has a relatively sparse vascularization in comparison with the marrow. Nevertheless, the characteristic capillary vessel anatomy remains that of a sinusoid, but in this case with an ordered Haversian system organized around it.

The veins that accompany the nutrient arteries outside the bone lack the venous values characteristic of veins that lie in intermuscular tissue planes. In diaphyseal marrow, the nutrient vein is continuous with a central longitudinal venous sinus and the latter is confluent with horizontal and radial collecting sinuses. These drain the profuse medullary sinusoids.

OSSEOUS ACTIONS OF ENDOTHELIN

Action on bone in organ culture

Endothelin-1 stimulates bone resorption in organ culture. Additionally, it influences the synthesis of collagen and non-collagen protein and phosphatidyl inositol turnover[4]. The enhancement of bone resorption is most evident in the neonatal mouse calvarial system. However, fetal rat limb bone cultures, which less capable of producing prostaglandins in response to a stimulus, do not respond similarly to endothelin. Furthermore, the resorptive effects of endothelin are inhibited by the cyclooxygenase inhibitor, indomethacin. These findings suggest an involvement of prostaglandins in the bone-resorptive action of endothelin. In contrast, the effects of endothelin on protein synthesis appear to be independent of prostaglandins.

Action on osteoblasts

Endothelin enhances the proliferation of MC3T3 osteoblast-like cells[5]. The peptide also stimulates DNA synthesis, but reduces cellular alkaline phosphatase activity in primary calvarial osteoblasts[6]. These activities are concentration-dependent and display the following rank order of potency for the three endothelin isoforms: endothelin-1 = endothelin-2 > endothelin-3. ^{125}I-endothelin binding studies and affinity cross-linking experiments have suggested the existence of a single class of endothelin-binding sites. These putative sites show a similar 10-fold greater affinity for the endothelins-1 and 2 in preference to endothelin-3. Furthermore, endothelins stimulate inositol phosphate production in a concentration-dependent manner, resulting in the mobilization of Ca^{2+} from intracellular stores. The relative potency of the three endothelin isoforms is similar to that obtained on receptor-binding assays. Findings of this kind indicate that bone-forming osteoblasts possess a functionally

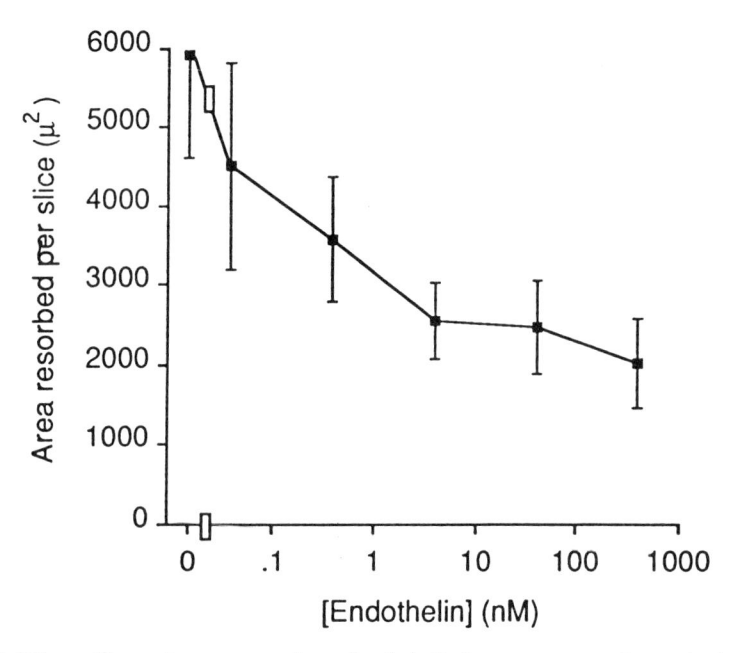

Figure 22.2. Effects of increasing concentrations of endothelin-1 on mean area of osteoclastic resorption per bone slice (means ± standard errors of the mean) (reproduced by permission, from Alam et al., 1992).

important endothelial receptor exhibiting a preferential affinity for the isoforms 1 and 2.

After binding to osteoclast receptors, endothelin activates phospholipase C thus causing a rapid increase in the intracellular concentration of inositol trisphosphate (IP$_3$) and 1, 2 diacyglycerol. This results in the release of Ca^{2+} from intracellular stores seen as a rapid initial, up to 10-fold, peak increase of cytosolic Ca^{2+}, followed by a fall to a plateau attributed to an entry of extracellular Ca$^{2+(5)}$. The cytosolic Ca^{2+} response to endothelin persists in the absence of extracellular Ca^{2+} providing further evidence for the release of intracellularly stored Ca^{2+}. However, the endothelin effect is resistant to the Ca^{2+} channel antagonist, nifedipine, and to the cyclooxygenase inhibitor, indomethacin[7]. Endothelin pretreatment significantly attenuates cytosolic Ca^{2+} responses to the agonists, α-thrombin and epidermal growth factor and significantly potentiates such transients induced by prostaglandin E$_1$. In contrast, pretreatment with either one of the above-mentioned factors does not alter the responsiveness of osteoclasts to endothelin-1[8]. Finally, endothelin does not increase cyclic AMP concentrations in osteoblasts[7].

Action on osteoclasts

Endothelin inhibits the activity of disaggregated rat osteoclasts[9] (Figure 22.2). These effects are seen at endothelin concentrations of 2.5 to 8 nM, similar to those required for vasoconstriction (3 to 100 nM)[10]. Although the local concentration of endothelin in

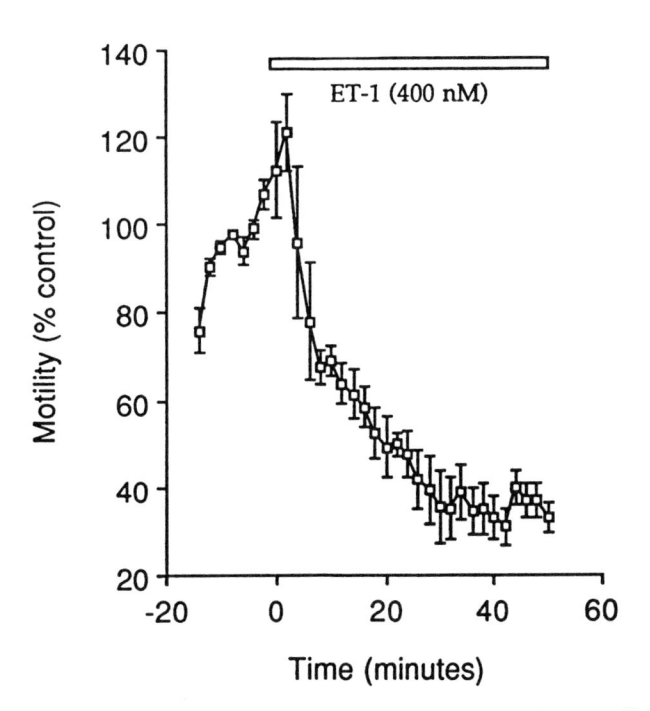

Figure 22.3. Time course of the effect of endothelin-1 on mean osteoclast motility (expressed as a percentage of motility at time zero) (modified from Alam et al., 1992).

bone is not known, these findings suggest that the action of endothelin might be of physiological importance.

Contrary to the classical observations in the vascular system, endothelin has been found not to elicit changes in cytosolic Ca^{2+} in the osteoclast. Exposure to endothelin nevertheless abolishes margin ruffling, a Q effect, without causing cell retraction (R effect) (Figure 22.3). Although osteoclastic quiescence (Q effect) is associated with activation of a cholera-toxin sensitive G-protein and cyclic AMP elevation, a direct coupling of endothelin receptors to adenylate cyclase has not yet been demonstrated. Thus, the second messenger regulation of the endothelin effect on the osteoclast remains unclear. Finally, it is worth mentioning that the other endothelial cell-derived product, NO, produces an R effect without elevating cytosolic Ca^{2+} [11].

Effects on parathyroid hormone secreting chief cells

Parathyroid hormone is one of the major hormonal regulators of circulating calcium concentration. Specific receptors for endothelin have been reported in human parathyroid tissue and endothelin appear to influence parathyroid hormone secretion from such cells[12]. ^{125}I-endothelin-1 binding studies have indicated that there is significant endothelin-1 binding to parathyroid membranes prepared from tissues from patients with hyperparathyroidism. Binding of ^{125}I-endothelin-3 is to these tissues is less marked than endothelins-1 and 2. Furthermore, there is evidence for the inhibition by endothelin of basal parathyroid hormone secretion from parathyroid adenoma cells *in vitro*. Again, endothelin-1 and 2 are much more potent than endothelin-3. These studies suggest the presence of functionally important endothelin receptor in human parathyroid tissue.

CONCLUSIONS

There is clear evidence for an action of endothelin on bone. Whilst the peptide seems to stimulate the osteoblast, it inhibits the osteoclast directly. In view of the low effective (nanomolar) concentrations of the peptide required to produce inhibitory effects, it is possible that endothelin may be relevant physiologically in the process of bone remodelling.

Acknowledgements

The studies described were supported by the Arthritis and Rheumatism Council (UK) and the Sandoz Foundation for Gerontological Research (Basel). The authors are grateful to Professor Iain MacIntyre for his continued support.

References

1. Zaidi, M., Alam, A. S. M. T., Bax, B. E., Shankar, V. S., Bax, C. M. R., Gill, J. S., *et al.* (1993) Role of the endothelin cell in osteoclast control: new perspectives. *Bone*, **14**, 97–102.
2. Zaidi, M., Alam, A. S. M. T., Shankar, V. S., Bax, B. E., Bax, C. M. R., Moonga, *et al.* (1993) Cellular biology of bone resorption. *Biological Reviews*, **68**, 197–264.

3. Brookes, M. (1971) The blood supply of bone. Butterworths. London.
4. Tatrai, A., Foster, S., Lakatos, P., Shankar, G., and Stern, P. (1992) Endothelin-1 actions on resorption, collagen and non-collagen protein synthesis, and phosphatidyl inositol turnover in bone organ cultures. *Endocrinology*, **131**, 603–607.
5. Takuwa, Y., Ohue, Y., Takuwa, N., and Yamashita, K. (1989) Endothelin-1 activates phospholipase C and mobilises Ca^{2+} from extra- and intracellular pools in osteoblastic cells. *American Journal of Physiology*, **257**, E797-E803.
6. Takuwa, Y., Masaki, T., and Yamashita, K. (1990) The effects of the endothelin family peptides on cultured osteoblastic cells from rat calvariae. *Biochemical and Biophysical Research Communications*, **170**, 998–1005.
7. Tatrai, A., Lakatos, P., Thompson, S., and Stern, P. H. (1992) Effects of endothelin-1 on signal transduction in UMR-106 osteoblastic cells. *Journal of Bone and Mineral Research*, **10**, 1201–1209.
8. Tatrai, A., and Stern, P. H. (1993) Endothelin-1 modulates calcium signalling by epidermal growth factor, α-thrombin, and prostaglandin E_1 in UMR-106 osteoblastic cells. *Journal of Bone and Mineral Research*, **8**, 943–952.
9. Alam, A. S. M. T., Gallagher, A., Shankar, V. S., Ghatei, M. A., Datta, H. K., et al. (1992) Endothelin inhibits osteoclastic bone resorption by a direct efect on cell motility: implications for the vascular control of bone resorption. *Endocrinology*, **130**, 3617–3624.
10. Haynes, W. G., and Webb, D. J. (1993) The endothelin family of peptides: local hormones with diverse roles in health and disease? *Clinical Science*, **84**, 485–500.
11. MacIntyre, I., Zaidi, M., Alam, A. S. M. T., Datta, H. K., Moonga, B. S., Lidbury, P. S., et al. (1991) Osteoclastic inhibition: an action of nitric oxide not mediated by cyclic GMP. *Proceedings of the National Academy of Sciences of the USA*, **88**, 2936–2940.
12. Eguchi, S., Hirata, Y., Imai, T., Kanno, K., Akiba, T., Sakamoto, A., et al. (1992) *Biochemical and Biophysical Research Communications* **184**, 1448–1455.

INDEX

Acetylcholine 83
Actinomycin D 127, 161
Acute renal failure 237
Adenylate cyclase 30
Adrenals 287
Aging 120
Airway epithelium 262
Airway smooth muscle 260
Alcohol dependency 30
Aldosterone 287
Alzheimer's disease 131, 186
Amnion 309
Amniotic fluid 312
Angiographic vasospasm 168
Anterior pituitary 120
Aortic cross-clamping 238
Area Postrema 149
Arginine vasopressin 71
Asthma 266
Atrial natriuretic peptide 71

Baroreceptor reflex 187
Barrel-rolling 129
Behavior 129
Blood–brain barrier 156
Bone 299
Bradykinin 74
Brain circulation 217
Brattleboro rats 222
Bronchoconstrictor 264

Calcitonin gene related peptide 72
Calcium flux 28
Cardiac transplantation 200
Cardiomyocytes 194
Cardiovascular effects 6
Carrageenin 342
Catecholamine 289
Cathepsin 55
Central cardiovascular 123
Central nervous system 101, 117, 143, 183

Central respiration 122
Cerebral infarction 188
Cerebral ischemia 128
Cerebral vasospasm 158, 172, 188
Cerebrospinal fluid 185
Cerebrovascular 125, 155
Chief cells 366
Children 334
Chimeric receptor studies 17
Chorion 309
Chronic renal failure 238
Chronotropic effect 195
Chymase 55
Circular dichroism 37
Classification 18
Conformational studies 37
Congestive heart failure 105, 198
Convulsions 130
Coronary angioplasty 203
Coronary artery disease 201
Coronary circulation 220
Cortisol 288
Cyclosporine 201, 238
Cytokines 75

Decidual cells 309
Delayed ischemic neurological deficits 174
Dementia 186
Depression 131
Depressive patients 189
Diabetes Mellitus 297
Diabetic nephropathy 241
Dialysis 238
Dopamine 84, 283
Drinking behavior 130
Ductus arteriosus 329
Dysfunctional uterine bleeding 308

Edema 343
Eisenmenger syndrome 197, 198
Elderly patients 206

Endocrinal disorders 106
Endocrine hormones 80
Endopeptidases 54
Endothelin-converting enzyme 6, 53
Endothelin receptors 41
Endothelin receptor subtypes 5, 16, 41
Endothelin release 254
Endothelin structure 37
Endothelin synthesis 252
Endothelium-derived relaxing factor 69
Endotoxin 353
ET non-selective antagonists 42
ET_A selective antagonists 42
ET_A selective compounds 18
ET_B selective antagonists 42
ET_B selective compounds 20
ET_B selective agonists 42

Fat storing cells 355
Fetal plasma 311
Feto-placental 313
Fetus 332

G-proteins 26
Gastrointestinal circulation 220
Glioma 189
Glomerular functions 235
Glomerulonephritis 239
Growth hormone 285
Guanylate cyclase 30

Heart 195
Hemoglobin 170
Hepatic circulation 221, 355
Hepatic disorders 108, 356
Hepatic glycogenolysis 356
Hyperalgesia 345
Hypertension 104, 124
Hypertensive nephropathy 239
Hypothalamo-neurohypophyseal 120
Hypothalamus 281

Indomethacin 343
Inflammation 339
Inotropic effect 195
Intracerebroventricular 145

Kupffer cell 354

Labor 311
Leukocytes 61, 205, 344
Lipoproteins 76
Liver 353
Liver cirrhosis 357
Liver transplantation 354, 358

Long Evans rats 222
Luteinizing hormone 284

Maternal plasma 311
Medulla 148
Menstrual cycle 317
Mesangial cell functions 235
Metabolism 255
Metalloprotease 58
Micturition 130
Migraine 131
Mitogenic actions 8, 76, 162
Mitral stenosis 206
Monocyclic analogues 40
Mucous glands 262
Multiple system atrophy 187
Myocardial cell hypertrophy 194
Myocardial infarction 105, 203

Na^+/H^+ exchange 30
Neuroendocrine system 101
Neurological disorders 107
Neuromodulator 118
Neuropeptide 7
Neurotransmitter 118
Neutrophils 205
New born 334
Norepinephrine 82
Nuclear magnetic resonance 37
Nucleus tractus solitarius 148

Obstetrics 316
Ocular effects 131
Ontogeny 120
Open chest operations 206
Orthostatic hypotension 187
Osseous actions 363
Osteoblasts 364
Osteoclasts 365
Ovaries 290
Oxyhemoglobin 161, 176
Oxytocin 286

Pain 344
Parathyroid 296, 366
Paraventricular nucleus 146
Pepsin 55
Pertussis toxin 27
Pheochromocytoma 289
Phosphoinositide hydrolysis 27
Phospholipase A_2 28
Phospholipase C 27
Phospholipase D 29
Phosphoramidon 36, 58, 127, 161
Pituitary 281

Placenta 308
Platelet activating factor 74
Postural change 199
Pre-eclampsia 239, 316, 332
Pregnancy 311, 331
Progressive renal disease 240
Prolactin 282
Prostaglandins 74
Pulmonary hypertension 196, 268
Pulmonary vascular smooth muscle 262

Radiocontrast nephropathy 241
Receptor affinity 14
Receptor densities 14
Regional circulation 217
Renal circulation 221, 234
Renal disorders 108
Renal ET receptors 233
Renal function 103
Renin-angiotensin system 73
Reproductive system 102
Respiratory system 102

Saphenous vein 218
Senile dementia of Alzheimer type 186
Septic shock 241
Serotonin 84
Sex 294
Skeletal homeostasis 361
Sodium exchange 236
Spinal cord 151, 183
Structure–activity relationship 38
Subarachnoid clot 175

Subarachnoid hemorrhage 126, 160, 167, 188
Subfornical organ 146
Substance P 85
Sudden infant death 123
Supraoptic nucleus 146
Sympathetic drive 124
Systemic hemodynamics 216

Testes 293
Thapsigargin 196
Thrombin 70
Thrombus 205
Thymidine incorporation 77
Thyroid 295
Thyrotropin 285
Transmembrane signaling 25

Ureteric obstruction 242
Utero-placental 308
Uterus 317

Valvular heart disease 197
Vascular diseases 106
Vascular permeability 342
Vasomotor tone 215
Vasopressin 286
Ventrolateral medulla 150

Water exchange 236
Wheal formation 345

Zymosan 342

NORTHERN MICHIGAN UNIVERSITY LIBRARY

3 1854 005 312 130

DATE DUE

Demco, Inc. 38-293